The Human Body
Its Function in Health and Disease

THIRD EDITION

Joanne Mambretti-Zumwalt, M.D., ALHC

Charles F. Belanger, Jr., M.D.

Marvin Goldstein, M.D.

Based on previous editions by
Walter S. Clough, M.D., CLU

Edited by
JoyceAbrams Fleming, J.D., FLMI,ALHC,ACS

INTERNATIONAL CLAIM ASSOCIATION

ISBN 1-877595-02-0

Library of Congress Catalog Card Number: 94-75802

Printed in the United States of America

Preface

The Human Body: Its Function in Health and Disease (3rd edition) is a project of the International Claim Association for use in its Claims Education Program. This textbook can also be used as a reference source for claim reviewers, underwriters, actuaries, and others in the insurance industry who must understand complex medical terminology and concepts. This book should provide the broad background necessary to allow these individuals to work knowledgeably and effectively as they deal with insurance claims, applications for insurance, and other insurance documents that contain medical information.

As an introductory text, *The Human Body* assumes no prior knowledge of medical terms and concepts. Each medical term is defined or explained when it is first used, and jargon and nonessential technical language have been kept to a minimum. Important medical terminology is highlighted in boldface italic type when the term is first used or defined. The book also includes a glossary of medical terms.

Acknowledgments

The authors recognize that other people provide valuable assistance that make publication of a book possible. Such is the case with *The Human Body.* We would especially like to thank Jon B. Meier, FLMI, ALHC, who served as the ICA's Project Coordinator for this book and provided assistance, advice, and encouragement throughout the project.

The members of the ICA's textbook review panel shared their knowledge and expertise in ensuring the book's clarity, completeness, technical accuracy, and adherence to current industry practices. The panel members read every chapter of the manuscript and carefully noted their corrections, comments, and suggestions. Our thanks go to each of them.

R. J. "Sam" Schwarztrauber, ALHC
Team Leader
General American Life Insurance Company

Lawrence L. Segel, M.D., C.B.I.M., FLMI, ALHC, ACS
Assistant Vice-President and Chief Underwriter
Crown Life Insurance Company

Kenneth R. Strasen, ALHC
Vice President
Independent Life & Accident Insurance Company

Donald Woodley, M.D.
Associate Medical Director
Lutheran Brotherhood

Many other people also contributed to this third edition. Harriett Jones, J.D., FLMI, ACS, copyedited the final manuscript and Iris F. Hartley, FLMI, ALHC, prepared the index. Sharon Bibee at LOMA compiled the glossary and provided invaluable editorial and production assistance throughout the project.

As co-authors of the third edition, we are indebted to Walter S. Clough, M.D., CLU, the author of the first and second editions of this text, and to Lillian Michael who provided the medical illustrations. Thanks also go to LOMA staff members Joyce Abrams Fleming, J.D., FLMI, ALHC, ACS, who edited the manuscript, and Katherine C. Milligan, FLMI, ALHC, who supervised the project.

Finally, we thank Bella Hickey, coordinator, and Gayle Sanders, word processing operator, who typed and retyped the initial drafts, and Lori Korkidis, medical department secretary, who provided invaluable assistance. We also gratefully acknowledge the physicians who reviewed the chapters in their specialty: Laurence Cignoli, M.D., hematology; Roger Epstein, M.D., gastroenterology; Steven Greenberg, M.D., psychiatry; and Michael Theerman, M.D., nephrology. Our thanks also go to Gary T. Athelstan, Professor and Counseling Psychologist at the University of Minnesota, for his contributions.

Joanne Mambretti-Zumwalt, M.D., ALHC
Charles F. Belanger, Jr., M.D.
Marvin Goldstein, M.D.

Worcester, Massachusetts
1994

Contents

List of Illustrations

1

Introduction

This third edition of *The Human Body: Its Function in Health and Disease* is an introduction to the structure and function of the human body and to the disorders affecting the body. This text is designed for people who work in life and health insurance companies. Applications for insurance, claim forms, attending physician's statements, and bills for medical services use the terminology of the medical profession. Life and health insurance company employees in claims, underwriting, and other areas need to develop a familiarity with the names and functions of organs in the body and to understand normal physiology and the effects of illness on the body. These employees also need to be familiar with the techniques and procedures used to diagnose and treat illnesses. Claim personnel must be able to recognize the usual course of illness and typical treatments and to determine if deviations require investigation. Unnecessary investigation of routine claims produces an unacceptable rise in company expense. On the other hand, failure to investigate invalid claims results in the insurer taking on an unacceptably high level of risk.

Health is the normal functioning of the human body. *Disease* is a condition in which the body, or part of it, deviates from health. Disease may involve structural, functional, or psychological disorder. This text will discuss both health and disease.

MEDICAL TERMINOLOGY

In order for you to understand and learn the information in this text, you must develop a scientific and medical vocabulary. Two shortcuts to the development of a medical vocabulary are available, and we recommend both. One shortcut is to make frequent use of a medical dictionary or glossary of medical terms. Few readers will be familiar with all the medical terms used in the chapters that follow. You should not pass over words that are unfamiliar, but should look up their meanings. A medical dictionary is an essential tool that should be kept close at hand. In addition, you should refer to the Glossary at the end of this book. It contains definitions of many of the words found in this text.

The second shortcut requires learning certain word elements or components commonly used in medical terminology. Most medical terms are derived from the combination of two or more word elements, known as roots, prefixes, and suffixes. A *root* is a more complex word element than is a prefix or suffix. A root can be used as a prefix, a suffix, or the body of a longer word that is formed by the combination of the root with a prefix, suffix, or both. A *prefix* is a letter or group of letters attached to the beginning of a root. A *suffix* is a letter or group of letters attached to the end of a root. Knowledge of the more common roots, prefixes, and suffixes will greatly enhance your ability to read medical literature with speed and understanding.

In many instances, you should be able to determine the meaning of a word by dividing the word into its component parts: prefix, root word, and suffix. For example, divide the word *myocarditis* into its component parts. "Myo" refers to muscle; "cardi" relates to the heart; and "itis" means inflammation. By putting these parts together, you get the meaning of myocarditis, an inflammation of the heart muscle. In the word *arthrotomy*, the root "arthr" pertains to joints and the suffix "otomy" means cutting into, and so arthrotomy refers to a surgical incision into a joint. As a third example, consider the word *cholecystostomy*. The root "chole" refers to bile, the root "cyst" to bladder, and the suffix "ostomy" to the surgical formation of a mouth or opening into an organ. Thus, cholecystostomy is a surgical procedure that creates an opening into the gallbladder for drainage of its contents. As you may have noticed from these examples, many of the word elements used in scientific and medical literature are derived from words that originated in Greek or Latin.

Commit to memory the meanings of the common roots, prefixes, and suffixes that are provided in the figures in this chapter. Figure 1–1 lists some of the common medical roots, Figure 1–2 lists some common medical prefixes, and Figure 1–3 lists common medical suffixes. Figure 1–4 lists some of the most common suffixes that refer

Figure 1–1.
Common Roots.

Root	Meaning	Example
arter(i)-	artery	periarteritis: inflammation of the outermost tissues in the wall of an artery
arthr-	joint	arthrotomy: surgical incision into a joint
bronch-	windpipe	bronchospasm: spasmodic contraction of muscles supporting the bronchus or windpipe
cardi-	heart	myocardium: the heart muscle
cerebr-	brain	cerebrovascular: pertaining to the blood vessels of the brain
chole-	bile	cholemia: the presence of bile or bile pigments in the blood
cyst-	bladder	cystitis: inflammation of the urinary bladder
gastr-	stomach	gastroscopy: inspection of the lining of the stomach by a viewing instrument
hepat-	liver	hepatomegaly: enlargement of the liver
myo-	muscle	myology: the scientific study of muscles
pneum-	air	pneumothorax: the presence of air in the pleural cavity
ren-	kidney	adrenal: a gland located adjacent to the upper pole of the kidney

Figure 1–2.
Common Prefixes.

Prefix	Meaning	Example
a-	deficient	anoxia: inadequate supply of oxygen
ante-	before	antepartum: before delivery
dys-	painful; difficult	dyspnea: labored breathing
endo-	within	endocarditis: inflammation of the inner lining of the heart
epi-	upon; outside	epidermis: outermost layer of skin
hyper-	above; excess	hypertrophy: abnormal enlargement or excessive growth of an organ or tissue
hypo-	under; below	hypoglycemia: low level of glucose in the blood
peri-	around; above	pericardium: membrane around the heart
post-	after; behind	postcibum: after meals
pre-	before; in front	prenatal: before birth

Figure 1–3.
Common Suffixes.

Suffix	Meaning	Example
-agra	seizure of acute pain	podagra: gouty pain in the great toe
-cid	kill	germicidal: a substance lethal to germs
-cis	cut	excision: removal of tissue by cutting
-flect	bend	deflection: a turning aside or bending
-fugal	travel away from	centrifugal: moving away from a central point
-gram	record	electrocardiogram: record of the heart's electrical activity
-itis	inflammation	appendicitis: inflammation of the appendix
-odynia	pain	pleurodynia: pain from irritation of the pleura
-oid	like or resembling	carcinoid: resembling carcinoma
-oma	tumor	adenoma: tumor of glandular structures

Figure 1–4.
Suffixes Indicating Surgery.

Suffix	Meaning	Example
-centesis	withdrawal of fluid	abdominocentesis: withdrawal of abdominal fluid with needle or aspirator
-ectomy	removal of	appendectomy: removal of the appendix
-oscopy	examination by means of a specialized viewing instrument	cystoscopy: examination of the urinary bladder through a cystoscope
-ostomy	the surgical creation of a mouth or opening	colostomy: surgical formation of an opening from the colon to the abdominal wall
-otomy	a surgical opening into an organ	tracheotomy: incision into the trachea
-plasty	an operative procedure	ureteroplasty: a surgical procedure which repairs or restores the ureter

Figure 1–5.
Anatomical Spatial Relationships.

Term	Meaning
anterior	toward the front
central	relating to the center; passing through the center
cephalad	toward the head
deep	at a location distant from the surface of the body or an organ, and the opposite of superficial
distal	further away from the beginning or from a stated point
dorsal	toward the back, or posterior, side of the body
inferior	lower, below, under; located at the lower part of an organ or below some other organ
lateral	at, belonging to, or pertaining to the side; situated on either side of the median vertical plane
medial	pertaining to the middle; closer to the midline of a body or structure
peripheral	pertaining to or placed near the edge or boundary
posterior	toward the back; the posterior surface of an organ faces the dorsal side of the body
proximal	nearer to the beginning or to a stated point, and the opposite of distal
superficial	at, on, or near the surface of an organ or the skin, and the opposite of deep; external or outward
superior	above, over, higher in location, and the opposite of inferior; situated at the upper part of an organ or above some other organ
ventral	toward the abdominal side of the body

to surgical procedures. These figures also provide examples of each word element's use.

To continue the development of a medical vocabulary, students should learn the meanings of the terms in Figure 1–5. These terms describe the spatial relationships between parts of the body or between a part of the body and its environment.

The Appendix to this text contains a more extensive list of common medical word parts.

SYMPTOMS, SIGNS, AND INDICATIONS

Medical terminology usually makes a distinction between two manifestations of disease known as symptoms and signs. A ***symptom*** is a subjective phenomenon of disease that leads to a complaint by the patient. On the other hand, a **sign** is objective evidence, a physical manifestation of disease that can be noted by someone other than the patient. The presence of a heart murmur is a sign—the physician can hear its characteristic sound through the stethoscope. The patient complains of pain in the lower right abdomen—a symptom; the physician notes the presence of tenderness in this area—a sign. Symptoms and signs assist the physician in establishing a diagnosis. The physician will need to perform other studies before establishing a firm diagnosis, since many conditions have similar manifestations. A **syndrome** is a set of signs and symptoms that occur together to characterize a certain abnormality.

A general term for a manifestation of disease is an indication. **Indications** are any symptoms, signs, or occurrences in a disease that provide directions toward the cause, treatment, or diagnosis for the condition. For example, the obstruction of the respiratory passage in the upper trachea may be an indication for performing a tracheotomy to open an airway and prevent suffocation. Indications can also lead to a **prognosis**, which includes both the probable course of a disease and the patient's prospect of recovery from the disease. **Contraindication** is evidence that warns against a particular procedure or treatment. For example, if the patient's medical records show a history of allergic reactions, certain medications should not be prescribed. For this particular patient, these medicines are contraindicated.

ACUTE AND CHRONIC DISORDERS

Throughout this text, you will learn about acute forms of disease and chronic forms of disease. **Acute diseases** of any type are generally characterized by a sudden onset and a relatively short course of illness. These disorders may or may not be severe. **Chronic diseases**, on the other hand, are generally characterized by a slow onset and a relatively long and progressive course of illness. Some chronic disorders result from multiple attacks of acute disease.

As noted before, the Glossary at the end of this text provides definitions of technical terms used in this book and the Appendix contains lists of medical roots, prefixes, and suffixes. The Appendix also includes a list of textbooks which will be helpful to insurance personnel. These textbooks describe and explain diseases, drugs, duration of disability for many common conditions, and other topics relevant for claims work.

2

Scientific Background for The Study of Disease

This chapter provides a brief introduction to the scientific background and investigative studies in medicine that contribute to the understanding of the human body and the disorders that affect it. Specifically, this chapter introduces anatomy and physiology, pathology, microbiology, pharmacology, anesthesiology, immunology, genetics, and mortality studies. The student should not attempt a mastery of the disorders discussed in the chapters that follow without first building a solid base of fundamental medical knowledge. Students should be able to apply the basic information presented in this chapter to information presented in subsequent chapters, and so develop a more complete understanding of the human body in health and disease.

ANATOMY AND PHYSIOLOGY

Human anatomy is the study of the *structure* of the human body, its cells, tissues, muscles, organs, blood vessels, and skeleton. ***Physiology*** is the study of the *function* of the various parts of the body, how the work of one part is interrelated with the work of other structures and systems, and how a structure or organ acts when it is healthy and when it is diseased. The structure of most of this book—its anatomy, if you will—is designed to give the student some basic knowledge of the anatomy and physiology of the various body systems. The text describes the disorders that can affect the parts of each system and some of the common diagnostic techniques and methods of treatment.

Cells and Tissues

All living organisms consist of minute structures called cells. *Cytology* is the microscopic study of cells, including a study of their origin, structure, function, and pathology. Cells possess properties that are commonly associated with life:

- Cells support the endless chain of chemical processes that occur in the body to keep it functioning and that are referred to as *metabolism*.
- Cells are able to nourish themselves, to grow, to reproduce, and to react or respond to stimuli.

The outside lining of the cell is a membrane which allows some substances to pass into and out of the cell. Contained within the cell are the *nucleus*, a spherical body located near the center of the cell that serves to direct all cell activities, and the *cytoplasm*, a colorless semiliquid substance in which many vital activities take place.

Histology is the branch of anatomy that deals with the microscopic study of tissues. A *tissue* is composed of a group of specialized cells of similar structure that are united for the performance of a particular function. Customarily, tissues are classified into four groups: (1) epithelial tissue; (2) connective tissue; (3) muscle tissue; and (4) nerve tissue. Knowledge of these different types of tissues will be particularly helpful in studying the classification, terminology, and tissue origin of tumors in Chapter 4.

Epithelial Tissues

Epithelial tissues cover or line most organs of the body. The four types of epithelial tissue are

- *squamous epithelium*, which is composed of thin, flat cells, and which covers the entire surface of the body and the orifices of cavities opening on it. For example, squamous epithelium covers the skin and forms the lining of the lungs.

- *columnar epithelium*, which is composed of long, cylindrical cells, and which is the chief secretory tissue of the body. Columnar epithelium comprises the inner lining of the stomach, intestine, gallbladder, larynx, trachea, and uterus.
- *cuboidal epithelium*, which is composed of cube-shaped cells, and which forms the lining of gland ducts, kidney tubules, and bronchi.
- *transitional epithelium*, which is composed of several layers of overlapping, large rounded cells that have the ability to stretch, and which can adapt to increases in the contents of the organs where this epithelium is found, including the ureter, bladder, and the pelvis of the kidney.

Connective Tissues

Connective tissues are those tissues that help to support the body. One important type of connective tissue binds tissues and organs to each other, forms the framework of most organs, and surrounds blood vessels. The ordinary connective tissue of the body is called *fibrous tissue*. When ordinary connective tissue contains many fat cells, it is called *adipose tissue. Tendons* are connective tissues that connect muscles to bone, and *ligaments* join bone to bone.

Cartilage is a specialized type of connective tissue that forms most of an embryo's temporary skeleton, providing a model in which most of the bones develop. In adults, cartilage is found in the nasal septum, larynx, trachea, bronchi, external ear, intervertebral disks, and at the ends of long bones.

Bone is a dense form of connective tissue that is made rigid by deposits of large amounts of calcium. Bone forms the supporting skeleton of the body. *Marrow* is a soft tissue that occupies the central cavity of bones. *Red marrow*, which is restricted to the vertebrae, sternum, ribs, cranial bones, and ends of long bones, is the chief blood cell forming organ of the adult body.

Muscle Tissues

The three types of muscle tissue are smooth muscle, skeletal muscle, and cardiac muscle.

Smooth muscle appears in the walls of blood vessels, the digestive tract, bronchi, trachea, and bladder—locations that are not under the voluntary control of the individual. The contraction of smooth muscle is slow and sustained. Smooth muscle is not as richly supplied with blood vessels as are skeletal and cardiac muscles. *Skeletal muscle* appears in the muscles that are attached to bone and in the eye and comprises the bulky muscles of the body that are under the individual's voluntary control. Skeletal muscle contracts rapidly and with great force but fatigues quickly. **Cardiac muscle** appears only in the heart and is not under the individual's voluntary control. Cardiac muscle has some features that are similar to smooth muscle and other features that are similar to skeletal muscle.

Nerve Tissues

Nerve tissues consist of nerve cells, which are called **neurons,** and connecting cells, which are called **neuroglia**. Nerve tissue exists in the brain, spinal cord, and the cranial and spinal nerves. Nerve tissue is very sensitive to injury and does not regenerate after injury from oxygen deficiency, trauma, infection, or other disease as rapidly or completely as does other tissue.

Organs

Organs are composed of tissues from the four major tissue groups. Each tissue serves a specialized function within the organ and all tissues work collectively for a common purpose. The heart, lungs, kidneys, brain, and pancreas are examples of organs. A group of organs that have a similar physiologic goal is known as an **organ system**. The kidneys, ureters, bladder, and urethra taken together are an example of an organ system—the urinary system. Sometimes "tract" is used instead of "system," so that the urinary tract, for example, is the same as the urinary system.

Membranes

A **membrane** consists of a surface epithelium layer supported by an underlying connective tissue that is invested with blood vessels and nerves. A membrane that lines the cavities and passages that communicate from internal structures to the exterior of the body is referred to as a **mucosa**, or *mucous membrane*. Mucous membranes play significant roles in various parts of the body. In their various locations, these membranes differ slightly in both structural details and in function. Most mucous membranes contain epithelial cells and other cells located just underneath the epithelial layer. These cells secrete a mucus that covers and moistens the membrane. However, the amount of mucus secreted by mucous membranes in different parts of the body varies. Those mucous membranes in the oral cavity and respiratory tract, for example, contain an abundance of mucus-secreting cells, whereas the mucous membranes of the bladder and ureter contain no mucus-secreting cells.

In contrast with mucous membranes, **serous membranes** line the walls of the closed body cavities, such as the peritoneal, pleural, and pericardial cavities. Serous membrane cells secrete a small amount of a watery fluid, which provides lubrication for organs as they move in contact with each other.

A third type of membrane is the **synovial membrane**, which forms the lining of movable joints. Synovial fluid acts as a lubricant facilitating the smooth gliding of joint surfaces.

PATHOLOGY

Pathology is the study of disease. Hospital pathologists perform autopsies and examine tissues that physicians remove from their patients during surgery. The diagnoses and opinions of hospital pathologists are often useful in managing a disease process. Pathology may be divided into two main branches: anatomic pathology and clinical pathology. **Anatomic pathology** involves the gross and microscopic study of changes in the structures of diseased organs. (*Gross* in this context means visible to the naked eye.) **Clinical pathology**, on the other hand, refers to the chemical, hematologic, bacteriologic, microscopic, and other laboratory analyses of blood, urine, and specimens from other tissues and fluids. Both divisions of pathology are concerned with **etiology**, which is the study of the causes of disease.

The prime function of the laboratory is to aid the clinicians— those people who are actually involved in the practice of medicine— in the diagnosis and management of their patients' diseases. The laboratory can help clinicians detect unsuspected disease, monitor known conditions, and determine if a disease is active, arrested, cured, or in a chronic stage. For example, chemical and microscopic examination of the patient's urine gives information both on an individual's general health and, more specifically, on the status of the patient's kidneys. Tests for glucose and albumin and microscopic analysis of the patient's urinary sediment form the core of every complete urine examination. A finding of **glycosuria**, which is an excessive amount of glucose in the urine, is often the first sign of diabetes. Similarly, urinalysis can indicate the presence of many other conditions in **asymptomatic** patients, who, by definition, do not experience symptoms of disease.

Many tests can be performed on whole blood, serum, and plasma. **Plasma** is the liquid portion of the blood in which the blood corpuscles are suspended. **Serum** is that portion of the blood that separates from the blood clot after clotting has occurred. Thus, serum is plasma from which **fibrin**, a protein blood component that is essential for blood coagulation, has been removed. When a lab technician runs a test on whole blood, he or she adds a small amount of anticoagulant to the blood specimen to prevent the cellular components of the blood from clotting. Modern laboratories that have automated equipment can perform a dozen or more chemical tests simultaneously for a relatively low cost.

"Normal values" for specific tests can vary among laboratories because of differences in testing techniques and other factors. Therefore, anyone interpreting a test result should refer to the reporting laboratory's listing of normal values for that test.

MICROBIOLOGY

Microbiology is the branch of biologic science that deals with the study of microorganisms such as bacteria, viruses, fungi, and protozoa. Only a small percentage of microorganisms cause disease in otherwise healthy people.

Bacteria

Bacteria are microscopic unicellular organisms that occur in several shapes. **Coccus bacteria** are round or oval. **Rod bacteria,** which are also called *bacillary bacteria,* have one axis markedly longer than the others and are cylindrical or rod-shaped. Spiral-shaped bacteria are called **spirochetes**.

The study of bacteria is **bacteriology**. Bacteria existed for many years before scientists suspected a relationship between bacteria and infectious disease. As bacteriologic knowledge increased, bacteriologists discovered that specific, identifiable bacteria cause certain diseases. Bacteriologists and other scientists then developed precise treatments and preventive medicines for bacterial diseases. These advances have largely eliminated the scourge of epidemics so that diseases such as typhoid fever, diphtheria, and whooping cough no longer present widespread health hazards in developed countries.

One method of identifying bacteria involves placing a tiny droplet of pus from infected tissue, or an equally small sample from a culture, on a glass slide and observing the staining characteristics of the sample. The Gram stain technique involves the use, in succession, of two dyes. Those bacteria that retain the color of the first dye are referred to as Gram positive. Those bacteria that lose the first dye during a decolorizing step and pick up the second dye of a contrasting color are known as Gram negative.

Some bacteria are difficult to stain by ordinary techniques but may be stained by the application of special dyes in the presence of heat. Once stained in this way, certain bacteria are "acid fast," which means that even if these bacteria are treated with a strong acid that customarily decolorizes other bacteria, acid-fast bacteria will retain their color. An example of an acid-fast bacterium is the tubercle bacillus, which is the reason tuberculosis is referred to occasionally as an "acid-fast" infection. A number of other staining techniques may also be used for identifying specific bacteria.

Bacteria are everywhere in nature. They are present in our drinking water, in our food, in the air we breathe, and on almost everything we touch. Why do some bacteria fail to produce disease in normal, healthy individuals? Why do other related and almost indistinguishable bacteria cause illness, even when introduced into a body in small numbers? Why do certain bacteria cause disease in some individuals and not in others? The answers to these questions involve a discussion of the properties that enable bacteria to cause disease, plus a consideration of host resistance. Full answers to these questions are beyond the scope of this text, although a brief description of some of the pathogenic properties of bacteria follows.

A **pathogen** is any disease-producing microorganism, but the material contained in this section will address only bacterial pathogens. The aggressive behavior of pathogenic bacteria is a result of their ability to produce toxins and to invade the host's bloodstream. Some bacteria possess both attributes, and others possess only one of these attributes. Toxin-producing bacteria multiply slowly and generally remain at the original site of introduction into the host's body. However, the toxin these bacteria produce travels rapidly through the host's bloodstream to all the tissues, where it interferes with normal tissue metabolism. The tissues of the nervous system are especially sensitive to bacterial toxins. Botulism, which is a type of food poisoning, and tetanus are examples of diseases caused by toxin-producing bacteria.

Non-toxin-producing bacteria multiply rapidly, invade the host's bloodstream, and spread in great numbers to all tissues of the host's body, where continued enormous multiplication of the bacteria occurs. When these invasive bacteria interfere with the normal functioning of the host's cells and tissues, disease results. Bacterial pneumonia and bacterial meningitis are examples of diseases caused by invasive bacteria.

As noted earlier, some bacteria are both invasive and capable of producing toxins. This **dual pathogenicity**, or the ability to cause

disease in two ways, is possessed by streptococcus and staphylococcus bacteria.

Not all bacteria, however, are harmful, especially if they remain in
the location in which they normally appear. On the other hand, if
certain bacteria invade a foreign location, they become pathogenic.
For example, certain bacteria present in the colon are useful in
assisting in the decomposition of food, but if these same bacteria
invade the urinary tract, they cause disease.

Other Pathogenic Microorganisms

Bacteria do not cause all infectious diseases. Fungi, protozoa,
viruses, and rickettsiae can also cause disease.

Fungi and Protozoa

Medical mycology is the study of fungi and how fungi may be
pathogenic for humans. Fungi can infect various parts of the body,
including a person's skin, hair, nails, vagina, lungs, and mucous
membranes of the mouth. *Athlete's foot* and *ring worm*, for example, are common fungal infections of the skin, hair, and nails. Other
common fungal infections include *monilial vaginitis*, which affects
the vagina; *histoplasmosis*, which affects the lungs; and *thrush*,
which affects the mucous membranes of the mouth.

Protozoa are small unicellular microorganisms. Some are parasitic and others can live free of a host. A few protozoa are pathogenic
for humans, and other protozoa live in humans without causing any
apparent ill effect. The more common protozoan diseases include
amebiasis, malaria, toxoplasmosis, and Trichomonas vaginalis
vaginitis.

Amebiasis is a condition which is typically characterized by
abscesses of the liver, and ulcers of the colon. Although amebiasis
may affect up to ten percent of people worldwide, most people who
harbor the parasite are carriers and are asymptomatic. *Malaria*,
probably the most widespread of all diseases, is characterized by
intermittent shaking chills and high fever. The main pathologic
changes resulting from malaria occur in the patient's liver, spleen,
and red blood cells. *Toxoplasmosis* may affect the central nervous
system and may lead to blindness, brain defects, and death. This
disease occurs worldwide and often is asymptomatic. *Trichomonas
vaginalis vaginitis* is characterized by a copious, greenish-yellow,
frothy vaginal discharge. This disease affects up to 20 percent of all
females during their reproductive years, and many of these affected

females receive the infecting organism from sexual intercourse with an asymptomatic male.

Viruses and Rickettsiae

Virology is the study of viruses, their identification, and the elaboration of their role as causative agents in disease. A *virus* is a submicroscopic organism that lacks the capacity to reproduce itself unless it gains entrance into a cell of another living organism. Once within the cell of another organism, the virus "borrows" the host cell's protein-making abilities to reproduce itself. Disease is the result of damage done to the host cell when the virus uses the host.

Although the size and shape of viruses are not uniform, most viruses are much smaller than the smallest bacteria and require an electron microscope for their measurement. The diameter of a red blood cell, which can be readily measured with an ordinary microscope, is 300 times the diameter of the virus responsible for poliomyelitis.

If the body develops a viral disease, immunity to that disease often follows. Immunity is the state of resistance to a particular infection and can result naturally from a spontaneous attack of the infection or artificially from the injection of a vaccine. The immunity that follows recovery from many viral diseases persists throughout life, as exemplified by measles and small pox. Immunity to other viral infections, including the common cold, herpes, and influenza, is of short duration.

Viruses abound in nature, and, therefore, many viral diseases exist. Figure 2–1 lists some of the more important diseases caused by viruses.

A few human infections arise from microorganisms that are intermediate in characteristics between viruses and bacteria. These microorganisms, known as *rickettsiae*, are readily visible with an

Figure 2–1.
Diseases Caused by Viruses.

AIDS	Measles	Shingles
Chickenpox	Mumps	Smallpox
Common cold	Poliomyelitis	Viral encephalitis
Hepatitis A, B, & C	Rabies	Viral pneumonia
Infectious mononucleosis	Roseola	Warts
Influenza	Rubella	Yellow fever

ordinary microscope. Immunity may follow rickettsial infections. Like some bacteria and viruses, some rickettsiae produce toxins that can be rapidly fatal. A few of the more common rickettsial diseases are epidemic typhus, Rocky Mountain Spotted Fever, and scrub typhus.

PHARMACOLOGY

Pharmacology is the science that studies properties of drugs and their actions in living organisms, whether or not the use of the drug is for therapeutic purposes. Throughout history, some ill people have completely recovered from their diseases regardless of the therapy used. As a result, pharmacologic activity has been credited to some substances that scientists have later learned have none. Many of the early effective drugs came from crude plant extracts, and people discovered the drug's therapeutic value only by pure chance. Modern pharmacologists have analyzed these extracts and have synthesized new compounds that provide greater reliability, potency, and safety than the original forms.

Most drugs are pharmacologically active in one of several ways:

- Drugs may exert their effects by interacting with an enzymatic process of normal cell functioning.
- Drugs may produce an effect by supplying an essential constituent to the cell.
- Drugs may be effective because they compete in the cellular metabolism of invading organisms.
- The effects of a few drugs are produced purely physically or chemically. For example, drugs such as creams and lotions that furnish surface protection by means of a coating action operate on a physical basis only, and an antacid that neutralizes stomach acid works only on a chemical basis.

The therapeutic and toxic effects of drugs in the body are determined by such factors as the rate and extent of the drug's absorption, the distribution of the drug in body tissues and fluids, inactivation of the drug, and the rate and route of excretion of the drug from the body. Repeated administration of a drug may result in either drug tolerance or a cumulative effect. **Drug tolerance** is a condition wherein repeated administration of the same quantity of a drug will produce a lessened pharmacologic effect. The lessened pharmacologic effect may arise from a change in the rate by which the drug is metabolized or by a change in the reactivity level of the affected tissues. A ***cumulative drug effect*** produces heightened pharmacologic action, and occurs when the rates of detoxification and excretion of the drug are lower than the rate of administration of the drug. This cumulative effect should not be confused with a ***sensitization effect***, an allergic effect that is characterized by the sudden appearance of toxic signs and symptoms.

Drugs may be given to a patient orally in the form of pills, tablets, elixirs, and syrups. As a supplement or an alternative to the oral route, a drug may be administered rectally, in the form of suppositories and liquids. Rectal administration of drugs is particularly valuable if the patient is unable to swallow orally-administered drugs or if the patient would not retain oral medications because of vomiting. Drugs (or other substances, for that matter) also may be administered ***parenterally***, which means by injection. The more common parenteral routes are

- ***intradermal***—between skin layers
- ***subcutaneous***—below the skin in subcutaneous fatty tissue
- ***intramuscular***—in muscle tissue
- ***intravenous***—in a vein

Intravenous injection is the most rapid method of introducing a drug into the organs and tissues of the body. In addition, drugs may be given by inhalation or by local application directly to the skin and mucous membranes.

Many types or classes of drugs exist. Some therapeutic formulations consist of combinations of drugs, in which each drug in the combination retains its own specific action. Other drugs have a broad therapeutic range of activity and quite properly could be, and often are, listed as belonging to more than one drug class. The antihypertensive drugs that control high blood pressure are examples of this latter type of drug. These drugs are considered ***antihypertensives*** because of their effect on reducing elevated blood pressure, but some of them also promote the excretion of urine from the body and so are classified as ***diuretics***, as well. Three names may be applied to a drug: a chemical name, a generic or common name, and a brand name given by the drug company that produced the drug.

ANESTHESIOLOGY

Anesthesiology is the study of ways of producing an absence of sensation. A general definition is the absence of sensation or feeling, especially of the sensation of pain. However, ***anesthesia*** has come to have the narrower meaning of an artificially induced insensibility to the pain caused by surgery, other painful procedures, injury, or disease. This text will use the narrower sense of the term.

Management of anesthesia is easier if the patient is cooperative and at ease. However, contemplation of surgery and anesthesia evoke apprehension and fear in many patients. Thus, most patients, before going to the operating room, receive pre-anesthesia medication to produce a drowsy state, decrease anxiety, raise the patient's pain threshold, and counteract some of the unpleasant side effects of the anesthetic agent.

Regional Anesthesia

Anesthesia can be regional or general. **Regional anesthesia** is the induced loss of sensation of a part of the body as a result of pharmacologic interruption of nerve conduction. This type of anesthesia is adequate for many operations, especially for those procedures that are performed on ambulatory patients.

Regional anesthesia can be administered topically, by local infiltration, or by blocking a particular nerve. **Topical anesthesia** results from the absorption of the anesthetic agent through an intact membrane. The conjunctiva and the mucous membranes of the mouth, throat, urethra, and bladder are examples of areas that respond well to topical anesthesia. An example of a topical agent for ear, nose, and throat (ENT) use is cocaine.

Anesthesia by local infiltration results from injecting the anesthetic agent into the patient's skin and subcutaneous tissues. Local infiltration produces an area of anesthetized tissue, called a field block, around the operative site. This anesthetic technique is appropriate for superficial biopsies, excision of moles, and suturing of lacerations. Drugs used for local infiltration include Novocain, Pontocaine, and Xylocaine.

If the anesthesiologist desires to eliminate the conduction of impulses in one of the patient's nerves, the physician injects the anesthetic agent close to that nerve to create a **nerve block**. Many nerves of the body can be blocked. Patients who have surgery on their hand or foot often receive nerve block anesthesia. The technique of blocking the spinal nerves after their emergence from the spinal cord is a special type of block, known as **spinal anesthesia**. Spinal anesthesia is used for many operations within the peritoneal cavity and on the lower extremities. The anesthetic drugs used for spinal anesthesia are similar to those used for local infiltration. This anesthetic technique is discussed more fully in Chapter 14, *The Nervous System*.

General Anesthesia

General anesthesia is a reversible, drug-induced depression of the central nervous system that renders the patient unconscious. General anesthesia may be produced by inhalation drugs, such as ether, nitrous oxide, cyclopropane, and halothane, or by intravenous drugs such as Pentothal. Most operations on a patient's upper abdomen, chest, head, and neck are performed while the patient is affected by a general anesthetic.

IMMUNOLOGY

The body's *immune system* defends the body against disease. The immune system includes the bone marrow, lymph nodes, spleen, thymus, tonsils, and other lymphoid tissue. *Immunology* is the study of the body's immune system in health and disease and focuses upon the body's responses to natural infection, immunization procedures, blood transfusions, organ transplantation, cancer, and numerous other conditions. If an individual's immune response mechanism works well, the person is protected from disease, especially infections and certain cancers. If an individual's immunity mechanism works poorly, immunologic disorders, which may vary in severity from very mild to fatal, occur. Not all protection from infection comes from immune responses, however. For example, although the skin is not considered to be part of the immune system, it uses physical methods to help prevent infection by providing a barrier that prevents harmful elements in the external environment from entering the body.

The Immune Response System

The immune system is composed of specialized cells and proteins that recognize a substance as being foreign to the individual and that respond to the substance thereby protecting that person. The foreign substance may be, for example, a bacterium or virus, a cancer cell, red blood cells of a different blood type, or a drug. Each foreign substance contains *antigens*, which are molecules or parts of molecules found on the surface of the substance and recognized by the immune system as being foreign. Under normal circumstances, individuals develop antibodies only for those antigens that do not normally inhabit their bodies. *Antibodies* are complex proteins that the body generates in response to the presence of antigens.

The cells that effect the immune response are lymphocytes, plasma cells, monocytes, and macrophages. *Lymphocytes* are white blood cells that originate in lymphoid tissue. A number of subtypes of lymphocytes perform different functions, and each is identifiable by certain proteins on its cell membrane surface. These proteins are labeled by the letters CD, which stands for Cluster of Differentiation, followed by a number. The lymphocytes that contain these specific surface molecules are also given the appropriate CD labeling. The two major groups of lymphocytes are T lymphocytes and B lymphocytes. *T lymphocytes* are so named because part of their development occurs in the thymus. The tasks of T lymphocytes include both controlling and modifying the immune response to, and some of the direct cellular actions against, foreign antigens.

B lymphocytes derive from bone marrow and are primarily involved with antigen identification and antibody production. When stimulated by an antigen, B lymphocytes undergo a series of cell divisions that increase their number. Eventually, many B lymphocytes transform into plasma cells, the highly specialized cells that manufacture immunoglobulins. *Immunoglobulins* are proteins secreted by the immune system that have antibody activity. Because plasma cells have a limited life span, the continued presence of the antigen is necessary to stimulate their replacement. If the antigen is removed, plasma cell manufacture diminishes and antibody production decreases. If the antigen returns, antibody stimulation will resume.

Scientists have identified only a relatively small number of antibodies and their specific actions. Some antibodies, such as the tetanus antitoxin, neutralize the offending antigen, in this case the tetanus toxin. Other antibodies, such as the rubella, which is the German measles antibody, mark past infections and, thus, current immunity. Some antibodies, including the HIV antibody, indicate the presence of disease. Antibodies, such as the ones used in pregnancy testing, may be synthetic. Furthermore, some antibodies do not yet have a recognized function.

Macrophages and monocytes are other specialized cells that are involved in the body's identification and destruction of antigens.

An individual can acquire immunity in several ways. *Passive immunity* is an acquired immunity that results when the individual receives a pre-formed antibody or specifically sensitized lymphoid cells. A fetus can acquire passive immunity before birth from its mother's antibodies. The injection of antibodies, such as the tetanus antitoxin, may also confer passive immunity. Passively acquired immunity usually is short-lived.

In order to acquire long-lasting immunity, the body must develop its own antibodies from inoculation with disease agents or from direct contact with the disease. Immunity resulting from the presence of either antibodies or immune lymphoid cells that were formed in response to an antigen is known as *active immunity,* and it often lasts for the person's lifetime.

Immune responses may not always be protective and beneficial to the body. Harmful responses to contact with certain antigens can occur, and these harmful responses may also last a lifetime.

Characteristics of the Immune Response System

Antibodies are produced by plasma cells. An initial encounter with a specific antigen stimulates the plasma cells to produce antibodies. The cells remain ready to produce more antibodies, and will produce the antibodies to an increased degree if the same antigen invades the body again. Thus, the immune system is said to have an immunologic memory because the system "remembers" past contacts with specific antigens.

The immune system also has specificity in that each antigen triggers the production of a specific antibody. Varicella antibodies, for example, will neutralize only the varicella virus, which causes chickenpox and shingles. These antibodies, however, will not protect the individual against other antigens.

The immune system also shows an enhanced response that is both faster and of greater degree to each subsequent exposure to a specific antigen. Generally, this enhanced response is sufficient to repulse subsequent encounters with the specific antigen without the development of the disease.

The Immune Response System in Action

Antigen-antibody reactions, in general, serve useful purposes, such as the life-long immunity that develops after attacks of the communicable diseases of childhood. Furthermore, the cellular response of the immune system continually destroys potentially cancerous cells by physical or chemical methods and cures most viral or fungal infections. The class of T lymphocytes identified as CD4, or T4, lymphocytes, is particularly crucial in this cellular immune process. These lymphocytes are also called "Helper T" cells because they facilitate the body's immune response in general.

On the other hand, not all antigen-antibody reactions are useful. Some antigens evoke detrimental responses and may actually contribute to disease. Transfusion reactions, for example, result when antigens located on the recipient's red blood cells react with incompatible antibodies present in a donor's serum.

Hemolytic anemia, which results from an abnormally shortened lifespan for mature red blood cells and the inability of the bone marrow to compensate for this occurrence, is another example of an undesirable antigen-antibody reaction. One situation in which this form of anemia occurs is when a pregnant woman's immunologic system considers fetal red blood cells to be foreign antigens. If, during pregnancy, Rh-positive fetal red blood cells enter an Rh-negative mother's bloodstream, the mother's body produces Rh-positive antibodies. These antibodies return through the placenta to the fetus to destroy fetal red blood cells. Usually, during a woman's first pregnancy, the anemia resulting in the fetus from the antigen-antibody encounter is mild and requires no specific treatment. However, each successive Rh-positive pregnancy will trigger early, rapid, and increased production of antibodies as a result of the enhanced response phenomenon. These Rh-positive antibodies destroy the fetal red blood cells, producing a profound fetal anemia that may be fatal to the baby. Fortunately, treatment that prevents most cases of hemolytic anemia in newborns is now available.

The Immune System and Immunoglobulins

Immunoglobulins are divisible into five major classes, designated IgG, IgM, IgA, IgD, and IgE. Each major class has special properties that enable it to do a specific type of work. The IgG class of antibody, which accounts for about 80 percent of serum immunoglobulins, is comprised mostly of antibodies from prior infections. Reexposure to an earlier infection will trigger the production of antibodies from this group to neutralize reinfection.

IgM immunoglobulins are antibodies that neutralize an infection that the body has not experienced before. IgM antibodies tend to disappear with time, but the IgG antibodies do not. IgE immunoglobulins are antibodies that develop in individuals who have allergies. IgA antibodies mostly appear on mucous membranes on the body's surface and are part of the body's initial surface protection against infection. IgD antibodies appear most prominently in the body on B lymphocytes and are involved in triggering the production of other antibodies.

Disorders of the Immune Response System

A normal immune response plays an important role in maintaining health. However, a normal response may not occur because of a deficiency or an excess of immunoglobulin or because some component of this very complex system fails to function in the normal, anticipated manner. Failure of the normal response leads to a number of recognized clinical problems. If the immune response is less than normal, the affected individual is more susceptible to infection or certain malignancies, and if the response is greater than anticipated, the individual will have a hypersensitivity reaction, which can vary in severity from mild to fatal.

Immune Deficiency Disease

In two general categories of immune deficiency states, either antibody production is reduced or cellular immune responses are defective. Primary immune deficiency diseases may result from a genetic disorder or from unknown causes. Secondary immune deficiency diseases result from acquired disorders that interfere with the production or function of one or more of the components of the immune system. Both categories of immune deficiency states are characterized by chronic and recurrent infections which generally do not develop if the person's immune response system works normally. A trivial infection to most people can develop into a life-threatening infection in an individual who has an immunodeficiency disease. However, primary and most secondary immune deficiencies are uncommon.

Hypogammaglobulinemia is the most common immunoglobulin deficiency disorder. *Hypogammaglobulinemia* is characterized by recurrent bacterial infections, especially of the lung. Complications include bronchiectasis, intestinal malabsorption, and atrophic gastritis with pernicious anemia. Treatment of this condition typically involves monthly gammaglobulin injections.

Severe combined immunodeficiency disease (SCID) is a heterogenous group of genetic disturbances of the immune system. This condition primarily affects infants, is often fatal, and is associated with various defects in the patient's T and B cell functions. SCID patients experience severe fungal and viral infections and chronic persistent yeast infections of the oral cavity, the skin, and the nails.

Secondary immune deficiency diseases result from some underlying cause, such as some other disease, condition, or drug. The patient's immune response may be suppressed by corticosteroids, chemotherapy, and radiation, either as a result of deliberate immunosuppression following organ transplantation or as an unwanted side effect of therapy for other purposes. A few of the many other causes of secondary immunodeficiencies are Hodgkin's disease, leprosy, leukemia, lymphoma, thymoma, certain fungus infections, malnutrition, sarcoidosis, severe burns, some viral infections, uremia, and AIDS.

Acquired Immune Deficiency Syndrome

The *acquired immune deficiency syndrome (AIDS)*, which was virtually unknown before mid-1981, is caused by the human immunodeficiency virus (HIV). AIDS causes both the suppression of the patient's immune system and in an irreversible defect in the patient's cell-mediated immunity. HIV produces increased susceptibility to infections and to neoplasms, such as Kaposi's sarcoma.

HIV is transmitted by most body fluids, especially blood and sexual secretions, but is not transmitted by tears, saliva, stool, or urine unless these substances have been contaminated by blood or sexual secretions. HIV infects cells that have the CD4 marker molecule on their surface and eventually destroys them. CD4 (T4) lymphocytes and certain monocytes or macrophages, especially within the nervous system, are HIV's main targets. The virus itself causes symptoms, but most symptoms result from the loss of CD4 cells and from subsequent secondary infections.

The classification definitions of HIV infection, including AIDS, have evolved over time. This text uses the 1993 Centers for Disease Control (CDC) definitions for HIV infections. As an overview, in up to 80 percent of HIV patients, initial infection with HIV is followed in three weeks to three months with a "flu-type" illness of several weeks' duration. Symptoms may include fever, sweats, aches and pains, diarrhea, disease of the lymph nodes, and, on occasion, *thrombocytopenia*, which is a reduction in the number of platelets in the blood. These symptoms generally resolve. The patient then enters a latent period of eight to ten years without obvious symptoms, during which time the patient is contagious. All or almost all HIV infected patients will acquire AIDS. Also during this latent period, the patient undergoes a progressive decrease in CD4 lymphocytes. AIDS occurs when the patient reaches a certain low level of CD4 lymphocytes or when certain opportunistic infections, such as pneumocystis carinii pneumonia or candidiasis of the esophagus, occur. Similarly, the onset of certain cancers, such as Kaposi's sarcoma or lymphoma of the brain, will define AIDS. Central nervous system symptoms, including dementia, gait problems, and peripheral or cranial neuropathy, may also define AIDS. The presence of any of the above conditions indicates the presence of AIDS in a person who is HIV positive only if no other identifiable cause for the symptoms can be found. The Appendix contains the CDC's list of disorders that indicate the presence of AIDS in patients who are HIV positive.

A positive HIV antibody test indicates an infection by the virus. This test can identify both HIV-1, which is overwhelmingly the more common cause of infection, and HIV-2. The most conclusive evidence of HIV infection is a positive antibody result on each of a series, or protocol, of three tests: two positive enzyme-linked immunosorbent assay (ELISA) tests and a confirmatory Western blot test. In an ***ELISA test,*** the pathologist places a blood serum or plasma sample from the person being tested in contact with antigen-coated cells, in this case with HIV antigen-coated cells. If antibodies are present in the sample, they link to the corresponding antigens in the prepared cells. The ***Western blot test*** is a technique in which the pathologist places a blood serum or plasma sample from the person being tested and HIV antigens on opposite sides of a medium and then subjects the sample and antigens to an electric field. If HIV antibodies are present in the sample, they will migrate toward the antigens. The Western blot test is definitive in diagnosing HIV infection, but requires a tremendous amount of pathologist skill, experience, and labor, and so is performed only after two positive ELISA tests. If the three positive test results are reported by a reliable laboratory that uses approved testing procedures, there is scant chance that the person is not infected with HIV. The effect of HIV on the patient's immune system can be monitored by checking the patient's level of CD4 (T4) lymphocytes.

The treatment for HIV occurs at many levels. Primary prevention involves avoiding contaminated secretions. The nation's blood supply, which at one time was a source of HIV transmission, is very unlikely to contain contaminated products now because donors are screened and their blood is tested. However, sexual transmission of the virus and HIV transmission by intravenous drug use with infected needles continue to be common methods of spreading the virus.

A number of antiviral agents, such as Zidovudine, or AZT, are available, but so far none are curative. Treatment of infections and tumors secondary to HIV infections is important, but such treatment will not cure the AIDS infection itself. For example, treatment with Bactrim or pentamadine may prevent pneumocystis carinii pneumonia, which is a very common lethal infection in AIDS patients.

The impact of HIV infection on the individual and the world is enormous. In the United States from 1981 through September 1993, 400,000 cases of AIDS were reported and 200,000 deaths have been attributed to AIDS. Worldwide estimates are that 1.5 million people either have AIDS or have died from the disease. The long asymptomatic period of HIV infection provides a great deal of time for people to unwittingly pass on the disease. In the United States, HIV infection initially affected only members of certain groups: homosexual and bisexual men, intravenous drug abusers, and patients who received contaminated blood. The disease now affects all ages and both sexes, and is increasingly being transmitted through heterosexual contact.

The incidence of AIDS in children who are contaminated at birth or prenatally is increasing.

A very small group of patients have a disease that looks like AIDS, but they are not infected by HIV-1 or HIV-2. These patients have low levels of CD4 lymphocytes and develop opportunistic infections and/or cancers, as do AIDS patients. The cause of this AIDS-like disease is unclear.

Immediate Hypersensitivity Reactions

Immediate hypersensitivity reactions typically manifest from seconds to minutes after an antigen-antibody encounter. These reactions occur in association with hay fever and allergic asthma and may also occur following insect stings or the administration of a drug or serum to which the individual is sensitive. Symptoms vary in severity. Common symptoms, which generally are mild to moderate in severity, include itching, sneezing, wheezing, and difficulty in breathing. The most dangerous manifestation of immediate hypersensitivity is the generalized systemic reaction known as *anaphylaxis*, which is an unusual or exaggerated allergic reaction to a foreign substance. Symptoms of anaphylaxis include *urticaria*, or *hives*, which is a skin condition characterized by widely scattered, intensely itchy, slightly elevated welts that are surrounded by an area of redness; wheezing; choking; chest tightness; and collapse. Acute pulmonary edema or obstructive edema of the larynx can lead to death in severe anaphylaxis cases. Fortunately, anaphylactic shock is an uncommon reaction. When anaphylaxis does occur, it usually follows insect stings or the injection of immune antisera, such as tetanus antitoxin, penicillin, or other drugs having a relatively high sensitizing risk. Rarely, anaphylaxis occurs following orally administered drugs and foods.

Most individuals who are at risk for anaphylaxis will initially experience only the urticaria and nasal symptoms. Emergency treatment with adrenaline and intravenous fluids may be life saving. Antihistamines and steroids may also be necessary for a short time. Those individuals who have severe allergies are encouraged to avoid the offending agent and to carry injectable adrenaline with them at all times for self-injection if necessary.

Cellular Immunity and Delayed Hypersensitivity Reactions

Some immune responses are not dependent on a circulating antibody, but result from the interaction of an antigen with sensitized lymphocytes or other sensitized cells. This type of interaction is known as

cellular immunity or *cell-mediated immunity*. Most antigen-lymphocyte reactions require 12 to 48 hours for the immune reaction to
develop, and, as a result, the reactions of cellular immunity are known
as *delayed hypersensitivity reactions*. A positive tuberculin skin test
and contact dermatitis are examples of delayed reactions.

Cellular immunity phenomena may also be of importance in viral
infection, prevention of malignant disease, rejection of a transplanted
organ, and autoimmune disease.

Immune Complex Reactions

Immune complexes are protein substances that are created by the
reaction of an antigen with an antibody and that usually are removed
from the person's system without harm or difficulty. These complexes are soluble in the blood and are free to travel throughout the
body, possibly causing damage to the blood vessels of the heart,
kidney, pancreas, liver, and skin. Circulating immune complexes play
a role in the origin of many diseases, including several types of
glomerulonephritis, systemic lupus erythematosus, and periarteritis
nodosa, each of which is discussed later in this text.[1] Symptoms
associated with immune complex reactions are varied and depend on
(1) the nature and severity of the reaction and (2) the area of the
body or the organ system that is primarily affected. Common symptoms of immune complex reactions include fever, enlarged tender
lymph nodes, painful swollen joints, and a rash.

Autoimmune Disease

The immune system is equipped to detect foreign antigens and attack
them. One of the characteristics of the immune response system
described earlier was that the body is able to discriminate between
foreign antigens and the body's own self-made antigens. As a general
rule, a healthy body produces antibodies only to foreign antigens, but
in certain disease states this system malfunctions. One theory is that
antigens from a foreign source, such as a bacterium, that are very
similar to the host's antigens "confuse" the host's immune system so
that it cannot distinguish between the foreign antigens and the
self-made ones. *Autoimmune disorders* are those diseases in which
the body attacks its own tissue. Sensitized lymphocytes and the
cellular immunity phenomenon are also important in the origin of

---

[1]*Glomerulonephritis* is discussed in Chapter 10, *The Urinary System; systemic
lupus erythematosus* is discussed in Chapter 5, *The Skin;* and *periarteritis
nodosa* is discussed in Chapter 14, *The Nervous System.*

autoimmune disorders. In many conditions, such as autoimmune hemolytic anemia, idiopathic thrombocytopenic purpura, Grave's disease, myasthenia gravis, primary myxedema, Addison's disease, pernicious anemia, rheumatoid arthritis and systemic lupus erythematosus, antibodies or sensitized cells react with self-made antigens.

Immunology is a rapidly expanding field of study, in part because many diseases that in the past were not suspected of having an immunological basis are now being linked to disorders of the immune system.

GENETICS

Genetics is the science concerned with the inheritance of traits, the study of chromosomal and gene abnormalities, and the contribution of chromosomes and genes to health and disease. A *chromosome* is a complex structure found in the nucleus of each cell in the body. Each chromosome is composed of *genes*, which are the basic units of heredity. More than 50,000 genes are present in each cell. Each gene holds the information for the transmission of a trait from one generation of living organisms to another. A gene provides a code for a single protein, which is the final expression of the gene. In humans, a gene resides at a specific location on a given chromosome. Tissue culture and special dye techniques permit the identification, counting, and grouping of human chromosomes.

All normal human cells, except the ovum and sperm, contain in their nuclei 46 chromosomes arranged in 23 pairs. One chromosome of each pair is derived from each of the individual's parents. Of these 23 pairs of chromosomes in each cell, one is a pair of *sex chromosomes*, so named because these chromosomes determine the gender of the individual. The paired *female* sex chromosomes are identical and both are called X chromosomes, whereas the *male* sex chromosomes are dissimilar and are designated X and Y chromosomes. Each member of a chromosome pair, with the exception of the male sex chromosomes, is the same as the other member of the pair.

The ovum, or egg, and sperm are the only cells in the human body that do not have 46 chromosomes. Each of these cells contains 23 chromosomes, or one chromosome from each of the 23 pairs. The sex chromosomes in the ovum are all X chromosomes. In contrast, the sex chromosomes in the sperm are either X or Y, but not both. When a sperm cell and an ovum unite at fertilization, the new cells produced by this union will have 46 chromosomes in 23 pairs, one of each pair coming from the ovum and the other from the sperm. When a sperm containing an X chromosome unites with an egg containing an X chromosome, then the offspring will be a female, because the resulting zygote has two X chromosomes. The union of a sperm containing a Y chromosome with an egg produces a male, because the zygote has an X and a Y chromosome. The sex chromosome pairs in females and males are designated XX and XY, respectively.

Although genes usually remain stable from one generation to the next, they may undergo a change, or mutation. Once produced, these mutations are transmitted in the altered form to the next generation. Gene mutations can occur spontaneously or can result from exposure to radiation, chemicals, or viruses. For reasons that are unknown, advanced maternal and paternal age at the conception of the fetus is associated with an increased risk of mutation.

Traits and Modes of Inheritance

A *trait* is any genetically determined characteristic and may be either dominant or recessive. A ***dominant trait*** requires the presence of a specific gene on only one of a pair of chromosomes in order to produce the trait. Each individual who has this gene will show the trait. A ***recessive trait***, in contrast, is one that requires the presence of the same gene on each chromosome of a pair—one from the father and one from the mother. A ***carrier*** is an individual who has a recessive gene on one chromosome and not on the other chromosome of a pair. The recessive trait does not appear in carrier individuals, but carriers can transmit the affected gene to their offspring.

The only exception to the statement that recessive traits require the presence of two affected genes on a chromosome pair occurs with recessive traits that are carried by genes located on the X chromosome in males. These traits are called ***X-linked traits,*** *sex chromosome-linked traits*, or *sex-linked traits.* Hemophilia is an example of an X-linked recessive trait. Whenever a male's X chromosome carries the hemophilic gene, the individual will show the disease because no corresponding gene on the Y chromosome can "neutralize" or offset the hemophilic gene. Because females have two X chromosomes, females have to possess the gene responsible for hemophilia on each of the pair of X chromosomes in order to have the disease. As a result, females are most often carriers of the hemophilic gene—and other X-linked recessive genes—but do not suffer from the disease themselves. In summary, the characteristics of a trait or disease carried by a gene on the X chromosome are

- Only a single gene is responsible for the appearance of the disease.

- The disease mostly affects males and rarely affects females.
- Affected males transmit the disease through their daughters to their grandsons.

Many other diseases, such as hypertension, diabetes mellitus, atherosclerosis, and schizophrenia, and many physical characteristics, such as height, weight, skin color, and intelligence, are not inherited in accordance with simple modes of genetic inheritance. Such traits and diseases result from *polygenic inheritance*, which involves the interaction of several, or many, genes that have been inherited from both parents. "Polygenic" means "many genes." Polygenic inheritance is sometimes influenced by environmental factors over which the individual can exert some control. For example, a person is more likely to be obese if his or her parents are obese than if the parents maintain normal weight patterns. However, the person inherits only the tendency, or predisposition, to obesity, and not the condition itself. By maintaining careful control over his or her diet and exercise regimens, the individual can avoid obesity.

Genetic Disorders

Genetic diseases fall into one of the following three categories:

- chromosome disorders
- disorders involving the inheritance of an abnormal gene
- polygenic, or multifactorial, disorders resulting from the interaction of many genes and the environment

Chromosome disorders arise from the presence of an abnormal number of chromosomes, or parts of chromosomes, indicating the excess or deficiency of hundreds or thousands of genes. Chromosome disorders are present in up to 50 percent of spontaneous abortions occurring in the first trimester of pregnancy. Thus, chromosomal diseases are fairly uncommon in living individuals, because the overwhelming majority of individuals who might have such disorders are not born.

The most common condition resulting from an abnormal number of chromosomes is *Down's syndrome*, which is also known as *mongolism*, and is characterized by mental retardation and a variety of physical malformations. Down's syndrome is caused by either the presence of three rather than the normal pair of a specific chromosome—called chromosome 21—or by abnormalities of chromosome 21's structure. No clinical difference exists between children who have the chromosomal structural abnormality form of Down's syndrome and children who have the extra chromosomal form of the disease.

Disorders resulting from the inheritance of an abnormal gene are classified into dominant, recessive, or X-linked diseases. Dominant diseases are caused by one abnormal gene. Most dominant disorders show two characteristics that usually do not appear in recessive disorders:

- The disorders do not become clinically apparent until the patient's adult life even though the abnormal gene was present at the person's birth.
- The trait is expressed in a wide range of severity.

Recessive disorders require the presence of two abnormal genes, one on each of the paired chromosomes, and affect males and females in equal proportions. Both parents of the affected person may have the disorder, both parents may be carriers, or one parent may have the disorder and the other parent may be a carrier. The severity of recessive diseases is not as varied as the range of severity of dominant diseases, and the initial appearance of the recessive disease often occurs early in the patient's life.

The genes responsible for X-linked diseases are located on the X chromosome. Hemophilia is an example of an X-linked disease.

Figure 2–2 lists common genetic diseases by category of abnormality.

Prenatal Diagnosis of Inherited Diseases

The scientific community has made tremendous advances in the ability to diagnose a selected number of inherited diseases in children before they are born. The number of conditions that can be detected prenatally by current diagnostic methods that are generally safe for both the mother and her fetus is increasing dramatically. Ultrasonography can detect major malformations of the fetus, and x-rays can disclose gross skeletal abnormalities. However, the most frequently used technique for the prenatal diagnosis of inherited diseases is amniocentesis.

Amniocentesis is a procedure by which amniotic fluid is withdrawn from a pregnant woman. The procedure is performed using a needle that passes through the woman's skin and subcutaneous tissues and advances into her uterus. For diagnostic purposes, amniocentesis is performed around the fifteenth week of pregnancy, because at that time an adequate amount of fluid is available for

Figure 2-2.
Genetic Diseases.

Diseases Resulting from Chromosome Abnormalities

Category of Abnormality	Example of Disease
Chromosome lack	Turner's syndrome (X,O)
Chromosome excess	Down's syndrome; Klinefelter's syndrome (X, X, Y)
Abnormal structure	Down's syndrome; variety of malformations; mental retardation

Diseases Resulting from Simple Inheritance Abnormalities

Category of Abnormality	Example of Disease
Dominant inheritance	Adult polycystic kidney disease; familial hypercholesterolemia; hereditary spherocytosis; idiopathic hypertrophic subaortic stenosis; neurofibromatosis; von Willebrand's disease; Huntington's disease
Recessive inheritance	Albinism; congenital deafness; cystic fibrosis; Friedreich's ataxia; phenylketonuria; sickle cell anemia
X-linked inheritance	Color blindness; hemophilia A; Duchenne form of muscular dystrophy

Other Genetic Disorders

Category of Abnormality	Example of Disease
Diseases resulting from multifactorial or polygenic abnormalities	Addison's disease; ankylosing spondylitis; cleft lip; congenital heart disease; coronary artery disease; diabetes mellitus; epilepsy; hypertension; hyperthyroidism; bipolar mood disorder; multiple sclerosis; myasthenia gravis; peptic ulcer; Reiter's syndrome; schizophrenia

chromosomal analysis. Some of the cells present in amniotic fluid derive from the fetus, and these cells are tested to determine if a genetic disease is present in the growing fetus.

Another prenatal diagnostic test, called ***chorionic villi sampling (CVS)***, involves the removal of some chorionic villi with a needle aspiration. ***Chorionic villi*** are thread-like projections that grow in tufts on the external surface of the membrane that surrounds the fetus. This procedure can be performed on a woman earlier in her pregnancy than an amniocentesis can be performed. A CVS may be done during the ninth through twelfth weeks of pregnancy.

For most pregnant women who do not have any known risk factors, the probability of their offspring's having serious birth defects that can be diagnosed before birth is very low. Therefore, because amniocentesis and CVS present a slight risk to both mother and fetus, these diagnostic procedures are reserved for those situations in which the percentage of fetuses that have genetic diseases is known to be higher than average. Such situations include

- previous delivery of an infant with a chromosome abnormality
- presence of a known chromosome abnormality in either parent
- the presence of a known maternal carrier state
- advanced maternal age—risk of Down's syndrome increases as the age of the pregnant woman increases beyond age 35
- possibility of single gene disorder—parents are carriers for Tay Sach's disease or parents have previously produced a child who has a significant single gene disorder

Prenatal testing has several purposes. By detecting birth defects early, a pregnancy can be terminated early, depending on the wishes of the parents. The earlier in the pregnancy a termination is accomplished, the lower the medical risk imposed on the mother. Furthermore, detecting birth defects early can make the parents and the physician aware that corrective procedures will need to be performed on the infant either while it is still in the womb or immediately after its birth. Because most prenatal testing produces normal findings, the procedure has the effect of enabling most couples at high risk to proceed with a pregnancy without undue anxiety.

The Importance of Family History

Each year scientists learn more about the hereditary nature of many common disorders. Investigation has produced evidence that many human diseases have important genetic components. For example, certain diseases run in families even though most members of the family do not develop the disease, indicating that the individuals inherit a "predisposition" to develop a disease. The process of inheriting a predisposition is complex because it involves multiple genetic factors. The abnormal genes interact in some combination or cumulative fashion with multiple environmental factors to produce the disease.

Physicians generally ask each patient questions with regard to family members affected with known genetic diseases. Sometimes the knowledge of the presence of an unusual disease in a patient's family member aids the physician in the investigation and diagnosis of a patient who has unexplained symptoms. For purposes of evaluating a family medical history, the individual who is first identified as having the abnormality is called the *index case. First degree relatives* are the affected individual's parents, siblings, or children.

MORTALITY STUDIES

The development of reliable mortality statistics is a by-product of the legal requirements to register all deaths and record the cause of each death. Even though identifying a single cause of death is sometimes difficult, especially when the deceased suffered from several chronic diseases, the accumulated statistics have been, and continue to be, of great medical and social interest. The comparison of causes of death in various time periods sheds light on society's progress in dealing with public health problems and points out areas of future concern.

Mortality Trends in the United States

Improved public health measures, especially in the areas of prevention of infectious diseases, better diagnosis, and more effective treatment, have greatly reduced death rates from most of the leading causes of death at the turn of the century. Of the ten leading causes of death listed for the United States in 1900, only heart disease, cancer, stroke, accidents, and pneumonia remain on the list today. The infectious diseases that were the top three leading causes of death in 1900 account for less than five percent of the deaths today.

The average age at death today is significantly higher than it was in 1900. As life expectancy has increased, heart diseases have taken on greater importance as leading causes of death. At present, diseases of the heart kill almost twice as many people as cancer—the second leading cause of death—does. The death rates from specific types of cancer have risen and fallen through the years, often for reasons that are not completely clear, but the overall cancer death rate has shown a slow, steady increase. At present, heart diseases, cancer, and cerebrovascular diseases account for slightly more than 70 percent of all deaths in the United States.

The relative and actual importance of specific causes of death varies with an individual's age. Cancer is a leading cause of death at any age, second only to accidents in the 1- to 14-year-old age group and second only to heart disease in older age groups. As individuals grow older, strokes assume greater mortality significance, rising from an uncommon cause in the younger age groups to third place after age 75. In the 15- to 34-year-old age group, suicide and homicide are the second and third leading causes of death, respectively, but these causes are responsible for relatively few deaths in older people.

HIV infection is the fourth leading cause of death in males 15 to 54 years of age. In fact, AIDS-related disease was the leading cause of death in males aged 25 to 44 in at least 5 states and 64 cities and accounted for approximately 19 percent of all deaths among males in that age category in the entire United States in 1991. This disease was the second leading cause of death in young males in at least eight other states in the same year. Furthermore, AIDS was the leading cause of death in black females in ten cities in 1991. These numbers regarding HIV-related deaths are expected to continue to rise pending effective treatment or reliable prevention. Figure 2–3 outlines the leading causes of death for all age groups in the United States.

Gender differences are also significant in ranking causes of death in

Figure 2–3.
Mortality, Leading Causes of Death, by Sex (United States, 1989).

Male		**Female**	
Total Number of Deaths 1,114,190		Total Number of Deaths 1,036,276	
Heart diseases	33.0%	Heart diseases	35.3%
Cancer	23.6%	Cancer	22.5%
Accidents	5.7%	Cerebrovascular diseases	8.5%
Cerebrovascular diseases	5.1%	Pneumonia, influenza	3.9%
Chronic obstructive lung diseases	4.3%	Chronic obstructive lung diseases	3.5%
Pneumonia, influenza	3.2%	Accidents	3.0%
Suicide	2.2%	Diabetes	2.6%
HIV infection	1.8%	Atherosclerosis	1.2%
Diabetes	1.8%	Septicemia	1.0%
Homicide	1.6%	Nephritis	1.0%

Adapted, with permission of the publisher, from Catherine C. Boring, et al., "Cancer Statistics, 1993," *CA: A Cancer Journal for Clinicians* 43 (1993) : 14.

the United States. Females have lower mortality rates than males throughout the life cycle until ages over 75, by which time the women have outlived many men. The greater longevity of women has been attributed to unknown biological factors. Fatal accidents are almost twice as common in males than in females in the 1- to 14-year-old age group and almost four times as common in males than in females in the 15- to 34-year-old group. Only after age 74 do accidents claim more female than male victims. The mortality from diabetes mellitus among females is somewhat higher than that for males at all ages combined. The mortality among women from respiratory diseases is less than that for men, but by the last decade of life this difference has become very slight. The mortality from cirrhosis among females is about half that for males. In the past, complications of pregnancy were an important cause of death in females in the 15- to 34-year-old group, but maternal mortality problems in women during childbearing years are no longer among the leading causes of death in the United States.

As factors contributing to death, the actual role of certain underlying chronic conditions such as hypertension, obesity, diabetes, and chronic obstructive pulmonary disease may not be apparent from a review of condensed mortality data. These conditions accelerate the aging process, especially as this process relates to coronary artery disease, other heart disease, and cerebrovascular accidents or strokes, but only infrequently are these underlying conditions listed as the primary cause of death. Nevertheless, their importance should not be underestimated.

In addition, mortality figures may understate the incidence of suicide. Deaths from suicide may be recorded as mortality from accidents, heart attacks, unknown causes, or other illnesses. For example, a diabetic who wishes to end his or her life needs only to stop self-administration of the daily insulin requirement. The person's suicidal intent probably will go undetected and the cause of death will be recorded as diabetes. The physician who completes a death certificate generally will not list suicide as the cause of the deceased's death unless the physician is certain of the diagnosis.

Mortality Trends in Canada

The two leading causes of death in Canada, as detailed in Figure 2–4, are the same as those in the United States—diseases of the circulatory system and cancer. Although the death rate from heart disease and stroke in 1993 is half the death rate for these disorders 20 years ago, heart disease continues to be the leading cause of death in Canada. On the other hand, mortality rates for cancer in Canada have increased in males and have not changed much in females over the past 20 years.

Cancer mortality for the entire Canadian population has shown a slow increase since 1973. Each of the other leading causes of death, including accidents, diseases of the respiratory system, diseases of the digestive system, diseases of the endocrine system, diseases of the nervous system, and diseases of the genitourinary system, account for significantly fewer deaths than do circulatory system diseases and cancer. In fact, circulatory system disorders and cancer account for approximately 70 percent of all deaths in Canada.

Although HIV infection is a growing concern in Canada, AIDS-related mortality rates do not seem to be increasing as rapidly in Canada as they are in the United States. In 1990, AIDS was the leading cause of death of men aged 20 to 45 in urban centers such as Toronto, Montreal, and Vancouver. Furthermore, the number of Canadian women who are HIV positive is growing rapidly. However, AIDS affected only about .16% of the adult Canadian population.

Furthermore, gender differences are much less significant in ranking causes of death in Canada than these differences are in ranking causes of death in the United States. As indicated in Figure 2–4, the rankings of causes of death in Canadian males and females

Figure 2–4.
Mortality, Leading Causes of Death, by Sex (Canada, 1988).

Male		Female	
Diseases of the circulatory system	39.5%	Diseases of the circulatory system	43.4%
Cancer	27.0%	Cancer	26.4%
Accidents & adverse effects	9.1%	Diseases of the respiratory system	7.6%
Diseases of the respiratory system	9.1%	Accidents & adverse effects	4.8%
Diseases of the digestive system	3.5%	Diseases of the digestive system	3.8%
Diseases of the endocrine system	2.2%	Diseases of the endocrine system	3.2%
Diseases of the nervous system	2.1%	Diseases of the nervous system	2.7%
Diseases of the genitourinary system	1.4%	Diseases of the genitourinary system	1.6%
All other causes of death	6.1%	All other causes of death	6.5%

Adapted from Statistics Canada, *Leading Causes of Death at Different Ages*, 1988.

3

Specialized Diagnostic Techniques

A careful review of the patient's medical history and a thorough physical examination are the cornerstones for the diagnosis of most medical conditions. Adjunctive diagnostic procedures often provide additional important and useful information to help arrive at or confirm a diagnosis. Diagnostic techniques and procedures can be invasive or noninvasive. An ***invasive*** technique or procedure involves the puncture of, or incision into, the patient's skin or the introduction of an instrument or foreign material into the patient's body. In contrast, a ***noninvasive*** technique or procedure does not involve the puncture of, or incision into, the patient's skin or the introduction of an instrument or foreign material into the patient's body.

Some diagnostic procedures are routinely performed on almost all patients each time they visit a doctor. For example, patients typically have their temperature and blood pressure measured by a nurse or medical assistant even before the doctor performs any type of examination. Furthermore, patients commonly provide blood and urine samples as part of an exam.

In addition to the many well-established diagnostic techniques, a host of specialized diagnostic procedures have been developed in recent years. Investigation with fiberoptic instruments, diagnostic ultrasonography, computerized tomography, magnetic resonance imaging, radionuclide imaging, and invasive radiology greatly assist physicians in making diagnoses. The purpose of this chapter is to describe these specialized techniques and to show their application in patients who have medical disorders.

INVESTIGATION WITH FIBEROPTIC INSTRUMENTS

Fiberoptic strands are tiny, flexible glass filaments having special optical properties. Each fiber transmits light, which, as it travels the length of a flexible fiber, can bend at acute angles without distortion and emerge at the fiber's end hardly diminished in intensity.

Endoscopy is an invasive technique that permits the visual inspection of a cavity or hollow organ with a specially designed tubular instrument, known as an endoscope, that incorporates fiber-optics. The endoscope has several longitudinal compartments, or channels, one of which contains a bundle of fibers for light transmission. The light comes from an external light source that is attached to the instrument. Another channel, which has its own fiberoptic bundle, is used for viewing. Lenses at either end of the instrument focus and magnify the viewed image. The endoscope provides an undistorted image, regardless of how looped the instrument becomes. The instrument is flexible throughout its length and has controlled bending capability at its tip so that the physician can view all surfaces of the tissue. The physician may view fiberoptic images directly or on a TV-like cathode-ray tube (CRT) screen, and the diagnostic information provided by the scope may be stored electronically.

The instrument may have additional channels for the instillation of air or water, for tissue biopsy, and for suction of mucus, fluid, or blood. Fiberoptic instruments are designed for specific purposes, such as inspection of the stomach, lung, joints, duodenum, or colon, and have modifications to facilitate their use for the specific purpose intended. In these specific modified versions, the instruments are known as gastroscopes, bronchoscopes, arthroscopes, duodenoscopes, or colonoscopes, respectively.

Endoscopy and other fiberoptic studies can also be combined with laser technology to remove diseased cells, tissues, or organs, tumors, or other materials. In addition, laser technology can be used alone to remove diseased cells or tumors in relatively easy-to-reach places in the body, such as a woman's cervix. In a combined laser and fiberoptic procedure, the laser is inserted into the patient through a small incision and is directed to the appropriate site by visualization through the fiberoptic scope. The surgeon then removes the tissue, organ, tumor, or other material by "zapping" it with the laser. Most types of laser surgery require that the patient receive general anesthesia. Many patients experience only a small amount of postoperative pain and do not take long to recuperate from the laser procedure. The primary benefit of the laser technique is that lasers are *self-cauterizing*, which means that they cause the patient's affected blood vessels to clot and seal, thus eliminating the need for internal stitches. Self-cauterization reduces the patient's risk of postoperative complications such as infection and bleeding.

This section will review a few applications of fiberoptic instruments in diagnosis and therapy, but more detailed discussions of fiberoptic instruments appear throughout this text in describing diagnostic and therapeutic techniques for specific organ systems.

Endoscopy of the Upper Gastrointestinal Tract

A physician may order an upper gastrointestinal (GI) tract endoscopy to:

- determine the source of a patient's gastrointestinal symptoms when x-rays of the upper GI tract have failed to do so
- determine the cause of bleeding from the patient's upper GI tract
- biopsy lesions that show up on x-ray
- remove polyps
- remove a foreign body
- dilate an esophageal stricture
- evaluate the results of surgery or the effects of radiation treatment
- treat certain conditions

Small, superficial ulcers that may not show up on a conventional upper GI series using a contrast medium such as barium may be seen by fiberoptic gastroscopy. Fiberoptic esophagogastroduodenoscopy identifies a bleeding site and other lesions more precisely than does x-ray. In more than 85 percent of patients who have GI bleeding and who undergo this diagnostic procedure, the endoscope provides an identification of the location of the bleeding site.

Upper GI endoscopy allows for the visualization and diagnosis of a number of common lesions. Figure 3–1 lists some of these lesions.

Essentially no contraindications to fiberoptic endoscopy of the

Figure 3–1.
Common Upper GI Lesions Visualized by Endoscopy.

Lesions of the Esophagus	Lesions of the Stomach	Lesions of the Duodenum
Hiatus hernia	Gastritis	Ulcer
Ulcerations and tears	Polyps	Duodenitis
Esophagitis	Leiomyoma	Polyps
Varices	Ulcer	Diverticula
Stricture	Cancer	Cancer
Cancer		

upper GI tract exist, and almost no morbidity or mortality is associated with the procedure. Complications from the procedure rarely occur.

Colonoscopy

Colonoscopy is the inspection of the interior of the large intestine by means of a flexible, fiberoptic colonoscope. This instrument is made in several lengths—the longer length scopes the entire colon and the shorter length scopes the left side of the colon only. A fiberoptic scope of the left side of the colon is called a *sigmoidoscopy*. Patients who undergo colonoscopies generally are not anesthetized, but they generally are mildly sedated. Colonoscopy represents a significant advance in the ability to diagnose colon cancers.

Colonoscopy is useful for investigating and evaluating:

- lower gastrointestinal tract bleeding
- inflammatory bowel disease
- abnormalities first seen in a barium enema examination
- the results of surgery on the colon

Colonoscopy also is useful for removing foreign bodies and polyps from the colon and for performing a biopsy on a suspicious lesion. Although colonoscopy is a relatively safe procedure, it probably should not be performed on a critically ill patient or on a patient who is experiencing an acute inflammation of the colon, such as acute diverticulitis or acute ulcerative colitis. Complications of colonoscopy are infrequent, but include perforation of the wall of the colon by the instrument, hemorrhage from trauma to the wall of the colon, and **bacteremia**, which is a transient bacterial invasion of the blood stream, in this case from bacteria that are normal inhabitants of the colon.

Bronchoscopy

A physician can examine the interior of the patient's trachea and bronchi with a conventional, rigid, hollow-tubed bronchoscope or with a flexible, **fiberoptic bronchoscope**. This text will consider only the fiberoptic instrument, although many of the indications for use and complications following bronchoscopy apply to both types of instruments. The purposes of bronchoscopy are the visualization of the endobronchial tree, the establishment of a tissue diagnosis by biopsy, and the collection of washings and other secretions for bacterial culture and cytology. Some of the indications for bronchoscopy include:

- malignant cells in the patient's sputum when the chest x-ray is normal
- unexplained bloody sputum
- pneumonia that fails to respond to therapy
- x-ray evidence of bronchial obstruction or suspected cancer

Flexible fiberoptic bronchoscopy causes minimal discomfort to the patient. Its major advantage over rigid bronchoscopy, however, is that it allows the physician to see more of the patient's internal tissues. The flexible bronchoscope permits biopsy of previously inaccessible tumors, resulting in the earlier detection of lung cancer and the hope of lengthening the patient's survival time from this disease. Possible complications of fiberoptic bronchoscopy include hemorrhage following biopsy, rupture of a bronchus permitting air to escape into the pleural cavity, and a reduction in oxygen tension in the blood, a condition known as **transient hypoxemia**.

Laparoscopy

Laparoscopy is the inspection of the patient's abdominal cavity by means of a special fiberoptic instrument that is designed for viewing, biopsy, and surgery and that the physician inserts through a small incision in the patient's abdomen. Laparoscopy is a simple and safe method for diagnosing intra-abdominal disease. The laparoscope enables the physician to examine the top and undersurface of the liver to determine if cirrhosis or cancer is present, and to locate small lesions of the liver that liver scans and needle biopsies miss.

Laparoscopes are also used to search the peritoneal cavity for the presence of metastatic disease, to obtain biopsies for a tissue diagnosis, to assist in the staging of Hodgkin's disease and other lymphomas, to determine the cause of abdominal pain, and to perform simple surgical procedures. Often laparoscopy makes major abdominal surgery unnecessary. For example, a surgeon can use laparoscopic techniques to remove a patient's appendix or gallbladder.

ULTRASONOGRAPHY, COMPUTERIZED TOMOGRAPHY, AND MAGNETIC RESONANCE IMAGING

Three other common diagnostic techniques are ultrasonography, computerized tomography, and magnetic resonance imaging. Although these procedures utilize different technologies, they can sometimes be used to diagnose similar conditions. Therefore, they are considered together in this section.

Ultrasonography

Ultrasonography, which is also called *echography*, is a noninvasive investigative method that utilizes sound vibrations to visualize organs by recording and displaying the reflections (echoes) of high frequency sound waves. An ultrasonic transducer, which translates one form of energy into another, is placed on the surface of the patient's body and focuses these sound waves into a narrow beam. As the sound waves penetrate the patient's body and strike tissues that have different densities, some of the transmitted sound waves are reflected to the transducer as an echo. The remainder of the sound waves continue deeper into the patient's tissues and are reflected by other echo-producing tissues. Because the amount of reflected energy varies with different surfaces, the size of the patient's organs and their relationship to each other are calculated by measuring the time it takes for the sound wave to travel from the transducer to the different reflecting surfaces and back to the transducer again. The echoes are amplified and displayed on an oscilloscope or on a strip chart recorder, thus producing an echogram. An *oscilloscope* is an instrument that displays images of electrical currents on the screen of a cathode-ray tube. A doctor or medical technician who has experience reading echograms can identify all structures represented on the oscilloscope or chart.

Uses of Ultrasound

Ultrasound is the most common diagnostic procedure for evaluating a patient's liver, gallbladder, and biliary system. Ultrasound also is useful in diagnosing female pelvic disease, often revealing ovarian cysts and uterine and other pelvic lesions. Because ultrasound does not expose the patient to radiation, this technique is used on pregnant women to determine fetal size and maturity, to diagnose fetal anomalies, to locate the placenta prior to amniocentesis, to monitor fetal distress, and to confirm fetal death. Moreover, ultrasound techniques can detect pregnancy as early as the fifth week of gestation.

A major application of ultrasonography is in the study of the heart and in the diagnosis and management of heart disease. Ultrasonography of the heart is called *echocardiography*. The section on cardiovascular disease in Chapter 7 contains a more detailed discussion of echocardiography. Figure 3–2 lists some of the cardiac uses of ultrasound.

Ultrasound is also used to determine the status and direction of the patient's blood flow through arteries and veins. It is useful for guiding a needle biopsy and increasing the accuracy of the biopsy of internal organs and/or tumors within those organs.

Advantages and Limitations of Ultrasonography

Ultrasound has many advantages:

- It is painless.
- It does not alter the physiology of the tissues studied.

Figure 3–2.
Some Cardiac Uses for Echocardiography.

For Evaluation of these Disorders:	For Obtaining these Measurements and Determinations:
Aortic stenosis	Size of the atrial cavity
Mitral stenosis	Valve motion
Atrial myxoma	Size of the ventricular cavity
Mitral valve prolapse	Ventricular function
Cardiomyopathies	Thickness of the ventricular wall
Pericardial effusions	Ventricular wall motion
Idiopathic hypertrophic subaortic stenosis	

- It does not cause immediate, delayed, or cumulative injury, and repeated examinations do not present a hazard to the patient.
- It does not require that the patient be moved around, because small, portable ultrasound machines can be used at the patient's bedside.

Thus, ultrasonography can be less physically and psychologically disruptive to the patient than are many other diagnostic techniques.

Ultrasound can also show changes in some diseased organs that are not functioning sufficiently. For example, x-ray following a contrast agent often will not outline the dilated biliary ducts and the gallbladder in patients who have obstructive jaundice. However, these ducts that are dilated with bile clearly show up on an ultrasonogram.

On the other hand, ultrasonic scanning does have several limitations. Its major drawback lies in the inability of the sound to penetrate gas and bone. When the sound beam hits gas or bone, most of the beam is reflected and is recorded as useless noise. Moreover, ultrasound waves do not always clearly delineate fat from other tissues and organs. As a result, markedly obese patients are not good candidates for ultrasound scanning.

Computerized Tomography

A very useful investigative tool available to a diagnostic radiologist is computerized axial tomography, popularly called a CT scan or CAT scan. *Tomography*, or *sectional radiography*, is a noninvasive technique that sends a very narrow x-ray beam through the tissue under examination and shows detail at a predetermined level of the body while blurring the images of structures above or below the desired level. *Computerized axial tomography*, a refinement of this tomographic or "sectioning" principle, is an examination of a section of the body in which a special machine that is linked to a computer records multiple x-ray images and then analyzes, reconstructs, and displays those images to give an accurate visualization of structures that are deep within the body and are inaccessible to conventional x-ray techniques. A CT machine employs sensitive crystal detectors in place of x-ray film and rotates around the patient to make multidirectional x-ray observations of tissues or structures. The images produced during a CT scan appear on a CRT screen as cross-sectional pictures of the area studied and provide much better detail than ultrasound images provide. Contrast media introduced into the patient's body either orally or intravenously can enhance the CT scan image. Although CT scans sometimes are performed in conjunction with the introduction of a contrast agent, the medical community typically considers this technique to be noninvasive. The disadvantages of CT scanning are cost, lack of portability, and risks inherent in exposing the patient to some radiation.

CT scanning can determine the size, shape, and position of many organs. Although the CT scan does not detect very small lesions or infiltrative lesions, it does demonstrate discrete defects produced by cysts, infarcts, and sharply defined tumors. CT scanning is the procedure of choice for evaluating problems in the patient's abdomen and chest. CT scanning also is useful for screening for aortic aneurysms, diagnosing masses in the patient's thoracic cavity, and differentiating hematomas from edema in neurological evaluations of head injuries. In fact, the CT scan is the most valuable method of detecting and determining the location of intracranial disorders. Figure 3–3 lists some of the conditions CT scans can identify.

Magnetic Resonance Imaging

Magnetic resonance imaging (MRI) is a diagnostic technique that utilizes strong magnetic fields, radio frequency waves, and a computer to obtain images of different cross-sections of a patient's body part. During an MRI exam, the patient lies on a flat surface within a capsule that is closed at one end. Usually, the patient's head rests at the closed end of the MRI machine, and the patient's feet are at the

Figure 3–3.
Selected Conditions Identified by CT Scan.

Organ or Area	Condition
Liver	Tumor, cyst, abscess
Biliary tract	Dilated ducts
Gallbladder	Stones, enlargement
Brain	Enlarged ventricle, tumor, hematoma, vascular anomaly
Spleen	Tumor, cyst
Pancreas	Calcification, pseudocyst
Kidney	Tumor, cyst, status of transplant
Retroperitoneal space	Tumor, aneurysm
Bone	Destruction, abscess, metastasis
Pleural cavity	Effusion, abscess, aneurysm

open end. The patient's body lies within only a few inches of the internal surface of the cylindrical shaft of the machine. The machine bounces radio waves off the patient's body, and a computer translates the reflected waves into video images, viewable on a CRT. The intravenous introduction of a safe nonradioactive contrast agent into the affected body part will provide an image that has even more details. Although some MRI studies are performed in conjunction with the injection of a contrast agent, they are generally considered to be noninvasive.

Full medical details and suspected diagnoses of the patient's condition may affect the radiologist's decision of which diagnostic technique to use, because MRI techniques are changing with improvements in technology and experience. MRI is very helpful in evaluating diseases of the central nervous system and has replaced some of the need for myelography. *Myelography* is a diagnostic technique in which an oily, radiopaque dye is injected into the patient's spinal canal, followed by an x-ray study of the movement of the dye through the canal. Good quality noninvasive studies of the heart muscle by MRI angiography are also available. MRI of the heart is now used primarily for studying congenital lesions, but this procedure is becoming increasingly useful for examining coronary artery disease. Furthermore, an MRI of the patient's knee can provide much of the same information arthrography or arthroscopy provide.

The disadvantages of MRI include cost, availability, and inappropriateness of use in patients who have contained metal devices, such as pacemakers and artificial joints. Also, approximately five percent of patients who have MRIs become claustrophobic while they are in the machine. However, some new MRI units are open at both ends and reduce these patients' anxiety.

Ultrasonography, Computerized Tomography, and MRI

A radiologist might choose ultrasonography, CT scanning, or MRI over the other investigative techniques for any one of many reasons. Chief among these reasons are the size, shape, consistency, and location of the lesion. The preference for any one of these techniques at a medical center, however, may depend more on availability, operator expertise, and the personal preference of the radiologist than on other factors. In some instances, one method of investigation will provide greater accuracy in diagnosing a patient's condition, but in other instances, one method may have little advantage in accuracy over another. If the results of one method are inconclusive, however, then another method can be used.

Ultrasound is widely available, comparatively inexpensive, fast, and flexible. On the other hand, ultrasound test results are somewhat difficult to interpret and ultrasonography requires a higher level of operator skill than do CT scanning and MRI. Computerized tomography and MRI provide superior image resolution, tissue specificity, and ease of performance and interpretation, as compared to ultrasonography. Furthermore, CT scanning and MRI require a lower degree of operator skill than ultrasonography, but the former are more expensive than ultrasonography.

RADIONUCLIDE IMAGING

A *radioisotope* is a radioactive substance, which means that as it undergoes decay, it emits radiation. A *radionuclide* is a type of radioisotope that has important diagnostic and therapeutic uses in clinical medicine and research. *Radionuclide imaging*, then, is a diagnostic and therapeutic procedure in which radionuclides are administered to patients orally or intravenously after which imaging devices record the distribution of radiation the radioisotope emits.

Two types of imaging devices are used for radionuclide imaging. *Scanning detectors*, or *scanners*, move back and forth across the area of the body that is under study, and radioactive patterns are recorded on paper or on x-ray film. *Scintillation cameras* are stationary devices that are aimed at the area of the body being studied and that display radioactive emissions on a screen or record them as a series of "stop action" photographs. In general, scintillation cameras provide better resolution of small images than do scanners.

Many radionuclides, including radioactive technetium, thallium, and iodine, are used for diagnosing diseases. The choice of radionuclide depends on the organ under investigation, because organs differ in their abilities to concentrate various radionuclides.

The physician can interface the scintillation camera with a computer for quantitative measurement of emitted radiation. Depending on the organ studied and the radionuclide used, an abnormal image, which indicates possible disease, may have either a higher or a lower concentration of radioactivity than is present in adjacent or comparable areas.

Radionuclide Evaluation of the Heart and Other Organs

Radionuclide imaging procedures can determine the openness of the coronary arteries, dilation and displacement of the aorta, the presence of fluid in the pericardial space, the volume of the cardiac chambers, the ability of the left ventricular wall to contract effectively, and the extent of damage to the myocardium. Technetium scans and thallium scans are two important nuclear medicine studies used in the investigation of suspected coronary artery disease and myocardial infarction and will be explained in Chapter 7, *The Circulatory System*.

Radionuclide evaluation of the liver and spleen depends on the removal, by certain cells lining the blood sinuses of these organs, of the injected radioactive isotope from the blood stream. Within a few minutes after the intravenous injection of a short-lived isotope into the patient, the scan will clearly delineate the anatomic features of the liver and spleen. A scan of the normal liver and spleen will show a uniform uptake of the isotope, whereas a scan of an abnormal liver will show variations in uptake. Thus, abnormalities associated with disease of these organs become readily apparent.

Radioisotope imaging procedures are also useful in the detection of disease in many other organs and tissues, including the thyroid gland, lung, kidney, bone, and pancreas.

Comparison of Radionuclide Imaging with Conventional X-ray

Both conventional x-ray and radionuclides expose the patient to some radiation. Radionuclide investigation, however, differs from conventional x-rays in several respects:

- The patient is exposed to less radiation with radionuclides than with x-rays.
- The emission images obtained by radionuclides are less sharp and show less detail than those obtained with x-rays.
- Radionuclide uptake in an organ can allow for a quantitative estimation of the functional activity of that organ, an estimation that x-rays generally cannot accomplish.

Great advances have been made in the development and refinement of imaging techniques, in instrumentation, and in uses for radionuclides. The coupling of the digital computer with the scintillation camera has increased the possibilities for evaluation of many organs. Although radionuclide studies usually do not diagnose the origin of a disease, they are very sensitive in detecting the location of pathologic conditions.

INVASIVE RADIOLOGY

A *catheter* is a hollow, flexible tube used for withdrawing fluids from or introducing fluids into a body cavity or blood vessel. *Invasive radiology* involves the catheterization of blood vessels and the injection through the catheter of *radiopaque contrast agents*, which are substances that provide visible images on x-ray film. The circulation of these contrast agents is observed by x-ray methods. Invasive radiology can also be used for therapeutic purposes.

An intravascular catheter may be useful for diagnostic or treatment purposes. *Interventional radiology* refers to any selective catheter technique adopted for treatment and includes the infusion through a catheter of *vasodilators* or *vasoconstrictors*—drugs that dilate or constrict blood vessels, respectively—and other therapeutic agents. The introduction into the patient's body of special catheters for dilating partially occluded vessels is another use of interventional radiology. This section will consider some invasive radiologic procedures used for diagnosis and treatment.

Angiography, Arteriography, and Venography

Angiography is a diagnostic technique involving the introduction of a contrast material into a patient's blood vessel, followed by a series of x-rays, usually taken in rapid sequence. *Arteriography* is a more specific term referring to the x-ray visualization of an artery after the injection of a radiopaque dye. The dye may be injected directly into the patient's blood vessel or into a catheter that has been inserted into the vessel. The catheter is used when the vessel or organ under examination is some distance from the site of the injection. *Venography* is the x-ray visualization of a vein after the injection of a radiopaque dye.

Arteriography of Peripheral Vessels and Organs

Arteriography is used in the diagnosis and treatment of obstructions in the peripheral vessels—arteries that carry blood through the trunk and extremities. For example, in patients who have arteriosclerosis of peripheral vessels, angiography is used prior to surgery in order to determine the precise location of the disease in the artery, the extent of the obstruction, and the status of arteries in the collateral circulation.

Arteriography can also be used to detect problems in various organs of the body. Not only can arteriography be used to diagnose problems of the arteries that serve the organs, but also it can be helpful in diagnosing nonartery problems within the organs themselves. Arteriography of the brain, for example, is an extremely valuable method for diagnosing obstructed cerebral arteries, but it may also be used in the diagnosis of brain tumors. When arteriography is performed on the brain, the physician inserts a needle, called a cannula, in one of the larger arteries of the patient's neck or introduces a catheter into the femoral artery in the patient's leg and advances the catheter into the patient's larger neck vessel or aorta. A dye is injected into the catheter so that the physician can view the cerebral arteries through x-ray and can note those vessels that are narrowed or obstructed. The physician may also be able to diagnose tumors or lesions of the brain by watching the dye as it proceeds through the vessels. If the circulation through the brain appears delayed at some point or if cerebral vessels are not in their usual place, these signs may indicate a tumor or other space-occupying lesion. Angiography cannot generally provide enough definition to distinguish between the various types of tumors that may be found in some organs and may not differentiate benign from malignant solitary tumors.

Uses of arteriography in various organs and systems will be addressed as they are discussed throughout the chapters of the text.

Computerized Intravenous Arteriography

The major difference between intravenous and standard arteriography is that in the former procedure the radiopaque dye is injected into a vein instead of an artery, thus avoiding the risk and discomfort associated with arterial puncture. Venous injection of the dye, which is usually performed through a catheter, causes a dilution of the contrast material as the dye passes from the venous circulation through the heart and out into the artery under study. The weak signal from the dye is amplified several times by image-intensification fluoroscopy, and a special computer further refines and sharpens the image.

Computerized intravenous arteriography is practically as safe as the noninvasive diagnostic methods and produces an image that has a clarity within ten percent of that obtained with standard arteriography. The use of computerized intravenous arteriography can indicate total occlusions, moderate stenosis, and flat areas in the blood vessels. This method produces clear visualization of intracranial and extracranial arteries, the aortic arch, the abdominal aorta and its branches, and the arteries in the arms and legs.

Catheterization of the Heart

Cardiac catheterization is the insertion of a catheter in order to obtain precise functional and anatomic information about the patient's heart prior to cardiac surgery. Only one side of the heart can be catheterized at a time. Catheterization of the right side of the patient's heart is accomplished by the introduction of a long, flexible radiopaque catheter into an arm or leg vein. The physician then guides the catheter into the patient's right atrium, right ventricle, and pulmonary artery.

Catheterization of the left side of the patient's heart is commonly accomplished by the insertion of a catheter into the femoral artery in the patient's groin. The physician guides the catheter into the patient's aorta and left ventricle.

During heart catheterization, physicians can obtain blood samples and can determine intravascular pressures from several intravascular locations and from the pulmonary artery and aorta. Furthermore, the physician can make several important measurements of heart function that are necessary in preparation for heart surgery.

Ventriculography and Coronary Arteriography

The route taken by the radiopaque catheter used in cardiac catheterization may give a clue to the presence of congenital anomalies in the patient's heart, aorta, or pulmonary artery. During a cardiac catheterization, the radiologist often will inject radiopaque dye at various sites within the patient's heart and great vessels. *Right and left ventriculography*, which is the x-ray visualization of the ventricles of the heart, is employed to define congenital and acquired lesions and to measure a patient's *stroke volume*, which is the volume of blood each contraction of the left ventricle pumps into the aorta.

Coronary arteriography involves the injection of a contrast medium through a catheter directly into each of a patient's coronary arteries. A radiologist makes an x-ray study of the patient's heart during and after the injection procedure. Selective injection of contrast media into the heart and coronary vessels combined with exposure of high-speed x-ray motion pictures, a procedure called *cineangiography*, permits accurate diagnosis of complex cardiac problems. Cineangiography using radionuclides is also possible. Cineangiography is more sensitive than exercise electrocardiography in detecting coronary artery disease.

Catheterization and angiography are used to make several important determinations of heart anatomy and heart function, including the

- extent of coronary artery obstruction
- severity of a heart valve lesion
- nature of other cardiac lesions
- identification of the cause of chest pain of cardiac origin
- identification of cardiac pathology amenable to surgery
- results of cardiac surgery

Although they are invasive procedures, cardiac catheterization and angiography are only infrequently associated with major complications, such as cardiac perforation, arrhythmia, hemorrhage, hypotension, thrombosis, myocardial infarction, and cerebral embolism. In the United States, the reported mortality arising from cardiac catheterization is at a rate of less than one-half of one percent. The rate is higher in individuals who are over age 60 or under age 1.

4

Tumors

This chapter will develop a working definition of tumors, and then will explain the systems medical professionals commonly use to classify tumors. Next, the chapter discusses the origins of many types of tumors and the staging systems for describing malignant tumors. The chapter concludes by addressing the diagnosis and treatment of various tumors and providing information on cancer rates and trends.

Because tumors arise from all types of human cells, developing a useful and specific definition that will be universally accurate and that will distinguish tumors from other masses is difficult. For the purposes of this text, we will define **tumor** and **neoplasm** synonymously as a disturbance in the normal growth of tissue characterized by an abnormal, excessive, and uncontrolled proliferation of cells. In general, to be considered a tumor, a new growth must have three characteristics. First, it must grow, respond, and react independently of the normal functions of the body. However, a tumor cannot exist totally independently, because it must depend on the body for its blood supply, oxygen, and other essentials for growth.

Second, the tumor's growth must be progressive within certain broad limits that vary with the type of tumor. Some tumors have the potential of growing to a substantial size, but others are more limited in their growth. Furthermore, progressive growth patterns may not occur at uniform rates over different periods of time.

Third, tumors do not provide the body with any added physiologic benefit. Most tumors do not secrete hormones and are devoid of all function. A few tumors retain the properties of their parent cells, and if these parent cells secrete hormones, the tumor cells also may do so. However, the hormones these tumors produce provide no physiologic benefit and actually may be detrimental to the body as a whole.

This chapter will take a general look at tumors. The more common tumors will receive specific consideration in the appropriate chapters that address the various organ systems in the human body.

CLASSIFICATION OF TUMORS

Tumors can be classified in several ways. They can be classified (1) as being either benign or malignant, (2) according to the type of tissue involved, and (3) according to the extent of the tumor's involvement in the patient's tissues.

The classification of a tumor as benign or malignant depends upon several important characteristics. In general, **benign tumors** are slow growing, do not invade neighboring tissues or spread to distant parts of the body, and do not recur after complete removal. During their growth, benign tumors are well circumscribed and often are encapsulated, meaning that they develop an enclosing capsule or shell. They grow in orderly patterns, and their cells resemble those of the parent tissues. As a general rule, benign tumors do not endanger the patient's life unless they develop in strategic locations, such as the patient's brain, heart, or spinal column. Moreover, benign tumors may produce symptoms if, by their growth and enlargement, they place pressure on important surrounding organs.

In general, **malignant tumors**, which are also known as *cancers*, grow autonomously, invade neighboring tissue, and spread beyond the organ originally involved. This spread may occur as a result of direct invasion into neighboring structures or by **metastasis**, which is the spread of malignant cells from the primary tumor to a distant location through lymph channels or blood vessels. In the new site, the malignant cells grow, multiply, and invade the distant tissue. By direct extension to adjacent tissues or by metastasis, the cancer cells cause destruction of normal cells and disturb the function of the invaded organ. Cancers may cause generalized body dysfunction, such as loss of appetite or weight, fevers, and fatigue. Malignant tumors may be difficult to remove completely from the patient's body and, if removed, sometimes recur. Cells of cancers can vary widely in size, shape, and staining characteristics from cells of the parent tissue and may bear little resemblance in structure and form to the cells of the tissue of origin. All malignant tumors endanger the patient's life, but some malignancies are much more life-threatening than others.

Sometimes classifying a tumor as benign or malignant is difficult, because not all benign or malignant tumors possess all the characteristics mentioned above. For example, in certain cancers, some malignant features may be absent at the time of the discovery of the tumor, but nevertheless the tumor retains the potential for the full development of all malignant characteristics.

Figure 4–1 lists the more common characteristics of benign and malignant tumors.

Some pathologic conditions have been designated as **precancerous**, meaning that they are not true cancers, but they have a tendency to develop into true cancers. In this large, heterogeneous group of conditions, the incidence of actual malignant transformation is low for certain conditions and nearly 100 percent for others. Examples of precancerous lesions include bladder papillomas, certain polyps of the stomach and intestines, and some skin lesions such as moles.

Carcinoma-in-situ, also known as *cancer-in-situ* or *intraepithelial cancer*, is a lesion that has all the characteristics of malignancy under microscopic analysis except that of invasion. By definition, a carcinoma-in-situ has not spread beyond the superficial epithelial layer of origin and has not passed the enclosing membrane. Given time, all in-situ lesions will progress to invasive cancer, but as long as

Figure 4–1.
Characteristics of Benign and Malignant Tumors.

Tumor Characteristics	Benign Tumor	Malignant Tumor
Endangers life	Rarely	Often
Growth rate	Often slow	Usually rapid
Local invasion	No	Frequent
Metastasis	No	Frequent
Tissue destruction	Little	Much
Disturbance of function	Usually little	Often much
Recurrence after removal	Rare	Sometimes
Encapsulation	Often present	Absent
Cellular pattern	Normal, orderly	Often bizarre

the carcinoma is restricted to the surface epithelium, metastases will not occur. Because carcinomas-in-situ are small tumors and generally are localized to a single epithelial focus, prompt and adequate treatment usually results in a complete cure. Carcinomas-in-situ are found most commonly in the cervix, breast, stomach, skin, oral cavity, larynx, bronchus, and vagina.

ETIOLOGY OF TUMORS

Many theories of the etiology, or cause, of tumors exist, but the basic cause remains unknown. Environmental factors that are suspected of predisposing an individual to the development of certain types of tumors include (1) prolonged exposure to smoke, radiation, sunlight, and toxic industrial chemicals and (2) chronic irritation from many sources.

Because some tumors have a higher incidence in certain families than would be expected in a normal population, a genetic predisposition to tumor formation also exists. A dominantly inherited predisposition is associated with certain sarcomas, brain tumors, leukemias, breast cancers, tumors of the retina, and colon cancers. Furthermore, scientists have identified certain genes, called *oncogenes*, that may facilitate cancer development. Other genes, called *tumor suppressor genes*, discourage the development of cancer, and loss of these suppressor genes may stimulate the development of certain cancers such as *retinoblastoma*, which is a malignant tumor arising in children from cells of the retina. Moreover, environmental factors may operate within the family in association with genetic factors. For example, a genetically predisposed group of smokers has a higher incidence of lung cancer than does either a similar group of nonsmokers or a group of smokers who have not inherited a cancer predisposition.

Age, gender, race, and occupation are other important factors in cancer predisposition. Early sexual contact may increase a female's risk of developing cancer of the cervix, and males who have been circumcised in early life have a lower incidence of cancer of the penis than either uncircumcised males or males who are circumcised later in life. The incidence of certain cancers differs in males and females, which may partially be explained by differences in lifestyles, exposure to industrial hazards or sunlight, or other factors. In addition, a true gender difference in predisposition to certain tumors may exist.

Age differences are significant factors in the development of certain cancers. For example, retinoblastoma and Wilms tumor develop exclusively in children, and cancer of the prostate rarely develops in patients under age 50.

Furthermore, certain viruses are causally related to cancer. For instance, hepatitis B carriers are at higher than normal risk for developing hepatoma, a primary liver cancer. Also, the Epstein-Barr virus is associated with nasopharyngeal cancer and Burkitt's lymphoma.

Scientists are now studying the possible immunologic aspects of cancer etiology. A disorder of the patient's immune response system may be responsible, at least in part, for the development of certain tumors. A number of immunological deficiency states, such as those resulting from AIDS and those resulting from immune suppression medications for transplant patients, indicate an increased risk of developing cancer. In fact, the human immunodeficiency virus (HIV) predisposes the patient to cancers such as Kaposi's sarcoma, lymphomas, and anorectal carcinomas.

The final way in which cancers may develop is by changes in the patient's cellular DNA brought about by some of the above-mentioned factors, perhaps in combination with other unknown or less recognized factors.

Tissue Origin of Tumors

Tumors may arise from any tissue in the body. Because organs are composed of several types of tissues, different tumors may arise in the same organ, although often one type of tumor predominates. Typically, the terms used to describe a tumor identify the type of tissue involved. For example, tumors in bone tissue will contain "osteo" in their name, and tumors in adipose, or fatty, connective tissue will contain "lipo." Figure 4–2 lists examples of benign and malignant tumors arising from various tissues.

Microscopic analysis of a tumor involves the study of (1) the shape and size of the tumor's cells, (2) the tumor's growth patterns, (3) the configuration and staining characteristics of the nuclei of the tumor's cells, and (4) the type of tissue from which the tumor arose. The significance of these cellular distinctions helps to determine the selection of treatment and the prediction for the patient's survival.

Nomenclature of Tumors

Suffixes, root words, and other terms used in the naming of tumors are not employed consistently, leading to confusion in tumor terminology. In some cases, "carcinoma" or "sarcoma" is part of the tumor's name, easily identifying these tumors as being malignant. But the names of some tumors do not reveal whether the tumor is benign or malignant or may even suggest a benign condition when the tumor is actually malignant.

Figure 4–2.
Examples of Tissue Origin of Tumors.

Type of Tissue	Benign Tumor	Malignant Tumor
Epithelial tissue		
Squamous	Papilloma	Squamous cell carcinoma
Columnar/cuboidal	Adenoma	Adenocarcinoma
Transitional	Papilloma	Transitional cell carcinoma
Connective tissue		
Adult fibrous	Fibroma	Fibrosarcoma
Adipose	Lipoma	Liposarcoma
Cartilage	Chondroma	Chondrosarcoma
Bone	Osteoma	Osteogenic sarcoma
Muscle tissue		
Smooth	Leiomyoma	Leiomyosarcoma
Striated	Rhabdomyoma	Rhabdomyosarcoma
Nerve tissue	Ganglioneuroma	Neuroblastoma

Frequently, the names of benign tumors end with the suffix "oma," but some malignant tumors, such as a melanoma, also end with that suffix. In addition, some swellings that have names ending in "oma" are not tumors at all. A *hematoma*, for example, is a collection of blood within the tissues.

Nomenclature of Benign Tumors

Papillomas and adenomas are examples of benign tumors. A *papilloma* is a polyp-like growth that has a layer of epithelium on its surface and a connective tissue stalk for support. Papillomas may be found in many of the locations in which epithelium is located. An *adenoma* is a benign tumor composed of glandular cells that may manufacture and secrete hormones and other substances. A *cystadenoma* is formed when these secretions from the glandular cells are retained within the tumor, leading to its dilation and cyst formation. Adenomas may be observed in many locations, including the breast, prostate, ovary, and thyroid glands.

Lipomas, which are growths arising from fatty tissue, and *osteomas*, which are growths arising from bone, are examples of benign tumors that originate in connective tissue.

Nomenclature of Malignant Tumors

The word "cancer" refers to all types of malignant tumors. Malignancies are further classified according to their tissue of origin. A malignant tumor that arises from epithelial tissue is known as a *carcinoma*, and one that originates from connective or muscle tissue is called a *sarcoma*.

The word "carcinoma" generally appears in the full name of malignant epithelial tumors, and other descriptive terms are also used in the designation of the tumor. For example, *adenocarcinoma* is a general name given to a group of malignancies derived from the epithelium of glands or ducts. An adenocarcinoma of the thyroid will differ in its microscopic appearance and in its clinical behavior from an adenocarcinoma of the breast, and both will differ from adenocarcinomas of the pancreas, ovary, and other organs. *Transitional cell carcinomas* are found in the bladder, ureter, and renal pelvis, sites of transitional cell epithelium. *Squamous cell carcinomas* arise from the skin and from other locations of squamous cell epithelium and most often develop on the patient's face and other exposed skin surfaces. A *malignant melanoma,* which is also known as a *melanocarcinoma* or sometimes simply as a *melanoma*, is a malignant, darkly pigmented epithelial cancer that usually arises from a preceding mole.

Malignancies arising in fat, bone, muscle, cartilage, and fibrous connective tissues are examples of sarcomas. A *liposarcoma* is a malignant tumor arising from adipose, or fatty tissue; a *fibrosarcoma* arises from fibrous connective tissue; and a *chondrosarcoma* arises from cartilage. Sarcomas occur less frequently than do carcinomas and have their highest incidence in younger age groups.

GRADING AND STAGING MALIGNANCIES

Grading and staging are two methods of evaluating cancers. Evaluating cancers is important because a physician can determine the prognosis for the patient or the effectiveness of various modes of therapy by comparing the patient's cancer with similar cancers. *Grading* a tumor refers to describing its microscopic appearance, as noted on the original surgical pathology report. On a scale of I through IV, a *grade I tumor*, or low grade tumor, has cells that closely resemble the normal parent cells, whereas a *grade IV tumor*, or *high grade tumor*, has bizarre cells that do not resemble the parent cell. In many tumors, the grade of the tumor has a relationship to the patient's prognosis. As the grade of the cancer increases from I to IV, the average survival time for these patients shortens.

The **staging** of a cancer is the evaluation of the extent of the cancer's spread from its primary site. The goals of staging are to assist in the selection of the most effective method of treatment—for example, surgery might be chosen for localized lesions, and radiation or chemotherapy might be appropriate for advanced disease—and to forecast the patient's prognosis. To achieve these goals, only cancers of a similar stage are grouped for comparison. The staging of a malignancy is performed independently of its grading. Staging is determined by clinical examination, x-ray, CT scans, MRI, lymphangiograms, gross inspection during surgery, microscopic examination of excised tissue, and other methods.

Two methods—one older and one more recently developed—are commonly used for designating the stage of malignancies. In general, clinical staging by the older method will approximate that shown in the following tabulation:

- **stage 0** carcinoma-in-situ
- **stage I** disease is limited to the organ in which the tumor originated
- **stage II** disease has spread outside the primary organ and into local lymph nodes but no other organ is involved
- **stage III** disease has metastasized to distant lymph nodes and/ or to distant organs

The newer method of staging, known as the TNM system, can be applied to most nonhematologic malignancies. The TNM system has three variables that indicate the size of the primary tumor, the presence of localized lymph node involvement, and the extent of distant metastases, respectively. The letter T represents the primary tumor, the letter N designates regional node involvement, and the letter M represents distant metastases. The TNM staging method is extended further by the designations shown in Figure 4–3. T2, N1, M0 is an example of a staging designation. In this example, the primary tumor has undergone moderate increase in size and involvement of neighboring structures; a slight degree of nodal involvement has occurred; and no evidence of distant metastasis exists.

Each tumor has its own unique biologic characteristics that in turn affect the staging criteria. In some tumors, such as tumors of the prostate, the grade of the tumor is included in the staging system.

Some tumors are classified by different staging systems. For example, hematologic tumors, such as leukemias, do not lend themselves to the typical staging systems but are evaluated by cell type and immunologic and other markers. Malignant melanoma is staged

Figure 4–3.
Cancer Staging by the TNM System.

Major Category	Clinical Stage	Explanation of Stage
Tumor (T)	T0	No tumor clinically
	TIS	Carcinoma-in-situ
	T1 to T4	Increasing degrees of tumor size and involvement of neighboring structures by direct extension
	TX	Tumor cannot be assessed clinically
Nodes (N)	N0	No regional nodes involved
	N1 to N4	Increasing degrees of regional node involvement
	NX	Nodal involvement cannot be assessed clinically
Metastasis (M)	M0	No evidence of distant metastasis
	M1 to M4	Increasing degrees of metastatic spread

by depth of invasion, called Breslow's thickness, for stage 0 and stage I tumors. The thickness of a malignant melanoma lesion is strongly related to the patient's prognosis—the thinner the tumor, the better the prognosis.

DIAGNOSIS AND TREATMENT OF TUMORS

Prevention and early detection of a cancer are two important goals. For example, avoidance of tobacco products helps to prevent cancers of the mouth, larynx, lung, and bladder, and decreased exposure to ultraviolet light decreases the risk of developing skin cancer. Furthermore, early detection of cancer by examination and screening procedures is very beneficial for treating and curing a number of malignancies. Mammography and regular breast self-examination, for instance, may lead to early detection of breast cancers, Pap smears may detect early cancer or "precancerous" lesions of the cervix, and routine complete skin exams may detect early skin cancer.

Once a tumor has been detected, it must be accurately diagnosed and properly treated. The determination of the prognosis for both the course of the disease and the patient's chances of recovery is dependent upon an accurate diagnosis of the tumor. Making an accurate diagnosis involves determining whether the tumor is benign or malignant, identifying the type of tissue involved, and evaluating the extent of involvement—the grade and the stage—of the tumor. The course of prescribed treatment also depends on the diagnosis.

Diagnostic Techniques

Palpation, which is the application of light pressure by hand to the surface of the body in order to feel the internal body parts and/or their movements underneath, or examination by x-ray will often indicate the presence of a mass and, to some extent, its size. Determination of malignancy requires that a sample of the tissue involved be subjected to examination under a microscope. Two techniques that are commonly used to obtain tissue samples are exfoliative cytology and biopsy.

Exfoliative Cytology

Cytology is defined in Chapter 2 as the microscopic study of cells, including a study of their origin, structure, function, and pathology. Cytologic examination can be made from body fluids and secretions, such as sputum, urine, washings taken from the bronchial tree, effusions from the pleural and peritoneal cavities, and secretions from the vagina and stomach. *Exfoliative cytology* is the study of cells normally shed from the skin and other body surfaces in order to detect malignant changes. The value of exfoliative cytology has increased tremendously in recent years and is of particular help in studying cells that come from an area in the body in which a biopsy is difficult to obtain. The diagnostic accuracy of cytology is high if the samples are collected correctly and examined appropriately.

The Pap smear test, also called the cancer smear test, is an example of an exfoliative cytologic procedure. The purpose of the test is to detect cell changes in a precancerous stage or a malignancy in a preinvasive stage. Pap smears are used in the investigation of cells from several locations of the body, but the area most commonly investigated by this test is the female genital tract. Samples containing cells obtained from the test site are placed on a glass slide, stained, and examined under a microscope. Chapter 11, *The Reproductive System*, addresses this topic more fully.

Prior to 1930, the death rate from cancers of the cervix and the body of the uterus was significantly higher than the death rate for cancer of the breast. By 1940, the death rate from uterine cancer had begun to decline, and by 1946 the death rate from cancer of the cervix had fallen below that for breast cancer. Currently the death rate from cervical cancer is less than one-half that for cancer of the breast. This favorable trend is attributable in large part to the emphasis placed on early detection of cervical cancer that occurred with the widespread adoption of the Pap smear in the early 1940s.

Biopsy and Frozen Section

Obtaining a small piece of tissue for pathologic study is known as a *biopsy*. A biopsy may be performed through a needle or by an open biopsy technique. The location of the lesion, its size, and its suspected diagnosis are the most important considerations in the selection of the biopsy method. The needle biopsy technique is used to make a tissue diagnosis of lesions located in areas of the patient's body such as the prostate, breast, lung, thyroid, liver, bone, kidney, and mediastinum. Small bore needles permit the physician to recover only a small amount of tissue, but large bore needles can obtain a more substantial tissue sample. Nevertheless, the drawback to all types of needle biopsy methods is that the amount of tissue obtained is small compared to the amount that can be obtained by open biopsy procedures.

Tissue material adequate to satisfy any diagnostic requirement may be obtained safely by either of two open biopsy methods. If the tumor is of small size, the surgeon usually will perform an *excisional biopsy* by removing the entire lesion for pathologic examination. This method has the advantage of being both diagnostic and therapeutic at the same time. Excisional biopsy is used for small skin lesions, intestinal polyps, and for any small lesion that can easily be removed in its entirety.

The second open biopsy method is the *incisional biopsy*, in which the surgeon removes a small piece of tissue, usually located near the periphery of the lesion, for tissue examination. The excised tissue is prepared for microscopic examination by either the paraffin block technique or the frozen section method. In the *paraffin block biopsy technique*, the physician or technician fixes the biopsy specimen in formalin to harden the tissue and embeds it in paraffin. From this paraffin block, the physician or technician obtains a very thin slice of tissue, mounts it on a glass slide, stains the tissue sample, and examines it through a microscope. The paraffin block process yields tissue specimens that can be interpreted with great accuracy. The disadvantage of this method is that, even though the fixation and staining procedures now are largely automated, the process takes about two days before the tissue slide is ready for interpretation.

If a patient is anesthetized in an operating room, and the surgeon, before proceeding with treatment, wants an immediate interpretation of the suspect tissue, the surgeon can use the *frozen section biopsy method* in which a biopsy specimen is removed, frozen by a special quick freezing method, stained, and promptly interpreted. The process takes only a few minutes. This frozen section method assists the surgeon in deciding the type and extent of further surgery that should be performed before the patient is released from anesthesia.

Frozen sections also are used during surgery to indicate if the surgeon has removed all the malignant tissue. The surgeon needs this information before closing the incision and terminating the anesthesia. The breast is one area commonly examined by the frozen section method of open biopsy.

The frozen section technique does not provide a permanent slide for later review and comparison, and, in many instances, the quality of the tissue preparation by the frozen section method does not equal that produced by the paraffin block technique. Nevertheless, in most cases the quality of the frozen section preparation is sufficient to permit the pathologist to make an accurate diagnosis. The sole advantage of the frozen section technique is the speed by which a tissue diagnosis can be made.

Cancer Therapy

The three main forms of treatment for cancer are surgery, radiotherapy, and chemotherapy. The choice of treatment depends on the type of cancer, its location and stage, and the general physical condition of the patient. For example, in a very obese patient or in a patient who has severe heart disease, surgery might carry greater morbidity or mortality risk than other forms of treatment.

Surgery

Surgery is an invasive operative procedure, and it usually involves the physical removal of tissue or organs. Because it is the most effective curative method for cancer, surgery is the preferred treatment for most primary, localized cancers. A malignancy is localized if it has not spread beyond its organ of origin.

Radiotherapy

Effective treatment of some cancers may be achieved by radiotherapy, either employed alone or in combination with surgery. *Radiotherapy* may take the form of x-rays produced by linear accelerators or of gamma rays given off by radioactive substances such as radioactive phosphorus, iodine, cobalt, and radium. In some cases, radiotherapy is as effective as surgery in producing a cure. It is useful in the treatment of Hodgkin's disease at an early stage in its development and in the treatment of lymphosarcoma and certain cancers of the uterine cervix, prostate, and thyroid. Newer dosage schedules, imaging techniques to define the site of tumors, and computer controlled radiation beams have improved cancer patients' prognoses and have decreased the harmful effects radiation may have on normal tissue. Long-term complications of radiotherapy, such as damage to the heart or lungs, or the development of leukemias or second solid tumors, can occur occasionally.

Chemotherapy

A significant percentage of cancers are being effectively treated by chemotherapy, which also may be used alone or in combination with surgery or radiation. *Chemotherapy* is the treatment of disease using chemical agents. Chemotherapeutic agents may be administered orally or intravenously. Chemotherapy is the main form of treatment responsible for the long-term survival associated with several types of widespread cancer, including leukemia, lymphoma, choriocarcinoma, lymphosarcoma, testicular cancer, and Wilms tumor. In the treatment of other malignancies, chemotherapy has been used in conjunction with surgery or radiation to reduce painful symptoms and to lengthen the patient's survival time. Over 30 useful chemotherapeutic agents for the treatment of malignancies are currently available.

Although chemotherapy has demonstrated its therapeutic value, it does have the drawback of toxicity, the type of which depends on the specific agent used. Many of the anti-cancer drugs produce bone marrow depression, nausea and vomiting, skin changes, and loss of hair. Some of these drugs cause liver, heart, or kidney damage.

In addition to being curative, surgery, radiotherapy, and chemotherapy may also be *palliative,* meaning that they may reduce or relieve distressing symptoms without providing a cure, for those patients who have advanced cancers and for whom cure is improbable or impossible. Additional forms of treatment, including hormonal treatment, such as Tamoxifen for breast cancer, and bone marrow transplantation after high dose chemo- or radiotherapy for treatment of certain leukemias and solid tumors, are becoming more widely available.

Scientists are investigating immunologic tools such as interferon and interleukin-2 as possible treatments for certain cancers. Treatment protocols have evolved over time through careful study of different types and combinations of treatment. The 50 percent cure rate of childhood leukemia, a disease that used to be uniformly fatal, is a good example of this evolution.

Figure 4–4.
The Estimated Cancer Incidence and Mortality Rates for 1993 by Site and Sex.

1993 Estimated Cancer Incidence by Site and Sex*

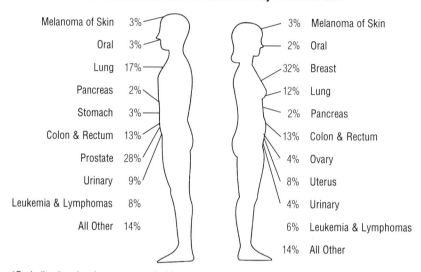

Melanoma of Skin	3%		3%	Melanoma of Skin
Oral	3%		2%	Oral
Lung	17%		32%	Breast
Pancreas	2%		12%	Lung
Stomach	3%		2%	Pancreas
Colon & Rectum	13%		13%	Colon & Rectum
Prostate	28%		4%	Ovary
Urinary	9%		8%	Uterus
Leukemia & Lymphomas	8%		4%	Urinary
All Other	14%		6%	Leukemia & Lymphomas
			14%	All Other

*Excluding basal and squamous cell skin cancers and carcinoma-in-situ.

1993 Estimated Cancer Deaths by Site and Sex

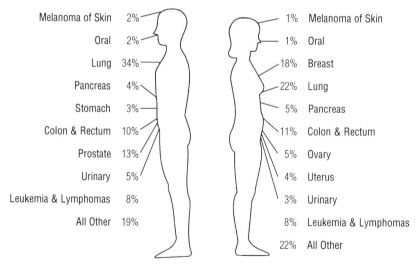

Melanoma of Skin	2%		1%	Melanoma of Skin
Oral	2%		1%	Oral
Lung	34%		18%	Breast
Pancreas	4%		22%	Lung
Stomach	3%		5%	Pancreas
Colon & Rectum	10%		11%	Colon & Rectum
Prostate	13%		5%	Ovary
Urinary	5%		4%	Uterus
Leukemia & Lymphomas	8%		3%	Urinary
All Other	19%		8%	Leukemia & Lymphomas
			22%	All Other

Reprinted with permission of the publisher from Catherine C. Boring, et al., "Cancer Statistics, 1993," CA: *A Cancer Journal for Clinicians* 43 (1993): 9.

Figure 4–5.
Leading Causes of Cancer Deaths in Men and Women as a Function of Age.

Mortality for the Five Leading Cancer Sites for Males by Age Group, United States, 1989

All Ages	Under 15	15–34	35–54	55–74	75+
Lung 33.8%	Leukemia 36.3%	Leukemia 19.6%	Lung 33.3%	Lung 39.3%	Lung 27.1%
Prostate 11.6%	Brain & CNS 24.3%	NHL* 12.7%	Colon & rectum 8.5%	Colon & rectum 10.2%	Prostate 20.2%
Colon & rectum 10.7%	Endocrine 10.6%	Brain & CNS 11.3%	Prostate 5.5%	Prostate 8.4%	Colon & rectum 12.5%
Pancreas 4.5%	NHL* 8.9%	Skin 7.4%	Pancreas 5.1%	Pancreas 4.8%	Pancreas 4.4%
Leukemia 3.8%	Connective tissue 4.8%	Hodgkin's disease 7.1%	Esophagus 4.7%	Esophagus 3.1%	Bladder 3.9%

Mortality for the Five Leading Cancer Sites for Females by Age Group, United States, 1989

All Ages	Under 15	15–34	35–54	55–74	75+
Lung 20.7%	Leukemia 33.6%	Breast 18.9%	Breast 31.8%	Lung 26.2%	Colon & Rectum 17.4%
Breast 18.4%	Brain & CNS 28.8%	Leukemia 13.4%	Lung 18.5%	Breast 18.3%	Lung 15.3%
Colon & rectum 12.5%	Endocrine 11.6%	Uterus 10.1%	Uterus 6.7%	Colon & rectum 10.4%	Breast 14.5%
Pancreas 5.4%	Connective tissue 6.7%	Brain & CNS 8.9%	Colon & rectum 6.7%	Ovary 5.9%	Pancreas 6.7%
Ovary 5.3%	Bone 4.0%	Ovary 5.5%	Ovary 5.9%	Pancreas 5.2%	NHL* 4.5%

*NHL = Non-Hodgkin's lymphomas
These numbers are derived by dividing the number of deaths involving the specific cancer site by the total number of cancer deaths for that age group.
Adapted, with permission of the publisher, from Catherine C. Boring, et al., "Cancer Statistics, 1993," *CA: A Cancer Journal for Clinicians* 43 (1993): 13.

Any cancer treatment requires careful follow-up in order to detect recurrences and complications of treatment. In addition, having one cancer may increase a patient's chance of developing a second cancer.

CANCER RATES AND TRENDS

A strikingly steady increase in the incidence of, and mortality from, lung cancer has affected both men and women, but the incidence of cancer of the stomach has decreased for both genders. Mortality caused by cancer of the colon, prostate, and bladder has increased slightly in men. However, the incidence of cancer of the cervix among women has declined. Figure 4–4 displays the estimated cancer incidence and mortality rates for 1993 by the site of the malignancy and the patient's sex.

The different sites of the cancers at different ages of the patients are significant, as are the mortality rates of lung and colorectal cancers in both genders, breast cancer in women, and prostate cancer in men. Figure 4–5 presents the five leading causes of cancer deaths as a function of age in men and women.

Scientists have made great advances in the treatment of certain cancers, which, until recent years, had a very grave prognosis. Hodgkin's disease is an example of a cancer which, with current methods of treatment, can be controlled in many instances, thus providing Hodgkin's disease patients with a much improved prognosis. Today, with modern methods of surgery, chemotherapy, and radiation, the outlook for many cancer patients has brightened.

5

The Skin

This chapter will first discuss localized skin diseases, and then will present other skin disorders which are manifestations of systemic diseases. We present these latter disorders in this chapter because many health insurance claims arise from medical treatment initiated by patients who noticed changes in their skin before they noticed other symptoms of the underlying diseases. The third section of this chapter addresses both benign and malignant skin tumors. Finally, we will look at miscellaneous skin-related topics, including burns and plastic surgery.

ANATOMY AND PHYSIOLOGY

Skin is a complex organ that provides a tough, flexible cover for the entire body. It is the largest organ in the body and comprises about 15 percent of an individual's total body weight.

The skin has two main portions: the epidermis and the dermis. The *epidermis* is the outermost, nonvascular portion of the skin. It consists of five layers of cells. Named from the outside inward, these epidermal layers are the stratum corneum, stratum lucidum, stratum granulosum, prickle cell layer, and basal cell layer. The basal cell layer is a single row of cells that forms the junction between the epidermis and the dermis. Cells in the basal cell layer actively multiply and, as new basal cells are formed, the older cells gradually pass up through the other layers to the skin surface where they eventually die and are shed.

The **dermis**, or *corium*, is the portion of the skin that lies beneath the epidermis. It consists of elastic white connective tissue and constitutes the bulk of the skin. The dermis is richly invested with blood vessels, nerves, glands, smooth muscles, and fat deposits that support and nourish the epidermis. The dermis varies in thickness depending on location, being thickest on the nape of the neck, back, palms of the hands, and soles of the feet. The dermis rests on *subcutaneous*, or beneath the skin, tissue composed mainly of fat.

Skin color, texture, thickness, and other characteristics vary considerably depending on the part of the body involved, as well as on the individual's age, gender, race, and occupation. The presence or absence of skin appendages also depends on these factors.

Sweat glands, sebaceous glands, hair, and nails are skin appendages. **Sebaceous glands** are glands that secrete an oily, thick, semifluid substance that is formed from the disintegration of cells in the central portion of the gland. Sebaceous glands are present everywhere except on the palms of the hands and soles of the feet. The largest concentration of sebaceous glands is on the head and face.

Figure 5–1 provides a cross-sectional view of the skin and its appendages.

Skin performs numerous functions that are vital to life. The most important function of skin is to provide a protective covering that prevents harmful forces in the external environment from entering and affecting the body. It slows the loss of water and electrolytes from the body, and it shields internal organs from temperature extremes, external trauma, and infectious diseases. Skin is a sense organ for touch, pain, temperature, and pressure. It plays an important role in the regulation of body temperature. When skin capillaries constrict, the quantity of blood that passes through the skin is reduced, conserving body heat. Sweating and dilation of skin capillaries, resulting in an increased flow of blood, cool the body. The average daily excretion of sweat totals about one pint. In addition, skin is a reservoir of water, vitamins, fat, protein, and carbohydrates.

Dermatologists use a number of terms to describe skin conditions. These terms include:

- *lesion*—any structural or functional alteration of tissue, including the skin, as a result of disease
- *macula*—flat skin lesion less than two centimeters in diameter
- *patch*—flat skin lesion greater than two centimeters in diameter

Figure 5–1.
A Cross-Sectional View of the Skin.

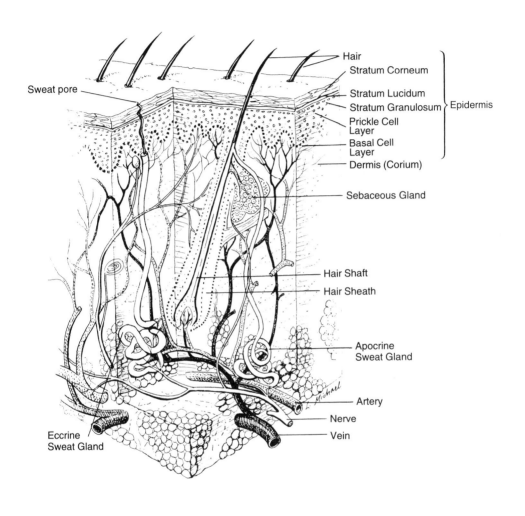

- *papule*—raised skin lesion less than one centimeter in diameter
- *plaque*—raised skin lesion greater than one centimeter in diameter that arises on any internal or external body surface, including the skin
- *polyp*—protruding growth from a mucous membrane
- *vesicle*—small skin blister

- *bullous lesion* or *bulla*—large blister
- *erythema*—redness
- *lichenification*—thickening of the skin
- *excoriation*—scratch mark
- *dermatitis*—general term for skin inflammation
- *pustule*—small irregular raised area containing pus
- *cyst*—any closed cavity or sac, normal or abnormal, lined by epithelium

Dermatologists are often able to diagnose skin disorders after examining the patient and reviewing the patient's medical history. On occasion, dermatologists use skin biopsy to aid in diagnosis. In a *punch biopsy*, a small metal punch removes a piece of tissue. In an excisional biopsy, abnormal tissue is partially or totally removed by a scalpel. After either of the biopsy procedures, a pathologist then examines the tissue sample under a microscope for final diagnosis.

DISORDERS OF THE SKIN

Localized Disorders of the Skin

Many disorders have manifestations limited primarily to the skin and sometimes to the subcutaneous tissue. The mechanism for these skin disorders is variable and in some cases is unknown. Although troublesome for cosmetic reasons or because of pain or itching, most skin and subcutaneous disorders are not life threatening in themselves. This section will review only the most common of these disorders.

The causes of localized skin lesions include

- friction, from tight clothing or parts of the body rubbing together
- contact with body fluids, such as sweat, urine, or feces
- contact with household or industrial irritants, such as cosmetics, soaps, or metals
- viral, bacterial, and fungal infections
- immune disorders and allergies
- response to hormones, such as the effect of any male hormone on the sebaceous glands, causing acne
- emotional factors
- aging processes, such as the loss of skin fullness and elasticity, which weaken the body's outer defense against bacterial invasion
- climatic elements, causing sunburn or frostbite

- drugs, which even in minute amounts will produce a rash in sensitized individuals

Contact Dermatitis

Contact dermatitis, one of the most common of all skin disorders, is a rash produced by contact with either a primary skin irritant or a sensitizing agent. A primary skin irritant will produce a rash on practically any skin. A sensitizing agent, such as nickel dermatitis and poison ivy, will produce a rash only on skin allergic to the agent. The skin response to the offending substance takes the form of redness, swelling, and the formation of liquid-filled blisters that ooze and crust. After the cause of the dermatitis is identified and the patient withdraws from or avoids the cause, the dermatitis usually clears. Treatment may also include the use of steroid creams.

Acne and Seborrheic Dermatitis

Acne, also called *acne vulgaris*, is a common skin condition character-ized by the presence of blackhead pimples, papules, pustules, and cysts. Acne results from a sebaceous gland disorder attributed to the hormonal changes associated with puberty. The lesions of acne commonly are found on the individual's face, back, and chest. Although acne may persist into the individual's thirties, most cases disappear spontaneously at an earlier age. Treatment with benzoyl peroxide, antibiotics, and retinoic acid, often in the form of tretinoin, can be very effective. Permanent scarring and pitting of the skin are possible complications of acne. Severe cystic acne may need treat-ment with isotretinoin, a potentially harmful drug to a developing fetus or the patient.

Acne may be secondary to (1) medications, such as iodine, corticosteroids, and Dilantin, (2) androgen excess, as occurs in Cushing's syndrome, (3) industrial exposure, or (4) polycystic ovary disease.

Acne rosacea affects people older than 30, and presents as a facial acne eruption and flushing. Severe rosacea may involve the patient's eyes and affect his or her vision. Tetracyclines often are effective treatment for this condition.

Seborrheic dermatitis is characterized by excessive oiliness of the individual's skin. The disorder may involve most areas of the body, but the greatest involvement is at sites, such as the scalp, in which sebaceous glands are highly concentrated. Clinically, the patient who has seborrhea demonstrates a greasy scaling accompa-nied by itching. Local remedies, especially topical steroids, are helpful in treating this condition. Seborrheic dermatitis is rarely associated with underlying diseases.

Atopic Dermatitis

Atopic dermatitis, which is also called *atopic eczema*, is a noncontagious inflammation of the skin that begins early in life and may be present intermittently in acute and chronic forms for many years, although many patients outgrow atopic eczema during childhood. The eczema lesions redden, ooze, scale, and crust. Intensive itching may induce scratching, opening the lesions to invasion by skin bacteria and secondary infection. Mild eczema will not interfere with the patient's activity, although severe cases may be disabling. Authorities suggest that atopic eczema may be related to immunological problems or to allergies such as asthma or hay fever.

Urticaria, Erythema Multiforme, and Erythema Nodosum

Urticaria, which is commonly called hives, is a common skin disorder manifested by the development of wheals. *Wheals* are sharply demarcated, raised, slightly pink, fluid-filled areas. The wheals develop quickly in large numbers, are very itchy, and generally remain only a few minutes to an hour or two, and then disappear without aftereffects. The torso is the most common location for the development of the wheals. Urticaria generally develops as an allergic response to the ingestion of certain foods and drugs, but it may also follow bee stings, emotional stress, or the inhalation of dusts. The cause of the reaction often is unknown, and the condition may occur once, repeatedly, or chronically.

Angioneurotic edema, or *giant hives*, involves swelling of deeper skin and fat. Angioneurotic edema that involves the mucous membranes may lead to respiratory tract obstruction.

Erythema multiforme is a skin eruption that involves different types of reddish skin lesions. The hallmark of erythema multiforme is a lesion that looks similar to a target. The cause is typically infectious, usually viral, or is related to medications or other allergens. Erythema multiforme is usually mild, but the severe form, the *Stevens-Johnson syndrome*, may be fatal. Fortunately, Stevens-Johnson syndrome usually does not recur if the person avoids the offending agent.

The characteristic lesions of *erythema nodosum* are painful, deep-seated, reddened nodules located chiefly on the front surfaces of the patient's legs, but the nodules may also occur on the arms, back, and other parts of the patient's body. The cause of erythema nodosum is often unknown but may be secondary to strep infections, tuberculosis, inflammatory bowel disease, or other diseases. The rash is usually self-limited, although it may require treatment with pain medications or steroids to ease the patient's discomfort.

Pyodermas

A *pyoderma* is an infection of the skin caused by pus-forming bacteria. This section will introduce several common types of pyodermas.

A *furuncle*, or *boil*, is an acute, tender, localized collection of pus, generally caused by a staphylococcus bacterium. A furuncle may be a solitary lesion or may be widespread. A collection of furuncles organized into one lesion is known as a *carbuncle*. A single boil is a self-limited condition. In most cases, no demonstrable cause can be found for chronic, repeated, furunculosis. Treatment for this condition typically involves an incision and drainage (I&D) procedure.

Impetigo is usually caused by either streptococcus or staphylococcus bacteria and is a common childhood disease. It is characterized by pustular, crusted eruptions and most frequently affects the patient's face and hands. Generally, impetigo is not a very serious condition, but it may cause acute poststreptococcal glomerulonephritis (AGN), a kidney inflammation which often heals completely.

Erysipelas is a more serious bacterial infection that primarily affects the patient's face and head with a red, hot, fluid-filled, spreading lesion that may involve large areas of the patient's skin. In severe cases of erysipelas, lymph vessel and blood stream invasion by the streptococcus can cause the infection to travel to other organs, especially the lungs and kidneys. Antibiotics will cure the infection.

Viral Infections of the Skin

Many types of viral infections primarily affect the skin. For example, *herpes simplex type I* is a virus that causes the common cold sore. Cold sores are often recurrent, but each episode is short-lived. Herpes simplex I may, in rare circumstances, infect the patient's brain or eyes with potentially serious consequences. *Herpes simplex type II* is a sexually transmitted disease that affects the external genitalia with painful vesicles and ulcers. It is recurrent and may be treated with, but not cured by, Acyclovir.

Shingles, a condition caused by the varicella zoster virus, is a painful vesicular and papular eruption which usually affects a local area of the patient's skin. Shingles is self-limited and rarely recurs. It may cause chronic pain or significant damaging inflammation of the eye in older patients. Acyclovir is often useful for treating shingles.

Pityriasis rosea is presumed to be of viral origin and causes an itchy papular dermatitis that lasts up to three months. It heals without ensuing lesion or disease.

Superficial fungal infections of the skin are very common and are easily treatable with topical agents. For example, tinea corporis, tinea capitus, and tinea pedis are medical names for ringworm of the body, head, and feet, respectively. Tinea versicolor is also a common superficial fungus infection. This chronic, noninflammatory and usually symptomless condition is characterized by discolored patches of skin.

Psoriasis

Psoriasis is characterized by itchy, raised, dull-red patches covered with thick, silvery-white scales. It affects about one percent of the United States population. Most psoriatic lesions are found on the patient's knees, elbows, scalp, upper back, nails, and face. These patches represent areas of rapid and exaggerated proliferation of epidermal cells. The cause of this increase in epidermal cell regeneration is unknown. Generally, psoriasis causes no interference with the patient's general health or activity and has no impact on the patient's mortality. Arthritis develops in approximately five percent of psoriasis patients and may be disabling.

No ideal method for treating psoriasis exists, although several treatment regimens are in current use. Most treatment regimens include use of topical steroid or coal tar cremes. The Goeckerman program consists of the topical application of crude coal tar ointment, followed by exposure to ultraviolet light. A treatment called *PUVA* consists of the oral administration of psoralen, a photosensitizing chemical, followed by exposure to high-intensity, long-wave ultraviolet light. An effective oral medication for severe psoriasis is methotrexate. Because methotrexate is potentially toxic and because PUVA may increase the risk of skin cancer, the effectiveness of these treatment programs must be measured against concern over their long-term health risks.

Skin Manifestations of Systemic Diseases

The skin is often the site of manifestations of systemic diseases. Space limitations make descriptions of all the internal diseases having cutaneous manifestations impossible, and so this text will discuss only a few of these diseases.

Infections

Viral Infections. Many viral diseases have skin manifestations. For example, several diseases of childhood, such as **rubeola**, which is commonly known as *measles,* and **rubella**, which is commonly known as *German measles*, cause reddened papules. These diseases are now rare because of prevention by immunization. **Varicella**, or *chicken pox*, a vesiculating disease, is usually mild in childhood, although it may be fatal for adults or children who have suppressed immune systems. **Erythema infectiosum**, or *fifth disease*, is a mildly contagious disease that is marked by a rose-colored macular rash. An attack of fifth disease is usually of short duration in children and may cause a brief noncrippling arthritis in adults. A fetus infected with fifth disease may be stillborn, and persons who have a hemolytic anemia, such as sickle cell disease, may develop a worsening of their anemia if they contract fifth disease.

Bacterial Infections. Certain of the streptococcal bacteria that cause "strep throat" produce a toxin that creates a red rash. This condition is **scarlet fever**, and it usually responds to penicillin or erythromycin.

Toxic shock syndrome (TSS) is indicated by a combination of fever, red rash, vomiting, diarrhea, and shock-like state which may be fatal. A staphylococcal infection of the genital tract, often related to tampon use, is the most common cause of TSS. Although this infection is serious, it usually responds to fluid and electrolyte replacement treatment and rarely recurs.

Lyme disease is caused by a tick-transmitted spirochete called Borrelia burgdorferi. The offending tick is small, and the initial bite is usually unrecognized. Lyme disease occurs worldwide. In the United States, it is mostly seen in the Northeast, Wisconsin, and Minnesota. The potential symptoms of Lyme disease are numerous and the testing is currently imprecise, which leads to both over- and underdiagnosis. Antibiotic treatment may cure or modify the illness.

Lyme disease is divided into the following three stages:

- **Stage 1** In up to 80 percent of the patients who have Lyme disease, an initial rash is seen within one month of the bite. This rash is called erythema migrans (EM or EMC). Fatigue may last a number of months and may be accompanied by fever, aches and pains, respiratory problems, swelling of the lymph nodes, or other complications. The other symptoms usually fade, but fatigue and lethargy may last.
- **Stage 2** Various neurologic abnormalities such as meningitis,

Bell's Palsy, radiculitis, or peripheral or cranial neuropathy,[2] occur in about 15 percent of Lyme disease patients weeks to months after the tick bite. These abnormalities may last for months or may become chronic. Cardiac involvement with first- to third-degree heart block occurs in up to ten percent of affected individuals and usually lasts several weeks. Such cardiac involvement may recur.

- **Stage 3** Up to 80 percent of untreated Lyme disease patients will develop arthritic symptoms from joint pains to frank destructive arthritis within two years of the bite. These symptoms may be recurrent or chronic, or they may disappear.

Treatment with oral antibiotics, such as penicillin, amoxicillin, erythromycin, or tetracycline, is especially effective in treating Lyme disease during stage 1. Intravenous antibiotics in very high doses may be necessary for treating neurologic or cardiac symptoms. With treatment, the majority of Lyme disease patients can expect complete recovery.

Collagen-Vascular Diseases

Collagen-vascular disorders, which are also called *connective tissue disorders*, are a diverse group of diseases that have in common widespread alterations of connective tissues. Because many of these diseases are suspected of having an immunologic basis, the term *autoimmune disease*, which refers to any one of several disorders in which the body attacks its own tissue, is used to describe this group. The connective tissue diseases generally include the following clinical entities: rheumatoid arthritis, lupus erythematosus, scleroderma, dermatomyositis, and mixed connective tissue disease. Rheumatoid arthritis is discussed in the chapter on musculoskeletal disorders. The other conditions are multisystem diseases with skin manifestations and are considered in this section.

Although collagen-vascular disorders are acquired diseases, their underlying causes are unknown. Because these disorders have many overlapping features, differentiation among them often is difficult. Common features include inflammation of the pleura, endocardium,

---

[2]*Bell's Palsy* is a unilateral facial paralysis of sudden onset, caused by a lesion of the facial nerve and resulting in characteristic distortion of the face; *radiculitis, meningitis*, and *neuropathy* are discussed in Chapter 14, *The Nervous System*.

myocardium, synovial membrane or kidney; characteristic and non-specific skin lesions; and alteration of connective tissue.

Lupus Erythematosus. *Systemic lupus erythematosus* (SLE) is a generalized connective tissue disorder that mainly affects women in the 20 to 40 age group. Its course ranges in severity from a benign illness to a fatal one. SLE shows great variability in its clinical manifestations. The most common initial manifestations of SLE are arthritis without deformity, a "butterfly" rash over the bridge of the nose and cheek bones, inflammation of the pleura and pericardium, and alopecia, which is the loss of hair. Other common manifestations include

- fatigue
- malaise
- sun sensitivity
- ***Raynaud's phenomenon***, which involves intermittent episodes of decreased bloodflow to the patient's fingers or toes and is marked by severe pallor, followed by blueness and then redness of the digits. It may be secondary to an underlying cause, such as connective tissue disease, repetitive trauma, emotional stimuli, or tobacco use
- neurologic symptoms
- an easily visible, purplish or brownish red discoloration, caused by hemorrhage into tissues in which the patient's platelet count is decreased
- prolonged low-grade fever
- nephritis with renal failure
- a biologic false-positive serologic test for syphilis

In all cases, remission of the manifestations is typical and may be followed by a symptom-free interval for years. Eventual recurrences are likely, with manifestations that may or may not be identical to those experienced before.

Laboratory findings in SLE patients often include the presence of high levels of antinuclear antibodies (ANA) and various other antibodies. These laboratory markers of SLE may be present in several other conditions, or sometimes with no disease, and so their greatest usefulness is to support the diagnosis when typical signs of SLE are also present.

Because SLE has such a highly variable course, the response to treatment is difficult to evaluate. Aspirin, nonsteroidal anti-inflammatory drugs (NSAIDs) such as ibuprofen, antimalarial drugs, and corticosteroids are useful in treating SLE. Cytotoxic drugs may be used to treat severe cases of SLE. Patients who have SLE are cautioned against exposure to strong sunlight.

Several drugs, including hydralazine, procainamide, isoniazid, and, rarely, birth control pills, may produce an SLE-like illness. This form of lupus is called drug-induced lupus erythematosus. Discontinuance of the medication usually leads to complete cure, although the cure may take several months.

The disorder known as ***discoid lupus erythematosus*** (discoid LE) is limited to the skin and is characterized by a scarring eruption with hair loss. Locations for the rash of discoid lupus erythematosus are the face, scalp, upper arms, or chest. Exposure to sunlight aggravates the condition. A "butterfly" rash is not seen in discoid LE.

The relationship of the discoid and the systemic forms of lupus erythematosus is unknown. Only four to five percent of patients who have discoid LE subsequently develop evidence of SLE. Although discoid LE has a tendency to relapse and is resistant to treatment, it offers no threat to the patient's life.

Scleroderma. Limited scleroderma often involves the skin exclusively and is characterized by skin that appears tightly drawn, bound, and fixed to underlying structures, especially in the fingers where contractures may occur. Frequently, the skin on the patient's face is also involved in limited scleroderma. Ulcers may develop over bony prominences and on the finger tips. Some patients may develop pulmonary hypertension, biliary cirrhosis, or hypertension.

Diffuse scleroderma, which is also known as *progressive systemic sclerosis (PSS)*, is a generalized disorder of connective tissue characterized by inflammatory, fibrotic, and degenerative changes in the patient's skin, esophagus, intestinal tract, heart, lungs, and kidneys. The cause and fundamental nature of PSS are obscure. Raynaud's phenomenon occurs in 95 percent of PSS patients and sometimes precedes other symptoms by as much as two years. However, most people who have Raynaud's phenomenon do not develop PSS.

The course of scleroderma is unpredictable and variable in severity. In those individuals in whom the disease is limited to mild skin involvement, scleroderma is only slowly progressive, and affected individuals may live a normal life span. Most patients, however, eventually show evidence of generalized involvement of the disease. The prognosis for scleroderma patients is significantly poorer when cardiac, pulmonary, or renal manifestations are present. In some scleroderma patients, the course of the disease may last many years, but other patients experience a rapid downhill progression to death. Treatment of scleroderma depends on the locale, extent, and severity of the disease. Aspirin, other NSAIDs, penicillamine, various chemotherapies, and steroids all have a potential place in treatment.

Morphea is a localized form of systemic scleroderma that is characterized by the formation of white or pink patches, bands, or lines. The lesions associated with morphea typically are firm but not hard. Other manifestations of this disease rarely occur.

Dermatomyositis. **Dermatomyositis** is a connective tissue disorder that affects the skin, subcutaneous tissues, and skeletal muscles. The cause of dermatomyositis is unclear. Weakness in the muscles of the hips, neck, and shoulders, and facial edema involving the eyelids are early signs of dermatomyositis. An erythematous rash over the patient's face, shoulders, and arms may also be present. Muscle wasting, weakness, and fatigue can occur at a variable rate of progression in dermatomyositis patients. Steroids and cytotoxic drugs are used in treating this disease. The prognosis for long-term survival is greater than 75 percent, and some patients may go into permanent remission with full recovery or only residual muscle weakness.

Mixed Connective Tissue Disorder. **Mixed connective tissue disorder (MCTD)** is a condition that presents with some manifestations of SLE, scleroderma, rheumatoid arthritis, and dermatomyositis. MCTD patients have very high levels of RNP antigen and ANA in blood testing. Symptoms of Raynaud's phenomenon, polyarthritis, myopathy, and esophageal and pulmonary involvement are common. Treatment of MCTD includes NSAIDs, aspirin, and low-dose steroids. The prognosis for MCTD patients is similar to that for SLE patients.

Tumors

As an organ, the skin is subject to both benign and malignant tumors, ranging in severity from harmless to life-threatening.

Benign Tumors

Benign tumors are very common and offer no threat to the life or health of the individual. An example of a benign epidermal tumor is the *verruca*, or wart, which is caused by a virus. Benign tumors of the dermis include the

- *nevus*, which is a common mole
- *lymphangioma*, which is a tumor composed of newly formed lymph spaces and channels
- *hemangioma*, which is a tumor composed of large, blood-filled spaces
- *fibroma*, which is a tumor composed of fibrous or fully developed connective tissue

- *neurofibroma*, which is a tumor of peripheral nerves
- *skin tag*, which is a small cutaneous appendage, flap, or polyp

Benign tumors of the skin appendages include adenomas of the sweat and sebaceous glands.

Neurofibromatosis type I, which is also called *von Recklinghausen's disease*, is a skin condition that has a dominant inheritance pattern and possibly involves the patient's nervous system. Multiple soft subcutaneous or nipple-like neurofibromas, which are often associated with multiple light brown spots, may be so numerous that they cover almost the entire body, or they may be very few. A small percentage of these neurofibromas undergo malignant transformation. Occasionally, neurofibromas are found in association with cranial or spinal nerves and may interfere with these nerves' function. If the neurofibromas occur in the patient's brain or spinal canal, significant neurologic impairment is possible.

Premalignant Tumors

Precancerous lesions located in the patient's epidermis may include leukoplakia, actinic keratoses, and dysplastic nevi.

Leukoplakia is a condition characterized by white patches on a mucous membrane. As the term is used clinically, leukoplakia includes any thickened, white patch of mucosa. Most cases of leukoplakia do not progress to malignancy. Hairy leukoplakia of the tongue is strongly associated with AIDS.

Actinic keratoses, which are the most common precancerous lesions of the skin, are irregular red patches of epidermis that are covered by rough scales. These lesions arise on chronically sun-damaged areas of the skin, in areas such as the face, ears, and back of the hands, and may lead to squamous cell carcinoma. Although most actinic keratoses do not progress to malignancy, most squamous cell carcinomas of the skin arise from actinic keratoses. Treatment by excision curettage, liquid nitrogen, or topical application of 5FU is almost always successful.

Dysplastic nevi are larger, more irregular in outline, and more variegated in pigmentation than other moles, and are precursors of malignant melanoma. An individual who has a positive family history of malignant melanoma and dysplastic nevi may have a greater than 50 percent chance of developing a malignant melanoma. The probability that an individual who has dysplastic nevi, but no family history of melanoma, will develop malignant melanoma is uncertain. Careful follow-up on dysplastic nevi to detect early malignant melanoma is important.

Malignant Tumors

Skin cancer is by far the most common type of malignant disease in humans. Because skin cancer grows slowly and is readily detected in an early stage of development, it is cured surgically in well over 95 percent of diagnosed cases. Malignant melanoma is an exception to this high cure rate.

Primary malignant skin tumors may arise from the epidermis, dermis, subcutaneous tissue, or from the skin appendages, such as sweat glands, sebaceous glands, and hair follicles. Chronic exposure to sunlight is the most important factor in the development of skin cancer. Other factors include prolonged industrial exposure to arsenic, tar, or other harmful substances. Malignant skin tumors also can occur as late sequelae of radiation, burns, and chronic skin ulceration. People who have fair skin that burns easily and tans poorly are more susceptible to the development of these tumors than are people who tan easily and do not burn. Blacks are much less likely than whites to develop these skin cancers.

Basal Cell Carcinoma. The most common skin malignancy in whites is the ***basal cell carcinoma***, sometimes referred to as the *basal cell epithelioma*. This tumor gets its name from the microscopic appearance of its cells, which resemble normal basal cells in size, shape, and arrangement. Basal cell carcinomas occur in the skin on any part of the patient's body but are most commonly found on the patient's face, as single or multiple lesions. Most patients who have this malignancy are middle-aged or older. Beginning as a smooth, slightly elevated papule, the basal cell carcinoma ulcerates centrally. These ulcerative lesions destroy tissue as they spread laterally. Basal cell carcinomas grow slowly. Distant metastasis is exceedingly rare, and local removal by excision, electrodesiccation, or irradiation generally effects a complete cure. For large or complicated tumors of the face, a special surgical technique, Moh's microscopically controlled surgery, is employed.

Squamous Cell Carcinoma. A squamous cell carcinoma, as defined in Chapter 4, is a malignant tumor that arises from the skin and other locations of squamous cell epithelium. This type of carcinoma is less common than basal cell carcinoma. A squamous cell carcinoma will most often develop on the patient's face and other exposed skin surfaces. Chronic exposure to sunlight is an even greater cause of squamous cell carcinoma than it is for other skin cancers. Sources of chronic irritation definitely predispose skin to squamous cell carcinoma. Pipe smoking, for example, may be seen in association with a lesion of the lower lip. Like basal cell carcinoma, squamous cell carcinoma may present as an ulcerated area and initially be only locally invasive, but unlike the former tumor, the squamous cancer may grow rapidly and may metastasize widely. The prognosis of squamous cell carcinomas if excised early in their development is excellent. The prognosis is somewhat more guarded when a squamous cell carcinoma is located on the patient's lip, mucous membranes, or on sites of previous burns or damage by ulcers.

Malignant melanoma. Malignant melanoma, as defined in Chapter 4, is a darkly pigmented cancerous tumor that usually arises from a preceding mole. Signs suggesting malignant melanoma are (1) mole size greater than six millimeters, (2) irregular borders or pigmentation, nodularity, ulceration, itching, scaling, or (3) awareness of the lesion. Based on microscopic characteristics, malignant melanoma is divided into the following four types:

- *lentigo-maligna melanoma*, which involves a large, flat, tan or brown mole that has irregularly scattered spots
- *superficial spreading melanoma*, which involves a noticeable enlargement or discoloration of a lesion
- *acro lentiginous melanoma*, which involves moles arising on palms or soles or under nails
- *nodular melanoma*, which involves a noticeably rapid enlargement of raised lesions

Malignant melanoma is noted for its rapid growth, early metastasis, and potentially poor prognosis. Metastasis occurs through lymphatics and blood vessels to the liver, lung, brain, and gastrointestinal tract.

Lesions of malignant melanoma are sometimes classified according to their invasiveness as determined microscopically. Invasiveness is recorded on a scale of I through V, and these levels are called Clark's levels. Level I refers to an in-situ lesion which, by definition, is confined to the original site and has not invaded neighboring tissues. Early invasion is present in level II, and deepening invasions are designated by levels III, IV, and V. Lesions are classified more commonly by Breslow's thickness, which measures the tumor's thickness in millimeters.

At present, the only curative treatment for melanocarcinoma is excision of the affected tissue at an early stage of the cancer's growth. Typically after initial excision, a reexcision is performed to be sure of complete removal of the cancerous tissue. Immunologic treatment for metastases is under active investigation, but so far has not been very successful.

Bowen's Disease. *Bowen's disease* is an intraepidermal in-situ squamous cell carcinoma usually occurring as a single lesion that spreads slowly by peripheral extension. It may occur anywhere on the skin of middle-aged or elderly patients. In the past, researchers theorized that Bowen's disease was associated with internal malignancy, but this hypothesis has been shown to be false. Complete surgical excision is curative for Bowen's disease.

Mycoses Fungoides. Mycoses fungoides, which are also called *cutaneous T cell lymphomas*, are rare, chronic lymphomas that are characterized by large, firm, reddish, painful, ulcerating tumors. Mycoses fungoides initially manifest in the patient's skin but often spread despite treatment. This disease may be difficult to diagnose by both clinical and microscopic exam. Diagnosis of mycoses fungoides may take six years from the initial skin lesion, at which time the median survival rate is less than five years. Treatment with radiation, chemotherapy, immunotherapy, and local excision do not greatly affect prognosis.

Kaposi's Sarcoma. Kaposi's sarcoma is a multifocal, metastasizing cancer that usually first presents as reddish blue or brownish soft nodules and tumors in the skin on the extremities. Until the AIDS epidemic, Kaposi's sarcoma was rare, and typically occurred in older males. Now, however, Kaposi's sarcoma occurs in up to 20 percent of all AIDS patients. The course in these patients is very aggressive and includes widespread metastases that can lead to death. Chemotherapy, radiotherapy, and immunotherapy with interferon have limited long-term benefits.

Burns

Burns are classified in three categories, according to the depth of the necrosis, which is the death of tissue. First-degree burns result from mild injury. The burned area shows redness and edema of the skin. Usually the superficial part of the epidermis will peel and then will heal completely without a scar.

Greater injury results from a second-degree burn. A second-degree burn is characterized by blister formation. Although the necrosis extends to varying depths in the dermis, enough viable epithelial remnants remain to permit regeneration of the epidermis, generally without the need for skin grafting. However, the healing process is much slower than for first-degree burns, and scarring may result.

In third-degree, or full thickness burns, the epidermis and most or all of the dermis is destroyed. Healing leads to scar formation. Underlying fat, muscle, and bone tissues may also be involved in third-degree burns.

Shock is one of the most serious consequences of an extensive second- or third-degree burn. Shock is caused by diminishing circulating blood volume resulting from the continuous seepage of plasma through damaged capillaries at the site of the burn. The fall in blood pressure impairs circulation to internal organs.

Infection is the second serious complication of a burn. The skin barrier is broken, and pathogenic organisms gain entrance to the body through the burned area. Infection not only delays healing but is the source of circulating toxins. Because of these serious complications, extensive third-degree burns frequently cause death.

No major treatment problems are involved with first- and second-degree burns, and local treatment with creams, lotions, and wet compresses is sufficient. Treatment of extensive third-degree burns represents a distinct therapeutic challenge. Analgesics are given for pain; intravenous fluids and whole blood are administered to replace plasma, to compensate for blood loss, and to maintain an adequate kidney circulation; and antibiotics are given to combat infection. Most full thickness burns require skin grafting to close the wound. Grafting is undertaken after the acute and critical phase of the extensive burn and its complications have passed and after the patient's condition has stabilized. Scar tissue is the long-term complication of burns and may have significant cosmetic or functional consequences regarding the patient's use of his or her hands and joint mobility.

Plastic Surgery and Skin Grafts

Plastic surgery involves the repair of deformities, usually superficial or external in location, in order to obtain improved appearance or function. Plastic surgery that is intended only to improve appearance and not to improve function is often called "cosmetic" surgery and generally is not covered by health insurance. Deformities can be congenital from intrauterine disease of the mother or from other causes of abnormal fetal development, or they may be acquired as a result of disease or trauma. To achieve a repair, the plastic surgeon modifies tissues, often with the use of grafts from other parts of the skin.

A skin graft should closely resemble the tissue it replaces. Characteristics such as thickness, color, texture, hairiness, and tension must be considered when transplanting skin. The continued viability of transplanted skin depends on obtaining a good blood supply to the host area and on the avoidance of infection in the host area.

6

Hematology

Hematology is the medical science that deals with the study of the origin, development, anatomy, and function of blood and blood-forming organs. The principal blood-forming organs are the bone marrow, liver, spleen, lymph nodes and, in fetal life, the thymus. Hematology includes the investigation and treatment of diseases of the blood-forming organs and is concerned with coagulation processes, blood groups, blood transfusions, and immune mechanisms. This chapter will first describe the normal anatomy and function of the various tissue and organ components of the hematologic system and then will consider some of the disorders that affect the components of the system.

ANATOMY AND PHYSIOLOGY

An understanding of blood and the lymphatic system provides an essential foundation for a study of hematologic disorders. This section will describe blood, focusing on its various components. We will look at how blood is formed and will discuss blood groups and coagulation processes. This discussion will then move to the lymphatic system and its component parts, including lymph channels, lymph nodes, and the spleen.

The Blood

Blood is the liquid that transports vital substances to body tissues and removes the waste products of the tissues' metabolism. Blood brings defensive forces to areas of disease and injury and plays a vital role in maintaining the proper water, salt, and acid-base balance in the body.

Blood Composition

Blood consists of plasma and cellular elements. *Plasma* is the faintly yellow liquid component of blood. Plasma is mostly water and contains mineral salts, fats, glucose, hormones, enzymes, and the waste products of cell metabolism. It also contains plasma proteins that contribute to the body's immunity, blood clotting, and anticlotting factors. The cellular elements of blood, which are called *blood corpuscles*, are suspended in the plasma and are of three types: (1) the *erythrocytes*, or red blood cells; (2) the *leukocytes*, or white blood cells; and (3) the *thrombocytes*, or platelets. Red corpuscles give the blood its characteristic tint and comprise about 45 percent of the total blood volume. Less than half the size of red cells, thrombocytes are irregularly shaped, colorless structures that have great adhesive power.

Erythrocytes. The function of the erythrocyte is to effect the exchange of oxygen from the inspired air with carbon dioxide from the body tissues. The red blood cell contains *hemoglobin*, a complex protein-iron substance that carries oxygen. In the lungs, the hemoglobin molecule combines with oxygen from the inspired air. This hemoglobin-oxygen combination is then transported within the red blood cell to the capillaries, where the oxygen is released. Carbon dioxide produced as a waste product of the metabolism of the cells of the body is transported to the lungs and is released into the expired air. A portion of the carbon dioxide is transported within the red cell and a portion is carried within the plasma.

The number of circulating red blood cells in normal individuals increases slightly from repetitive muscular activity, living at high altitudes, and from any condition of climate or lowered barometric pressure that results in a reduced supply of oxygen to the tissues. The average life span of a mature red blood cell is about 120 days.

Leukocytes. The leukocytes, or white blood cells, include several different cell types. These types differ in size, shape, nuclear structure, and function. The most numerous leukocytes are the *polymorphonuclear*, or multi-lobed nucleus, *neutrophils*. The "polys," as these leukocytes are called, account for 50 to 70 percent of the total leukocytes and are responsible for various important defensive functions. Polys engulf harmful bacteria, rendering them harmless, and act as scavengers for the body. ***Lymphocytes***, or "lymphs," are another common type of leukocyte. Lymphs have single nuclei and are involved in the production of antibodies and the destruction of cancerous cells, bacteria, and other infectious agents (see the section in Chapter 2 on Immunology). The polys and the lymphs comprise most of the circulating white cells. Other types of leukocytes exist in small numbers. The functions of these other leukocytes are not as well understood as the functions of polys and lymphs.

White blood cells are intimately involved with inflammatory responses to infections and injuries. The leukocytes travel by bloodstream to the site of an infection or injury and then exit from the capillaries to the damaged tissue.

An increased number of leukocytes is called ***leukocytosis*** and is seen most commonly in association with infections. ***Leukopenia***, on the other hand, is a decrease in the number of white blood cells and is most often a temporary condition during a viral infection, but it may be secondary to bone marrow damage or other conditions. ***Neutropenia*** is a decrease in the number of neutrophils and is typically present in association with viral infections. Persistently decreased numbers of white blood cells may increase the body's risk for infections. Furthermore, the cause of a persistent decrease in white blood cells may indicate malignancy, AIDS, bone marrow damage, or other serious problem.

Thrombocytes. Within seconds after an injury to a blood vessel, the thrombocytes begin to aggregate at the site of the injury to seal the leak. In addition, platelets assist the very complex process of blood coagulation by releasing blood-clotting substances.

Blood Formation

Blood cells are constantly lost from circulation because of aging, cell death, bleeding, and maintenance functions such as control of infection. To maintain the required quantities of blood cells, each cell type must have the capacity for self-renewal. In early fetal life, the spleen is responsible for the manufacture of erythrocytes. In later fetal life, the liver is the main organ involved in red cell formation, and the bone marrow and thymus are involved in white cell formation. Gradually, the bone marrow takes over the manufacture of all blood corpuscles. After birth, under normal conditions, the bone marrow is responsible for most blood formation. During early post-natal life, most bones participate in blood cell manufacture, but by age 18 this function is largely confined to the vertebrae, ribs, sternum, skull, and hip bones.

The formation of blood cells outside the bone marrow—in the

spleen, liver, and lymph nodes—occurs in post-fetal life generally only in association with disease. Bone marrow can be evaluated by a needle biopsy. The microscopic evaluation of a bone marrow biopsy sample provides information about diseases of the red or white cells and platelets, especially anemias or malignancies.

Blood Groups

Researchers have long recognized that red blood cells contain antigens and that plasma contains antibodies. Collectively, blood groups represent systems of antigens found in the surface of the red cells. These antigens are inherited according to the laws of gene and chromosome inheritance. The major antigens in the erythrocytes are those named "A" and "B." Red blood cells may contain one, both, or neither of the major antigens.

Testing to determine which antibodies and antigens are present, and so which blood group a person's blood belongs to, is called *blood typing*. Anti-A antibodies attack and destroy red cells containing A antigens, and anti-B antibodies destroy red cells containing B antigens. Normally, an individual's plasma does not contain antibodies that will destroy its natural red cells but may contain antibodies that will destroy transfused red cells. A *transfusion reaction* is the destruction of the donor's red cells by antibodies in the recipient's plasma and occurs when blood is improperly matched for transfusion. A transfusion reaction is an example of an antigen-antibody reaction. Antigens and antibodies, and additional examples of antigen-antibody reactions, are discussed in the section on Immunology in Chapter 2.

Another example of an antigen found in blood that is of great clinical significance is Rh. Rh designates an inherited factor that may be present in a person's red cells. About 85 percent of the population has this Rh factor, and so is Rh positive. Those individuals who do not have the factor are Rh negative. A problem may arise during pregnancy if the mother is Rh negative, the father Rh positive, and the fetus Rh positive. In this situation, the mother's antibodies may pass through the placenta into the fetus, where these antibodies attack and destroy the fetal erythrocytes, leading to severe fetal anemia or even fetal death. Appropriate testing and treating of women during their pregnancies can prevent these results.

Blood Volume

The blood volume of a young, healthy adult comprises seven to eight percent of that person's total body weight. Total blood volume relative to body weight is greater in males than in females, primarily because males have a greater red blood cell volume. Also, total blood volume is more closely related to physical size than to age. At birth, a person's total blood volume is about 300 milliliters. This volume increases gradually until puberty when the volume increases more rapidly.

Hemostasis and Coagulation

Hemostasis is defined as the arrest of bleeding, either spontaneously or by surgical means. Spontaneous hemostasis results from three processes: (1) the contractions of blood vessels; (2) the aggregation and adhesion of platelets at the bleeding site, forming a platelet plug; and (3) the coagulation of blood. Totally efficient hemostasis requires all three processes, but hemostasis compatible with maintaining life will occur even if one component is deficient.

Substances in plasma, known as *coagulation factors*, are essential to the clotting process. These factors are designated by roman numerals I through XIII. Some of the better known factors are I, VIII, and IX. Factor I is *fibrinogen*, a plasma protein that is converted to fibrin in a complex sequence of steps in the clotting process. Fibrin forms the essential portion of all blood clots. The clotting process is contained or limited by a number of opposing forces. Without these balancing forces, a beneficial clot could enlarge and cause harm.

Factor VIII is the *antihemophilic factor*. Deficiency of this factor causes a type of hemophilia, called hemophilia A. (Hemophilias are defined and discussed later in this chapter.) Factor IX is called the *plasma thromboplastin component*. Deficiency of this factor results in hemophilia B, or Christmas disease.

Deficiencies of the various factors can be detected by coagulation studies. Specialized testing measures the levels of specific factors that are typically expressed as a percent of normal.

Plasmapheresis

A technique known as plasmapheresis can remove soluble compounds or cellular elements from the circulation. In *plasmapheresis*, blood is removed from a vein and transported through tubing to a blood cell separator which filters out undesirable blood components that may contribute to disease. In some patients, the blood is returned to the donor's body through a vein. Plasmapheresis can also separate out normal blood components, such as white blood cells or platelets, that may then be transfused into patients who need the blood product.

The Lymphatic System

The lymphatic system consists of (1) lymphocytes; (2) lymph nodes scattered throughout the body and located at various points in the lymphatic capillary system; (3) an extensive network of tiny, thin-walled capillaries and collecting vessels; (4) the thoracic duct, which carries lymph from the lymphatic capillaries to the bloodstream; and (5) the spleen.

Lymphocytes, a type of white blood cell and a component of the lymphatic system, contribute to the functioning of the body's immune mechanism. Additional information on the immune system and the lymphocytes' role in that system is presented in Chapter 2, *Scientific Background for the Study of Disease.*

The *lymph nodes* are round or oval structures situated along the large blood vessels of the body. Lymphatic capillaries connect the lymph nodes with larger lymphatic ducts. The lymphatic ducts, in turn, eventually empty into the thoracic duct, which drains into the venous circulation.

The pressure of the blood in the arteriolar capillaries forces some of the fluid portion of the blood—but not the blood cells—through the capillary walls into the tissue spaces surrounding the cells of the body. This fluid surrounding the body's cells carries nutritive substances to the cells and takes away the cells' waste products. Much of the fluid bathing the cells gets reabsorbed into the bloodstream, but the remainder, a colorless, watery fluid known as *lymph*, drains from between the cells into the lymphatic collecting system, passes through regional lymph nodes, which act as bacterial filters, and eventually reaches the bloodstream.

The *spleen* is a fairly large organ that lies in the left upper quadrant of the abdominal cavity just below the diaphragm. The spleen is so well covered by the rib cage that normally it cannot be felt externally, except in the very thinnest of individuals. As a general rule, then, the spleen can be felt only if it is enlarged. The spleen increases in size slightly during digestion and varies in size according to the state of nutrition of the body, being somewhat larger in overweight individuals.

The spleen has many functions:

- It assists in the destruction of aged, abnormal, and damaged red cells and platelets.
- It acts as a reservoir for platelets, lymphocytes, red blood cells, and some leukocytes.
- It participates in the production of lymphocytes.
- It is involved in antibody production.

- It filters bacteria, other microorganisms, and particulate antigens from the bloodstream.
- In certain diseases of the bone marrow, the spleen can take over much of the bone marrow's function.

Nevertheless, the spleen is a nonessential organ and an individual can survive without one.

HEMATOLOGIC DISORDERS

A **hematologic disorder** is any abnormal or pathological condition of the fluid, chemical, or cellular components of blood or of the blood-forming organs. This section will first address the diagnosis of hematologic disorders and then will consider some of the more important of these disorders.

Diagnosing hematologic disorders requires a study of the affected individual's blood cells. To obtain a patient's blood cells for study, a medical professional uses a needle and syringe to withdraw a sample of blood from a vein or uses a small, sharp, pointed "razor" to prick the patient's finger and then collects the blood in a small tube.

Laboratory methods for the evaluation of blood cells are

- Counting the number of red cells.
- Determining the volume of packed red cells, known as the hematocrit. The hematocrit, or "crit," is determined by adding an anticoagulant to the blood, centrifuging it, and noting the volume of packed cells as a percent of the total blood volume.
- Determining the blood hemoglobin concentration. Hemoglobin concentration is readily determined by a variety of methods.
- Measuring the red blood cell indices. The three red blood cell indices are the mean corpuscular volume (MCV), mean corpuscular hemoglobin concentration (MCHC), and mean corpuscular hemoglobin (MCH).[1] The MCV is the most useful red cell index, and its value will help the diagnosis of anemia. (Anemias are discussed below.)
- Evaluating the blood smear. The smear evaluation is a microscopic look at the red cells, platelets, and white cells. A smear is helpful in evaluating diseases of red blood cells, platelets, and white blood cells, as well as in measuring the percentages of the different types of white blood cells.

---

[1] "Mean" in this discussion refers to "average."

- Measuring the reticulocyte count, or retic count. The reticulocyte count is a percentage measurement of the young red blood
cells compared with the total number of red cells. The retic
count decreases when the rate of red blood cell production
decreases, and it increases when the rate of red blood cell
production increases.

A complete blood count (CBC) usually includes the first five of
these methods. In evaluating an insured's test results, the claim
reviewer should always refer to the normal values used by the
laboratory performing the test under review.

Anemias

An *anemia* is a condition in which the amount of hemoglobin or the
number of erythrocytes in the blood is below the normal level.
Anemia may also refer to a reduction in the packed red cells, or
hematocrit.

Test results may be skewed by the method of blood collection.
For example, a blood sample taken from a vein is more likely to be
accurate than is a sample taken from a finger. Elapsed time from
blood collection to testing may also lead to abnormal results.
Retesting with attention to these details often "cures" an anemia.

Iron-Deficiency Anemia

Iron-deficiency anemia is a blood disorder characterized by low or
absent iron stores, low iron concentration in the blood, low hemoglobin concentration, low hematocrit, and other abnormalities. It is the
most common type of anemia. The most frequent cause of iron
deficiency leading to anemia in adults is blood loss. In females who
menstruate, excessive menstrual flow and pregnancy are the usual
causes of iron deficiency. In females who do not menstruate and in
males, the principal causes of blood loss are bleeding from peptic
ulcers, hiatus hernias, excessive aspirin intake, hemorrhoids, diverticulitis, or intestinal tumors. Inadequate diet and impaired absorption of iron following gastric surgery are other reasons for iron
deficiency. The extent of symptoms, such as weakness, easy fatigability, or shortness of breath, depends on the severity of the anemia,
although most anemic people have no symptoms. Oral iron therapy
is often effective in reversing the anemia, especially if the cause of the
iron deficiency is corrected. Rapid loss of blood may require a blood
transfusion in order to prevent shock.

Megaloblastic Anemia

A *megaloblastic anemia* is a type of anemia in which abnormally large oval red blood cells appear in the peripheral blood and large immature red blood cells appear in the bone marrow. The abnormally large oval red blood cells in the blood are known as *macrocytes* and the large immature red blood cells in the bone marrow are *megaloblasts*. Megaloblastic anemias usually arise from a deficiency of folic acid, vitamin B_{12}, or both. Folic acid deficiency is usually caused by inadequate dietary intake, and is especially common in alcoholics. Also, pregnant women have an increased need for folic acid. Vitamin B_{12} deficiency is usually related to a specific abnormality in the absorption of this vitamin. The MCV in megaloblastic anemia patients is often elevated, but the serum value of folic acid or vitamin B_{12} is often low.

Pernicious anemia is an example of a megaloblastic anemia that results from a deficiency of vitamin B_{12}. It is characterized by atrophy of the stomach lining, nausea, vomiting, weight loss, a faint yellow skin tint, lack of coordination, irritability, forgetfulness, dementia, and other neurologic difficulties. *Paresthesia*, which involves abnormal skin sensations that have no obvious cause, is another manifestation of pernicious anemia. Pernicious anemia has its highest incidence in persons in late adult life. Treatment with vitamin B_{12}, which must be continued for the patient's life, will arrest the progression of the disease and will restore the composition of the blood to normal. The neurologic symptoms, however, may be permanent. Some patients may have primarily neurologic symptoms without evidence of anemia. Folic acid deficiency anemia presents symptoms that are similar to those B_{12} anemia presents, but without the neurologic findings.

Hemolytic Anemia

Hemolytic anemias, which were discussed in Chapter 2, result from *hemolysis*—an increased rate of red blood cell destruction. The destruction of red cells may be chronic and ongoing, or the destruction may be intermittent and sudden in the form of repeated "hemolytic crises." Hemolysis may have many causes, and, as a result, many different hemolytic anemias are medically recognized. Correct identification of the cause of the hemolysis is essential, because proper treatment often varies with the cause.

Hemolytic anemias resulting from red cell enzyme defects are usually not problematic and are rare. Hemolysis is usually triggered by specific foods or medications. Avoidance of the triggering agent should prevent the condition. Similarly, the medical significance of hemolytic anemias resulting from infection depends on the underlying infection. For example, anemia arising from an HIV infection is far more serious than anemia arising from a self-limited infectious agent.

Sickle cell anemia is a chronic hemolytic anemia caused by abnormalities in hemoglobin manufacture and associated with increased red blood cell destruction. In this disease, which affects blacks almost exclusively and typically first manifests in childhood, red cells assume an abnormal sickle shape. The anemia usually is severe. Other manifestations of sickle cell disease include recurrent pain, gallstones, leg ulcers, heart enlargement, and signs of pulmonary embolism or thrombosis of major vessels. The prognosis for patients who have sickle cell disease varies, but many sickle cell sufferers live into adulthood. However, the morbidity among these patients usually is significant. Advances in general health care, plus careful medical attention to painful episodes, have improved sickle cell patients' morbidity and mortality. The hemoglobin abnormality is a single gene defect and may prove to be treatable with genetic therapy. Sickle cell trait, in which the sickle cell gene appears on only one of a chromosome pair and is recessive, is very common, but, unlike sickle cell disease, is associated with essentially no excess morbidity or mortality.

Thalassemia is a hemolytic anemia caused by abnormalities in hemoglobin manufacture. The disease occurs in people who have ethnic origins in countries bordering the Mediterranean Sea. It presents in several forms. The anemia associated with thalassemia major is severe. The prognosis for this condition is poor, although it can be improved with chronic transfusion treatment. Individuals who have thalassemia minor generally have no symptoms and experience no shortening of life expectancy or morbidity, although they often have a very mild anemia and decreased MCV. Intermediate forms of thalassemia have variable severity.

Hereditary spherocytosis is a dominant-gene hemolytic anemia. The condition gets its name from the presence of abnormal, small globular red cells known as *spherocytes*. The anemia and mild jaundice seen with this condition often are accompanied by gallstones and an enlarged spleen. The anemia is usually mild or moderate but may temporarily and episodically worsen. Removal of the spleen often cures hereditary spherocytosis.

Aplastic Anemia

Aplastic anemia is a disorder characterized by *pancytopenia*, which is a reduction in the number of red cells, white cells, and platelets. The percentage reduction for these three cell types, however, may not be uniform. In aplastic anemia, the bone marrow loses its capacity for normal cell renewal.

About one-half the aplastic anemia cases occur spontaneously without known cause. Other cases of bone marrow depression result from exposure to chemicals, drugs, or radiation that causes either temporary or permanent aplastic anemia. Anti-neoplastic drugs, for example, typically cause a temporary effect and the patient's bone marrow returns to normal when the patient stops taking the affecting medication. Aplastic anemia has also been associated with lupus erythematosus, viral infections such as hepatitis, and other diseases. Furthermore, an aplastic anemia-like illness occurs when the bone marrow is the site of tumor or infection.

Aplastic anemia, regardless of its cause, may be fatal. Bleeding can lead to death, because the abnormally small number of platelets prevents proper coagulation and clotting. Similarly, the reduced number of white blood cells characterizing aplastic anemia leaves the patient more susceptible to, and less able to fight, infections. Therefore, in some patients severe infections may lead to death.

The anemia, or its cause, may also lead to significant morbidity. The patient's prognosis depends on the successful identification and removal of the offending agent. Treatment, if necessary, may include anabolic steroids, bone marrow stimulatory factors, immunotherapy, or, in an extreme case, a bone marrow transplant.

Polycythemia

Polycythemia presents in two forms: polycythemia vera and secondary polycythemia. Although both forms involve an increase in the number of circulating red blood cells, several important differences exist between the two forms of polycythemia.

Polycythemia Vera

Polycythemia vera is a disorder of unknown cause characterized by an increase in the number of red cells, white cells, and platelets. Men are affected more often than women are. Typically this disorder arises in patients after age 50. Polycythemia vera's symptoms and signs, which probably result from increased blood cell mass and blood thickness, include a ruddy or bluish discoloration of the skin, especially of the face, an enlarged spleen, labored breathing, headache, and arterial and venous blood clots and hemorrhage. Repeated removal of blood and the use of radioactive phosphorus or chemotherapy to suppress the bone marrow manufacture of blood cells are important treatments of this condition. Secondary leukemias commonly arise in polycythemia vera patients, particularly those who receive chemotherapy. The course of polycythemia vera is variable, but many individuals live 12 to 15 years after the diagnosis is established. Blood clots in the coronary artery and strokes are the common causes of death in persons who have polycythemia vera.

Secondary Polycythemia

Secondary polycythemia, which is also known as *erythrocytosis*, is a condition marked by an increase in the number of circulating red blood cells as a result of some other condition or factor. Secondary polycythemia may be a compensatory response in people living at high altitudes or may arise in association with congenital heart disease, emphysema, pulmonary fibrosis, certain tumors, and some forms of kidney disease. Smokers sometimes have a mild polycythemia because of a relative lack of oxygen to their tissues. Stress erythrocytosis may arise in overweight, hypertensive, anxious men and generally has little medical significance of itself. Management of erythrocytosis from any cause involves a consideration of the underlying disease or condition.

Platelet Abnormalities

Thrombocytopenia is a condition characterized by a reduction in the number of platelets in the circulating blood. Thrombocytopenia results from deficient platelet production, acceleration of platelet destruction, or abnormal pooling of platelets in the spleen. This condition may be short-lived or chronic, severe or mild, and idiopathic or secondary to significant illnesses. Thrombocytopenia is the most common cause of *purpura*, which is a hemorrhage into the skin and subcutaneous tissues. Purpuric lesions occur in a variety of sizes and shapes. Minute, dot-like, red hemorrhages into the skin are called *petechiae*. Larger hemorrhages are called *ecchymoses* and are recognizable "black and blue" marks. Bleeding from the nose, gums, gastrointestinal tract and genitourinary tract also occurs with thrombocytopenia. Occasionally thrombocytopenia causes bleeding into the brain.

A common form of thrombocytopenia is *idiopathic thrombocytopenic purpura (ITP),* which can exist in acute and chronic forms. Acute ITP often occurs after a viral illness, most commonly in children. More than 90 percent of acute ITP patients recover spontaneously. An acute attack of purpura may last a few weeks or many months. Chronic ITP occurs more often in adult females than in other groups. The condition may last months or years if untreated, and spontaneous remissions are not common. Corticosteroids assist in the control of the disease, and splenectomy, if necessary, results in a complete cure in a majority of patients.

Thrombocytopenia may be caused by certain drugs and is usually corrected by discontinuing the use of the drug. Thrombocytopenia may result from bone marrow destruction, infiltration by malignancies, metabolic storage diseases, or an enlarged spleen. Thrombocytopenia may be the initial manifestation of HIV infections or systemic lupus erythematosus.

A relatively rare form of thrombocytopenia of unknown cause is **thrombotic thrombocytopenic purpura (TTP).** TTP is characterized by hemolytic anemia and renal and central nervous system abnormalities. Generally, TTP runs a rapid downhill course, and untreated patients experience a mortality rate of more than 80 percent. However, the introduction of plasma and whole blood exchange procedures and plasmapheresis have improved the outlook for patients who have this condition. High-dose steroid therapy is also used to combat TTP. An individual who has recovered from TTP may experience residual renal or central nervous system defects.

Thrombocytosis is a condition in which a patient's blood contains increased numbers of platelets. This condition often is secondary to inflammation, splenectomy, iron deficiency, neoplasms, polycythemia vera, or acute bleeding and may be temporary. Essential thrombocytosis has no known cause and can degenerate to leukemia. Very high platelet counts can lead to spontaneous bleeding or blood clots. Strokes, transient ischemic attacks,[2] gastrointestinal bleeding, and excessive bleeding following trauma or surgery are also possible results of extremely high platelet counts. Symptomatic patients who have elevated platelet counts often receive chemotherapy treatment.

Hereditary Coagulation Disorders

Hereditary coagulation disorders result from a deficiency of, or abnormality in, one of the blood coagulation factors. These disorders can produce abnormal and excessive bleeding that occurs spontaneously or from trauma. The range of symptoms resulting from these disorders is wide. For example, Factor XII deficiency does not cause clinical bleeding and is identified only as a lab test abnormality. On the other hand, Factor XI deficiency is associated with spontaneous and excessive bleeding only after significant trauma or surgery.

---

[2]Transient ischemic attacks are discussed in Chapter 7, *The Circulatory System.*

Hemophilia A

Hemophilia A, a common hereditary, sex-linked coagulation disorder, affects males far more often than females and is caused by a decreased level of Factor VIII. Three categories of hemophilia A severity are defined based upon the percent of Factor VIII present:

- Severe: Factor VIII is less than one percent of normal.
- Moderate: Factor VIII is one to five percent of normal.
- Mild: Factor VIII is five to twenty-five percent of normal.

Symptoms, which vary from mild to heavy bleeding, depend on the severity of the disease. Spontaneous or excessive bleeding generally occurs in moderate and severe cases.

In the severe form of this disease, repeated episodes of spontaneous bleeding into joints occur and sometimes result in crippling arthritis. An episode of spontaneous bleeding into a joint is called a *hemarthrosis*. The spontaneous development of hematomas, which involve bleeding under the skin and within muscles, is frequent in hemophilia A patients. Hematuria, nosebleeds, and gastrointestinal tract hemorrhages also occur. The most-feared hemorrhage is intracranial bleeding, because it can result in significant intellectual, motor, or sensory impairment. In moderate and mild hemophilia A cases, hemarthroses occur less frequently and less severely, and impairment is less common.

The treatment of an acute bleeding episode consists of the administration of Factor VIII concentrate. Many patients who have moderate or severe forms of this disease receive periodic treatments of Factor VIII concentrate to prevent hemarthroses and other spontaneous bleeding. Unfortunately, some earlier Factor VIII concentrate was produced from contaminated blood, and diseases such as HIV and hepatitis were inadvertently transmitted to some hemophilia A patients. Better screening procedures for blood products and their donors and improved sterilization procedures have reduced the likelihood that contaminated transmissions will occur in the future. In addition, genetically engineered Factor VIII is not obtained from blood, and, therefore, carries no risk of infecting a recipient.

Other Forms of Hemophilia

Hemophilia B, which is also called *Christmas disease*, is clinically similar to hemophilia A and occurs almost exclusively in males. The severity of the symptoms of hemophilia B may range from mild to severe. A deficiency of Factor IX causes this condition, which is usually treated with replacement therapy of Factor IX. However, hemophilia B may be more difficult to treat than hemophilia A.

Hemophilia C, or *von Willebrand's disease*, results from a deficiency or the abnormal functioning of a specific blood coagulation factor, which is called the von Willebrand coagulation factor. Usually patients experience an associated reduction in Factor VIII activity. Hemophilia C is the most common of the inherited coagulation disorders, affecting one in every 800 to 1,000 people. Most affected individuals have very mild forms of this disease and experience no spontaneous bleeding. Most patients experience excessive bleeding only as a result of surgery or severe trauma. Treatment, if necessary, is with cryoprecipitate, which is a blood product, or DDAVP, which is not a blood product. Only rarely do hemophilia C patients have symptoms as severe as those found in severe hemophilia A.

Acquired Coagulation Disorders

This section will review only two of the many forms of acquired coagulation disorders: vitamin K deficiencies and diffuse intravascular coagulation.

Vitamin K Deficiency

The liver manufactures several of the blood coagulation factors by a process that depends on vitamin K. A **vitamin K deficiency** usually occurs in individuals who fail to get an adequate amount of the substance from their diets or who suffer from poor vitamin K absorption from their intestinal tracts. Malabsorption of vitamin K can occur in association with several disorders of the digestive system. When bleeding occurs in vitamin K deficient individuals, it may be severe, but it is readily controlled by the administration of vitamin K. Infants are born with a relative deficiency of vitamin K. Injection of vitamin K at birth prevents vitamin K deficiency and bleeding.

Vitamin K-dependent coagulation factors are impaired by anticoagulant drugs, such as Coumadin, that are used to treat disorders such as some heart diseases. Disorders, such as cirrhosis, that impair liver function also affect vitamin K-dependent coagulation factors.

Disseminated Intravascular Coagulation

Disseminated intravascular coagulation (DIC) is an acquired disorder in which fibrin is abnormally generated in circulating blood. DIC is typically secondary to an underlying disease. The disorder may present either in acute form with massive bleeding or in chronic form in which abnormal bleeding is uncommon. Manifestations of DIC result from widespread blood clots throughout the body and from a depletion of platelets and clotting factors. Migratory clots, hemorrhages of the skin and mucous membranes, and arterial blood clots are common in DIC patients.

The most common causes of DIC are obstetrical complication, malignancies, bloodstream infections, shock, burns, and crush injuries. Therapy is generally sequential. First, the physician must identify and correct the underlying cause of the DIC. Then, anticoagulation therapy may be used to dissolve the intravascular blood clot. Replacement treatment with platelets, fibrinogen, or clotting factors may then be necessary.

Neoplastic Disorders

Leukemias and lymphomas are malignant neoplastic[3] diseases of unknown origin affecting blood cell formation. Many types of leukemias and lymphomas exist. This text presents a simplified discussion of some of the more common leukemias and lymphomas.

Leukemia

Leukemia, a cancer of the blood-forming tissues, exists in acute and chronic forms. Chronic leukemias are more common in adults, whereas acute leukemias occur more often in children. Leukemias are also classified as myeloid or lymphoid, which identifies the general abnormal cell type. *Myelocytes* are white blood cells that contain granules. Lymphocytes, as we discussed earlier, are white blood cells that contain a single nucleus.

Common signs of leukemia include enlargement of the liver, spleen, and lymph nodes. Because the normal cellular elements in the patient's bone marrow are replaced by an uncontrolled multiplication of abnormal white cells, anemia, hemorrhage, or infection often occur in leukemia patients. Leukemia may present with nonspecific, "flu-like" symptoms or with more specific complaints of discomfort in the joints, central nervous system, or other location.

Chemotherapy as a treatment for the leukemias continues to evolve. Long-term disease-free results after treatment are seen in more than 50 percent of children who have acute lymphoid leukemia (ALL). Without treatment, death occurs within months in patients

---

[3]As defined in Chapter 4, a neoplasm is any new and abnormal growth, particularly if the growth is uncontrolled.

who have this type of leukemia. Acute myelogenous leukemia (AML) and chronic myelogenous leukemia (CML) have variable responses to treatment. Chronic lymphocytic leukemia (CLL) is a disease that usually affects people over age 60. CLL patients often experience long-term survival of more than ten years, even without treatment. Thus, therapy is generally not initiated until active progression of CLL occurs. For CLL patients, overtreatment is often more dangerous than undertreatment.

Newer chemotherapeutic strategies, bone marrow transplantation, and immunotherapy are under active investigation to improve treatment results for all leukemia patients.

Malignant Lymphomas

Malignant lymphomas are a group of diseases showing neoplastic growth of the cells of the lymphatic system. Classification of malignant lymphomas is difficult because, although some of the diseases are pathologically and clinically distinct, others show considerable overlapping of features. The two main types of lymphomas are known as Hodgkin's disease and non-Hodgkin's lymphoma. Physicians usually first detect lymphomas by biopsy of enlarged lymph nodes. However, lymphomas also may produce enlargement of the patient's liver or spleen and may cause lesions in the patient's skin or bone marrow or in the patient's cardiovascular, nervous, gastrointestinal, or genitourinary systems.

Hodgkin's Disease. Hodgkin's disease is a malignant condition characterized by painless, progressive enlargement of the lymph nodes, spleen, and general lymphoid tissue. It presents in one of four cellular patterns. The prognosis in this disorder correlates well with the cellular pattern, the stage of the disease (see Figure 6–1) at the time treatment begins, and the presence or absence of systemic symptoms. Such symptoms include fever, night sweats, fatigue, and weight loss.

The overall prognosis of Hodgkin's disease is quite good. High-dose radiation treatment to the affected and adjacent areas produces long-term cures in more than 90 percent of those patients who have either stage IA or stage IIA Hodgkin's disease. Radiation and chemotherapy yield 80 to 90 percent long-term cure in either stage IB or stage IIB disease. Chemotherapy with or without radiation will cure more than 50 percent of patients whose Hodgkin's disease is in stages III or IV. Sometimes treatment for Hodgkin's disease causes long-term complications. Solid tumors, leukemia, radiation pulmonary fibrosis, or pericarditis can occur many years after treatment.

Non-Hodgkin's Lymphomas. Non-Hodgkin's lymphomas are a

Figure 6–1.
Staging of Hodgkin's Disease.

Stage I	Disease limited to the lymph nodes of one anatomical region
Stage II	Disease limited to lymph nodes of more than one region on the same side of the diaphragm
Stage III	Disease limited to the lymph nodes on both sides of the diaphragm or localized extranodal and/or spleen involvement
Stage IV	Diffuse involvement of one or several organs or isolated extranodal involvement with distant nodal involvement

Each stage is usually further categorized as being either type A, in which the patient does not experience any systemic symptoms, or type B, in which the patient does experience systemic symptoms, such as fever or night sweats.

heterogeneous group of malignant diseases that are characterized by the neoplastic proliferation of lymphoid cells that often spread throughout the body. Non-Hodgkin's lymphomas differ histologically from Hodgkin's disease. The peak frequency of the non-Hodgkin's lymphomas occurs in patients who are in their 50s. Hodgkin's disease, on the other hand, has its peak frequency in patients who are in their 20s. Like Hodgkin's disease, the lesions of non-Hodgkin's lymphoma can be found in the patient's skin, bone marrow, nervous system, gastrointestinal tract, liver, spleen, or lymph nodes.

The clinical staging system used for Hodgkin's disease is also applicable to non-Hodgkin's lymphoma. In addition, non-Hodgkin's tumors fall into three general grades: low, intermediate, and high grade. Each grade of tumor also has subtypes. Low-grade tumors that are not treated may take years to develop fully. High-grade tumors that are not treated generally have a short course that is defined in months.

Radiation is used much less frequently in treating non-Hodgkin's lymphomas than in treating Hodgkin's disease. Combination chemotherapy is the mainstay treatment for most types of non-Hodgkin's lymphomas. Cure with chemotherapy may be greater than 50 percent for patients who have high-grade tumors such as diffuse large cell lymphoma (DLCL), even for stages III or IV. Survival with low-grade stage I or stage II lymphoma tumors is likely to be greater than ten years after five disease-free years. Stage III or stage IV low-grade lymphoma tumors have a worse prognosis. New treatment protocols continue to improve the prognosis for lymphoma patients. Long-term complications of treatment for non-Hodgkin's lymphomas are uncommon.

Figure 6–2 outlines all the hematologic disorders discussed in the previous sections.

Disorders of the Spleen

One of the most common signs of many hematologic disorders is an enlargement of the spleen, a condition known as *splenomegaly*. Pain is not a prominent feature of disorders of the spleen, and, in many instances, splenomegaly may produce only a dull ache. Rupture of a normal spleen does not occur spontaneously, but results from extensive, direct trauma to the abdomen. However, an enlarged spleen may rupture either spontaneously or as a result of a slight injury.

Splenomegaly

A normal adult spleen is about the size of a closed fist. Splenomegaly is never normal, although it may not be medically serious and may

Figure 6–2.
Hematologic Disorders.

Anemias
    Iron-deficiency anemia
    Megaloblastic anemias, including vitamin B_{12} deficiency and folic acid
        deficiency
    Hemolytic anemias
    Aplastic anemias

Polycythemia
    Polycythemia vera
    Secondary polycythemia, erythrocytosis

Disorder of Platelets
    Thrombocytopenia
    Thrombocytosis

Hereditary Coagulation Disorders
    Hemophilia A
    Hemophilia B, Christmas disease
    Hemophilia C, von Willebrand's disease

Acquired Coagulation Disorders
    Vitamin K deficiency
    Disseminated intravascular coagulation

Neoplastic Disorders
    Leukemia
    Lymphoma

occur in association with many conditions. Figure 6–3 lists some of these conditions. The cause of splenomegaly is important in determining the medical significance of the condition.

Acute systemic viral and bacterial infections, such as infectious mononucleosis, can cause splenomegaly. Chronic infections of the spleen from tuberculosis, histoplasmosis, malaria, and abscess also cause splenic enlargement.

Congestive splenomegaly is an enlargement of the spleen resulting from an engorgement or "back-up" of blood within the portal veins that connect the spleen with the liver. These veins are the passageway through which blood from the spleen and other abdominal organs returns to the major vein leading to the heart. An obstruction in the venous pathway raises the individual's blood pressure within this system and produces portal hypertension. The obstruction causing portal hypertension may be located (1) within the liver as a result of cirrhosis, (2) outside the liver as a consequence of the compression of a vein from a pancreatic tumor or aneurysm or as a consequence of a thrombosis of the portal vein, or (3) from the inability of a heart weakened by congestive heart failure to pump the normal volume of blood returning to it.

Figure 6–3.
Causes of Splenomegaly.

Infectious
    Viral infections
    Subacute bacterial endocarditis, an inflammation of the endocardium or
        heart valves
    Infectious mononucleosis
    AIDS

Congestive
    Cirrhosis of the liver
    Thrombosis of the portal vein
    Cardiac failure

Neoplastic
    Cysts
    Lymphoma
    Metastatic tumors
    Leukemia

Miscellaneous
    Hemolytic anemia
    Idiopathic thrombocytopenia purpura
    Thyrotoxicosis, a condition resulting from overactivity of the thyroid gland
    Polycythemia vera

Hypersplenism

The term *hypersplenism* refers to a condition characterized by an enlarged spleen and a reduction of circulating red cells, white cells, and/or platelets in any combination. This reduction of cells results from an abnormally functioning spleen that destroys the cells too rapidly. The bone marrow, however, continues to function in a normal and undiminished manner. In many cases the cause of hypersplenism is unknown, although it may be secondary to lymphoma, congestive disorders, sarcoidosis, lupus erythematosus, or other disorder. Surgical removal of the spleen is an effective treatment for hypersplenism in some patients.

Infectious Mononucleosis

Infectious mononucleosis, also known as *mono* or *glandular fever,* is a systemic illness that is caused by the Epstein-Barr virus and that generally affects young adults between the ages of 17 and 25. Mono rarely affects persons over age 40. Symptoms of mono include fatigue, which may be severe and may last for months, sore throat, headache, and loss of appetite. Signs of mono often include generalized lymph node and liver enlargement, fever, pharyngitis, and splenomegaly. Evidence of self-limited mono-hepatitis is nearly universal in cases of mononucleosis. Laboratory findings in infectious mononucleosis patients include an elevated white cell count and the presence of many atypical lymphocytes on a stained smear of the peripheral blood. Other tests that are used to diagnose this disease include a mono spot test and an EBV blood test.

Complications of infectious mononucleosis are rare. However, rupture of the spleen, hemolytic anemia, ECG changes, and neurologic manifestations sometimes occur. No specific treatment for infectious mononucleosis exists, although steroids may be used to treat severely enlarged glands that obstruct airways. The prognosis for complete recovery from mono is virtually 100 percent, and the illness may last from several weeks to six months.

Treatment with Splenectomy

Splenectomy is the surgical removal of the spleen. Indications for splenectomy include

- rupture of the spleen
- hereditary spherocytosis
- idiopathic thrombocytopenic purpura
- hypersplenism

- many hemolytic diseases
- certain lymphomas
- some localized diseases, such as cysts

Splenectomy in patients who have other diseases is controversial, but may be indicated under special circumstances. Also, removal of the spleen is sometimes performed for diagnostic purposes, such as for staging Hodgkin's disease.

The possibility of increased susceptibility to bacterial infection following splenectomy is a concern, because the normal spleen plays a role in the body's defense against bacterial invasion of the blood-stream. The risk of infection is greatest in young children who had splenectomies because of hematologic malignancy or blood disorders. Some increased risk of infection after a splenectomy probably persists throughout the patient's life, but that risk is lower in all adults than in children. Risk of infection is minimally increased in those adults who had their splenectomies because of significant trauma rather than because of some underlying disease of the spleen.

7

The Circulatory System

This chapter first describes the components of the circulatory system and their functions. Then we address specialized procedures available for diagnosing circulatory system disorders. This chapter concludes with a discussion of disorders that commonly affect the circulatory system.

ANATOMY AND PHYSIOLOGY

The **circulatory system**, which is also called the *cardiovascular system*, consists of the heart and blood vessels and is responsible for the flow of blood throughout the body. After describing the heart and blood vessels, we will look more closely at their functions within the circulatory system.

The **heart** is a hollow, muscular organ that pumps blood to all parts of the body. About two-thirds of the heart's area lies to the left of the midline of the breastbone between the lungs in the area known as the *mediastinum* of the thoracic cavity. The muscular tissue of the heart is called the **myocardium**. A two-layered, white, fibrous sac known as the **pericardium** encases the heart and the cardiac junctions of the major blood vessels. Between the two layers of the pericardium is a very small amount of fluid that serves as a lubricant and prevents friction as the pericardial surfaces slide over one another.

The heart is divided into four distinct chambers. The chambers are lined by a thin, strong membrane called the **endocardium**. The two upper chambers, the right and left **atria**, are separated by a thin, muscular septum. The right atrium is larger than the left. Opening into the right atrium are two major veins, the superior vena cava and the inferior vena cava. The inferior vena cava is larger than the superior vena cava. Another, thicker septum separates the two lower chambers of the heart, the right and left **ventricles**. Between the right atrium and ventricle and between the left atrium and ventricle are valves that permit the blood to flow in only one direction. Because these valves are situated between an atrium and a ventricle, they are called A-V valves.

The heart serves as a pump for the two circulatory systems: systemic circulation and pulmonary circulation. **Systemic circulation** includes the blood vessels that carry oxygenated blood from the left ventricle of the heart to the various organs and tissues of the body (except the lungs) and back to the heart. **Pulmonary circulation** involves the network of blood vessels that transport oxygen-depleted blood from the right ventricle of the heart to the lungs for oxygenation and back again to the heart.

Figure 7–1 shows a cross-section of the interior of a healthy heart.

Functioning of the Heart

To better understand the complex workings of the circulatory system, we will look more closely at the process by which the heart pumps blood and the blood moves through the rest of the circulatory system. We will then look at how the heart rate and rhythm are regulated in a normal heart and will discuss how blood pressure is maintained in a healthy individual.

The inferior vena cava and the superior vena cava are the veins through which the right atrium receives blood from all parts of the body. During a contraction, the atrial-ventricular valves open to allow blood to pass into the next heart chamber and then close to prevent backflow. Each contraction of the right atrium pumps blood through the right A-V valve, which is also called the tricuspid valve, into the right ventricle. From the right ventricle, the blood moves through the pulmonary valve into the pulmonary artery. The pulmonary artery branches to the right and left lungs, and these branches carry blood to the lungs to receive oxygen. Most of the oxygen in the blood is carried in the red cells, but a small amount is carried in the plasma.

Figure 7–1.
A Cross-Sectional View of the Interior of the Heart.

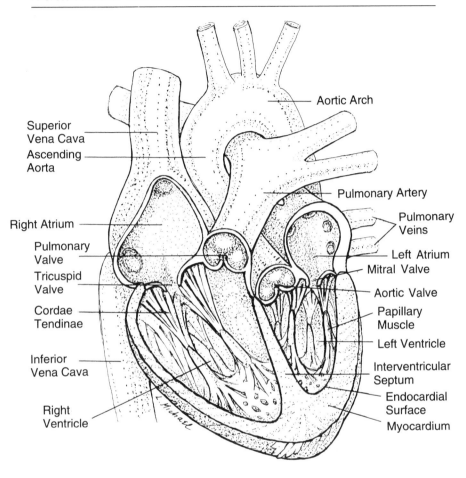

Oxygenated blood from the lungs returns through the right and left pulmonary veins into the left atrium. From this location, the blood moves through the mitral valve into the left ventricle. The mitral valve has two leaflets or cusps, but all other cardiac valves have three leaflets. The muscular walls of the left ventricle are about three times thicker than those of the right ventricle, because the left ventricle is responsible for pumping blood, through the aortic valve, into the systemic circulation.

In order to function properly and to meet its own oxygen and nutrition needs, the heart muscle needs a blood supply. The myocardium receives oxygen and nutrition from the blood in the right and left coronary arteries. These arteries arise from the first portion of the aorta just outside the heart and supply blood to all parts of the heart. The left main coronary artery subdivides into the left anterior descending coronary artery and the left circumflex coronary artery. The right coronary artery and the two branches of the left coronary artery provide the heart with a three-artery blood supply.

Figure 7–2 illustrates the flow of blood in the normal circulation.

Regulation of Heart Rate and Rhythm

In a normal heart, the electrical stimulus for each heartbeat originates in a functionally independent and specialized piece of neu-

Figure 7–2.
The Flow of Blood in Normal Circulation.

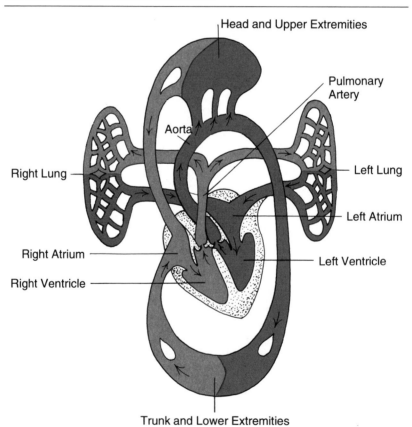

Head and Upper Extremities

Pulmonary Artery

Aorta

Right Lung

Left Lung

Left Atrium

Right Atrium

Left Ventricle

Right Ventricle

Trunk and Lower Extremities

romuscular tissue called the sinoatrial (SA) node, or simply the ***sinus node***. When the sinus node is controlling the rhythm of the heartbeat, the heart is said to be beating in normal sinus rhythm (NSR). Between 70 and 80 times each minute, an electrical impulse leaves the SA node and spreads down through the muscles of both atria, causing them to contract. Continuing down the heart, the stimulus travels within atrial fibers to reach the atrioventricular (AV) node, another specialized piece of neuromuscular tissue located high in the intraventricular septum. From the AV node, the stimulus travels into other specialized nerve fibers known as the Bundle of His. These fibers divide into right and left bundle branches that fan out over both ventricular walls. The transmission of the electrical impulse over this bundle branch network produces the muscular contractions of the ventricles. An electrocardiogram (ECG or EKG) provides a record of the origin of the electrical stimuli and shows the sequence by which they are transmitted to other parts of the heart. Figure 7–3 illustrates the heart's electrical conduction system.

Figure 7–3.
The Heart's Electrical Conduction System.

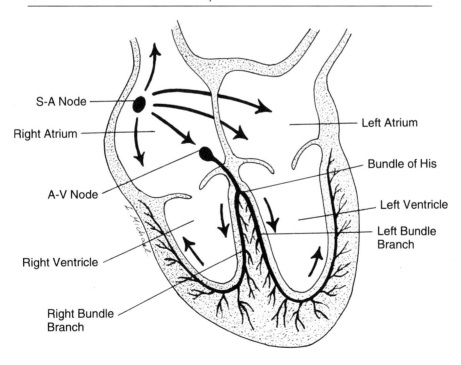

The Heart Sounds

Two heart sounds, which often are described as "lub-dub," occur during each complete heart cycle, or atrial-ventricular contraction. The start of the first sound begins the period of the heart cycle known as *systole*, during which the ventricles contract. The start of the second sound begins the period known as *diastole*, during which the ventricles relax and fill with blood. A complete heart cycle occurs approximately 100,000 times in 24 hours. The heart pumps the equivalent of approximately 2,000 gallons of blood through the body each day. Figure 7–4 illustrates the normal cardiac cycle.

The closure of the mitral and tricuspid valves contributes to the first heart sound. The closure of the aortic and pulmonic valves produces the second sound. The only other normal heart sound is a third sound that frequently occurs in young patients and that is created by the rapid inflow of blood into the ventricles in the early part of diastole. In adults, this third sound is always considered abnormal.

Blood Pressure

During each contraction, the heart provides the force necessary to propel blood through the arteries. The pressure that the blood exerts on the walls of the arteries is known as *blood pressure*. The weaker force the blood exerts on the walls of the veins is called *venous pressure*.

Blood pressure in an artery is dependent on the force of the heartbeat, the amount of resistance in the arteries caused by elasticity or atherosclerotic changes, the quantity and viscosity of the blood, and the timing of the blood pressure measurement in relation to contraction.

The customary method of measuring blood pressure is by means of the *sphygmomanometer*, or blood pressure cuff, encircling the upper arm of a seated and relaxed patient. The medical technician uses a stethoscope to listen to the patient's pulse. The medical technician inflates the blood pressure cuff until the patient's artery is blocked, as indicated by the disappearance of the pulse sound. As the technician releases the pressure in the cuff, the pulse sound returns. The pressure at which the force during a contraction is just sufficient to overcome the pressure in the cuff and produce a sound is the *systolic pressure*. As the pressure in the cuff falls, the sound disappears. The point at which the sound produced by the systolic pulse disappears is the *diastolic pressure*.

The blood pressure cuff gives readings, which are expressed as a ratio of systolic to diastolic pressure, in millimeters of mercury. The

Figure 7–4.
The Normal Cardiac Cycle.

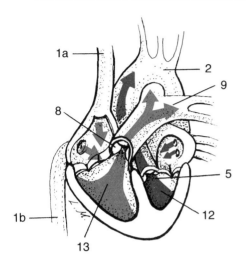

In *systole*, the aortic and pulmonary valves are open. With each ventricular contraction, blood passes into the aorta and pulmonary artery. Both atria relax and fill with blood. The mitral and tricuspid valves are closed.

1a - Superior Vena
    Cava
1b - Inferior Vena Cava
2 - Aorta
3 - Right Atrium
4 - Left Atrium

5 - Aortic Valve
6 - Mitral Valve
7 - Tricuspid Valve
8 - Pulmonary Valve
9 - Pulmonary Artery

10 - Right Ventricle
11 - Left Ventricle
12 - Oxygenated Blood
13 - Nonoxygenated
     Blood

In *diastole*, the mitral and tricuspid valves are open. With each atrial contraction, blood passes into the ventricles. This is a period of ventricular relaxation during which time the aortic and pulmonary valves are closed.

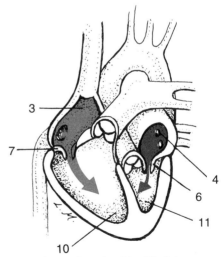

The term *cardiac systole*, or simply, *systole,* unless otherwise identified, is synonymous with ventricular systole. Similarly, *diastole* is synonymous with ventricular diastole.

higher pressure, represented by the numerator, is the pressure in the arteries during a ventricular contraction, which is the systole. The lower pressure, represented by the denominator, is the pressure between contractions when the heart is relaxing, which is the diastole. An individual's blood pressure is not constant and may vary widely with exercise, sleep, illness, excitement, and stress.

Functioning of the Blood Vessels

As mentioned earlier, the blood vessels involved in the systemic circulation carry oxygenated blood from the left ventricle to the various organs and tissues of the body (except the lungs) and back to the heart. The blood vessels involved in the pulmonary circulation transport oxygen-depleted blood from the right ventricle to the lungs for oxygenation and back again to the heart. We will now look more closely at these two types of circulation.

Systemic Circulation

The aorta is the main trunk that conveys oxygenated blood to the body. Ascending for a short distance after it leaves the left ventricle, the aorta arches backwards and to the left and then descends through the thoracic and abdominal cavities.

The *carotid arteries* furnish the principal arterial blood supply to the head and neck. On the left, the carotid artery arises directly from the aorta. On the right, the carotid artery is a branch of the innominate artery, the largest branch of the arch of the aorta. The subclavian (beneath the collarbone) arteries and their branches supply blood to the upper extremities. Like the carotid arteries, the subclavian arteries arise directly from the aorta on the left and as a branch of the innominate artery on the right.

The descending aorta is divided into two portions, the thoracic and abdominal sections, which are named in relation to the two major body cavities in which the aorta is situated. Branches from the aorta supply blood to the various organs located in these cavities. At its lower end, the abdominal aorta divides into the left and right common iliac arteries. These vessels and their branches supply blood to the lower extremities.

Throughout its length, the aorta divides into branches, and these branches divide into smaller branches, which also divide into smaller branches. This branching continues until the blood vessels are microscopic in size. Microscopic blood vessels are called *capillaries*. Oxygen and nutrients pass from the blood into other cells and tissues in the body through the walls of the capillaries. Similarly, carbon dioxide and other waste products of cellular metabolism pass from the cells and tissues into the blood through these same capillary walls.

Veins convey blood from the organs and tissues back to the heart. The superior vena cava returns blood to the right atrium from the upper half of the body, and the inferior vena cava returns blood to the right atrium from the lower half of the body. The main veins that feed into the superior vena cava are the jugular veins, which drain blood from the head and neck, and the subclavian veins, which carry the blood returning from the upper extremities. The veins that drain the thighs, liver, and kidneys are major contributories to the inferior vena cava. Figure 7–5 depicts the principal arteries and pulmonary veins in the body.

Pulmonary Circulation

The pulmonary artery transports oxygen-depleted blood to the lungs from the right ventricle. In the lungs, the blood releases the carbon dioxide it acquired in the tissues, gathers oxygen, and returns to the left atrium through the pulmonary veins. Notice that in the pulmonary circulation, veins carry oxygenated blood back to the heart and arteries transport oxygen-depleted blood to the lungs. The pulmonary circulatory system is the only place in the body in which veins carry oxygenated blood, and arteries carry oxygen-depleted blood. In all other locations, arteries carry oxygenated blood and veins carry oxygen-depleted blood. Figure 7–6 illustrates the principal veins and pulmonary arteries in the body.

TREATMENT AND DIAGNOSTIC PROCEDURES

The medical profession has made advances in cardiac surgery for correcting complicated congenital heart problems, replacing valves, and bypassing obstructions in the coronary arteries. Cardiac pacemakers can control the heart's pacing and conducting functions. *End-stage heart disease* is a condition of chronic intractable congestive heart failure no longer amenable to drug therapy. For end-stage heart disease patients, cardiac transplantation is now a common therapeutic option. Cardiac transplantation has achieved a one-year survival rate of 85 percent, a five-year survival rate of 75 percent, and a ten-year survival rate of 65 percent. Currently, fewer than 2,000 heart transplants are performed each year because of the underavailability of replacement hearts.

Figure 7–5.
The Principal Arteries and Pulmonary Veins.

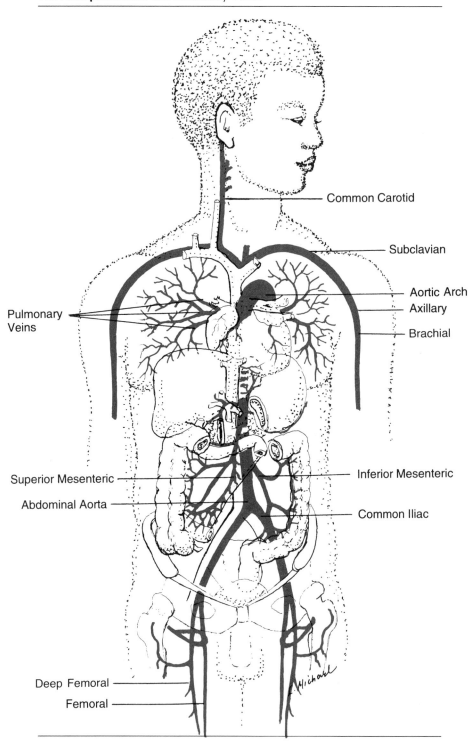

Common Carotid

Subclavian

Aortic Arch

Axillary

Pulmonary
Veins

Brachial

Superior Mesenteric

Inferior Mesenteric

Abdominal Aorta

Common Iliac

Deep Femoral

Femoral

Figure 7–6.
The Principal Veins and Pulmonary Arteries.

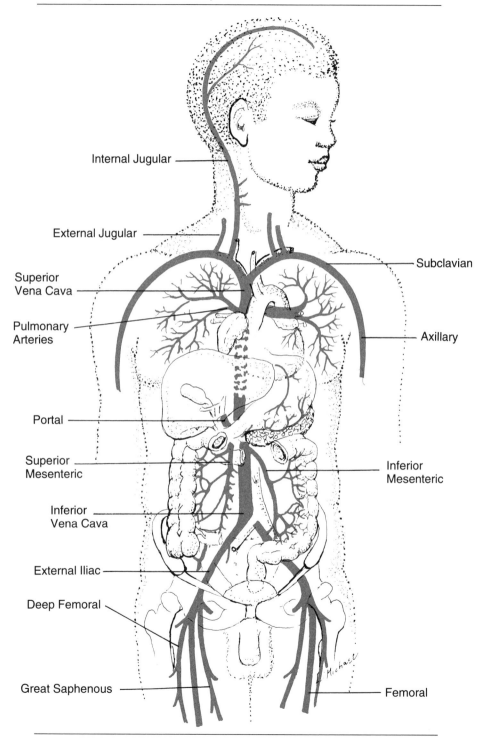

Internal Jugular

External Jugular

Superior
Vena Cava

Pulmonary
Arteries

Portal

Superior
Mesenteric

Inferior
Vena Cava

External Iliac

Deep Femoral

Great Saphenous

Subclavian

Axillary

Inferior
Mesenteric

Femoral

The concepts and management of coronary artery disease have also advanced. For example, *angina pectoris*, which is chest pain of cardiac origin, results from an inadequate supply of oxygen to the myocardium, usually because of an obstruction in a coronary vessel. Angina may also arise from coronary artery spasm, which reduces bloodflow in the absence of any organic obstruction in the coronary vessels. This new understanding of the causes of anginal pain has assisted in the management of chest pain.

Cardiovascular drug therapy has also changed dramatically. For example, drugs that were not available before can now control and treat atherosclerosis, hypertension, congestive heart failure, and arrhythmias.

The number and variety of techniques available for use in the diagnosis of circulatory system disorders has increased tremendously in recent years. This section will discuss several of the more common noninvasive and invasive techniques physicians use to detect heart disease.

Noninvasive Techniques

Noninvasive diagnostic techniques carry less risk of harm to the patient and are more likely to be used than invasive diagnostic techniques. We will discuss the noninvasive diagnostic techniques of electrocardiography, exercise testing, chest x-ray studies, and echocardiography.

Electrocardiography

An *electrocardiograph* is an instrument that records the electrical current generated by the heart muscle, and an *electrocardiogram* is the recording produced by this instrument. With each heartbeat, electrical currents spread throughout the entire body. Electrodes placed on the patient's arms, legs, and chest record these currents on the body surface, which then are displayed in a 12 lead format, each lead reflecting a different electrical circuit in the recording device or anatomic position.

The electrocardiograph is the single most important tool in the investigation of heart disease. It can detect *hypertrophy*, which is an enlargement of any tissue, in this case of the heart muscle; myocardial infarction, which is commonly called a heart attack; *arrhythmia*, which is any alteration in the pattern or rate of normal cardiac sinus rhythm; and *pericarditis*, which is an inflammation of the pericardium.

Exercise Test

Certain abnormalities, especially those created by *cardiac isch-*
emia, which is a reduced bloodflow to the heart, can show up on an
electrocardiogram. Even if a cardiac abnormality is not detectable
when the patient is at rest, the abnormality may appear during the
stress of exercise. An exercise test, which is also called a stress test,
involves the taking of an electrocardiogram during strenuous exercise and the following recovery period.

One popular exercise test utilizes a treadmill. This procedure uses
progressively increasing exercise levels that are individualized for
different types of patients. The treadmill test is able to identify many
individuals who have coronary artery disease, because about 75
percent of patients who have coronary artery disease produce
abnormal test results. The test is most sensitive in patients who have
multivessel disease. The electrocardiographic exercise test is
approximately 70 to 75 percent sensitive for detecting the presence
of coronary artery disease and 70 to 75 percent specific that an
abnormal reading truly indicates the presence of this disease. The
exercise test is notoriously insensitive and nonspecific in women,
patients who hyperventilate, and patients who have mitral valve
prolapse.

An exercise ECG is performed using a protocol that reflects
different levels of activity that are required of the patient. The most
popular protocol for exercise testing is the Bruce protocol, which is
presented in Figure 7–7. Protocols typically provide exercise levels in
metabolic equivalents, which are called METs. At rest, the human
body requires approximately 3.5 milliliters of oxygen per kilogram of
the person's weight. Exercise physiologists call this minimal level of
oxygen consumption one MET. From exercise testing, the physician
can determine the patient's safe capacity for physical activity.

METs can be translated into specific types of physical activities.
Figure 7–8 outlines some physical efforts and their metabolic equivalents.

The exercise ECG test can also monitor the progression of disease; the patient's response to therapeutic interventions, such as
drug therapy, coronary artery bypass surgery, and angioplasty; and
the patient's prognosis. Finally, the exercise test can assess the
physical capacity of patients who have valvular and other forms of
heart disease.

Echocardiograms, which will be described below, are often used
in conjunction with exercise tests. Furthermore, radionuclide studies, which will be described in detail later in this chapter, are often

Figure 7–7.
The Bruce Protocol for Exercise Testing.

Stage	Speed (mph)	Grade (%)	Duration (min.)	METs (units)
0[a]	1.7	—	—	—
1/2[a]	1.7	5	—	—
1[b]	1.7	10	—	4
2	2.5	12	3	6–7
3	3.4	14	3	8–9
4	4.2	16	3	15–16
5	5.0	18	3	21
6	5.5	20	3	—
7	6.0	22	3	—

[a]Stages in the "modified" Bruce protocol.
[b]The starting point of the full Bruce protocol.

performed either in conjunction with or instead of exercise tests. Pharmacological radionuclide stress tests pose less danger than the traditional exercise stress tests do to those patients for whom exercise is risky.

In general, patients' maximal heart rates, or pulse rates, are predictable, within certain age ranges. The most common method for determining a patient's maximal heart rate is to subtract the patient's age from 220.

Chest X-Ray

A chest x-ray can confirm the clinical suspicion of an enlarged heart or of congestive heart failure. Congestive heart failure is manifested by evidence of pulmonary vascular congestion and/or pleural effusion. The physician can measure the size of a patient's heart by studying the posterior-anterior (PA) x-ray film of the patient's chest. The cardio-thoracic (CT) ratio is the transverse, or crosswise, diameter of the heart divided by the internal diameter of the thorax at its widest point above the diaphragm. The physician measures the patient's heart directly from the film. Normally, the CT ratio should be less than .50. A value larger than .50 suggests heart enlargement.

Many insurance company medical directors use the Ungerleider-Clark table to determine the degree of heart enlargement from an x-ray of the chest. This table gives predicted values, based on the

Figure 7–8.
Metabolic Equivalents for Specific Physical Efforts.

Number of METs	Physical Efforts
1$^{1}/_{2}$ to 2	working at a desk, driving a car, typing, standing, walking (1 mph), playing cards, sewing, knitting
2 to 3	repairing a car, radio, or television; bartending; performing maintenance work; level walking (2 mph); level bicycling (5 mph); using a riding lawnmower; playing billiards, shuffle-board, or golf (with an electric cart); bowling; canoeing (2$^{1}/_{2}$ mph); driving a power boat; playing piano and many other musical instruments; horseback riding (walking)
3 to 4	brick laying, cleaning windows, steering a wheelbarrow with a 100 lb. load, walking (3 mph), cycling (6 mph), golfing (pulling a wheeled bag cart), handling a small sailboat, pushing a light power mower, horseback riding (trotting without "posting"), fly fishing (standing wearing waders), playing badminton (social doubles)
4 to 5	painting; hanging wallpaper; performing light carpentry; walking (3$^{1}/_{2}$ mph); cycling (8 mph); playing table tennis, golf (carrying clubs), badminton (singles), tennis (doubles); raking leaves; hoeing; performing many types of calisthenics
5 to 6	digging in garden, shoveling light earth, walking (4 mph), cycling (10 mph), canoeing (4 mph), horseback riding (trotting while "posting"), stream fishing (walking in light current), ice or roller skating (9 mph)
6 to 7	shoveling for 10 min. (10 lbs.), shoveling snow, hand lawn-mowing, splitting wood, walking (5 mph), cycling (11 mph), playing badminton (competitive), or tennis (singles), folk (square) dancing, light downhill skiing, water skiing
7 to 8	digging ditches, carrying 80 lbs., sawing hardwood, jogging (5 mph), cycling (12 mph), horseback riding (galloping), mountain climbing, vigorous downhill skiing, canoeing (5 mph), playing basketball, ice hockey, touch football, paddle-ball
8 to 9	shoveling for 10 min. (14 lbs.), running (5$^{1}/_{2}$ mph), ski touring (4+ mph in loose snow), playing handball or squash, cycling (13 mph), fencing
10 or more	shoveling for 10 min. (16 lbs.), playing competitive handball or squash, ski touring (5+ mph in loose snow), running (6+ mph)

Adapted with permission from Samuel M. Fox III, MD, et al., "Physical Activity and Cardiovascular Health—III. The Exercise Prescription: Frequency and Type of Activity," *Modern Concepts of Cardiovascular Disease*, XLI (1972): 25–30.

patient's weight and height, for the transverse diameter of the heart. Using the actual measurement of the transverse diameter obtained from the PA film, the degree of cardiac enlargement can be read directly from the table.

Both the CT ratio and Ungerleider-Clark values provide only rough estimates of heart size. On deep inspiration, the diaphragm descends and the heart assumes a more vertical position within the thorax. If the individual does not take a deep breath at the moment the chest x-ray is taken, the heart will lie in a more transverse position. Measurements taken when the heart is lying transversely are greater than when the heart is vertical. Thus, transversely positioned hearts may create an impression of heart enlargement that does not exist. Although a large amount of data available to an insurance company derives from x-ray studies, in modern clinical practice, the echocardiogram, which provides specific measurement of heart chamber size and heart chamber wall thickness, has become the "gold standard" method for evaluating the size of a patient's heart.

Echocardiography

Echocardiography has become a tool second only to electrocardio-graphy in frequency of use and as a source of information about a patient's heart. An *echocardiograph* consists of an ultrasound machine that directs high-frequency sound waves into the patient's body and a mechanism that records the sound waves as they reflect off the patient's heart walls, chambers, valves, and red blood cells. Viewing the patient's heart during echocardiography is done in "real time" on an oscilloscope, and the image is also recorded for further viewing and study. The recorded image is called an *echocardi-ogram*.

Currently, medical personnel can study sound waves for the Doppler effect created by reflections from the moving red blood cells in order to determine myocardial mechanical function. To further enhance the data from Doppler studies, computers color-code the Doppler shifts and produce colorful images of the patient's beating heart for "real-time" imaging and recording.

The enormous value of echocardiography is self-evident. In some instances, this technique has eliminated the need for cardiac cathe-terization prior to valve surgery. Most physicians now use electrocar-diography to measure heart size and wall thickness secondary to hypertension and to analyze segmental wall abnormalities secondary to ischemia or infarction. Echocardiography is the definitive tool for identifying pericardial effusion, prosthetic valve dysfunction, cardiac tumors, and valve abnormalities.

Physicians also use the echocardiograph in conjunction with the electrocardiograph exercise test. In this application, the physician performs the echocardiograph immediately before and after the patient's exercise test, looking for segmental wall changes that result from exercise-induced ischemia. These segmental wall changes consist of varying degrees of poor to absent contractions of segments of the heart wall during systole.

Invasive Techniques

This section will discuss the invasive techniques of cardiac catheterization, technetium imaging, thallium imaging, and ventriculography.

Cardiac Catheterization

Cardiac catheterization, as defined in Chapter 3, *Specialized Diagnostic Techniques*, is the insertion of a catheter into a patient's heart in order to obtain precise functional and anatomic information about the heart. This information can be used to make a diagnosis of the patient's condition and to perform certain types of therapy. Cardiac catheters are useful in determining blood pressures within the heart and can measure those pressures in the atria, ventricles, and pulmonary and peripheral arteries. Because resistance to bloodflow is several times greater in the systemic arteries than in the pulmonary arteries, the pressure of the blood within the heart is significantly higher in the left side of the heart than in the right.

A cardiac catheter can also be useful in determining the level of oxygen in the patient's blood in various blood vessels. Measuring blood oxygen content is important, because total cardiac output (CO) in liters per minute may be found from the oxygen content of the blood in the pulmonary artery and in the left systemic circulation. The CO is expressed as the cardiac index (CI) when it is standardized to body surface area. The CI data measures the heart's ability to pump adequate amounts of blood to the peripheral tissues.

Furthermore, cardiac catheterization can be used to perform corrective surgery. One specific type of corrective surgery that involves cardiac catheterization is a percutaneous transluminal coronary angioplasty. ***Percutaneous transluminal coronary angioplasty (PTCA)*** is a procedure that is used to dilate partially occluded coronary arteries by introducing a balloon-tipped catheter into the large artery in the patient's thigh and advancing the catheter into the patient's aorta and then into the narrowed coronary artery. An elongated balloon at the tip of the catheter is inflated, pressing the atherosclerotic plaque in the coronary artery against the arterial wall. The widening of the vessel channel allows for an increase in the patient's bloodflow. The procedure is successful if the vessel is less constricted than before the procedure, if a follow-up to a prior abnormal stress ECG is normal, or if the patient experiences relief from angina pectoris.

The PTCA procedure has the potential for technical problems. For example, a catheter will not enter a blood vessel if the vessel is too narrowed, or the vessel may be injured by the balloon's inflation. The PTCA procedure is most useful for treating lesions located in the initial segment of the patient's coronary arteries at or near their origin from the aorta, because lesions in this location are most accessible.

In addition, the PTCA procedure has its dangers. For instance, PTCA carries a risk of unintentionally dislodging blood clots and of causing arterial wall damage at the site of plaque compression, leading to rupture of the vessel. The PTCA is performed on a patient who is under local anesthesia, but a surgical team is on standby, ready to perform coronary artery bypass surgery if complications arise.

Technetium Imaging

Technetium myocardial imaging uses radioactive technetium to locate abnormal coronary bloodflow or damaged heart tissue. The imaging follows an intravenous injection of technetium into the patient. Because technetium will concentrate in dead myocardial tissue, a person who has had a myocardial infarction will have an increased accumulation of radioactivity, called a "hot spot," in the area of myocardial injury. Images are most likely to be abnormal for two to ten days following the infarct.

Technetium imaging is most useful when other indicators of infarction, such as an abnormal electrocardiogram and elevated enzyme levels, are not diagnostic or are difficult to evaluate. Most cases of acute myocardial infarction are not difficult to diagnose, but in some instances, ECG changes and enzyme studies provide confusing results. In these cases, the demonstration of a hot spot offers evidence of a recent infarct. The technetium method also assists in diagnosing a recurrent infarction in patients who show preexisting evidence of an old infarction. In addition, for patients such as alcoholics, who show enzyme elevations for reasons other than acute infarction, a technetium scan may clarify the problem. Technetium scans can also clarify various forms of myocarditis.

Thallium Imaging

Thallium myocardial imaging, which is also called a *perfusion test*, utilizes radioactive thallium to locate ischemic heart tissue. The thallium concentrates in normal myocardial cells that receive an adequate blood supply. After a thallium injection, an area of myocardium that has an impaired blood supply appears as a "cold spot" on a radionuclide image. The cold spot is a region of diminished activity or lack of activity that indicates that the cold spot area did not receive or extract the radionuclide in the same way that the surrounding myocardial tissue that had a good blood supply to normal myocardial cells did.

The majority of stress tests do not require supplementation with radionuclide imaging. However, if a stress electrocardiogram fails to clarify a diagnostic problem, as might occur if the patient has a preexisting ECG abnormality, or if a patient's treadmill test results are suspicious, thallium stress radionuclide imaging often is helpful in identifying those areas of the myocardium that receive an adequate blood supply at rest but do not receive a sufficient blood supply during exercise. In order to test for exercise- or stress-induced myocardial oxygen insufficiency, the patient may undergo two imaging procedures, one immediately after treadmill exercise and one at rest, typically four hours later. Cold spots that develop as a result of exercise, but fill in after rest, indicate that myocardial ischemia is stress-induced.

Single photon emission computerized tomography (SPECT) is a diagnostic technique that is similar to radionuclide imaging but that utilizes different radioactive materials. The SPECT technique provides more detail to abnormalities of bloodflow than the standard thallium scanning technique does.

Ventriculography

Right and left ventriculography, the x-ray visualization of the heart ventricles, was first discussed in Chapter 3, *Specialized Diagnostic Techniques*. An analysis of the left ventricular cavity silhouette on a ventriculogram may show areas of absent contraction, called ***akinesia***; reduced contraction, called ***hypokinesia***; outward expansion during systole, called ***dyskinesia***; or ventricular aneurysm. An ***aneurysm*** is an expansive sac or dilation that forms from a weakened section in the wall of an artery, a vein, or the heart. A patient who has a normal heart will exhibit a relatively symmetrical contraction during a ventriculographic study.

Ventriculography can also measure a patient's stroke volume. Stroke volume, as defined in Chapter 2, is the volume of blood each contraction of the left ventricle pumps into the aorta. The *ejection fraction* is the ratio of stroke volume to the volume of the left ventricle at the end of diastole. A reduced ejection fraction often indicates the presence of a poorly contracting left ventricle. A patient's ejection fraction can also be measured by radionuclide imaging and echocardiography.

DISORDERS OF THE CIRCULATORY SYSTEM

Many syndromes that affect the circulatory system were once virtually unknown, but now are commonly diagnosed. Correspondingly, in the last 20 years, the death rate from total major cardiovascular disease has declined more than 25 percent. Circulatory system disorders, however, still constitute the leading cause of death in both the United States and Canada. Some of these disorders are relatively rare, but those that involve the coronary and cerebral arteries are, unfortunately, fairly common. Hypertension and arteriosclerosis and its consequences, which include coronary artery disease, ischemic heart disease, and strokes, account for most of the deaths.

Arterial Hypertension

A certain level of blood pressure is necessary to move blood through the circulatory system, but an individual's blood pressure is high if it exceeds a normal range. Because transient elevations occur in many people, the diagnosis of *hypertension*, which is also known as *high blood pressure*, is reserved for persistently elevated blood pressure levels as determined on at least three separate occasions.

Although all physicians consider a blood pressure reading of 120/80 to be normal and 220/120 to be elevated, no universal agreement as to the dividing line between normal blood pressure and hypertension exists. Complicating the problem is the fact that an individual's blood pressure is not constant and varies normally with exercise, excitement, and anxiety. Most authorities consider sustained blood pressures above 140 systolic and 90 diastolic to be hypertensive in individuals younger than 50. Some physicians adopt slightly lower levels as the dividing line in much younger persons and slightly higher persistent levels in individuals over the age of 50.

However, some people maintain a relatively unchanged blood pressure as they grow older, so a rise in blood pressure is not an invariable accompaniment of advancing age. Moreover, although hypertension is more common in females than in males, hypertensive heart disease is reported more frequently in males than in females.

Essential Hypertension

In 95 percent of hypertension patients, the cause of high blood pressure is unknown. Hypertension of unknown cause is called *essential hypertension*, or *primary hypertension*. In the United States, about 60 million people have essential hypertension. Heredity predisposes a person to the development of high blood pressure, but the specific genetic factors are unknown and probably multiple. A family history of premature deaths from hypertension, heart attack, or cerebrovascular disease is an especially unfavorable risk factor.

Essential hypertension produces no specific symptoms and is called the "silent killer" because it rarely produces warning manifestations of its presence, even in the presence of marked blood pressure elevation. The higher the patient's blood pressure, however, the greater the likelihood that the patient will develop early cerebral, cardiac, renal, and peripheral vascular signs. These manifestations reflect the effects of high blood pressure upon the arterioles in the brain, heart, kidney, and other organs.

Long-standing hypertension of a moderate or marked degree frequently will lead to *hypertensive heart disease*, a condition of heart hypertrophy that is secondary to systemic hypertension. Recent studies have shown that this same correlation is also present for isolated systolic hypertension. Changes in the patient's chest x-ray or echocardiogram, or electrocardiographic patterns of hypertrophy or "strain" may indicate cardiac enlargement. If hypertensive heart disease develops, additional symptoms, including labored breathing, weakness, and fatigue, which are the hallmarks of congestive heart failure (CHF), may be present.

Some specific clinical forms of hypertension include

- *accelerated hypertension*—markedly and increasingly elevated blood pressure accompanied by vascular changes in the retina
- *malignant hypertension*—a markedly elevated diastolic blood pressure accompanied by swelling of the optic nerve
- *hypertensive encephalopathy*—headache, confusion, and coma resulting from accelerated or malignant hypertensive effects upon the brain

- *hypertensive crisis*—severe hypertension that may go on to hypertensive encephalopathy
- *complicated hypertension*—the presence of hypertension and one of its common complications, such as stroke, congestive heart failure, myocardial infarction, and renal failure

The prognosis of essential hypertension varies with the level of the patient's blood pressure. Higher pressures have a poorer prognosis than do lower ones. A better correlation exists between blood pressure and mortality if the patient's blood pressure is measured while the patient is subjected to the usual variety of mild daily stresses than if the patient is resting. Ambulatory blood pressure readings may be the best markers for possible hypertension complications and may provide the definitive measurement of persistent hypertension. Even trivial hypertension appears to increase the risk of cerebral vascular accident.

People who have unrecognized and untreated essential hypertension may die from congestive heart failure, myocardial infarction, cerebral hemorrhage, or uremia. *Uremia* is a toxic condition characterized by the retention in the blood of excessive amounts of metabolic by-products. It can result from renal involvement in the hypertensive process. Ophthalmologic findings of retinal hemorrhage, exudates, and swelling of the optic nerve are other unfavorable prognostic signs.

The objective of high blood pressure treatment is to reduce the patient's blood pressure levels, which in turn will reduce the rate of progression of organ deterioration from the effects of hypertension. The beneficial effects of the antihypertensive drugs are impressive. The effectiveness of early drug therapy directed towards moderate and severe hypertension is well-established. Furthermore, recent evidence suggests that early therapy directed toward the milder forms of the disease will extend the patient's life expectancy, even for elderly patients.

Secondary Hypertension

Secondary hypertension results from a known cause, which can often be treated successfully. For this reason, secondary hypertension is sometimes referred to as "curable hypertension." Secondary hypertension occurs in less than five percent of all hypertension patients. Because secondary hypertension occurs infrequently, expensive diagnostic testing is limited to certain situations, for example, hypertension occurring in patients under age 30, suddenly appearing in the elderly, or worsening in any age group.

Coarctation of the Aorta. Coarctation of the aorta is a congenital narrowing of the aorta just beyond the point at which the arteries that supply the upper extremities leave the aorta. Coarctation of the aorta is characterized by elevated blood pressure in the patient's arms and low or normal blood pressure in the patient's legs. The treatment is the surgical removal of the narrowed section of the aorta and a rejoining of the remaining ends. The patient's prognosis is best if the coarctation is corrected during the patient's childhood. Balloon dilation of the aorta is an alternative therapy. Nonetheless, all coarctation patients require monitoring for late long-term complications of coarctation recurrence and/or hypertension. Coarctation of the aorta is also discussed later in this chapter in the section entitled "Congenital Heart Disease."

Pheochromocytoma. **Pheochromocytoma** is a rare tumor that secretes adrenalin and usually grows in the adrenal medulla, but occasionally arises in other locations. The tumor can occur at any age, but the incidence is highest in young adults. The associated hypertension results from tumor cells' production of an excessive amount of a hypertensive substance known as a catecholamine. Often the hypertension caused by a pheochromocytoma appears suddenly and transiently and occurs in association with headaches, excessive sweating, a flushed appearance, palpitations[1], and a drop in blood pressure upon standing. Approximately half of all pheochromocytoma patients experience these symptoms, and the other half experience manifestations of fixed, or persistent, hypertension. Surgical removal of the tumor will cure the secondary hypertension.

Aldosteronism. **Primary aldosteronism** is a condition that is caused by agents within the adrenal gland. It is characterized by increased secretion of aldosterone. The classical symptoms of primary aldosteronism are attributable to a low blood level of potassium: muscle weakness; frequent urination, especially at night; excessive thirst; muscular spasm; and headache. Aldosteronism is discussed more fully in Chapter 12, *The Endocrine System.*

Renovascular Hypertension. Renovascular hypertension is the most common form of secondary hypertension. In one-third of renovascular hypertension patients, and predominantly in young females, the disorder is caused by fibromuscular disease of the renal arteries. In two-thirds of the patients, particularly older patients who have high systolic blood pressure, renovascular hypertension results from atherosclerotic disease of the renal arteries. A narrowing of either small or large renal arteries results from one of these two causes, producing an ischemia which in turn leads to renal secretion of renin. The resulting cascade of the renin-angiotension-aldosterone

---

[1]Palpitations are subjective sensations of unduly rapid or irregular heart beats.

system causes elevated blood pressure. Typically, treatment of renovascular hypertension involves angioplasty, surgical revascularization of the stenotic lesion, or both.

Other Endocrine Causes. Secondary, and usually correctable, hypertension can also occur with Cushing's syndrome and congenital adrenal hyperplasia. These conditions are discussed in greater detail in Chapter 12.

Congenital Heart Disease

One baby in every 100 live births has a congenital heart problem, the single most common congenital anomaly in newborns. Approximately 25 percent of these babies born with heart problems will die in their first year. The cause of these congenital heart problems is thought to lie in a combination of genetic and environmental factors, rubella infections, or teratogenic drugs. *Teratogenic drugs* are drugs that a pregnant woman ingests that produce physical defects in her fetus before its birth. Congenital heart abnormalities usually involve absent vascular channels to and from the heart, defects in the walls of the atria and ventricles, obstructions to valves or vessels, and abnormal connections between the chambers of the heart, and/or their entering and exiting vascular connections. These abnormalities result in a complex series of combinations of almost infinite number. Fortunately, the simplest abnormalities represent two-thirds of all congenital heart defects at birth. These abnormalities include

- ventricular septal defects
- patent ductus arteriosus
- pulmonary stenosis
- atrial septal defects
- coarctation of the aorta
- aortic stenosis
- tetralogy of Fallot

These malformations are clinically characterized as being (1) shunt lesions if they cause the patient's blood to be abnormally diverted from the left side to the right side of heart, or vice versa, (2) obstructive lesions with or without shunts, or (3) obstructive and regurgitant lesions if blood is impeded in its forward flow or is abnormally driven backward.

The treatment of these lesions begins with identifying them from (1) the appearance of symptoms, such as failure to thrive and grow, bluish discoloration of skin from the shunting of deoxygenated blood from the venous circulation directly into the systemic circulation, recurrent pulmonary infections, labored breathing, collapse, and (2) indications appearing during physical examination and upon special studies, such as electrocardiogram, echocardiogram, cardiac catheterization, and angiography.

Congenital heart abnormalities are now recognized earlier in a patient's life, so that most of these lesions can be corrected while the patient is still an infant. Occasionally patients develop complications from the surgical correction of a congenital abnormality decades after the original surgery. Echocardiography has played a significant role in the earlier diagnosis of these lesions—sometimes while the fetus is still in the womb—and in many cases has eliminated the need for later cardiac catheterization. Many congenital heart defects are mild and are compatible with long-term survival, never needing surgical correction and requiring only antibiotic preventive therapy.

Ventricular Septal Defects

The most common congenital defect, a *ventricular septal defect (VSD)*, is an abnormality that affects the septum that separates the right and left ventricles. A VSD is often small and closes without intervention by the age of three in more than 30 percent of all patients who have congenital heart abnormalities. Larger VSDs do require surgery to prevent the development of pulmonary hypertension secondary to abnormal shunting of large volumes of blood from the left side of the heart to the right side.

Patent Ductus Arteriosus

Patent ductus arteriosus is a shunt of blood from the aorta to the pulmonary artery through an arterial connection that is normal before birth but abnormal after birth. The shunt, or ductus, usually arises opposite the left subclavian artery and inserts into the pulmonary artery at the point at which it branches into right and left pulmonary arteries. Signs and symptoms of patients who have this disorder will vary with the volume of shunted blood. This lesion was the first congenital heart disease abnormality to be surgically corrected. Surgery on these lesions is performed on all patients who are children. Small lesions in adults may be left uncorrected, because of the attendant surgical risk.

Pulmonary Stenosis

Stenosis is an obstruction to or narrowing of a blood vessel or other hollow channel in the body. *Pulmonary stenosis* is the narrowing of the opening between the pulmonary artery and the right ventricle. Pulmonary stenosis may be mild, moderate, or severe in degree, as defined by the actual pressure gradient across the valve. Mild cases require only observation and antibiotic treatment to prevent infection. Moderate and severe cases are usually treated by balloon catheter dilation. Only very deformed valves require surgery.

Atrial Septal Defects

An *atrial septal defect (ASD)* is an opening in the atrial septum allowing an abnormal shunt between the two atria. These defects vary in their location and size, the latter factor determining the volume of the shunt. All ASD lesions in children are surgically corrected, preferably when the child is age three or four. Surgery is still the suggested treatment for ASD, even for patients in their 60s, provided that severe pulmonary hypertension has not developed. Atrial septal defects in patients over the age of 40 frequently present with congestive heart failure and atrial arrhythmias, developments that do not preclude surgical repair.

Coarctation of the Aorta

Coarctation of the aorta, as discussed earlier in this chapter, is a congenital narrowing of the aorta. It occurs more commonly in males than in females, and approximately 25 percent of these defects have associated congenital cardiac abnormalities, usually of the aortic valve. The narrowing of the aorta causes hypertension above the defect and all its attendant problems. The coarctation also results in blood deficiency problems, including diminished pulses and blood pressure and coolness and intermittent claudication in the legs. *Intermittent claudication* is a condition characterized by pain in a limb when it is exercised and relief from pain when the limb is at rest.

Clinical symptoms and signs suggest the diagnosis of coarctation. Echocardiography can confirm the diagnosis, and treatment can be effected by angioplasty or surgery. Despite relief of the congenital defect, however, coarctation patients require prolonged follow-up, because many of them develop recurrent stenosis or hypertension in adult life.

Aortic Stenosis

Aortic stenosis is an obstructive lesion of the aorta that is usually secondary to an abnormal valve. It presents in childhood or in later life as the valve undergoes progressive degeneration, fibrosis, and calcification. Once diagnosed, aortic stenosis may be treated by angioplasty, or more commonly, by surgical removal of the valve and the insertion of a prosthetic one. The latter requires life-long anticoagulation therapy to prevent the formation on the valve of blood clots that can dislodge and move into the peripheral circulation. After correction of the defect, the patient will be able to function normally. Life-long antibiotic treatment to prevent bacterial endocarditis is necessary for all aortic stenosis patients, before and after valve replacement.

Tetralogy of Fallot

Tetralogy of Fallot consists of a combination of four defects: (1) pulmonary stenosis, (2) ventricular septal defect, (3) an overriding aorta that is positioned over both right and left ventricle outlets, and (4) right ventricular hypertrophy. First described by Fallot in 1888, this condition is the most common congenital heart lesion that causes bluish discoloration, called cyanosis. In patients over the age of two, three out of four cyanotic congenital heart cases arise from this lesion. This condition usually is surgically corrected during the patient's infancy, but in severely oxygen-deficient infants, a temporary shunt of blood from the left to the right circulation first is created and then later the definitive correction is performed.

Many other congenital lesions exist, and nearly all are amenable to surgical correction in varying degrees. Surgical correction, however, does not always restore the heart to physiologic normality. Abnormalities may show up in the patient's later years in the form of circulatory limitations. Furthermore, most patients who have congenital heart lesions require life-long antibiotic treatment to prevent infection of residual abnormalities.

Arteriosclerosis and Atherosclerosis

Arteriosclerosis is the thickening, with loss of elasticity, of small, medium and large arteries. Although arteriosclerosis accounts for some clinical illness, far more common is *atherosclerosis*, a disease of lipid, or fat, in the medium and large muscular and elastic arteries. Atherosclerosis accounts for myocardial and cerebral infarctions, which are major causes of death in our society. This condition affects males far more often than females.

The etiology of atherosclerosis remains unclear, but studies have identified major risk contributors to its development. These risk factors include

- cigarette smoking
- elevated cholesterol and triglyceride levels
- hypertension
- physical inactivity
- diabetes mellitus
- obesity
- emotional stress
- genetic predisposition

Hyperlipoproteinemia is the abnormal elevation of certain normal physiologic lipid elements in the body. *Lipids* are fats and fat-like substances that serve as fuel sources and important components of cell structure. Cholesterol is an essential factor in cell wall integrity and endocrine hormone synthesis. The presence of cholesterol in the blood reflects both its synthesis in the liver and its absorption from food. The other major lipid, *triglyceride*, is a major metabolic component in the energy cycle of all cells and is stored as adipose, or fatty, tissue. The presence of triglyceride in the blood reflects that it was absorbed from food in the intestines. Both cholesterol and triglyceride are transported in the body as components of lipoproteins because neither is soluble in plasma alone. Lipoproteins are compounds of proteins, phospholipids, cholesterol, and triglyceride. Absorbed cholesterol and triglyceride are carried from the intestines as chylomicrons to the liver and the peripheral tissues. Chylomicrons are substances that are found in the intestinal lymph vessels and blood during and after meals and that contain triglyceride, cholesterol, other lipids, and protein. Chylomicrons are converted to very low density lipoprotein (VLDL) and in turn to low density lipoprotein (LDL), a form particularly rich in cholesterol. High density lipoprotein (HDL) has a fairly specific carrier role in this complex carrier system, shuttling back and forth between liver and peripheral tissues carrying triglyceride and cholesterol.

Studies have shown that cholesterol has a quantifiable risk relationship to atherosclerosis, and the United States National Cholesterol Education Program, an offshoot of the National Heart, Lung and Blood Institute, has established these parameters:

	Total Cholesterol	**LDL Cholesterol**
Desirable	<200 mg/dl*	<130 mg/dl*
Borderline risk	200–239 mg/dl*	130–159 mg/dl*
High risk	>240 mg/dl*	>160 mg/dl*

---

*milligrams per deciliter

Thus, a healthy individual has a total cholesterol level below 200 mg/dl, and a high percentage of that total level should consist of HDL. Sometimes HDL is called "good cholesterol." Triglycerides remain a somewhat uncertain risk factor for atherosclerosis, although markedly elevated values do seem to carry some such risk.

The presence of elevated lipids and the risk of associated vascular disease warrants specific therapeutic response. One response is a diet that restricts cholesterol and saturated fat intake and that allows the patient to obtain and maintain proper body weight. If these measures fail, then drug therapy is commenced. Drug therapy is progressively directed at inhibiting lipid absorption from the intestines and inhibiting cholesterol synthesis in the liver with enzyme-blocking drugs.

The pathologic consequence of failure to control lipid abnormalities is an atherosclerotic lesion. The lesion first appears as a "fatty streak" which is a cholesterol infiltration of the artery wall. The fatty streak lesion is very common, appearing in even young children. The lesion progresses by developing "fibrous plaque," which arises from an irregular proliferation of smooth muscle cells, other types of cells, and cholesterol, all of which may progress to fibrosis and calcification. Fibrous plaque may also develop independently of fatty streaks.

If the surface of the fibrous plaque, which intrudes into the artery, degenerates with ulceration, cracks, or fissures, then a "complicated lesion" has developed. The complicated lesion is in open contact with the blood stream, and, by virtue of its composition, predisposes the patient to platelet adherence, aggregation, and thrombosis. Thrombosis in an already narrowed vessel creates partial or total obstruction to bloodflow. Partial obstruction limits bloodflow to distal tissue and may result in transient changes. It manifests as angina or intermittent claudication. Total obstruction results in death of the distal tissue, and it manifests as myocardial or cerebral infarction.

Associated Disorders of the Coronary Arteries

Atherosclerosis is the major disease of the coronary arteries that feed the heart muscle, but other conditions may compromise the circulation through these arteries.

Angina Pectoris

Partial obstruction of a coronary artery may lead to angina. Each episode of angina typically lasts less than 15 minutes and is secondary to inadequate blood supply. Angina usually appears after physical exertion, a large meal, or emotional excitement. Angina typically begins suddenly and is felt as a tightness or constriction in the center of the patient's chest. The discomfort may radiate to the patient's neck or jaw or to the left shoulder and arm. Angina is often associated with labored breathing and sometimes with a chilling perspiration. It is promptly relieved by physical rest or nitroglycerine administration. The patient's medical history is a highly sensitive and specific marker for angina in a high-risk candidate. The diagnosis of angina is confirmed by electrocardiograph or exercise test. The exercise test may include isotope or echocardiographic studies that confirm either impaired bloodflow or segmental wall abnormalities. Cardiac catheterization may show no disease or may show varying degrees of stenosis. If cardiac catheterization indicates an absence of disease, the physician may make a diagnosis of nonatherosclerotic causes of chest pain, such as coronary vasospasm, which is also called Prinzmetal angina or "Syndrome X," which is angina that occurs in "normal" coronary arteries. Of all patients sent to cardiac catheterization for evaluation of chest pain, more than 30 percent are found to have normal coronary arteries. Obstruction is considered to be minimal if it blocks less than 30 percent of the channel's cross-section area, moderate if the channel is 30 to 50 percent obstructed, and severe or critical if the obstruction is greater than 50 percent.

Angina is classified as stable or unstable, based on the patient's clinical history, and therapy will vary accordingly. Patients who have unstable angina are usually hospitalized for intensive observation and care, including anticoagulation treatment. Drug therapy is used in all patients initially, and, depending upon clinical circumstances, may be the only mode of treatment. For other patients, further testing and observation may indicate that interventional therapies, such as PTCA or coronary artery bypass grafting (CABG), are appropriate. PTCA, as described earlier in this chapter, is catheter balloon dilation of a stenotic lesion. It is less traumatizing than a CABG, requires a shorter hospital stay, and may be repeated if necessary. Its major drawback is that approximately 30 percent of dilated lesions become stenotic again within six months.

Coronary artery bypass grafting, on the other hand, involves an incision into the patient's chest to allow for the insertion of a graft, usually consisting of a segment of a leg vein, from the ascending aorta to a coronary artery. The graft bypasses a stenotic segment in the coronary artery. Surgeons attempt to provide as many bypass grafts as possible, to ensure the optimum revascularization of the myocardium. Figure 7–9 provides illustrations of both the major coronary arteries in a healthy person and a vein bypass graft.

Figure 7–9.
The Major Coronary Arteries and a Vein Bypass Graft.

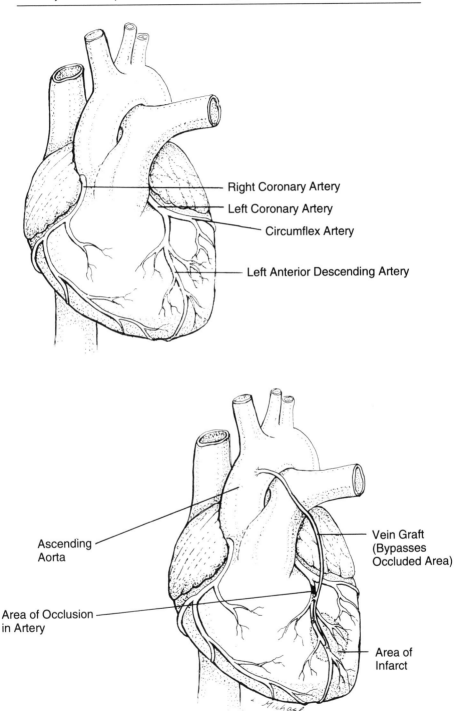

Right Coronary Artery

Left Coronary Artery

Circumflex Artery

Left Anterior Descending Artery

Ascending
Aorta

Vein Graft
(Bypasses
Occluded Area)

Area of Occlusion
in Artery

Area of
Infarct

Sometimes an internal mammary artery is taken from the chest wall and is used as the bypass vessel, particularly for the left anterior descending artery. This bypass vessel is not likely to develop subsequent blockage. Vein grafts develop blockage postoperatively at the rate of ten percent in the first year, and then at two to five percent per year for the next ten years. After ten years, 50 percent of vein grafts will have failed.

Despite these problems, both angioplasty and CABG do relieve angina, thus improving the patient's quality of life. Despite total operative morbidity and mortality for PTCA and CABG of five to ten percent, these procedures prolong life, especially in patients who have

- critical left main coronary artery disease
- three vessel disease and reduced ejection fractions of 30 to 50 percent (normal is 55 to 75 percent)
- multivessel disease, including the proximal left anterior descending artery
- post-heart attack angina

In the United States, well over 300,000 patients per year have a CABG procedure, and another 300,000 have a PTCA. These numbers for PTCA and CABG stand against the background of an estimated 6,000,000 people living in the United States who have angina and who have survived myocardial infarction. About 75 percent of CABG and PTCA patients return to work, as compared to about 50 percent who return to work after a heart transplantation.

Myocardial Infarction

Myocardial infarction, commonly called a *heart attack*, is the death, or necrosis, of myocardium tissue resulting from inadequate blood supply. The amount of tissue at risk is proportional to the involved arteries. Localized ischemia produces segmental wall abnormalities, but a ten percent loss of myocardium may affect ventricular function, as measured in the ejection fraction. A 40 percent loss of myocardium may lead to intractable congestive heart failure and death. Acute thrombosis superimposed upon atherosclerotic plaque is the final precipitating event leading to complete or near complete blockage of the coronary artery, and thus to myocardial infarction.

Acute myocardial infarction (AMI) is characterized by the sudden onset of severe, persistent chest pain, often associated with excess perspiration, pallor, restlessness, and a sense of impending doom. An AMI is usually secondary to coronary artery atherosclerosis. Twenty to thirty percent of all AMIs are "silent" and are only detected on subsequent, unrelated examination. AMIs lead to an estimated 750,000 hospital admissions in the United States per year and over 500,000 deaths per year. In fact, 70 percent of AMI mortality victims die within one hour of the attack. Eight percent of AMI patients are under age 45, and these patients are 40 times more likely to be male than female. Forty percent of heart attacks occur in patients under age 65, and the male-to-female ratio is three to one. Approximately 50 percent of all AMIs occur in patients who are over 65, and the male-female ratio is five to four in this group.

AMIs are divided into "Q wave" (transmural, or literally "across walls") and "non-Q wave" (subendocardial) infarctions. This distinction is based on the presence or absence of a pathologic Q wave in the electrocardiogram and reflects the difference between a total, persistent, thrombotic occlusion, which is a Q wave infarction, and a transient, incomplete thrombotic occlusion, which is a non-Q wave infarction. Prior to the 1960s, in-hospital mortality for AMI patients was 30 percent, but the advent of coronary care units (CCUs) reduced the death rate to 15 percent by providing prompt treatment for lethal arrhythmias. The current use of drug therapy to dissolve the occluding coronary artery blood clot, thereby restoring blood-flow to the endangered myocardium and forestalling AMI, has reduced heart attack mortality even further. Other details of AMI treatment in the CCU are beyond the scope of this book. Relief of pain, support of the heart's rhythm and pumping action, maintenance of blood pressure and oxygenation, and emergency PTCA or CABG are some of the components of modern therapy.

A patient who has experienced a typical uncomplicated AMI, with an absence of shock, congestive heart failure, major arrhythmia, cardiac rupture, or recurring angina and myocardial infarction, is hospitalized for seven to ten days, the first two to three days in the CCU. Prior to discharging the patient, the physician determines a risk stratification for the patient. The physician may administer a modified exercise test on the patient prior to discharge or within four to six weeks after discharge to determine if the patient requires further study and/or intervention. Non-Q wave AMI patients have a better in-hospital survival rate than Q wave AMI patients, but a worse late-term prognosis, and so non-Q wave patients receive more intensive long-term study.

The infarct patient who has been discharged from the hospital will undergo therapy to reduce secondary risks. This therapy often includes control of hypertension, reduction of blood cholesterol levels, elimination of smoking, physical re-conditioning, and lifestyle alterations relative to work and stress. Drug therapy frequently involves (1) antiplatelet drugs, such as aspirin and dipyridamole, and anticoagulants, such as Coumadin, to forestall subsequent coronary artery thrombosis; (2) angiotensin converting enzyme (ACE) inhibitors; (3) beta-blockers to control arrhythmia and angina; and (4) antianginal agents and/or coronary vasodilators, such as nitroglycerin and calcium channel-blockers. If congestive heart failure is present, *diuretics,* which are drugs that promote the excretion of urine, are also prescribed.

Heart Failure and Shock

Heart failure, which is also called congestive heart failure, and shock are imbalances in the normal dynamics of the pumping heart, its cardiac output, and the vascular channels receiving the cardiac output. *Congestive heart failure* is the inability of the heart to pump an adequate supply of blood to the peripheral tissues for their metabolic needs, leading to vascular congestion. It may be further classified as acute or chronic, right or left heart failure, high or low output, or as systolic or diastolic dysfunction. The left ventricle is the most common and most serious site of heart failure. The causes of left ventricle heart failure run the gamut of cardiovascular disease—hypertension, ischemic heart disease, valvular heart disease, cardiomyopathies, inflammatory heart disease, or infiltrative disease. Failure of the left ventricle manifests as a diminished cardiac output, cardiac enlargement, and elevated filling pressures. These manifestations are in turn transmitted to the lungs, causing pulmonary vascular congestion and presenting symptoms of fatigue and weakness, difficulty in breathing in some circumstances, and acute pulmonary edema. These problems may develop acutely or chronically and are recognizable from the patient's medical history, physical examination, and changes, such as cardiac enlargement and pulmonary vascular congestion, in the patient's chest x-ray. An echocardiography or a cardiac catheterization indicating (1) left ventricular enlargement, (2) diminished ejection fraction, (3) elevated filling pressures, and (4) diminished cardiac output also suggests left ventricle failure.

Right heart failure is usually secondary to left heart failure. Other major causes of right heart failure include acute pulmonary embolization, chronic obstructive pulmonary disease, and large left to right intracardiac shunts, either congenital or acquired. These changes may be acute or chronic and result in symptoms of weakness, fatigue, and peripheral edema. They are recognizable from signs of cyanosis, abnormal heart sounds and murmurs, and peripheral congestion, such as systemic venous congestion, hepatomegaly, pleural effusion, ascites, and peripheral edema. Common to patients who have either right or left advanced heart failure are anxiety and *cachexia*, which is a condition of general ill health and malnutrition.

Heart failure may develop from (1) pressure overloads resulting from pulmonary and systemic hypertension or valvular stenosis, (2) volume overloads arising from valvular incompetence or intracardiac shunts, or (3) true failure of myocardial cell function as a result of primary or secondary cardiomyopathy. The heart accommodates to the specific insult by dilating, enlarging, and increasing its rate of contraction. When these reactions no longer suffice, clinical congestive heart failure presents.

One recent development in the understanding of heart failure has been the recognition that both systolic and diastolic actions of the myocardium are metabolically active processes. Systolic dysfunction is the most common mechanism of heart failure, occurring in two-thirds of all cases, and results in increased heart size and diminished ejection fraction. Diastolic dysfunction is most likely to occur in association with normal-sized hearts, normal ejection fractions, and changes in cardiac catheterization, echocardiography, and nuclear studies showing elevated diastolic filling pressures and abnormal diastolic flow patterns within the patient's heart.

The treatment of heart failure requires the recognition of its presence and the determination of its origin. Therapy is designed to (1) improve pump performance; (2) reduce the heart's work load through rest, weight control, and vasodilator drugs; and (3) control salt and water retention, by limiting dietary sodium intake and using diuretics. Frequently, open-heart surgery to correct anatomic abnormalities, such as septal defects and valve abnormalities, or to restore coronary artery circulation is the definitive therapeutic response. Valves may be resculptured or replaced, or angioplasty or CABG may restore coronary artery function. All such interventions carry some risk of morbidity and mortality, but overall, they have contributed to improved care of chronic congestive heart failure patients.

Chronic intractable congestive heart failure remains a major medical problem, estimated to afflict more than three million people in the United States, with a projected 50 percent four-year mortality rate. For these patients, cardiac transplantation has become a significant therapeutic measure.

Shock is a complex failure of the circulatory system involving multiple organs including the brain, heart, lungs, liver, and kidneys. It arises from multiple causes which can broadly be classified as follows:

- hypovolemic—resulting from major blood loss, dehydration, or internal extravascular sequestration

- cardiogenic—resulting from acute myocardial infarction, congestive heart failure, cardiomyopathy, or arrhythmias
- obstructive vascular catastrophes—resulting from acute pulmonary embolism or aortic dissection
- vasomotor dysfunction—resulting from sepsis, hypoxia,[2] anaphylaxis, drugs, toxins, or endocrine abnormalities

Unless counteracted by specific therapy, once the shock process is initiated, it typically progresses rapidly through deteriorating bloodflow stages that end in hypotension, pallor with cool perspiration, impaired thinking, diminished cardiac output, and diminished renal function. Advanced cases of shock require team therapy in a CCU to provide circulatory and organ support and treatment for the initiating injury. The prognosis for shock patients is always guarded.

Cardiac Arrhythmias

Any alteration in the pattern or rate of normal cardiac sinus rhythm (NSR) is an arrhythmia. Arrhythmias may be as simple as **sinus bradycardia**, in which NSR is less than 60 beats per minute, or **sinus tachycardia**, in which NSR is greater than 100 beats per minute. These variations are common and occur in normal hearts under various circumstances, such as during sleep or exercise or if the individual experiences excitement or fever. Sinus arrhythmia is a normal phasic increase and decrease in heart rate related to respiration and is particularly common in young people.

More significant arrhythmias may present as clinical problems. These problems usually manifest as palpitations or as a sense of difficulty in breathing. In severe forms, arrhythmias may compromise the patient's cardiac output and lead to fainting, congestive heart failure, or death.

Arrhythmias are classified by site of origin, mode of mechanism, and timing of heartbeats. The basic mechanisms of arrhythmia involve (1) abnormalities of impulse generation, such as

- sinus bradycardia
- "sick sinus syndrome," in which patterns of sinus bradycardia alternate with abnormal atrial tachycardia
- premature atrial contraction (PAC)
- premature ventricular contraction (PVC)

---

[2]*Sepsis* is a toxic condition resulting from the presence in the blood of chemical products of disease-causing microorganisms; *hypoxia* is a reduction of oxygen below levels necessary for proper tissue functioning despite adequate blood supply to the tissue.

and (2) abnormalities of impulse conduction, such as

- A-V heart block, in which conduction of the electrical impulse arising in the atria and its transmission into the ventricles is abnormal. A-V heart block is graded into three levels: first-degree A-V heart block, second-degree A-V heart block, and third-degree, or complete, A-V heart block.
- supraventricular tachycardia, in which electrical impulses re-enter the atria and ventricles through dual pathways in the A-V node, or through aberrant accessory connecting tissue between the atria and ventricles.
- ventricular tachycardia, in which electrical impulses recycle within the ventricle through a pathway within the ventricle itself.

The rest of this section will describe the more common and clinically significant arrhythmias.

Premature beats occur in the majority of individuals and in practically every older person. They are more common in men than in women and are usually not associated with heart disease. PVCs are far more common than PACs, but are not considered frequent unless they exceed ten per hour. Treatment is not necessary unless the patient is symptomatic. Once treatment becomes necessary, it must be tailored to the individual patient. For example, some patients will need to stop using tobacco, alcohol, or caffeine, and other patients will require treatment for an underlying disease. Still other patients will need to take anti-arrhythmic drugs.

Atrial flutter is a regular supraventricular tachycardia that rarely occurs in normal hearts and is more common in children than is atrial fibrillation (which is discussed below). Atrial flutter may be acute or chronic and represents a re-entrant rhythm alteration in the atria. Because of the rapid ventricular response to the increased frequency of generated atrial electrical impulses, the ventricular rate must be slowed by drug therapy. Conversion of an atrial flutter to NSR is accomplished by drug therapy or by electrical cardioversion. Electrical cardioversion, which is the more common conversion method, involves the application of direct current, low electrical energy across the patient's thorax through two contact paddles that put the entire heart to rest, allowing the patient's natural atrial pacemaker to initiate NSR. Atrial flutter can be converted to NSR in over 90 percent of patients.

Atrial fibrillation is an irregular, chaotic rhythm in the atria with a rapid irregular ventricular response. It is the most common atrial tachyarrhythmia. Atrial fibrillation rarely occurs in normal hearts and is usually secondary to hypertensive cardiovascular disease. The condition may be acute or chronic. An atrium fibrillating appears to be beating like a "bag of worms." Restoration to NSR is difficult to impossible, depending upon the left atrial chamber size. The larger the atrium, the less likely NSR will be reestablished.

Chronic atrial fibrillation doubles overall cardiovascular morbidity and mortality and leads to a five-fold increase in cerebral vascular accidents and a seventeen-fold increase in cerebral vascular accidents in patients who have rheumatic heart disease. Modern therapy for atrial fibrillation includes life-long anticoagulation treatment to prevent strokes. Anticoagulation treatment has been shown to reduce strokes by two-thirds. The restoration of atrial fibrillation to NSR is achieved in the same manner as in atrial flutter—by drug therapy and/or direct current cardioversion—but the success rate is much lower for fibrillation patients than for atrial flutter patients.

Both chronic atrial flutter and chronic atrial fibrillation are detrimental to cardiac output, even in the presence of controlled ventricular rates, because of the absence of synchronized atrial contribution to diastolic ventricular filling. This lack of synchronized atrial contribution has serious implications for a patient who has congestive heart failure.

Atrial-ventricular block is designated as first degree, second degree, or third degree, which is complete heart block, depending upon the degree of impulse delay or block from atrium to ventricle. The effects of the level of heart block will vary from patient to patient, and the therapeutic response depends upon given circumstances. Complete block was the initial medical problem that led to the development of mechanical cardiac pacemakers in the early 1960s.

Pacemakers replace the electrical components of the heart by originating electrical impulses to the atria or the ventricles, or both, in a synchronized fashion. Currently, most pacemakers run on lithium batteries that are designed to last four to fifteen years. The rate of "firing" can vary in response to physiologic demands, such as body movement, respiratory rate, and blood temperature. A pacemaker today can stimulate or pace both atria and ventricles, inhibit or trigger both chambers' electrical responses, and vary the rate of contraction according to the physiologic stimuli.

The criteria for pacemaker insertion have broadened over the years. Currently over 300,000 pacemakers are implanted in patients in the United States each year, and all are implanted without a surgical incision into the patient's chest wall. The surgeon utilizes a transvenous approach to the heart for the wire leads that connect the pacemaker, which is implanted beneath the skin on the patient's chest wall, to the endocardium of the right atrium and right ventricle.

Delay in conduction below the A-V junction in the right and left bundle branches may be sufficient to alter a normal electrocardiogram and produce recognized patterns of right bundle branch block (RBBB) or left bundle branch block (LBBB). LBBB is also susceptible to variations of left anterior hemiblock (LAHB) or left posterior hemiblock (LPHB). These changes may reflect primary abnormalities in the conducting tissues alone, but more commonly, these changes coexist with primary disease, such as hypertrophy, myocardial infarction, or ischemia, in the heart muscle itself.

Ventricular arrhythmias consist of PVCs, ventricular tachycardia, and ventricular fibrillation. Ventricular tachycardia is most often related to ischemic heart disease. Although ventricular tachycardia is sometimes tolerated transiently by the patient, it is treated as a medical emergency. This condition requires prompt conversion back to NSR by drug therapy or electrical cardioversion before it produces bloodflow complications or deteriorates into ventricular fibrillation. In ten percent of ventricular tachycardia patients, no underlying heart disease can be found for the abnormal rhythm. Physicians make a diagnosis of idiopathic ventricular tachycardia with caution because some of these cases eventually manifest themselves as unusual forms of cardiomyopathy. The appearance of ventricular tachycardia has an ominous prognosis—approximately 40 percent of these patients die within the first year. Effective drug therapy or the use of automatic implanted cardioverter/defibrillators (AICDs) decreases the mortality rate of ventricular tachycardia patients to about five percent per year. AICD is discussed in more detail in the "Sudden Death" section below.

Ventricular fibrillation is a rapid, chaotic electrical rhythm of the ventricles that leads immediately to the cessation of cardiac output, shock, and death. The only treatment for ventricular fibrillation is electrical cardioversion, although cardiopulmonary resuscitation (CPR) may sufficiently prolong the life of the patient to allow for the application of electrical cardioversion. The majority of ventricular fibrillation victims have ischemic heart disease, but less than 50 percent have a demonstrable acute myocardial infarction on subsequent postmortem study. Ventricular fibrillation accounts for at least 75 percent of all out-of-hospital cardiac arrests or sudden deaths.

Some arrhythmias arise by virtue of an anomalous or aberrant connecting tissue bridge between the atria and ventricle which, in conjunction with the normal A-V junction conduction system, allows for a re-entry circuit tachyarrhythmia. One particular form of this type of arrhythmia pattern is the Wolff-Parkinson-White syndrome, which has a characteristic electrocardiographic contour when in NSR. Patients who have this syndrome are predisposed to tachyarrhythmias. At times, the syndrome can lead to atrial fibrillation, ventricular fibrillation, and death. An electrophysiologic study (EPS) is a widely used technique for diagnosing and treating arrhythmias. In this procedure, multiple lead wires are placed in the patient's heart to record the site and/or pathway of arrhythmias. The identified anatomic sites can be treated with radio-frequency alternating currents, thus curing the patient and avoiding the need for life-long drug therapy. In other situations, the EPS is used to evaluate ventricular tachyarrhythmia and guide the selection of specific drug therapy. EPS is also valuable for locating an arrhythmogenic site before corrective surgery. The use of surgery will probably diminish as the use of AICD increases.

Sudden Death

Sudden cardiac death is defined as death within one hour of the appearance of acute cardiovascular symptoms. In 25 percent of patients dying from coronary artery disease, these acute symptoms are the first manifestations of the underlying disease. Approximately 350,000 sudden death cases occur each year in the United States, constituting one-half of all cardiovascular deaths and almost one-quarter of all deaths. Eighty percent of sudden cardiac deaths result from ventricular tachycardia and/or ventricular fibrillation, and twenty percent arise from severe bradycardia or asystole. Sudden cardiac death is obviously a major public health concern, but it has proven difficult to anticipate. When ventricular extra beats, called *ventricular ectopy*, are present, preventing deterioration to ventricular fibrillation is difficult, despite drug therapy. Automatic implanted cardioverter/defibrillators are battery-energized implanted devices that can sense changes in heart rhythm and then deliver a defibrillating current through a two-patch epicardial electrode system. The life expectancy of the battery itself is five years. The implantation requires an incision into the chest wall, a procedure called a *thoracotomy*, but transvenous leads are being developed, as are other capabilities, such as pacing and antitachycardia therapy. Early follow-up studies indicate a significant reduction in the sudden death rate in the at-risk patient population.

Valvular Heart Disease

A generation ago this discussion would have been principally one of acute rheumatic fever and its late, long-term valvular residual. However, the incidence of acute rheumatic fever in the Western world has decreased dramatically, as evidenced by a drop of over

90 percent in mortality from acute rheumatic fever and rheumatic heart disease in the United States since 1945. In the Third World, on the other hand, rheumatic heart disease constitutes 20 to 40 percent of all cardiovascular disease. Acute rheumatic fever remains a prevalent disease in the Middle East, Africa, the Indian subcontinent, and South America.

Acute rheumatic fever is a delayed, non-pus-producing, inflammatory reaction that occurs principally in the joints, heart, and subcutaneous tissues and is secondary to a streptococcal oropharynx infection. Rheumatic fever rarely occurs in patients under age four. It typically attacks patients in the five to fifteen age group. This disease usually arises during the colder months and varies in its epidemiology, sometimes occurring in sporadic cases and other times in large outbreaks.

Major manifestations of acute rheumatic fever are migrating polyarthritis, carditis, subcutaneous nodules, erythema marginatum, which is a particular skin lesion, and *chorea*, which is characterized by involuntary, purposeless muscle movements and/or personality changes. Minor features of rheumatic fever are fever, arthralgia, and changes in the patient's electrocardiogram. The diagnosis of this condition can be made with these criteria only in conjunction with supporting evidence of an acute streptococcal infection.

A typical attack of rheumatic fever lasts one to five weeks, and the factor of greatest concern is the degree of inflammatory change in the heart valves producing scarring and deformity. The appearance of heart murmurs indicates varying degrees of deformity and malfunction in the mitral, aortic, and tricuspid valves. These murmurs reflect either an incompetence of the affected valve in closing, a condition called insufficiency, or stenosis resulting from scarring and constriction. The risk of residual valve disease primarily depends upon the clinical evidence of carditis at the time of the episode of acute rheumatic fever. For example, in patients who do not have carditis, only six percent eventually have rheumatic heart disease. Patients who have mild carditis have a 30 percent incidence of rheumatic heart disease, and patients who have severe carditis have a 40 to 70 percent incidence of rheumatic heart disease.

A patient who develops acute rheumatic fever is at added risk of a repeated attack and of subsequent rheumatic heart disease. Current medical practice includes antibiotic preventive treatment against recurrent streptococcal infections. For patients who have rheumatic heart disease, this preventive treatment is necessary for the remainder of the patient's life. For patients who do not develop rheumatic heart disease after acute rheumatic fever, the preventive antibiotic treatment may be discontinued in adult life.

Aortic Stenosis

Aortic stenosis, as discussed earlier in this chapter, is an obstructive lesion that causes the left ventricle to hypertrophy. The hypertrophy is a compensatory response of the ventricle in adapting to the obstruction. The major indicator of aortic stenosis is a systolic murmur at the aortic area. The patient may complain, at a relatively late stage in the development of this condition, of chest pain, symptoms of heart failure, and fainting spells. The appearance of these symptoms indicates a two- to five-year life expectancy. The principle causes of aortic stenosis are a congenitally abnormal valve, rheumatic heart disease, and tissue degeneration with calcification in aging patients.

Once suspected on clinical examination, the diagnosis of aortic stenosis is confirmed by echocardiography and/or cardiac catheterization, which can define aortic valve square area and pressure gradients. For some older patients, valve angioplasty is the suggested treatment for aortic stenosis, and for children a valvuloplasty may delay the need for a prosthetic valve until the patient's body has developed in size. For most aortic stenosis patients, the implantation of a prosthetic valve is the operation of choice. Some of these patients receive a porcine, or pig-derived, valve that requires no subsequent anticoagulation therapy. The porcine valve has about a ten-year life expectancy before deterioration. However, most patients receive a mechanical prosthetic valve. Mechanical prosthetic valves do require life-long anticoagulation therapy to prevent clotting in and around the valve, because clots can compromise the valve's function or can lead to emboli. Operative mortality for valve implant patients is well under five percent. The life survival of mechanical valves is measured in decades. Late complications of valve replacement therapy, including problems relating to anticoagulation therapy, average five percent per year.

Aortic Regurgitation

Aortic regurgitation, or aortic insufficiency, is failure of the aortic valve to close properly in diastole, thus allowing blood from the aorta to flow back into the left ventricle and leading to excessive blood volume in that chamber. The left ventricle compensates for this bloodflow imbalance by dilating and then enlarging.

The clinical course of aortic regurgitation depends upon the cause of the condition. In the chronic form of this disease, slow, progressive deterioration takes place, often years before the patient becomes symptomatic. Chronic aortic insufficiency arises from rheumatic heart disease or a connective tissue disease, such as Marfan's syndrome, ankylosing spondylitis, rheumatoid arthritis, or Reiter's syndrome.[3] Acute aortic insufficiency, on the other hand, can result from endocarditis or aortic dissection and can rapidly lead to acute congestive heart failure. The recognition of aortic insufficiency begins with the appearance of an aortic diastolic murmur along the left or right parasternal border and is confirmed by echocardiography.

Medical therapy for congestive heart failure and treatment for preventing endocarditis are necessary in the presence of aortic regurgitation. Optimally, the abnormal valve will be surgically replaced before irreversible impairment of left ventricular function has occurred. The timing of valve replacement surgery is a clinical judgment, as is the determination of the type of valve—porcine or mechanical prosthetic—used. Operative mortality for valve replacement patients is less than five percent. The late, long-term ill-effects from anticoagulation therapy following valve replacement for aortic regurgitation are the same as those following valve replacement for aortic stenosis.

Mitral Stenosis

Mitral stenosis is a narrowing of the mitral orifice that impedes the flow of blood from the left atrium into the left ventricle. As the valve surface area narrows, symptoms, such as labored breathing during physical exertion, appear. Progressive narrowing results in severe symptoms, even if the patient is at rest. This mitral valve narrowing is secondary to scarring of the valve commissures and results from the inflammatory reaction of acute rheumatic fever. A *commissure* is the juncture between one valve leaflet and another. The original episode of acute rheumatic fever is followed by the appearance of a mitral diastolic murmur some ten years later, with symptoms usually appearing between the ages of 25 to 30. Mitral stenosis is twice as common in females as in males.

After the initial appearance of mitral stenosis symptoms, a period of increasing symptoms ensues. These symptoms of mitral stenosis include diminished exercise capacity, palpitations, and coughing. Meanwhile, the left atrium dilates in response to the increased pressure necessary to maintain the flow of blood from the atrium to

---

[3]*Marfan's syndrome* is a congenital disorder of connective tissue characterized by abnormal length of the extremities, especially of fingers and toes, cardiovascular abnormalities, often dilation of the ascending aorta, and other abnormalities. *Ankylosing spondylitis, rheumatoid arthritis,* and *Reiter's syndrome* are defined and discussed in Chapter 13, *The Musculoskeletal System.*

the ventricle. Eventually, atrial fibrillation develops. This arrhythmia further compromises cardiac function and makes the patient's symptoms worse.

Medical therapy counteracts the effects of atrial fibrillation with digitalis and beta-blockers and counteracts the effects of congestive heart failure with a sodium-restricted diet and diuretics. Treatment also attempts to reduce the significant incidence of systemic embolization associated with mitral stenosis and/or atrial fibrillation through anticoagulation therapy. Eventually, for most patients, surgery is the therapy of choice. The timing of surgery depends upon the patient's clinical picture and findings on the patient's echocardiograph and cardiac catheterization. The echocardiogram can indicate the valve's cross-sectional area and the pressure gradient across the valve, so that many patients undergo surgery without also undergoing cardiac catheterization. The surgical procedure varies with the patient's clinical situation. For some patients, valvuloplasty is feasible, but for most patients a prosthetic valve replacement is necessary. Life-long anticoagulation therapy is required for valve replacement patients.

Mitral Regurgitation

Mitral regurgitation is the result of failure of the mitral valve to close properly at the onset of systole, allowing blood from the left ventricle to flow back into the left atrium. Common causes of mitral regurgitation are mitral valve prolapse, rheumatic heart disease, connective tissue diseases, coronary artery disease, and any condition that results in enlargement of the left ventricle and distortion of the mitral valve apparatus. Mitral regurgitation may occur acutely and result in acute congestive heart failure, but the more common form of this condition is chronic mitral regurgitation.

Increasing volumes of regurgitant blood causes the left atrium to dilate, then leading the left ventricle to dilate and hypertrophy. When these compensatory changes no longer allow the system to maintain an adequate cardiac output, congestive heart failure ensues, resulting in symptoms of fatigue, exertional dyspnea, and orthopnea. Acute congestive heart failure can result in pulmonary edema.

The diagnosis of mitral regurgitation initially arises from the patient's medical history and a physical examination that indicates cardiac enlargement and a mitral systolic murmur. The diagnosis is confirmed by the patient's electrocardiogram, chest x-ray, echocardiogram, and cardiac catheterization. Therapy for mitral regurgitation consists of the usual measures for preventing congestive heart failure, but if congestive heart failure has developed, surgery is a prime consideration. The timing of surgery is a clinical decision based upon variables in the findings of the patient's echocardiograph and cardiac catheterization. Corrective surgery can take the form of a valvuloplasty or of a valve replacement with porcine or mechanical prosthetics. For patients who receive mechanical prosthetic valves, life-long anticoagulation therapy is mandatory. The overall operative mortality rate for corrective mitral regurgitation surgery varies from five to ten percent, depending upon the severity of the patient's condition at the time of surgery.

Mitral valve prolapse deserves special attention because of its frequent diagnosis and because many people have heard of the condition. This valve abnormality results from a fibrous degeneration of the valve that usually is idiopathic. Mitral valve prolapse seems to have a genetic origin and occurs in females more than in males.

The diagnosis of mitral prolapse is indicated by the finding of a "click" sound in systole, accompanied by a systolic murmur, and is confirmed by echocardiography. Most patients who are diagnosed as having mitral valve prolapse remain asymptomatic. A small number of mitral valve prolapse patients experience palpitations and chest pains, a smaller number develop significant mitral regurgitation, and a very small percentage develop peripheral emboli, endocarditis, or sudden death. From the clinician's viewpoint, the anxiety created in the public at large by this diagnosis is almost as major a problem as the pathologic features associated with the condition. In fact, the anxiety associated with the diagnosis of mitral valve prolapse has caused this factor to be considered a feature of the disease itself.

Diseases of the Myocardium

Primary diseases of heart muscle are not associated with any other disease of the heart and are termed *cardiomyopathies*. They are classified into three types according to certain characteristics.

Dilated cardiomyopathy, the most common of these entities, is defined as an increase in the internal diameter of the ventricles, principally the left ventricle, without a corresponding increase in the size of the chamber wall. The major functional change resulting from dilated cardiomyopathy is systolic dysfunction, which manifests as a decreased ejection fraction. This change leads to the clinical appearance of congestive heart failure, with associated complications of peripheral emboli and sudden death. In the vast majority of these dilated cardiomyopathy cases, no specific origin of the condition is determinable, although researchers think that viral myocarditis is the main culprit. A specific virus, Coxsackie virus group B, can be identified as the precipitating factor in some dilated cardiomyopathy patients. Noninfectious causes of dilated cardiomyopathy include toxins, such as alcohol or chemotherapeutic agents; genetic diseases, such as hereditary dilated cardiomyopathy, progressive muscular dystrophy, or Friedreich's ataxia; autoimmune diseases; transplantation rejection; peripartum; and certain metabolic diseases.

Treatment of dilated cardiomyopathy is directed to the specific cause of the condition, if known. Heart transplantation is the principal treatment for the end-stage congestive heart failure patient, and, in fact, half of all cardiac transplantations are performed to treat dilated cardiomyopathy. Sudden death accounts for about half of all deaths in these patients.

Hypertrophic cardiomyopathies are characterized by hypertrophy of the left ventricle, and most cases arise as a genetic autosomal[4] dominant disease. These cardiomyopathies show normal or reduced chamber size, an increased ejection fraction, and diastolic dysfunction, which is manifested by an elevated end diastolic pressure in the left ventricle. Hypertrophic cardiomyopathies commonly present as congestive heart failure and chest pain in patients aged 20 to 40.

The echocardiogram is the most common procedure for diagnosing hypertrophic cardiomyopathy, although a physical examination and an electrocardiograph can point to the diagnosis. Treatment of hypertrophic cardiomyopathies consists of drug therapy, using a beta adrenergic-blocker or a calcium channel-blocker to reduce ventricle muscle contraction, thereby preventing potential left ventricle outflow obstruction. Sometimes surgery is performed on hypertrophic cardiomyopathy patients to remove hypertrophic muscle tissue in the septum. Most patients who have a hypertrophic cardiomyopathy show a gradual deterioration over decades.

Restrictive cardiomyopathies, the least common of the cardiomyopathies, are characterized by a diastolic filling impairment and a normal, or near normal, systolic function and chamber size. A restrictive cardiomyopathy may arise from endocardial thickening and loss of compliance that results from radiation injury, drug therapy for a tumor, or endomyocardial fibrosis. The myocardium may be functionally impaired by idiopathic restrictive cardiomyopathy thus causing a mechanical impediment to diastolic relaxation. The common form of restrictive cardiomyopathy is an infiltrative phenomenon, such as amyloid or hemochromatosis, and the treatment for a given patient will depend upon the patient's specific cardiomyopathy.

---

[4]An *autosome* is any ordinary paired chromosome, as distinguished from a sex chromosome. Humans have 22 pairs of autosomes.

Infections of the Heart

Infections of the heart may involve the endocardium, myocardium, or pericardium and may present as acute or chronic illness. These conditions can run a course from a benign, asymptomatic, unrecognized illness to a rapidly lethal and painful disease.

Bacterial endocarditis is an infection that primarily affects the endocardium overlying the heart valves. Although the valves may have been normal before the infection, more often they were abnormal, which clearly predisposed them to this bacterial complication. Therefore, patients who have abnormal heart valves routinely receive preventive antibiotic treatment prior to surgery to protect these patients against the possibility of bacteremia that follows any invasive procedure.

The clinical course of bacterial endocarditis may be acute or subacute, depending principally upon the virulence of the infectious agent. In the days before antibiotics, the *mortality* rate of bacterial endocarditis patients was 100 percent, but today the *survival* rate is 80 to 90 percent. Survivors of bacterial endocarditis are sometimes left with deformed valves that require surgical relief. The left heart valves are the most common sites of this type of infection, but intravenous drug abuse has resulted in a growing number of right heart endocarditis patients.

Myocarditis is predominantly a viral infection problem and was previously discussed in relation to dilated cardiomyopathies. Myocarditis is not uncommon and, for the most part, is benign.

Pericarditis is an infection or inflammation of the pericardium. It may present as an acute or chronic illness, and it may involve complications, such as effusion or late-term constriction. The specific origin of the pericarditis may arise from

- infectious agents, including viruses, tuberculosis, and fungi
- physical agents, including trauma and radiation
- metabolic diseases of the liver, kidney, or thyroid gland
- a variety of connective tissue diseases

Acute pericarditis may present with chest pain mimicking pleurisy or myocardial ischemia. The diagnosis is established by a physical examination of the patient that identifies a pericardial friction rub and electrocardiographic changes. Coexistent effusion usually requires no medical response. However, effusion that compromises cardiac diastolic filling necessitates drainage, usually by needle aspiration. This effusion is called the cardiac tamponade syndrome.

Constrictive pericarditis has the same clinical picture as restrictive cardiomyopathy, and making the clinical distinction is sometimes quite difficult. Constrictive pericarditis is often idiopathic or neoplastic, but this condition also may result from radiation, trauma, or connective tissue disease. In the past, tuberculosis was the principal cause of constrictive pericarditis. Regardless of the cause of the condition, surgical removal of the pericardium will usually cure constrictive pericarditis that significantly inhibits bloodflow.

Other Heart Problems: Direct and Indirect

Prior sections of this chapter have discussed the major heart diseases. This section will address some other heart conditions, their causes, and their prognoses.

Although cardiac tumors occur relatively rarely, echocardiography indicates their presence and seriousness. Secondary tumors of the heart occur 20 times more often than do primary tumors. Of the primary tumors, benign atrial myxomas are the most common, occurring three times more often in females than in males and usually arising in the left atrium. The symptoms of atrial myxomas sometimes mimic valvular congestive heart failure, or the symptoms may include fever, joint pains, or traveling blood clots. Surgical removal of these myxomas is a successful treatment for most patients. The most common primary malignant tumor of the heart is sarcoma, which has little potential for cure.

Secondary tumors of the heart primarily arise from melanoma, leukemia, or metastasized cancers of the breast or lung. The treatment of secondary tumors depends on their underlying causes and on any local mechanical ill effects, such as pericardial effusion.

Cardiac manifestations of various systemic diseases have been mentioned previously. The heart participates in connective tissue diseases—including systemic lupus erythematosus, rheumatoid arthritis, and scleroderma—metabolic-endocrine disorders, and infiltrative diseases.

Finally, traumas to the heart, direct and indirect, are not uncommon. Direct trauma resulting from bullet wounds or knife stabs can lead to cardiac perforation with hemorrhage, valve disruption, conduction abnormalities, and other problems. Indirect traumas to the heart from chest wall contusion and/or sudden deceleration may result from auto accidents, sports injuries, or industrial accidents. Such indirect traumas are also capable of causing bruising and disruption of the cardiac walls, coronary arteries, or valves. Cardiac traumas, direct or indirect, are not always easily recognized. Nonetheless, a trauma may be serious, resulting in acute cardiovascular collapse that requires prompt surgical intervention.

An individual who has a cardiac diagnosis is not automatically uninsurable and is not necessarily dealing with a major medical impairment. Many patients who have mild congenital heart disease lead physically vigorous lifestyles, and never require medical care more extensive than preventive antibiotic treatment. Patients may live 20 to 30 years with acquired heart disease before clinical symptoms appear. With modern drug therapy and surgical techniques, these patients may be restored to a physical status that allows for strenuous activity. Furthermore, drug and surgical measures have lessened the ischemic effects of coronary artery disease to the point that some patients have participated in marathons. Moreover, cardiac pacemakers can adapt to patients' changing physiologic needs by varying the patients' heart rates. In short, a cardiac diagnosis alone is insufficient for an underwriter or claim examiner to assess a client—the functional status of the patient must also be considered. The insurer's employee, therefore, should refer to the clinical functional assessment of the patient that the attending physician or the independent medical examiner has made. The New York Heart Association classification is one system medical professionals use to evaluate the level of a patient's cardiovascular impairment. The results of exercise tests play a large role in the objective measurement of this evaluation. Figure 7–10 presents a comparison of two commonly used disability assessment classifications and a specific activity scale.

Diseases of the Aorta and Peripheral Vessels

Aneurysms of the aorta are classified as being either congenital or acquired and are further classified by location and complication. They may be identified on routine examination or may present as acute vascular emergencies. The most common aneurysm is the abdominal aortic aneurysm, which appears in one to three percent of autopsy studies, is six times more likely to occur in men than in women, and usually appears above the renal arteries. Atherosclerosis is the usual cause of abdominal aortic aneurysms, but trauma and inflammation may also produce them. They may be found during a physical examination, can be viewed by ultrasound, and are best treated by preventive surgery when they attain significant size—more than five centimeters in diameter, as determined by ultrasound or CT scan. Unrecognized, these aneurysms may rupture and/or may lead to dissection of the aortic wall and further vascular compromise. In either case, mortality is high. Dissection of the aorta usually arises in the thoracic aorta, and its principal association is with hypertension. Certain congenital diseases and pregnancy are often underlying causes of aortic dissection that are not associated with hypertension. Early recognition of the dissection is critical to avoid vascular catastrophes and death.

Figure 7–10.
Methods of Assessing Cardiovascular Disability.

	New York Heart Association Classification	Canadian Cardiovascular Society Functional Classification	Specific Activity Scale
CLASS I	Patients who have cardiac disease but without resulting limitations of physical activity. Ordinary physical activity does not cause undue fatigue, palpitation, dyspnea, or anginal pain.	Ordinary physical activity, such as walking and climbing stairs, does not cause angina. Angina with strenuous or rapid or prolonged exertion at work or recreation.	Patients can perform to completion any activity requiring >7 METs, e.g. can carry 24 pounds up eight steps; carry objects that weigh 80 pounds; shovel snow or spade soil; ski, jog/walk at 5 mph, or play basketball, squash, handball.
CLASS II	Patients who have cardiac disease resulting in slight limitation of physical activity. They are comfortable at rest. Ordinary physical activity results in fatigue, palpitation, dyspnea, or anginal pain.	Slight limitation of ordinary activity. Walking or climbing stairs rapidly, walking uphill, walking or stair climbing after meals, in cold, in wind, or when under emotional stress, or during the few hours after awakening may be problematic. Walking more than two blocks on the level and climbing more than one flight of ordinary stairs at a normal pace and in normal conditions may also be problematic.	Patients can perform to completion any activity requiring >5 METs, but cannot, and do not perform to completion activities requiring >7 METs, e.g. can rake, weed, roller skate, walk at 4 mph on level ground.
CLASS III	Patients who have cardiac disease resulting in marked limitation of physical activity. They are comfortable at rest. Less than ordinary physical activity causes fatigue, palpitation, dyspnea, or anginal pain.	Marked limitation of ordinary physical activity. Walking one to two blocks on the level and climbing more than one flight of stairs in normal conditions is problematic.	Patients can perform to completion any activity requiring >2 METs, but cannot and do not perform to completion any activities requiring >5 METs, e.g. can shower without stopping, make a bed, clean windows, bowl, golf, dress without stopping, walk at 2.5 mph.
CLASS IV	Patients who have cardiac disease resulting in inability to carry on any physical activity without discomfort. Symptoms of cardiac insufficiency or of the anginal syndrome may be present even at rest. If any physical activity is undertaken, discomfort is increased.	Inability to carry on any physical activity without discomfort—anginal syndrome may be present at rest.	Patients cannot or do not perform to completion activities requiring >2 METs. Cannot carry out activities listed above (Specific Activity Scale, Class III).

Adapted with permission from L. Goldman, et al.: "Comparative Reproducibility and Validity of Systems for Assessing Cardiovascular Functional Class: Advantages of a New Specific Activity Scale," *Circulation* 64 (1981): 1227.

Atherosclerosis may also involve the more distal aorta in the abdomen and its major subdivisions in the legs, leading to bloodflow deficiency, called ***arteriosclerosis obliterans***. Clinically, arteriosclerosis obliterans often leads to intermittent claudication. The majority of claudication patients can lessen or eliminate the symptoms of that condition by avoiding tobacco, engaging in regular physical activity, and controlling the underlying atherosclerotic-producing illness. For the minority of patients who have rest ischemia and its complications, surgical interventions, including angioplasty and bypass graft, are available. Peripheral vascular disease (PVD) is a major complication in diabetic patients, and amputations of diabetic ischemics' digits or limbs frequently are necessary.

Obstruction in the peripheral vessels may occur without atherosclerosis, as a consequence of inflammation of segments in the small and medium arteries and veins. This condition is termed *thromboangiitis obliterans*, or ***Buerger's disease***, and its cause is unknown. Buerger's disease primarily affects young male smokers, and, unlike arteriosclerosis obliterans, frequently involves the upper extremities as well as the lower extremities. The treatment for this condition is similar to that for arteriosclerosis obliterans, and unless the patient stops using tobacco completely, his or her condition will progressively worsen.

Nonfixed arterial obstruction of the peripheral vessels is secondary to abnormal vascular smooth muscle constriction of a transient, but repetitive, nature. Sixty percent of all such nonfixed arterial obstruction cases are idiopathic. ***Raynaud's disease*** is a condition of unknown cause which involves intermittent episodes of decreased bloodflow to the patient's fingers or toes. This disorder is marked by severe pallor, followed by blueness and then redness of the digits. It occurs most commonly in young women. Raynaud's phenomenon, as described in Chapter 5, *The Skin*, is an obstruction that is secondary to an underlying cause, such as connective tissue disease, repetitive trauma, emotional stimuli, or tobacco use. Regardless of the condition's origin, arterial obstructions almost always involve the patient's upper extremities. The characteristic episodes of obstruction go through classic serial color changes of the skin, showing pallor or whiteness, cyanosis, and redness. The attacks are often brought on by cold or emotion and generally respond to warmth. The ischemic color changes are often associated with skin changes, such as abnormal sweating, hair and nail changes, ulceration, and pain.

Treatment of Raynaud's disease is directed to relaxing smooth muscle constrictions by the avoidance of tobacco, the use of calcium channel-blocking agents or alpha-adrenergic blocking agents, and/or injection or surgery to block sympathetic nerve activity. The prognosis in Raynaud's disease is good and results in no mortality and little morbidity. More than 50 percent of Raynaud's phenomenon cases improve or subside spontaneously over several years, although a small percentage later show evidence of an underlying connective tissue disease, particularly scleroderma. The treatment and prognosis for Raynaud's phenomenon depends upon the underlying primary disease.

Inflammation of an arterial wall, called **arteritis**, is a major pathologic lesion that occurs in a number of diverse diseases mostly of unknown cause. Giant cell arteritis, temporal arteritis, polyarteritis nodosa, and Takayasu's disease are examples of specific primary arteritis. Secondary arteritis occurs in various autoimmune diseases, including systemic lupus erythematosus and rheumatoid arthritis; connective tissue diseases, such as scleroderma; infections; and allergic reactions.

Veins and lymphatic vessels are common sites of diseases which are, for the most part, acquired. An inflammation in a vein is called **phlebitis**, and an inflammation in a lymphatic vessel is called **lymphangitis**. Phlebitis and lymphangitis are usually secondary to (1) direct infection of the skin, (2) trauma, or (3) stasis as may arise from prolonged bed rest. Segmental dilation of a vein represents a congenital weakness of the vein wall. In a patient's leg, the segmental dilation presents as a varicosity and in a patient's rectum, as a hemorrhoid. Varicosities and lymphatic vessel disease may cause marked symptomatic swelling of the legs. Clots may occur within the varicosities and may break off and travel to the lung in the form of pulmonary emboli. Pulmonary emboli are frequent causes of morbidity and mortality, occurring in some 600,000 patients each year in the United States. Autopsy studies reveal that pulmonary emboli play a major role in 10 to 20 percent of all hospital deaths and 15 percent of operative deaths. Chapter 8, *The Respiratory System*, provides more details about the recognition and treatment of pulmonary emboli. Localized chronic venous obstruction secondary to varicosities that are associated with clot formation is the cause of the **post-phlebitic syndrome**, which is characterized by a swollen leg with skin changes, following phlebitis. This condition is sometimes called "milk leg" and may occur in women just after childbirth or may occur in association with obesity, leg fractures, and prolonged bed confinement. Surgical therapy for varicose veins in the lower extremities consists of removal by stripping the superficial venous channel, allowing the venous circulation to be sustained by the deeper patent venous channels, and/or by tying off—ligating—connecting veins between the superficial and deep venous channels.

8

The Respiratory System

Respiration is a group of processes concerned with the exchange of gases between the body and its environment. Among these processes are

- ***Breathing***—the process by which air, with its supply of oxygen, is taken into the lungs during inspiration and is expelled with carbon dioxide during expiration
- ***Diffusion of gases in the lungs***—the process by which oxygen from the inspired air crosses the alveoli to enter the blood in the lung's capillaries, and carbon dioxide, a product of cellular metabolism, is released from the blood to become part of the expired air
- ***Diffusion of gases in the tissues***—the process by which oxygen is released to the cells and carbon dioxide enters the small peripheral capillaries
- ***Control of breathing***—the process by which the rate and depth of ventilation is maintained (1) during periods of exercise, rest, and stress, (2) in environments having reduced atmospheric pressure, and (3) in the presence of changing metabolic needs

The ***respiratory system*** consists of a group of organs and structures that work to exchange gases between the air we breathe and our bloodstream. The organs and structures that comprise the respiratory system are the nasal cavity, pharynx, larynx, trachea, lungs, and the bronchi and alveoli. Figure 8–1 illustrates these organs and structures. This chapter will discuss these components of the respiratory system and their functions. It will then address many of the diseases and disorders that affect the respiratory system.

ANATOMY AND PHYSIOLOGY

The Nasal Cavity

The **nasal cavity** is the area in the skull between the cranial cavity and the roof of the mouth and is divided by a thin-walled, vertical nasal septum into approximately equal halves. The chief functions of the nasal cavity involve the preparation of air for use in the lungs. These functions, which rest largely on the mucous membrane that lines the nasal cavity and produces changes in the inspired air to protect the lungs, are

- *Humidification*—Before going into the lungs, the air must be moistened.
- *Temperature adjustment*—Generally, the temperature of the inspired air must be raised. The necessary heat comes from blood vessels located in, and just below, the mucous membrane.
- *Air cleaning*—Particulate matter will adhere to the mucous membrane as the particles come into contact with it. This matter may be removed by sneezing. The inspired air is also partially filtered by coarse hairs found in the nasal passages.

The nasal cavity has another important function. In the upper portion of this cavity is the olfactory region, where the mucous membrane has receptors for the sense of smell.

The **paranasal sinuses** are irregular air cavities that are adjacent to the nose. The sinuses vary in size and configuration. Approximately 24 sinuses are located in the facial bones. Each sinus is lined with a mucous membrane and communicates through a small opening with the nasal cavity. The sinuses lighten the weight of the skull, but they have no obvious function. They are of medical importance because of the diseases that affect them.

The Pharynx

The **pharynx**, or throat, is a vertical, muscular, tubular structure about five inches long extending from the nasal cavity to the esopha-

Figure 8–1.
A Cross-Sectional View of the Organs and Structures of the Respiratory System.

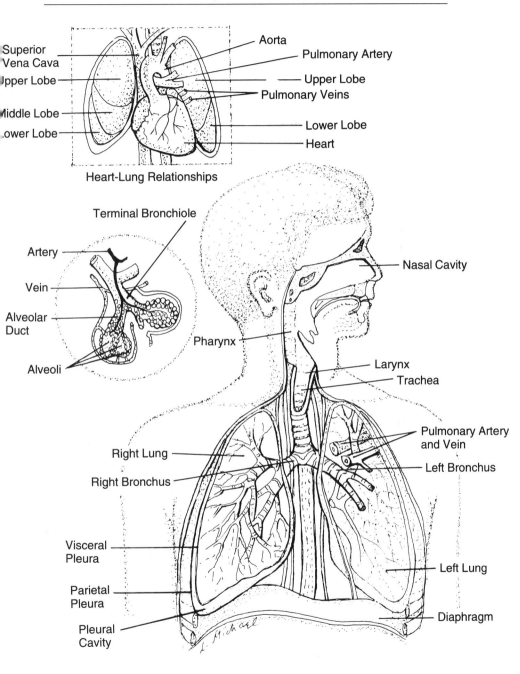

Superior Vena Cava

Upper Lobe

Middle Lobe

Lower Lobe

Aorta

Pulmonary Artery

Upper Lobe

Pulmonary Veins

Lower Lobe

Heart

Heart-Lung Relationships

Terminal Bronchiole

Artery

Vein

Alveolar Duct

Alveoli

Nasal Cavity

Pharynx

Larynx

Trachea

Pulmonary Artery and Vein

Left Bronchus

Right Lung

Right Bronchus

Visceral Pleura

Parietal Pleura

Pleural Cavity

Left Lung

Diaphragm

gus. The pharynx, which functions as a passageway for food and air, is divided into the following three parts, each of approximately equal length:

- The **nasopharynx** is the pharyngeal section located behind the nose and in back of and above the soft palate. The nasopharynx connects to the nasal cavity, contains the tonsils, and has one opening for each eustachian tube on either side. A **eustachian tube**, which is also known as an *auditory tube,* is a canal leading from the middle ear to the nasopharynx. This tube equalizes the air pressure on the inner surface of the eardrum with the air pressure existing outside the drum. The eustachian tube opens during the act of swallowing.
- The **oropharynx** is the portion of the pharynx located behind the mouth between the soft palate and the epiglottis, which is a part of the larynx. The oropharynx is important clinically because the back wall of the pharynx is the site of certain acute and chronic inflammations.
- The **laryngopharynx** is the lower third of the pharynx. The laryngopharynx is located behind the larynx and extends downward to the esophagus.

The Larynx

The **larynx**, or voice box, is a tubular structure that connects the oropharynx and trachea. It consists of nine cartilages that are joined by an elastic membrane. The "Adam's apple" is one such cartilage. Another cartilage is the **epiglottis**, which, during swallowing, forms a lid over the opening to the larynx to prevent the entrance of food or other material into the larynx and trachea. The larynx contains two **vocal cords,** which are white fibrous bands of tissue located on the lateral walls of the larynx.

The larynx performs several functions, the most important of which are:

- Protection of the trachea, bronchi, and lungs—The epiglottis closes the laryngeal airway to avoid the intrusion of foreign substances. By initiating the cough reflex, the larynx helps to expel substances that do gain entrance.
- Phonation—The intrinsic muscles of the larynx regulate tension on the vocal cords for the production of sounds.
- Air transportation—The larynx serves as a passageway for air to the trachea.

The Trachea

The *trachea*, or windpipe, is a hollow, tubular structure located in front of the esophagus. It extends from the larynx to the bronchi and is the passageway through which inspired air reaches the bronchi and lungs. The trachea measures approximately 11 centimeters in length and is supported by 16 to 20 C-shaped cartilage rings and muscle fibers.

The Lungs

The *lungs*, which are the most important organs of respiration, effect the exchange of carbon dioxide and oxygen by the blood. The two lungs are situated in the thoracic cavity and are separated from one another by the contents of the mediastinum. The *thoracic cavity* is the conical-shaped cage that contains and protects the principal organs of respiration and circulation. The mediastinum extends back from the breastbone to the spinal column and contains the aorta and other large blood vessels, the heart, the esophagus, and the bronchi. The *diaphragm* is a thin, dome-shaped muscle that is attached to the spinal column and to the lower ribs and rib cartilages and forms the lower boundary of the thoracic cavity. The diaphragm is the major muscle of the respiratory system.

The left lung is divided into two lobes, and the right lung is divided into three lobes. The left lung has less capacity than the right lung because the heart lies on the left side of the body. The right lung is shorter than the left because the diaphragm rises higher on the right side to accommodate the liver.

Each lung is covered by an exceedingly delicate, two-layer membrane called the *pleura*. One layer, the *parietal pleura*, lines the inner surface of the chest wall, and the other layer, the *visceral pleura*, covers the lung. In a healthy patient, these two layers are in contact with one another. A thin film of fluid lubricates the two pleural layers so that these surfaces move without friction during breathing. The potential space between these two pleural layers is known as the *pleural cavity*. The potential cavity becomes a real one only following penetrating chest wounds and in certain disease states in which air or fluid collects between the two pleural layers.

The Bronchi and Alveoli

A *bronchus* is a large air passage in the lungs. The trachea divides into a right and a left mainstem bronchus, extending into the right and left lungs, respectively. (Figure 8–2 shows the relationships among the larynx, trachea, and bronchi.) The mainstem bronchi have

Figure 8–2.
The Spatial Relationships among the Larynx, Trachea, and Bronchi.

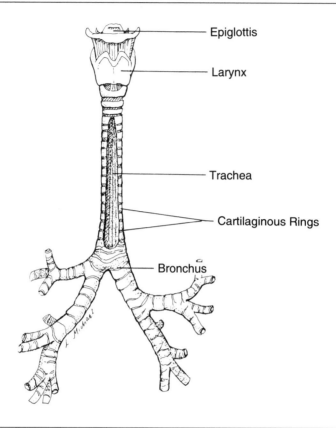

cartilaginous rings similar to those on the trachea. Upon entering the lung, each bronchus divides into smaller bronchi. These bronchi continue to divide within the lungs into smaller and still smaller bronchi until the surrounding protective cartilages disappear, leaving only tiny air tubes, called ***bronchioles***. The bronchioles divide repeatedly, eventually forming fine branches, the ***alveolar ducts***, which lead into numerous rounded projections, called the air spaces or ***alveoli***. In the alveoli, an exchange of gases occurs between the surrounding blood capillaries and the inspired air. The trachea and bronchi are lined with a thin mucous membrane that continues to warm and humidify the inspired air. Certain cells in this membrane have microscopic hair-like structures, called ***cilia***, which protrude into the air passages. By their constant sweeping action, the cilia help move excess secretions to the throat to be expelled from the body.

THE MECHANISM OF RESPIRATION

The nervous system controls respiration. The respiratory center is located in the brain and is stimulated by certain forces, such as

- lack of oxygen in the blood, a condition called *hypoxemia*, which causes an increase in the rate and volume of respiration, with a corresponding increase in oxygen intake
- an elevation of carbon dioxide in the blood, which causes increased respiration
- heat, from fever or high external temperature, which causes an increase in the respiratory rate, thus cooling the body
- physical work, exercise, and hypermetabolic states, all of which create a need for more oxygen
- emotions, such as fear, anxiety, and elation, which may increase the respiratory rate

External and Cellular Respiration

At rest, the air pressure within the thoracic cage of the normal adult is lower than the atmospheric pressure. When the diaphragm and chest muscles contract, elevating the ribs and sternum during inspiration, the negative pressure becomes even more negative, thus causing an influx of air into the lungs. During expiration, the diaphragm and muscles relax, the chest wall returns to its original position, the pressure within the thoracic cavity increases and becomes less negative, and air is expelled.

Respiration also takes place at the cellular level. As cells use oxygen, energy is released, and carbon dioxide and water are formed. The circulating blood gives oxygen to the cells as it takes away the carbon dioxide and water from the cells. Oxygen cannot be stored in the body, and so it must be constantly replenished through the mechanisms of respiration and blood circulation.

Vital Capacity

A person's *vital capacity* is the total volume of air that the person can exhale after a maximum inspiration. The vital capacity consists of three parts:

- *Tidal air*—the volume of air that moves during each respiration when the individual is at rest
- *Inspiratory reserve volume*—the volume of air that with maximum effort can be inhaled in excess of the tidal air

- *Expiratory reserve volume*—the volume of air that, after a maximum inspiration, can be exhaled with maximum effort in excess of both tidal air and the inspiratory reserve volume air

Vital capacity decreases both with age (as the mobility of the thoracic cage decreases) and in certain respiratory diseases. Training can increase vital capacity.

The basic method for studying the lungs' function is the *forced vital capacity (FVC)* measurement. FVC is the volume of air expired as forcefully and completely as possible after maximum inspiration. Males have approximately 25 percent greater FVC than females of comparable age and height. Aging produces a decline in FVC that generally cannot be improved with training, although athletes have higher FVCs than nonathletes. The FVC declines more rapidly with age in smokers than in nonsmokers. Differences in height produce the greatest difference in FVC. A ten-inch increase in height will produce up to a 30 percent increase in FVC.

In any individual, the observed FVC (FVC_o) is expressed as a percentage of the predicted FVC (FVC_p) as obtained from a pulmonary (lung) function chart: FVC_o/FVC_p. In a normal individual, this value should be at least 80 percent. Values below 60 percent indicate severe restrictive airway disease.

Another important pulmonary function study is the timed vital capacity (TVC). As usually measured, the most important volume of air is that expired during the first second of the total FVC measurement. This volume is called the forced expiratory volume at one second (FEV_1). This measurement is of greater value when expressed either as a percentage of the predicted FEV_1 as obtained from pulmonary function tables or as a percentage of the observed FVC.

In a healthy person, the observed FEV_1 to predicted FEV_1 ratio should be at least 80 percent, and the ratio of FEV_1 to the FVC should be 75 percent. Values on either ratio below 50 percent indicate severe obstructive pulmonary disease.

Reduced vital capacity may arise from many organic causes, including

- skeletal deformity of the chest or any condition that limits chest expansion
- restrictive lung diseases that produce a low total FVC and FEV_1
- conditions that interfere with lung function
- conditions that interfere with the downward movement of the diaphragm

Sometimes values for pulmonary function tests are low even without organic pathology. Lack of interest or motivation on the part of the individual being tested or that person's failure to understand instructions may affect test results. If the individual is tired, worried, tense, or distracted, the test results will be affected. Persons who live sedentary lives, who are not in good physical condition, or who are unaccustomed to deep breathing often produce low results on pulmonary function tests.

DISORDERS OF THE RESPIRATORY SYSTEM

Any part of the respiratory system can be affected by disease. Disorders of the upper respiratory tract are the most common of these conditions but generally are not serious. Disorders of the bronchi and lungs occur less frequently but tend to have more serious consequences.

Diseases of the Upper Respiratory Tract

The upper respiratory tract consists of the nose, nasal cavity, paranasal sinuses, and pharynx. Although infections of the upper respiratory tract usually are not serious, they constitute a leading cause of minor disability and absenteeism from work because they occur frequently.

Colds and Allergies

The most common upper respiratory infection (URI) is acute rhinitis, which is also called the common cold. *Acute rhinitis* is a condition caused by one of many viruses that produce well-known manifestations, including: inflammation of the mucous membrane of the nose with large amounts of nasal discharge, mild fever, sore throat, headache, and a general feeling of discomfort. Unless complications arise, the common cold is a self-limited condition of short duration.

An *allergy* is a hypersensitive reaction to a particular antigen. Hay fever and allergic rhinitis are common allergic disorders affecting the upper respiratory tract. Allergic manifestations of sneezing and nasal discharge may occur after contact with windborne pollens, house dust, animal dander, food, or other allergens.

Pharyngitis and Tonsillitis

Pharyngitis is an inflammation of the pharynx. The most common pharyngitis results from infection by either a virus or bacterium. Viral infections are more common than bacterial ones. However, the streptococcus bacterium is a common cause of bacterial pharyngitis. During a bout with pharyngitis, the patient's pharynx is red and swollen, and the patient often complains of a hot, dry sore throat and pain upon swallowing. Acute pharyngitis may precede or accompany the common cold or it may arise from an extension of infections located in the nose, sinuses, or tonsils.

Tonsillitis is an inflammation of a tonsil. Acute bacterial tonsillitis is an acute infection of the tonsil, generally caused by a streptococcus bacterium, that affects children more often than adults. The swollen, red tonsils may be coated with an inflammatory exudate.[1] Sore throat, pain in swallowing, fever, and chills are common manifestations of tonsillitis.

Acute pharyngitis and tonsillitis generally are self-limited disorders which respond to gargling and analgesics. An *analgesic* is an agent that relieves pain without causing a loss of consciousness. Aspirin, acetaminophen, and ibuprofen are common analgesics. Antibiotics cure pharyngitis and tonsillitis caused by bacteria. Untreated streptococcal infections may be dangerous. The infrequent complications of these infections include inflammation of the middle ear, mastoiditis, rheumatic fever, and glomerulonephritis. These diseases are discussed elsewhere in this book.[2]

Sinusitis

Sinusitis is a sinus infection. It may occur alone or may accompany the common cold or other URI. In addition, sinusitis may result from an extension of a dental infection or from an allergy. Frequently, an obstruction to the normal drainage from the sinus—which may be produced by a nasal polyp or deviated septum—causes this condition. Headache is a common symptom, and its location depends on which sinus is involved. Pressure on the involved sinus may elicit pain.

---

[1]An exudate is any material, such as fluid, cells, or cellular debris, which has escaped from blood vessels and has been deposited in tissues or on tissue surfaces, usually as a result of inflammation.

[2]Inflammation of the middle ear and mastoiditis are discussed in Chapter 15, *The Sense Organs*; rheumatic fever is discussed in Chapter 7, *The Circulatory System*; and glomerulonephritis is discussed in Chapter 10, *The Urinary System*.

Treatment of sinusitis includes decongestants, antihistamines, and/or antibiotics. If the sinusitis results from an allergy, treatment focuses upon the identification and removal of the offending allergen. Complications of sinusitis have decreased in incidence since the introduction of antibiotics. Stubborn cases of sinusitis that do not respond to medical therapy may require an operation to provide drainage. A *Caldwell-Luc procedure* to relieve chronic sinusitis involves the creation of a window in the affected sinus for drainage and removal of the diseased contents.

Diseases of the Larynx and Trachea

Laryngitis is an inflammation of the larynx, and *tracheitis* is an inflammation of the trachea. Upper respiratory infection, such as the common cold, is the most frequent cause of acute inflammation of the larynx and trachea. Laryngitis and tracheitis also may occur in the course of bronchitis, pneumonia, influenza, and other viral and bacterial infections, or they may follow excessive use of the voice, excessive smoking, or inhalation of irritating substances. Hoarseness is the most prominent symptom if the infection involves the larynx.

   Acute laryngotracheobronchitis is an acute respiratory infection in which the mucous membranes of the larynx, trachea, and bronchi are acutely inflamed and swollen. This condition is characterized by high fever, hoarseness, cough, and shortness of breath. If the swelling is so marked as to produce respiratory obstruction, a tracheotomy is necessary. A *tracheotomy* is the surgical creation of an opening in the patient's trachea to relieve airway obstruction and allow for ventilation. Tracheotomy also permits the suction removal of the mucus secreted during the course of this disease.

   One specific type of laryngeal infection is epiglottitis. *Epiglottitis* is an inflammation of the epiglottis that is usually caused by the bacteria Hemophilus influenza. A pediatric emergency, and occasionally an adult emergency, epiglottitis begins abruptly in children and presents with severe sore throat, fever, and difficulty in swallowing. This condition rapidly progresses to a stage requiring hospitalization and *intubation*, which is the insertion of a tube into a body canal or hollow organ. In the case of epiglottitis, the tube is inserted into the patient's larynx.

   The most common tumor of the larynx is the benign *singer's nodule*, which is an enlargement of the edge of the vocal cord. It generally occurs as a solitary nodule, is easily removed, and rarely recurs. The singer's nodule is also called a *vocal cord polyp*.

   Carcinoma of the larynx develops most commonly in individuals who are in their 60s. This cancer is ten times more common in men than in women and is related to tobacco abuse. Laryngeal malignancies are generally classifiable into intrinsic cancers and extrinsic cancers, depending on their location. Intrinsic cancers of the larynx arise in the vocal cords. Seventy percent of all laryngeal cancers are intrinsic. Extrinsic cancers of the larynx extend beyond the vocal cords. Hoarseness is an early symptom of the intrinsic lesions, but is a late symptom of the extrinsic lesions. Cancers in the supraglottic (above the vocal cords) area and in the hypopharynx (below the pharynx) area can be silent. These cancers present at a more advanced stage of malignancy and are more likely to spread to other tissues than are laryngeal carcinomas.

Radiation may be an appropriate treatment for cancer-in-situ of the larynx. This treatment has the advantage of preserving a normal voice. Early lesions also may be treated by removing one side of the larynx and thus preserving a useful, albeit not normal, voice. For more advanced lesions, the removal of the larynx in a *laryngectomy* and the creation of a tracheotomy are preferred to radiation treatments. Laryngectomy is accompanied by the loss of natural voice, but about two-thirds of laryngectomy patients develop effective esophageal speech after the surgery. The cure rate for early stages of cancer of the larynx is high, but the rate decreases with advanced disease.

Disorders of the Pleura and Pleural Cavity

As noted earlier in this chapter, in a healthy patient, the pleural cavity is only the *potential* space between the two layers of the pleural membrane. In diseased states, air, fluid, or pus accumulates in this space. Disorders of the pleura and pleural cavity include pleurisy, pleural effusion, and empyema.

Pleurisy is a condition characterized by inflammation of the pleura. It may occur with or without fluid in the pleural space. The most common cause of pleurisy is a bacterial pneumonia, but the condition may complicate viral pneumonia, pulmonary infarction, pulmonary malignancy, trauma to the chest wall, pericarditis, and other pulmonary and nonpulmonary diseases. Chest pain, aggravated by deep inspiration, is the major symptom of pleurisy. The movement of the pleural surfaces during breathing produces a friction rub in a patient who has pleurisy. A crackling or grating noise may be heard by listening to the pleurisy patient's chest.

Pleurisy may resolve or may progress to pleurisy with effusion. *Pleural effusion* is a condition characterized by the development of fluid in the pleural cavity. It usually indicates pleural infection, but may also accompany pulmonary infarct or a malignant process.

Figure 8–3 lists the types of pleural effusion, the characteristics of the fluid, and a few of the primary conditions that may produce or accompany the pleural effusion.

The manifestations of pleural effusion depend on the signs and symptoms of the primary disease and the amount of fluid in the pleural cavity. Very large collections of fluid will compress the lung, producing a marked shortness of breath. A chest x-ray can generally detect fluid in the pleural cavity. A *thoracentesis*, the removal of pleural fluid through a needle, has both diagnostic and therapeutic value. The fluid removed by thoracentesis may be clear, a condition known as *hydrothorax*; pus-filled, a condition called *pyothorax*; or bloody, a condition called *hemothorax.* Hydrothorax may accompany severe congestive heart failure, cirrhosis, and certain types of kidney disease. A thoracentesis often includes a biopsy of the pleura. This biopsy may reveal cancer or tuberculosis.

Empyema is a condition that is characterized by the presence of pus in the pleural cavity. This disorder results from bacterial infection and may be acute or chronic. Empyema occurs as a complication of pneumonia, lung abscess, bronchiectasis (which will be discussed later in this chapter), or tuberculosis. Empyema also may result from the introduction of bacteria into the pleural cavity as a result of penetrating wounds of the chest wall. Empyema is treated with antibiotics and/or drainage of the pus.

Disorders of the Bronchi and Lungs

Many of the disorders affecting the bronchi or lungs tend to spread from one to the other. Nearly all disorders of the bronchi and lungs

Figure 8–3.
Types and Characteristics of Pleural Effusion.

Type of Pleural Effusion	Character of Pleural Fluid	Associated Conditions
Hydrothorax	Clear yellow	Cardiac failure, cirrhosis with ascites, nephrotic syndrome
Pyothorax	Cloudy with pus	Bacterial pneumonia, lung abscess
Hemothorax	Blood-tinged or bloody	Carcinoma, pulmonary infarction

have at least the potential of serious consequences. Some of the most common diseases of the bronchi and lungs are acute diseases, but other pulmonary disorders are chronic. As defined in Chapter 2, *Scientific Background for the Study of Disease*, an acute disorder is generally characterized by a sudden onset and a relatively short course of illness, and a chronic disorder is generally characterized by a slow onset and a relatively long and progressive course of illness.

Acute and Chronic Bronchitis

Acute bronchitis is an acute inflammation of the tracheobronchial tree and is often a part of a general acute URI. It may result from the inhalation of irritating chemicals. Early symptoms of the URI are followed by a cough, which indicates the beginning of the bronchitis. The condition is generally followed by complete healing with a return to normal function. Acute bronchitis is the most common disease of the tracheobronchial tree.

Chronic bronchitis is a chronic inflammation of the tracheobronchial tree and is a distinct pathological entity. The chronic form does not refer merely to repeated attacks of acute bronchitis, although repeated acute attacks may lead to chronic bronchitis. The diagnosis of chronic bronchitis is made on the history of a chronic cough that produces sputum. *Sputum* is mucus-like matter that is ejected from a person's lungs, bronchi, and trachea through the mouth. Mild forms of chronic bronchitis may exist for years as a "smoker's cough." The disease commonly progresses slowly, and patients experience increases in both cough and sputum production. Pulmonary function tests for chronic bronchitis show early and progressive changes.

Cigarette smoking is the most important predisposing factor for this disease, although air pollution, certain occupations, and untreated bacterial infections also contribute to the onset of chronic bronchitis. Recurrent severe bronchial infections can lead to more serious disorders. Mortality depends on whether generalized obstructive changes develop in the bronchi.

Influenza

Influenza is an acute viral disease that has predominantly respiratory manifestations. It is characterized by fever, muscle aches, headaches, runny nose, cough, and malaise. Three viruses, each of which may be associated with several strains, cause influenza. The disease may occur sporadically in a localized distribution, or it can occur as a major epidemic with frequent, severe complications that occasionally lead to death.

The most common complication of influenza is pneumonia. Life-threatening pneumonia is most common in persons at high risk: the elderly, pregnant women, and individuals who have heart, kidney, or lung disease. Myocarditis occasionally occurs as a complication of influenza. Furthermore, Reye's syndrome, which is discussed in Chapter 14, *The Nervous System*, has been reported as a complication of influenza in children, especially those children who are given aspirin for flu symptoms.

Influenza vaccine is the mainstay of influenza prevention. Unfortunately, a "flu" vaccine offers little cross-protection if its virus strain is not the same as the virus to which a person is exposed. Rest and supportive care are the principal treatments for individuals who have influenza. Antibiotics treat secondary bacterial respiratory complications. Amantadine, which is an antiviral compound, can be an effective preventive agent against several strains of influenza, especially for the elderly and other patients at risk for complications of influenza. However, Amantadine users sometimes experience side effects on their central nervous systems. Fortunately, these side effects generally are mild and disappear promptly when use of the drug is discontinued.

Pneumonia

Pneumonia is an acute infection of the alveolar spaces of the lung and may be caused by many different types of bacteria, viruses, and other microorganisms. If the bacterium causing the pneumonia is known, its name is commonly used to describe the patient's condition. For example, if a streptococcus bacterium is causing the illness, the patient is suffering from streptococcal pneumonia. Pneumonias caused by viruses are known simply as viral pneumonias.

Infectious organisms which are neither viruses nor bacteria may also cause pneumonia. For example, pneumocystis carinii pneumonia is caused by a protozoa. This unusual type of infection, which is usually lethal if left untreated, has emerged as a complication of intensive immunosuppressive therapy and end-stage HIV infection. Intensive immunosuppressive therapy alters the body's immune response and is used for treatment of cancer.

In most instances, an upper respiratory infection will precede pneumonia. Most pneumonia patients experience chills, fever, chest pain, coughing, and they cough up sputum mixed with blood. Generally, patients who have pneumonia are acutely ill. Complications of pneumonia include the presence of liquid in the pleural cavity, the collection of pus in the chest, inflammation of the pericardium and endocardium, lung abscess, and meningitis. Other organs, including the liver, spleen, kidney, and gastrointestinal tract, may be involved if the infection process is severe. Generally, the clinical manifestations and complications of pneumonia depend on the specific microbe causing the infection.

With appropriate antibiotic therapy, most individuals who have bacterial pneumonia recover. The prognosis may be affected adversely by infancy, old age, pregnancy, and the presence of other disease, particularly a debilitating one. Vaccination with an antipneumococcic vaccine has some benefit for selected persons in certain groups that demonstrate increased mortality from pneumococcal pneumonia despite appropriate therapy. Most viral pneumonia patients recover completely once the disease has run its course.

Asthma

Bronchial asthma is a symptom-complex that is characterized by shortness of breath and wheezing and is caused by constriction of the smaller bronchi and bronchioles. Asthma occurs in one to two percent of the population, and allergic or presumed allergic factors are responsible for most cases. Because inflammation of the bronchial mucous membrane plays a significant role in triggering bronchospasm, treatment is directed at this element.

In the course of a severe bronchial infection, some individuals develop asthma-like signs and symptoms. The term *asthmatic bronchitis* is used to designate asthma-like attacks that occur during the course of a bronchitis or other respiratory tract infection. Figure 8–4 compares extrinsic asthma and intrinsic asthma. A clear separation between extrinsic and intrinsic asthma, as Figure 8–4 suggests, often is not possible because clinical manifestations typically are the same. However, the treatments of intrinsic asthma and extrinsic asthma differ.

Bronchoconstriction causing asthma symptoms also may occur in response to psychologic stress in individuals whose bronchi are already hyperactive from some other cause. Fatigue and cold air inhalation may also influence the frequency and severity of asthmatic attacks.

Symptoms of an asthmatic attack, including chest tightness, coughing, wheezing, and labored breathing, may last a few minutes to several hours and may have a wide range of severity. In rare cases, symptoms may persist as status asthmaticus[3] for several days. Between attacks the patient may be well.

---

[3]*Status asthmaticus* is also known as asthmatic crisis or asthmatic shock and is characterized by a sudden, intense, and continuous state of asthma and the lack of response to normal therapeutic efforts. Status asthmaticus can lead to death.

Figure 8–4.
Comparison of Extrinsic Asthma and Intrinsic Asthma.

	Extrinsic Asthma	Intrinsic Asthma
Also known as	Bronchial asthma Allergenic asthma Noninfective asthma	Asthmatic bronchitis Nonallergenic asthma Infective asthma
Age at onset	Youth	Middle age
Family history of allergy	Usually present	Usually absent
Evidence of allergy in patient	Usually present	Usually absent
Cause	An allergen, such as dust or pollen, or a food, drug, or chemical	Common cold, acute bronchitis, or exercise

The following criteria may be helpful in classifying asthmas:

- Mild asthma—no time lost from work; hospitalization not required; seasonal; lungs clear between attacks; no more than six attacks per year
- Moderate asthma—occasional brief disability; more than six attacks per year; attacks treated by adrenalin (epinephrine) or aminophylline
- Severe asthma—frequent disability and/or occasional hospitalization required; wheezing or rhonchi[4] present between attacks; treatment with cortisone or other steroids

Customarily, asthmas that begin during childhood become less severe and attacks become less frequent as the child grows older. The attacks may disappear completely in late adolescence. Nevertheless, if attacks do persist into adult life, especially if the attacks are frequent and severe, pneumothorax, chronic airway obstruction, and other lung conditions associated with severe disability may result. Treatment of asthma typically includes the relief of bronchial and bronchiolar constriction, the identification and avoidance of allergens, and the use of antibiotics for any accompanying pulmonary infection. Furthermore, severe asthma may require treatment with corticosteroids.

---

[4]A rhonchus (pl. rhonchi) is a dry, coarse rattling in the bronchial tubes caused by a partial obstruction.

Emphysema

Emphysema is an irreversible condition of the lung characterized by an increase in the size of the alveoli with destructive changes in their walls. The walls between adjacent alveoli gradually thin, then are ultimately destroyed. The alveoli fuse together to form air cysts of varying sizes. Emphysemic destruction of lung tissue can be localized or diffuse. The main symptom of emphysema is shortness of breath upon limited physical exertion.

Chronic bronchitis can be associated with emphysema. The destruction of the alveolar walls leads to the loss of associated pulmonary capillaries, thus reducing the ability of the lungs to exchange oxygen and carbon dioxide and leading to elevated blood pressure in the pulmonary artery, which is a condition called *pulmonary hypertension*. Localized, large solitary air cysts, in a condition known as *bullous emphysema*, occasionally occur in the absence of generalized emphysema of the lung. Pneumothorax is a common complication of bullous emphysema.

The degree of pulmonary emphysema is far greater among cigarette smokers than among nonsmokers and generally increases with age. Death rates from emphysema are far higher among cigarette smokers than among nonsmokers. A congenital absence or low amount of the enzyme alpha$_1$-antitrypsin is a cause of progressive emphysema in a young person. The structural integrity of the lung depends upon alpha$_1$-antitrypsin because it protects the lung from enzymes released from leukocytes.

As a result of the changes of aging, the walls between adjacent alveoli may become stretched and thin. In the past, this condition was referred to as senile emphysema, but unlike pulmonary emphysema, the changes produced by aging do not include rupture of lung tissue or bronchial obstruction. Aging will produce alveolar overinflation, but will not significantly reduce respiratory function.

Chronic Obstructive Pulmonary Disease

Chronic obstructive pulmonary disease (COPD) is a varied group of chronic respiratory disorders that are associated with varying degrees of obstruction to the flow of air during expiration. Increased airway resistance which results from increased mucus secretions represents a low degree of obstruction. A thickened bronchial wall from edema represents a higher degree of obstruction. Finally, a constricted bronchial wall from chronic inflammation with fibrosis represents severe obstruction. COPD results from chronic bronchitis, emphysema, or the combination of chronic bronchitis and emphysema, and it is closely associated with cigarette smoking. COPD is a major cause of disability in older people and is an increasingly important cause of mortality. The condition usually first appears in patients between ages 55 and 65 and is more common in men than in women.

Labored breathing upon physical exertion is the most common complaint of COPD patients. Other manifestations include a productive cough, wheezing, morning tightness in the chest, difficult breathing except in an upright position, weight loss, and recurrent respiratory infections. Right heart failure occurs in the end stages of COPD.

The chest x-ray is a poor guide to the early diagnosis and differentiation of COPD. The chest film is often normal in persons who have asthma and chronic bronchitis, and emphysema can be moderately advanced before it becomes apparent on the x-ray. FVC and FEV_1 are much more accurate measurements of the severity of COPD. The airways of patients who have pulmonary bronchial obstruction become so narrow as to limit the rate of air flowing out of the lung. These patients experience a slow, progressive reduction in ventilation function. Labored breathing and impairment of work capacity are related to moderately severe and severe airway obstruction.

The development of resting tachycardia and weight loss in individuals who have COPD are negative prognostic indicators. The development of right heart failure is another negative sign for COPD patients. Risk to the life of a patient who has COPD occurs with the development of (1) sudden airway obstruction from an acute increase in bronchial secretions, (2) heart failure, and (3) progressive cerebral oxygen deficiency, which is manifested by drowsiness, disorientation, and coma.

Bronchiectasis

Bronchiectasis is a chronic inflammatory pulmonary disease characterized clinically by a cough productive of large amounts of foul-smelling or bloody sputum, chest pain, and shortness of breath. Bronchiectasis is characterized pathologically by the localized destruction of the smaller bronchi, bronchioles, alveolar ducts, and alveoli. As a result of the weakening of the walls of the smaller bronchi from chronic infection, irregular dilation of these walls occurs, with resultant damage to the epithelial lining, thus interfering with drainage. As a result, infected bronchial secretions that perpetuate the destructive process are retained in the lung.

The destructive process of bronchiectasis may be confined to a small segment of one lobe, or the process may be widespread, involving the entire lung. Bronchitis with necrosis of the bronchial wall is a principal cause of bronchiectasis, which may also appear as a sequel to a severe pneumonia or infected obstructive atelectasis, a condition that is discussed later in this chapter. Another group of bronchiectasis patients have cystic fibrosis, a congenital disorder which also affects the gastrointestinal tract. (Cystic fibrosis is discussed more fully in Chapter 9, *The Digestive System.*)

Bronchography, in which a radiopaque dye is introduced into the bronchial tree and is followed by a chest x-ray, may confirm the diagnosis, extent, and location of bronchiectasis. However, CT scans are now being used more often than bronchography to diagnosis this disorder. Bronchiectasis patients usually receive antibiotic treatment. More severe cases of bronchiectasis, however, may require the surgical removal of the affected segment or lobe if the condition is localized and is causing bleeding or if the condition is not responding to medical therapy.

Pulmonary Fibrosis

Pulmonary fibrosis is a pathologic condition resulting from an increase in the fibrous connective tissue in the lung. It may be a localized lesion occurring in association with a single tubercular lesion, a localized pneumonia, lung abscess, or bronchiectasis. On the other hand, the fibrosis may be a diffuse process involving both lungs. Diffuse fibrosis most commonly occurs secondarily to chronic bronchitis, widespread tuberculosis, or other pulmonary disease, such as a pneumoconiosis, which is discussed below. Another clinical form of the diffuse disease, idiopathic pulmonary fibrosis (IPF), has no known cause.

Diffuse fibrosis is characterized by a reduction in lung vital capacity because the blood vessels surrounding the alveoli are replaced by dense connective tissue. Symptoms and signs of pulmonary fibrosis depend on the extent of fibrous infiltration. The key manifestation of diffuse fibrosis is progressive shortness of breath. At first this symptom occurs only during exercise, but as the process advances, the shortness of breath occurs with less and less physical exertion, and finally, in a few instances, the patient experiences labored breathing even at rest. A nonproductive cough and a low-grade fever also are common manifestations of diffuse fibrosis. As the process continues, the attending physician monitors the patient's arterial blood gases (ABG). Continuous oxygen therapy is required for patients who have severe oxygen deficiency.

Pneumoconioses

Pneumoconioses are a group of lung diseases resulting from inhalation of mineral or vegetable dusts from occupational exposure. Inorganic dusts generally do not cause observable biologic effects until the lung has retained the dusts for many years. The end result of a pneumoconiosis is pulmonary fibrosis, the extent and character of which depend on the type, size, and number of particles inhaled. For example, the inhalation of iron and carbon dusts are characterized by very little fibrosis. Silica and asbestos, on the other hand, cause extensive tissue reaction with a large amount of fibrosis. This fibrosis may be sufficient to reduce vital capacity and to predispose the patient to, and alter the course of, infections such as tuberculosis and pneumonia.

The pneumoconioses are classified by the type of dust inhaled:

- Coal dust causes *anthracosis*
- Silica causes *silicosis*
- Asbestos causes *asbestosis*
- Cotton dust causes *byssinosis*

A patient's symptoms depend on the type of dust inhaled and the degree of fibrosis; symptoms frequently include labored breathing, irritated dry cough, and occasional chest pain. In long-standing cases, the symptoms of COPD may be present. For those pneumoconiosis patients who show little tissue reaction and no symptoms of COPD, the life expectancy may be normal, especially if exposure to the irritating dust ceases.

Lung cancer is common among people who have worked with asbestos and is frequently found in asbestos workers who smoke. *Mesothelioma*, which is a malignant tumor of the pleura, is another type of cancer that occurs mainly in people exposed to asbestos dust.

Lung Abscess

Lung abscess is a localized infection that results in the destruction of tissue and the formation of pus. If the abscess ruptures into a bronchus, some of the pus may leave the lung through coughing. This action will create a cavity that is partially filled with pus, fluid, and air.

The most common cause of lung abscess is the inhalation of infectious material when the patient is unconscious or dulled from acute alcoholism, convulsions, anesthesia, diabetic coma, or other conditions such as esophageal dysfunction. Bronchial obstruction may lead to the compression of a bronchus, and this compression may lead to the development of an infection behind the compressed area. Abscess formation frequently follows staphylococcal pneumonia. Septic emboli in the lungs also may produce tissue death and lung abscess.

The diagnosis of lung abscess is made on the basis of a medical history of a cough productive of foul-smelling or bloody sputum and other nonspecific symptoms of pulmonary infection. Fluid in a cavity may show on x-ray examination. Typically, full recovery from lung abscess occurs following treatment with antibiotics. However, healing often results in scarring and fibrosis in the involved area.

Pneumothorax

Normally the pleural cavity contains no air or fluid. The presence of air or gas in the pleural cavity is a condition known as **pneumothorax**, and it produces some degree of lung collapse. Symptoms of pneumothorax include sudden chest pain and marked shortness of breath. Symptoms depend on the speed of the condition's development and the degree of lung collapse. Pneumothorax may be traumatic or spontaneous in origin. **Traumatic pneumothorax** is the presence of air in the pleural cavity caused by perforation of the chest wall, fractured ribs, crushing chest injuries, or any injury that permits air to gain access to the pleural cavity.

Spontaneous pneumothorax, on the other hand, may result from the rupture of a superficial emphysematous air cyst or may occur in the course of some other lung disease, such as bronchiectasis, lung abscess, or tuberculosis. In addition, spontaneous pneumothorax may occur in apparently healthy individuals. If no cause of this condition is discovered, the spontaneous pneumothorax is said to be idiopathic. Fifty percent of individuals who have spontaneous pneumothorax can expect a recurrence.

Spontaneous pneumothorax may not require any special treatment, other than that directed at the specific cause. Severe spontaneous pneumothorax is treated with a chest tube placed in the patient's pleural space to remove the air. Re-expansion of the lung, collapsed by the presence of air in the pleural space, will occur as the air in this space is removed.

Atelectasis

Atelectasis is a condition of airlessness resulting from a collapse of lung tissue. The process may be confined to a small area or may involve the entire lung. Collapse of lung tissue may occur when a bronchus is obstructed or may result from (1) pressure in the pleural cavity from large quantities of air, as occurs in pneumothorax; (2) fluid, as occurs in pleural effusion or hydrothorax; or (3) pus, as occurs in empyema. Obstruction of a bronchus may be caused by a thick plug of mucus or other secretion, a foreign body, or a tumor. Collapse of lung tissue occurs because the air entrapped in the alveoli is absorbed and, because of the obstruction, cannot be replenished.

The sudden development of atelectasis produces pain on the patient's affected side and labored breathing. If the area of involvement is large, cyanosis and shock may supervene. The patient's prognosis depends on the cause of the atelectasis and the extent of lung involvement. Successful removal of the obstruction allows air to enter the affected segment, and generally the lung returns to its normal state.

Pulmonary Edema

Pulmonary edema is a swelling of the lungs as the result of the escape of serous fluid from the capillaries surrounding the alveoli. This fluid may remain between the alveoli, a condition called *interstitial edema*, or it may enter the alveolar space, a condition called *alveolar edema*. The principal factor responsible for causing pulmonary edema is increased pressure in the pulmonary venous circulation as the result of the failure of the left ventricle to adequately pump the blood volume load placed upon it. Acute myocardial infarction, hypertension, and aortic valve disease are common causes of left ventricular failure. Mitral stenosis also causes an increased pressure in the pulmonary circulation by obstructing the emptying of the left atrium. Pulmonary edema also may follow or complicate kidney disease, inhalation of irritating gases, sudden administration of large amounts of blood or intravenous fluids, pneumonia, anemia, nutritional deficiency states, and certain lesions of the brain.

The diagnosis of pulmonary edema is made from the patient's history of labored breathing and orthopnea. *Orthopnea* is difficult breathing except in an upright position. Moist, bubbling sounds are heard in the pulmonary edema patient's chest, and diffuse shadows are seen on a chest x-ray. Pulmonary edema interferes with the efficient exchange of oxygen and carbon dioxide between the alveoli and the pulmonary capillaries. In a severe, acute attack, death may result from oxygen deficiency unless the patient receives adequate treatment.

Acute pulmonary edema is the chief characteristic of a lung condition known as adult respiratory distress syndrome (ARDS).

ARDS can result from (1) acute local lung injury, (2) massive nonthoracic trauma with shock, (3) pneumonia resulting from the entrance of foreign matter, such as food particles, into the bronchi, (4) embolism of tiny fragments of fat that have entered the bloodstream, often following fractures of long bone, and (5) overwhelming infection. A common aggravating factor in the development of this disorder is the overloading of the circulation with blood and fluids used in the treatment of shock. The principal signs of ARDS are severe, rapidly progressive labored breathing and cyanosis. The mortality from ARDS is about 50 percent.

Pulmonary Thromboembolism and Infarction

A *thrombus* is a blood clot. A thrombus may form in a patient's leg or pelvic veins, right atrium, or right ventricle. When a clot develops in a vein, the condition is called a *phlebothrombosis*. An *embolus* is a blood clot, bubble of air, tumor, or piece of fat, infected tissue, or other material that travels in the bloodstream to a distant location where it obstructs circulation. An *embolism* is a circulatory system obstruction resulting from an embolus becoming lodged in a blood vessel. A *thromboembolism* is the obstruction of a blood vessel by a blood clot, or a fragment of a blood clot, that has broken away from its initial site and has traveled through the bloodstream. The pulmonary arteries are common sites for thromboemboli to lodge. Pulmonary thromboembolism is also called pulmonary embolism (PE).

PE may develop in patients following surgery, trauma, congestive heart failure, atrial fibrillation, previous PE, use of oral contraceptives, malignancy, prolonged bed rest, respiratory failure, the postpartum state in new mothers, and pancreatitis. PE may also occur as a result of phlebitis of the deep venous system. Sometimes PE occurs without known cause.

An embolus lodged in a pulmonary artery interferes with the blood supply to the segment of lung tissue that vessel serves. If a major artery is totally obstructed, an infarction of lung tissue will occur. However, this major complication does not always follow embolism, especially if the obstructed blood vessel is small. Symptoms and signs of PE depend on the location of the embolus and the extent of tissue death, if any. Chest pain behind the breastbone or in the pleural cavity, expulsion of bloody sputum, cough, pleural effusion, fainting, and rapid shallow breathing are common manifestations of PE.

A ventilation perfusion scan is a highly sensitive test for diagnosing PE and actually consists of two scans. A *lung perfusion scan* involves gamma camera imaging of the patient's lungs to determine the distribution of intravenously injected radioactively tagged proteins in the patient's pulmonary circulation. A *lung ventilation scan* involves gamma camera imaging of the patient's lungs to determine the distribution of inhaled radioactively tagged gas in the pulmonary alveoli. The two scans are then compared to identify areas of mismatch. A normal finding virtually excludes the diagnosis of PE when the scans are performed soon after the suspected embolic event. However, the ultimate diagnostic study for PE is a pulmonary angiogram or arteriogram. The injection of the radiopaque material is accomplished through a cardiac catheter that has been advanced into the pulmonary artery.

Pulmonary embolism, with or without infarction, is an important cause of morbidity and mortality and is one of the most common pulmonary lesions hospitalized patients experience. Anticoagulants are the mainstay treatment for PE patients. A patient's prognosis depends on the extent of the infarction, the general health of the patient, and the degree of success in the prevention of subsequent emboli. The development of recurrent emboli may require the placement of a filter in the patient's inferior vena cava if anticoagulation treatment alone is not curative. In a small percentage of cases, death results from the original or recurrent emboli.

Tuberculosis

Tuberculosis (TB) is a relatively common communicable disease usually affecting the respiratory system and caused in humans by the tubercle bacillus, which is a mycobacterium.[5] In the United States and Canada, tuberculosis almost always results from the inhalation of infectious material. In some other parts of the world, the infection may also result from the ingestion of milk and other bovine products that have been contaminated by the bacillus. Furthermore, a recent increased prevalence of tuberculosis is associated with AIDS patients' weakened immune systems.

TB is characterized by inflammatory infiltrations, and although it usually affects the respiratory system, tuberculosis may also involve the bones, the central nervous system, the gastrointestinal and genitourinary systems, and the skin. TB may progress throughout one or both lungs. The formation of cavities in the lung, the development of tuberculous pleuritis, and the accumulation of pus are common complications of pulmonary TB. Advanced disease may

---

[5]Mycobacteria, unlike other bacteria, resist decoloration by an acid-alcohol solution following an initial Gram positive staining, and so tuberculosis is referred to as an acid-fast infection.

involve the patient's larynx, pericardium, bone, liver, peritoneum, and meninges. Healing following tuberculosis may involve considerable fibrosis and some calcification. The disease is classified as active during any period—and for three months thereafter—when tubercle bacilli are present in the patient's sputum. The tubercle bacilli may be present but dormant if the disease is not completely treated and can reactivate months to years after the initial attack.

A major tool in the diagnosis of tuberculosis infection is a tuberculin skin test. Infection by the tubercle bacillus results in skin sensitivity to tuberculin, which is a biologic product derived from cultures of tubercle bacilli. An incubation period of six to eight weeks between infection and the appearance of the skin sensitivity is typical. The preferred and most sensitive tuberculin test is the **Mantoux test**. The test is performed by the intradermal injection of a purified protein derivative (PPD) of tuberculin. A positive skin reaction in 48 to 72 hours, reflecting an allergic reaction to the tuberculin protein, indicates that the individual now has, or had in the past, active tuberculosis. Thus, the test's chief value is in screening out those who have not been exposed to the disease. The attending physician must perform further tests on individuals who show a positive reaction to the skin test. For example, a chest x-ray following a positive skin test will distinguish disease from infection without disease. Furthermore, the positive identification of the tubercle bacilli on a culture proves the presence of TB.

The discovery of several drugs that have significant antitubercular activity has revolutionized the treatment of tuberculosis. A common treatment program includes isoniazid (INH), a drug central to all treatment programs, in combination with rifampin (RIF) daily for 9 to 12 months. This program has a favorable outcome in 99 percent of tuberculosis patients. Daily therapy with INH and ethambutol for 18 months is an alternative treatment. This latter program is the least toxic, is suitable for patients who have minimal disease, is the regimen of choice in pregnant women, and is 90 to 95 percent effective. However, researchers are discovering an increased number of tuberculosis strains that are drug-resistant.

Sarcoidosis

Sarcoidosis, which is also known as *Boeck's sarcoid*, is a predominantly respiratory disorder that is characterized by the presence of microscopic, rounded tumor-like masses of tissue in the lungs or lymph nodes. These masses of tissue contain inflammatory cells and minute blood vessels. Sarcoidosis is a chronic disease of unknown cause, although genetic factors and hypersensitivity phenomena may play a part in its development. The most common symptoms of this disease are cough, bloody sputum, and labored breathing. Sarcoidosis most commonly affects certain lymph nodes and the lungs. However, it may also involve the patient's skin, peripheral lymph nodes, liver, spleen, salivary glands, eyes, and myocardium. Furthermore, elevated blood calcium, which could lead to the development of kidney stones, may occur in connection with sarcoidosis.

Sarcoidosis most commonly affects individuals between the ages of 20 and 40 and affects men twice as often as women. In the United States, blacks develop the disease about ten times more often than do whites. The earliest stage of this intrathoracic disease is symmetrical, bilateral hilar lymph node enlargement. The **hilus** of the lung is that area of the mediastinum in which the blood vessels, bronchus, and nerves enter the lung. The diagnosis of sarcoidosis is strongly suspected when the patient's chest x-ray shows characteristic hilar shadows. Patients who have sarcoidosis often have an elevated blood level of certain enzymes. A Kveim test is a diagnostic procedure in which a sarcoid antigen is injected into the patient's skin. A Kveim test is positive if a red papule develops at the site of the injection. A positive Kveim test strongly suggests the presence of sarcoidosis. Biopsy of an accessible lymph node or of the lung establishes the pathologic diagnosis of sarcoidosis.

The course of sarcoidosis is usually benign, characterized by remissions and flare-ups. Approximately 70 percent of sarcoidosis patients recover completely or with minimal residual disease, and about 30 percent progress into a chronic phase with extensive pulmonary fibrosis. The prognosis in chronic cases depends on the organs involved and the extent of the involvement. Common causes of death from sarcoidosis are (1) an irregular heartbeat produced by involvement of the disease in the heart's electrical conduction system and (2) pulmonary hypertension with **cor pulmonale**, which is a form of heart disease caused by high pressure in the pulmonary blood vessels, secondary to increased pulmonary vascular resistance.

Tumors of the Lung

The lung is the site of many types of tumors, most of which are malignant. Because benign tumors of the lung occur very infrequently, they will not be described in this section. Malignant tumors of the lungs may be either metastatic or primary. Lung cancer constitutes 16 percent of all malignant tumors and is the most common malignant neoplasm in men. In the United States and Canada, lung cancer is the leading cause of death from cancer in both sexes. Although mortality from other solid tumors has been declining, mortality from lung cancer has continued to rise, especially in women.

The most common tumor of the lung is metastatic carcinoma. Metastatic lung disease commonly originates in cancers of the kidney, thyroid, breast, prostate, testis, stomach, or intestine. Most often the tumor cells arrive at the lung through the pulmonary arteries, although some malignancies spread through the lymphatic system or by direct invasion. Lesions in the lung may be single or multiple. Multiple lesions and lesions that affect both lungs usually result from metastatic disease. Generally, the source of the metastasis is not determinable from a chest x-ray.

Primary lung cancers are divided into two subtypes: small-cell carcinoma and non-small-cell carcinoma. Small-cell carcinoma occurs in 25 percent of all primary lung cancer patients. This type of tumor usually is centrally located and is already large at discovery. Generally, metastatic spread has occurred at the time of the discovery of the lung lesion. Non-small-cell carcinoma includes (1) adenocarcinoma, (2) squamous cell carcinoma, and (3) large-cell carcinoma. Adenocarcinoma is the most common primary lung cancer, occurring in 35 percent of all these cases, and tends to be peripheral but may present with hilar or mediastinal involvement. A subtype of adenocarcinoma is bronchoalveolar cell carcinoma, which commonly appears as a peripheral nodule or with symptoms that are similar to a pneumonia. Squamous cell carcinoma, which occurs in 25 percent of primary lung cancer patients, tends to be central but can present as a peripheral cavitary lesion. Large-cell carcinomas, which appear in 15 percent of primary lung cancer cases, tend to be peripheral, poorly defined, lobular masses.

Pulmonary malignancies have no unique symptoms and frequently appear in the presence of other intrathoracic disease. When symptoms of lung cancers do occur, often advanced disease is present. Cough is present in 40 percent of lung cancer patients and arises from bronchial irritation. Bloody sputum, which results from the ulceration of the tumor, is present in 60 percent of these patients. Other common manifestations of lung cancers are wheezing, chest pain, labored breathing, weight loss, weakness, recurrent pneumonia, and hoarseness.

Tools for Diagnosing Lung Cancer. Physicians and medical technicians may use one, or a combination, of several methods for determining the presence and extent of malignancy in a patient's lung or bronchus. These diagnostic tools include chest x-rays, computerized tomography (CT) scans, cytology, and fiberoptic bronchoscopy.

An x-ray is the best and most practical first step in the detection of a lung tumor. The finding of an abnormal shadow on the patient's chest x-ray suggests a lung malignancy. Some lesions will produce a shadow close to the hilum, whereas other tumors will create a rounded "coin lesion" in the periphery of the lung. If the tumor mass obstructs a bronchus, the chest x-ray may disclose signs of atelectasis. Computerized tomography is extremely useful in clarifying the nature of lesions that are hidden by mediastinal structures on conventional x-rays, because the scans show the area in question without the overlying structures. CT scans are also sometimes useful for guiding biopsies.

Cytologic examination of biologic material obtained during a fine needle biopsy can provide important information for diagnosing lung cancer. Fine needle biopsy is practical, safe, reliable, and accurate. In fact, this method is 95 percent accurate for diagnosing peripheral carcinoma. Moreover, biopsy of a lymph node located above the collarbone provides positive results in 90 percent of lung cancers when the nodes are enlarged enough to be felt externally. Cytologic examination of a patient's sputum can also reveal malignant cells that indicate the presence of a tumor.

Fiberoptic scoping is useful for visual exploration of internal organs and spaces. For example, physicians can introduce a fiberoptic bronchoscope into the patient's trachea and bronchus during a **bronchoscopy** prior to surgery to assess the presence and extent of endobronchial carcinoma lesions. Because many cancers originate in the bronchial epithelium, bronchoscopy is also useful for direct visualization of the lesion and for obtaining a biopsy specimen. Furthermore, if the patient's x-ray indicates the presence of a malignant lesion, but the results of other tests are negative, direct inspection of the mediastinum by a mediastinoscopy and the biopsy of suspicious nodes may provide important diagnostic information. Often, a mediastinoscopy spares the patient more extensive exploratory thoracic surgery. Also, because mediastinal spread of the carcinoma is an unfavorable sign, mediastinoscopy is valuable in judging the operability of the cancer.

Staging Lung Cancers. After the physician diagnoses a patient as having a lung carcinoma, the physician then stages the disease in order to assess the extent of the cancer's infiltration, determine the patient's prognosis, and select the appropriate treatment or therapy. Small-cell carcinoma is staged as being either *limited*, which means it is confined to the patient's thorax, or *extensive*, which means it has metastasized outside the patient's thorax.

The tumor-node-metastasis (TNM) classification system is used for staging non-small-cell carcinomas. The prognosis is best, with a five-year survival rate of 50 percent, in those patients who have non-small-cell carcinoma and pathological stage I (T1, N0, M0 or T2,

N0, M0). Stage I includes those lesions that have not metastasized to regional nodes. Patients whose cancer has reached stage II (T1, N1, M0 or T2, N1, M0) have a five-year survival rate after surgery of 30 percent. Stage II includes those cancers that involve at least one hilar or tracheobronchial lymph node. The five-year survival rate for patients who have stage IIIa (T3, N0, M0 or T2, N2, M0) lung cancer is 17 percent, after surgery. Cancers that have reached stage IIIb (T3, N3, M0 or T4, any N, M0) or stage IV are considered to be inoperable. Stages IIIb and IV include those lesions that involve distant metastasis. The five-year survival rates for stages IIIb and IV are zero. Figure 8–5 lists the stages of the TNM classification system for non-small-cell lung cancer and their descriptions.

Treatment of non-small-cell carcinoma depends upon the cancer's diagnostic stage. The best long-term results of treatment have occurred with patients who have stage I small primary tumors. Surgery for this condition may involve the removal of a lobe from the lung if the patient has peripheral lesions or of the affected lung tissue if the patient has central lesions. Patients who have a stage II tumor in the hilum or mediastinum may be eligible for surgery, but the surgery is more extensive and the prognosis is poorer than for patients who have stage I tumors. Radiation treatment following surgery does not prolong survival in non-small-cell carcinoma. Chemotherapy is helpful therapy for small-cell carcinoma patients but is still experimental for non-small-cell carcinoma patients.

Figure 8–5.
TNM Classification for Non-Small-Cell Lung Cancer.

Stage	Description
T1	Lesions are smaller than or equal to three centimeters in diameter
T2	Lesions are larger than three centimeters in diameter
T3	Tumor invasion of the chest wall, mediastinum, or diaphragm
T4	Tumor invasion of the heart or great vessels, or malignant pleural effusion
N0	No lymph node involvement
N1	Tracheobronchial or hilar lymph node involvement
N2	Same side mediastinal lymph node involvement
N3	Opposite side or supraclavicular lymph node involvement
M0	No metastasis
M1	Systemic metastasis

9

The Digestive System

The **digestive system**, which is also called the *digestive tract*, is the group of organs that converts food into chemical substances that the body can absorb and assimilate. The chief functions of the digestive system involve: (1) breaking down solids into a liquid mass; (2) breaking down large insoluble molecules from complex foods into smaller, soluble molecules; (3) absorbing these soluble molecules into the bloodstream to transport them to the cells for immediate use or storage; and (4) eliminating the waste products of digestion from the body. This chapter introduces the organs that comprise the digestive system and then explains how these organs function. The chapter then addresses the major diseases that affect each component of the digestive system and concludes with a discussion of other disorders that are associated with this system.

ANATOMY AND PHYSIOLOGY

The digestive system consists of the organs of the gastrointestinal (GI) tract and certain accessory glands and other organs. The term "gastrointestinal" refers to the stomach and intestines. The organs of the gastrointestinal tract include the

- mouth, tongue, and teeth
- pharynx and esophagus
- stomach
- small and large intestines
- rectum and anus

The accessory glands and organs that contribute to the digestive process are the

- salivary glands
- liver
- gallbladder
- pancreas

Figure 9–1 illustrates the major organs of the gastrointestinal system.

The Mouth, Tongue, and Teeth

The **mouth**, which is also called the *oral cavity*, is located at the beginning of the digestive tract and includes the lips, cheeks, gums, and teeth. The hard and soft palates form the roof of the mouth, and the tongue forms the floor. The teeth reduce the size of food particles to make swallowing easier. The tongue begins the swallowing action and is the site of the taste buds. It also moves food around, facilitating enzyme action by mixing the food with **saliva**, a secretion of the salivary glands that is 98 percent water and that contains small quantities of enzymes. The enzymes start the breakdown of some sugars that are found in the food.

The salivary glands secrete two to three pints of saliva daily. The three pairs of salivary glands are the (1) parotid glands, (2) submandibular glands, and (3) sublingual glands. The **parotid glands** are the largest of these glands, and they lie upon either side of the face immediately below and in front of each external ear. The parotids communicate with the oral cavity by means of the **parotid ducts**, which are also called *Stensen's ducts*. The **submandibular glands** lie beneath the base of the tongue in the floor of the mouth. The ducts through which the submandibular glands communicate with the oral cavity are called **Wharton's ducts**. The **sublingual glands** are the smallest of the three types of salivary glands. The sublinguals are located beneath the tongue, in front of the submandibular glands. They have several ducts through which they communicate with the oral cavity.

Figure 9–1.
The Major Organs of the Gastrointestinal System.

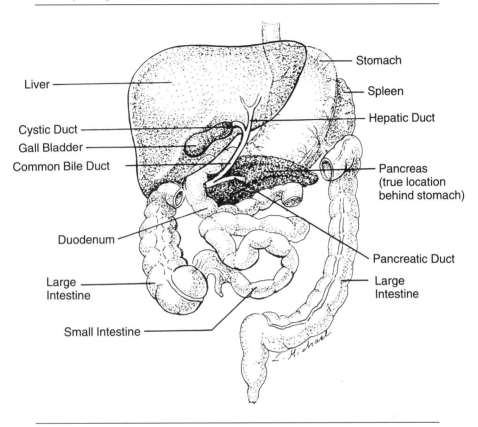

Stomach

Liver

Spleen

Hepatic Duct

Cystic Duct

Gall Bladder

Common Bile Duct

Pancreas
(true location
behind stomach)

Duodenum

Pancreatic Duct

Large
Intestine

Large
Intestine

Small Intestine

The Pharynx and Esophagus

The *pharynx,* as described in Chapter 8, is a passageway for air and food. The discussion of the pharynx in Chapter 8 focused on its function as a passageway for air, but the discussion of the pharynx in this chapter will focus on its function as a passageway for food. The **esophagus** is a muscular canal that is about ten inches long and that extends from the pharynx and connects the oral cavity with the stomach. (Figure 9–2 depicts the spatial relationships among the pharynx, esophagus, and trachea.) The lower portion of the esophagus, which lies at the junction with the stomach, is known as the **gastroesophageal junction**. At the gastroesophageal junction is the lower esophageal sphincter. A **sphincter** is a ring-like muscle. The

Figure 9–2.
The Spatial Relationships among the Pharynx, Esophagus, and Trachea.

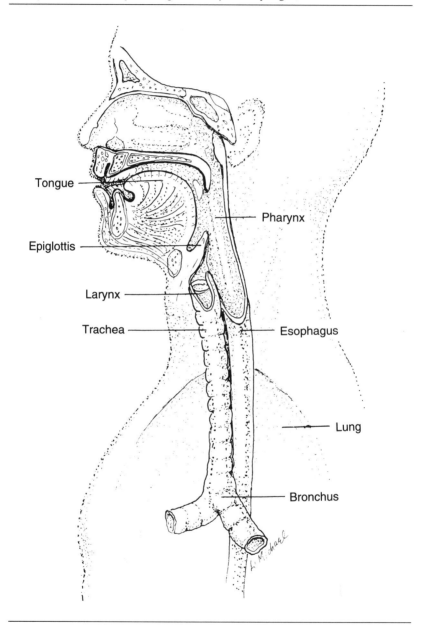

gastroesophageal sphincter relaxes—opens—to permit the passage of food into the stomach and constricts—closes—to prevent the reflux of gastric juice into the lower esophagus.

Deglutition is the act of swallowing. Once the food passes beyond the tongue into the pharynx, the process of swallowing is beyond voluntary control. Liquids and solid foods, chewed and lubricated with saliva, pass into the oropharynx, triggering the involuntary swallowing reflex. During this reflex, the soft palate closes off the nasopharynx to prevent nasal regurgitation, the larynx elevates, the epiglottis closes to prevent passage of food into the larynx and the lungs, and breathing momentarily stops. The constrictor muscles of the pharynx propel food into the esophagus where esophageal muscles move the food along by successive, involuntary, coordinated contractions. These contractions can occur in any hollow structure and are known as *peristaltic waves. Peristalsis* is the process by which peristaltic waves propel the contents of the hollow organ. The involuntary reflex that promotes peristalsis in the esophagus and the involuntary reflex that opens the lower esophageal sphincter assist swallowing. In the stomach and intestines, peristaltic waves move ingested solids and liquids through the entire gastrointestinal tract.

Liquids pass rapidly down the esophagus into the stomach, but solids take slightly longer. When the individual is upright, gravity contributes substantially to the passage of ingested material through the esophagus.

Organs of the Abdominal Cavity

The *abdomen* is the largest cavity in the body. The abdomen contains the greater part of the digestive tract, some of the accessory organs of digestion, the spleen, the kidneys, and the adrenal glands. The *pelvis* is the lower portion of the abdominal cavity, and it contains the urinary bladder, sigmoid colon, rectum, and some of the reproductive organs. Most of these structures, and the inner wall of the abdominal cavity, are lined by the *peritoneum*, the largest serous membrane in the body. For this reason, the abdominal cavity usually is known as the *peritoneal cavity*. Peritoneal fluid lubricates the cavity, reducing friction between organs. Figure 9–3 provides a cross-sectional view of the relationship between the peritoneum and the abdominal organs.

The Stomach

The *stomach*, the most dilated part of the digestive tube, lies just below the diaphragm and is a roughly J-shaped organ. The stomach's

Figure 9–3.
A Cross-Sectional View of the Spatial Relationship of the Peritoneum and the Abdominal Organs.

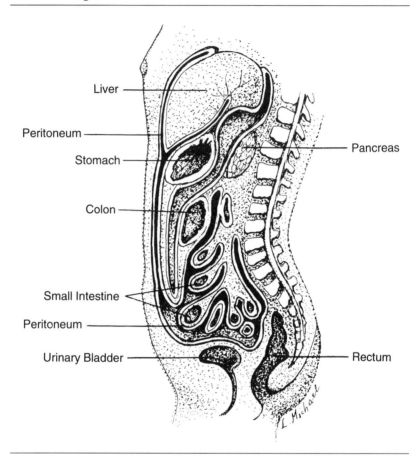

shape and position undergo continual modification depending on the amount of food in the stomach, the stage of digestion of that food, and the pressure from surrounding organs, especially the adjacent intestines. In addition, the position of the stomach may vary depending on the individual's body build. For example, the stomach may assume a lower position in tall and thin individuals than in short and heavy people.

The stomach has three main parts: (1) the **fundus**, which is the upper, expanded portion of the stomach, lies above and to the left of the esophageal opening, (2) the **body**, which is the largest part of the stomach, lies between the fundus and the pylorus, and (3) the

pylorus, which is the outlet of the stomach that communicates with the upper part of the small intestine through the pyloric sphincter. Other segments of the stomach include the ***cardia***, which is that part of the stomach that surrounds the esophagogastric junction, and the ***gastric antrum***, which is the distal portion of the body of the stomach that ends at the pylorus. (Figure 9–4 illustrates the parts of the stomach.) The stomach performs four functions:

- storing food during the digestive process
- digesting insoluble food by enzyme action
- manufacturing and secreting water, acids, enzymes, and mucin
- absorbing iron

Food enters the stomach through the cardia. Salivary enzymes begin the process of digestion in the fundus. ***Gastric juice***, which is a liquid secreted by the stomach lining that contains hydrochloric acid and digestive enzymes, assists the digestive process. The taste, smell, and sight of food and the distention and chemical stimulation of the stomach by food activate the release of gastric juice.

The process of digestion gradually liquefies the food in the fundus so that peristaltic waves can move the food into the upper part of the small intestine. Alcohol is absorbed through the mucous membrane

Figure 9–4.
The Parts of the Stomach.

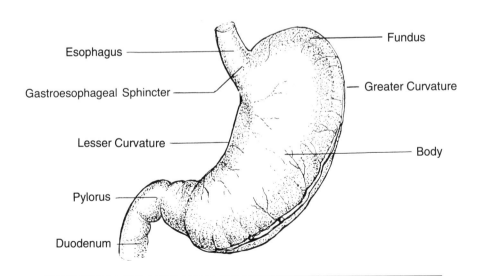

that lines the stomach, but only negligible amounts of water and glucose pass through the gastric mucosa. The average emptying time of the stomach is three to five hours, although fried and fatty foods that are irritating or difficult to digest may take longer. Fluids leave the stomach more rapidly than do solids. Emotional stimuli, such as fear, anger, and anxiety, also influence the emptying time of the stomach.

The Intestines

The *small intestine* is the tubular organ that extends from the pylorus of the stomach to the large intestine. Nearly all the soluble end products of digestion are absorbed into the body from the small intestine. The length of the small intestine varies from person to person, but is typically about 25 feet. The small intestine is divisible into three continuous, arbitrarily distinguished portions: the duodenum, the jejunum, and the ileum. The *duodenum* is the shortest, widest, most fixed part of the small intestine, and it is connected to the stomach. The *jejunum* is the upper two-fifths of the small intestine beginning after the duodenum and ending before the ileum. The *ileum* is the last section of the small intestine, and it connects with the large intestine.

The process of digestion that starts in the stomach continues as food enters the small intestine. Bile and pancreatic enzymes that aid digestion pass into the duodenum through the common bile duct and the pancreatic duct. *Bile* is an orange-brown or greenish-yellow solution that contains bile pigments, bile salts, cholesterol, minerals, and other organic substances. Bile salts break down fats, thus facilitating subsequent enzyme action. In addition, bile salts combine with dietary fats to form a water-soluble, easily absorbed compound.

The *large intestine*, which is also called the *colon,* is a tubular organ that extends from the ileum to the anus. It is about five feet long and has a larger diameter than the small intestine does. The large intestine begins in the lower right side of the abdomen in a dilated pouch known as the *cecum*. The *appendix* is a long, narrow, worm-like tube that arises from the cecum. The large intestine ascends from the cecum as the *ascending colon*. In the area of the liver, the large intestine bends and, as the *transverse colon*, crosses horizontally to the left side of the body. Then the large intestine extends downward as the *descending colon*. At the pelvis, the large intestine assumes an S-shaped loop, called the *sigmoid colon*, which averages about 15 inches in length. The sigmoid colon continues as the *rectum*, a somewhat dilated segment of the large intestine that measures about five inches in length. The rectum terminates in the *anus*, the distal opening of the digestive system to the outside of the body. (Figure 9–5 provides an illustration of the intestines.)

Figure 9–5.
The Small and Large Intestines.

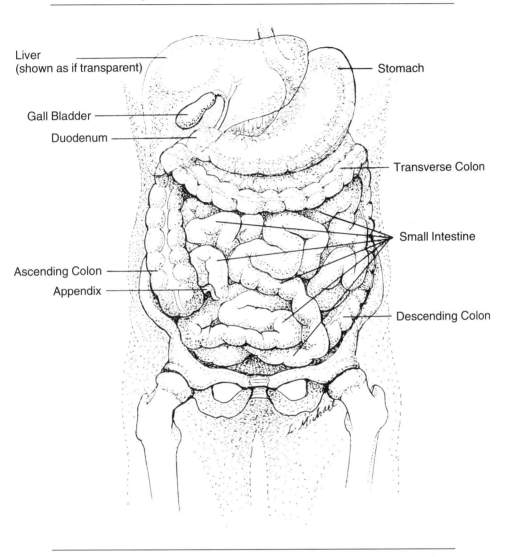

The main functions of the large intestine include

- absorbing water, thus reducing the waste products of digestion to a solid or semisolid state
- storing *feces*, which are excretions from the bowel consisting in part of indigestible matter and bacteria

- evacuating feces from the body
- producing certain vitamins

Food passes slowly through the large intestine, propelled by strong, slow contractions that originate in the cecum. In the large intestine, the digested food mixes with bacteria that are normally present in this location. The digested food may remain in the colon for 24 hours or more before peristalsis and voluntary muscle contractions result in evacuation. Only minute amounts of foodstuffs, mainly water and inorganic salts, are absorbed from the large intestine.

The Liver

The *liver* is the largest gland in the body, weighing about three to four pounds and measuring eight to ten inches at its greatest width. The liver lies in the upper right of the abdominal cavity and has four lobes. The right lobe of this gland is much larger than the other three lobes.

The liver is a vital organ, without which an individual would die within days. The liver has many important and diverse functions, among which are

- providing intermediate metabolism of amino acids and carbo-hydrates
- synthesizing and breaking down proteins and glycoproteins into less-complex compounds
- regulating lipid and cholesterol metabolism
- manufacturing and secreting bile, which assists in the digestion and assimilation of fats
- detoxifying harmful substances, such as drugs
- acting as a filter of bacteria
- manufacturing fetal blood cells, and after the person is born, the liver, as well as the spleen, acts as a reservoir for blood
- producing and storing certain proteins essential for blood clotting
- assisting in blood glucose regulation by converting large carbo-hydrate molecules to glycogen, which is stored in the liver for later use

The Gallbladder

The *gallbladder* is a four-inch-long pear-shaped sac that stores bile and is located under the right lobe of the liver. Bile leaves the liver through the hepatic ducts, which joins the cystic duct from the gallbladder to form the common bile duct. Bile may be stored in the gallbladder or it may pass directly through the common bile duct into the duodenum. The gallbladder stores bile so that a supply will be available to assist in the digestion of fatty foods. The gallbladder concentrates bile by reabsorbing water. In abnormal circumstances, the gallbladder's water reabsorption ability is a factor in the production of gallstones.

The Pancreas

The *pancreas* is a relatively long, narrow, and somewhat irregularly shaped gland that is located below the liver and stomach. The pancreas is both an exocrine gland and an endocrine gland. Glands are classified as being *exocrine* if they have ducts or *endocrine* if they do not have ducts. The secretions of *exocrine* glands exit the manufacturing gland and enter the body through a duct. On the other hand, the secretions of *endocrine* glands empty directly into the body's blood or lymph. (This subject is addressed more fully in Chapter 12, *The Endocrine System.*) The pancreas secretes pancreatic juice and insulin. *Pancreatic juice* is an exocrine substance that moves through the pancreatic duct to the duodenum and contains enzymes that assist in the digestion of protein, fat, and carbohydrate. *Insulin* is an endocrine substance that regulates the metabolism of sugar.

Digestive Enzymes

Digestive enzymes are secreted by exocrine glands. An *enzyme* is an organic substance capable of accelerating or producing by catalytic action some chemical change in another substance. Enzymes are often specific. Digestive enzymes convert complex foodstuffs into forms that are easily absorbed into the bloodstream. Figure 9–6 lists some of the more important digestive enzymes.

DISORDERS OF THE DIGESTIVE SYSTEM

Disorders of the digestive system are common. Although some of these disorders produce severe discomfort but do not have lasting consequences, others are extremely serious diseases. Many of the disorders discussed in the following sections have similar presenting symptoms and may require sophisticated investigative techniques for proper diagnosis. Furthermore, disorders affecting the upper part

Figure 9–6.
The Digestive Enzymes.

Name of Secreted Enzyme	Gland Producing Enzyme	Substances Acted Upon	End-Products of Enzyme Action
Ptyalin	Salivary glands	Starch	Simple carbohydrates and maltose
Pepsin*	Stomach	Protein	Soluble proteoses and peptones
Trypsin	Pancreas	Proteoses and peptones	Amino acids
Amylase	Pancreas	Starch	Simple carbohydrates and maltose
Lipase	Pancreas	Fat	Fatty acids
Maltase	Small intestine	Maltose	Glucose

*Hydrochloric acid needed for enzyme action.

of the digestive system, including the mouth, tongue, and teeth, are largely the province of dentistry and other specialties and will not be discussed in this text.

Disorders of the Esophagus

The esophagus is the site of many disorders, some of which are mild and some of which are serious. Moreover, disorders of the esophagus may indicate the presence of serious disease elsewhere in the digestive system.

Dysphagia

Dysphagia is difficulty in swallowing from any cause and is often associated with discomfort or mild pain beneath the breastbone. Dysphagia may be temporary and intermittent, or it may be constant. Often it is a symptom of another disorder. Some common causes of dysphagia include

- congenital narrowing or closure of the esophagus
- obstruction from lower esophageal rings, carcinoma, or strictures

- muscular dysfunction
- nervous system disease
- local irritation
- emotional disorders

Esophagitis

Esophagitis is an inflammation of the lining or mucosa of the esophagus. The chief symptoms of esophagitis are pain, dysphagia, and heartburn. *Heartburn*, which is also called *pyrosis*, is typically described as a burning or fiery sensation located beneath the sternum or in the upper middle area of the abdomen and is caused by disease of the esophagus. Esophagitis may result from swallowing irritating substances, frequent vomiting, or the reflux of gastric juice. A *reflux* is a backward flow. Incompetence of the lower esophageal sphincter that is located at the junction of the esophagus and stomach often results in the reflux of gastric contents, including digestive juices, from the stomach into the lower esophagus, a condition known as *reflux esophagitis* or *gastroesophageal reflux*. Neutralization of stomach acid by drugs reduces the tendency of the refluxed juices to irritate the esophageal mucosa. Keeping the upper part of the body raised above the level of the stomach, even at night, will decrease the reflux.

Long-term or repeated bouts of esophagitis may produce a fibrous narrowing at the lower end of the esophagus. Stricture of the esophagus also results from swallowing corrosive chemicals, which cause dense scarring. Above the constricted portion, a dilated segment of esophagus may develop.

Hiatus Hernia

A *hernia*, commonly called a *rupture*, is the protrusion of any organ or tissue from its normal location through a weakened place, or actual opening, in the wall of the cavity that contains the organ or tissue. A *hiatus hernia*, which is also called a *diaphragmatic hernia*, is a condition in which a portion of the patient's stomach extends upward into the thoracic cavity through a weakened and dilated opening in the diaphragm. Normally, this opening, through which the esophagus passes from the thoracic cavity into the abdominal cavity, surrounds the esophagus tightly, preventing the stomach from sliding up into the chest cavity. In a majority of people, a hiatus hernia produces no symptoms. However, some individuals experience heartburn, bleeding, and pain after eating. Sometimes the symptoms of a hiatus hernia mimic those of ischemic heart disease, cholecystitis, or peptic ulcer. Cholecystitis and peptic ulcers will be discussed later in this chapter.

Medical management of hiatus hernia with gastroesophageal reflux includes

- modification of the patient's diet, such as the elimination of spicy foods or a reduction in the quantity of food consumed
- elevation of the patient's head when sleeping
- antacid therapy
- medicines that inhibit acid production and that decrease gastroesophageal reflux
- avoiding caffeine and nicotine

Persistent heartburn or pain under the sternum despite medical management, or the development of significant complications, such as esophageal stricture or ulceration and bleeding, may require surgical treatment to secure the stomach on the abdominal side of the diaphragm to prevent reflux.

Achalasia and Diffuse Spasm of the Esophagus

Achalasia is a disorder in which the esophageal contracture is markedly ineffective and the lower esophageal sphincter over-contracts and is unable to relax and permit food to enter the stomach. The cause of achalasia is unknown. Achalasia used to be known as "cardiospasm," but the medical community now considers the latter term to be inaccurate and misleading. Treatment of achalasia by forced dilation of the esophageal sphincter is effective in 80 percent of patients who have this disorder. Surgery, which is performed on patients for whom forced dilation is not effective, is successful in 85 percent of these patients.

Diffuse spasm of the esophagus is a condition that is characterized by repetitive, nonperistaltic, and often powerful contractions of the esophagus. This condition affects patients in all age groups, but its cause is obscure. Dysphagia and pain beneath the sternum are the major symptoms of diffuse spasm and are usually intermittent. The diagnosis of diffuse esophageal spasm can be confirmed by a barium swallow study of the patient's esophagus. The treatment for esophageal spasm includes drug therapy, sometimes with nitroglycerine, and medical treatment of esophagitis, if the latter condition is present.

Esophageal Rings and Esophageal Varices

A lower *esophageal ring* is a thin ridge of mucosa that projects into the channel of the lower esophagus, usually at or near the gastroesophageal junction. Some rings go undetected because they cause no symptoms, but others cause marked dysphagia. Various theories have attempted to explain the development of esophageal rings, which affect both genders equally, but the origin of the rings is still unknown. Patients who have dysphagia resulting from esophageal rings are often under emotional stress, eat hurriedly, and complain that food sticks when they attempt to swallow. The clinical course of esophageal rings is relatively benign, and so surgery is rarely necessary. In fact, many individuals who have this condition adjust by learning to eat more slowly and by chewing their food thoroughly before swallowing. However, some of these patients will require dilation treatment.

Esophageal varices are dilated, or varicose, veins that surround the lower part of the esophagus and that are prone to rupture. They develop from the slowing or stoppage of normal bloodflow and from pressure on the venous system resulting from the obstruction of veins serving the liver. The most common cause of this venous obstruction is cirrhosis of the liver. Manifestations of esophageal varices depend on the degree of bleeding from the rupture. For example, small leaks may produce a slight anemia, but massive hemorrhage can cause irreversible shock and death. Vein shunting operations have met with limited success in treating the varices.

Carcinoma

Carcinoma of the esophagus is a major cause of dysphagia in older people. Most esophageal carcinomas occur in patients over the age of 50, and men are 7 times more likely to develop esophageal cancer than are women. Esophageal carcinoma is also associated with alcohol abuse, tobacco use, and chronic reflux esophagitis. Many of these cancer patients exhibit early symptoms of dysphagia, substernal pain, weight loss, and pulmonary problems. The carcinoma lesion is detectable by an x-ray study after a barium swallow or by esophagoscopy. The latter procedure allows for the direct visualization and a biopsy of the lesion. The usual treatment for carcinoma of the esophagus is surgical removal of the affected tissue, followed by supervoltage x-ray therapy. Unfortunately, the prognosis for these cancer patients is very poor, in large part because in a significant number of them, the cancer has spread to the pleura, pericardium, or lymph nodes.

Procedures Used in Diagnosing Esophageal Disorders

Physicians can study the patient's esophagus by performing (1) a barium swallow followed by an x-ray, (2) fiberoptic endoscopy, or (3) esophageal manometry. The barium swallow procedure is generally the first part of an upper gastrointestinal (upper GI) series and requires that the patient drink some radiopaque barium liquid. The x-rays that are taken of the patient's digestive tract immediately following the swallow indicate the path of the barium through the patient's body.

Fiberoptic endoscopy is a diagnostic procedure in which the physician directly views the patient's esophagus through a fiberoptic endoscope that has been inserted through the patient's mouth. The physician may also use endoscopy to determine the extent and location of a narrowing of the patient's esophagus and to dilate the narrowed section. Furthermore, endoscopy is valuable in evaluating the severity of esophageal varices. In addition, the physician can perform an endoscopy to obtain a tissue sample of an esophageal lesion in order to determine if the lesion is malignant or benign.

Esophageal manometry is a procedure that measures muscular pressures and dysfunctions of peristalsis in the patient's esophagus. This procedure is useful in diagnosing achalasia, diffuse spasm, and lower esophageal sphincter disorders. Physicians also use esophageal manometry to evaluate the effectiveness of therapeutic procedures such as antireflex surgery and forced dilation.

Disorders of the Stomach

The stomach is the site of several disorders, many of which are not serious and merely cause temporary discomfort. Other gastric disorders are quite serious and have significant morbidity and mortality implications. This section will address a few disorders of the stomach, including dyspepsia, gastritis, hypochlorhydria and achlorhydria, peptic ulcers, and gastric tumors.

Dyspepsia

Dyspepsia, or *indigestion*, is a common nonspecific designation for discomfort resulting from a wide variety of diseases that originate in the gastrointestinal tract, other abdominal organs, or elsewhere in the patient's body. Individuals who have dyspepsia experience (1) nausea, (2) heartburn, (3) abdominal pain or discomfort that typically is relieved by drinking milk, eating food, or taking antacid medication, and/or (4) belching, bloating, or gaseous distention with a sense of fullness.

Dyspepsia usually occurs after an individual eats too much or too rapidly, drinks excessive amounts of carbonated beverages, smokes excessively, or is under emotional stress. Persistent indigestion can be symptomatic of a serious disease, such as a peptic ulcer, gallbladder disease, malignancy, or heart disease. The severity and chronic nature of the symptoms of indigestion are important factors in determining the seriousness of the cause of the discomfort.

Gastritis

Acute gastritis is an acute inflammation of the lining of the stomach. It often results from the hypersecretion of acid by the patient's stomach. This disorder may also arise from the patient's overindulgence in alcohol, ingestion of spicy foods, consumption of certain drugs, such as aspirin or nonsteroidal anti-inflammatory drugs (NSAIDs), or use of tobacco. Acute gastritis may also result from food poisoning, acute infections, bacterial toxins, or uremia. Manifestations of gastritis include abdominal pain and dyspepsia. If the inflammation of the stomach lining leads to multiple minute erosions and ulcerations, the patient may also experience *hematemesis*—bloody vomiting—and *melena*—the passage of stools darkened by blood. Episodes of acute gastritis are usually of short duration. The identification and elimination of the causative agent of the gastritis is an important factor in the management of this condition.

Hypochlorhydria and Achlorhydria

The mucosa of the stomach, which is also called the gastric mucosa, normally produces hydrochloric acid and pepsin in amounts sufficient to maintain the normal digestive processes. Pepsin is a digestive enzyme. *Hypochlorhydria* is a condition in which the patient's gastric mucosa produces reduced amounts of hydrochloric acid. *Achlorhydria* is a condition in which the mucous membrane of the patient's stomach fails to produce any hydrochloric acid. Atrophy of the gastric mucosa results in reduced production of pepsin and acid, which in turn leads to pernicious anemia.

Peptic Ulcers

A *peptic ulcer* is a general term for any erosion of the lining of the stomach, duodenum, or esophagus that involves a single, small, circumscribed area resembling a crater in appearance. The ulcer results from the erosive effects of pepsin and hydrochloric acid. Males who frequently use cortisones, aspirin, NSAIDs, alcohol, or tobacco have a higher incidence of ulcers than do females and infrequent or non-users of these substances. Heredity is also associated with peptic ulcers. In fact, close relatives of individuals who have ulcers are three times more likely to develop these lesions than are individuals who have no family history of ulcers. Evidence also indicates a bacterium called Heliobacter pylori may cause some ulcers.

Peptic ulcers arise three times more often in the patient's duodenum than in the stomach, and they rarely occur in the esophagus and jejunum. Duodenal ulcers are usually benign and possess no potential of developing into a malignancy. Gastric ulcers, which are peptic ulcers that arise in the stomach, are also usually benign. However, gastric carcinoma also forms ulcers, and so a physician will need to perform a biopsy to distinguish a benign gastric ulcer from a malignant one. Symptoms of peptic ulcers are often intermittent and sharply localized. These symptoms tend to recur in spring and fall months. Common symptoms of these lesions include upper abdominal pain, heartburn, "hunger pains," nausea, excessive salivation, and other symptoms of indigestion. These symptoms may occur several hours after the patient has eaten or may precede meals. During an acute phase of a peptic ulcer, the pain may be severe enough to waken the individual from sleep. A patient who has a duodenal ulcer may find temporary pain relief by ingesting food, milk, or antacids, but a gastric ulcer patient will generally experience more pain after eating.

The main complications of peptic ulcer are (1) hemorrhage, (2) perforation of the affected tissue, and (3) obstruction. Symptoms of hemorrhage include weakness, fainting, vomiting blood or material the color of coffee grounds, or passing loose, large black stools. Hemorrhage occurs because a blood vessel at the base of the ulcer erodes from contact with stomach acid and pepsin. Another complication of peptic ulcers is perforation of the wall of the stomach or, more commonly, the duodenum. The perforation allows gastric juices and other stomach and duodenal contents to escape into the peritoneal cavity. This condition is a surgical emergency and necessitates the prompt closure of the perforation. The third common complication of peptic ulcer is obstruction at the pylorus. The obstruction may be partial or complete and may result from a temporary spasm of the pylorus, a condition called **pylorospasm**, or from a permanent narrowing of the pylorus, a condition called **pyloric stenosis**, as a result of scarring.

The diagnosis of peptic ulcer disease may be established by upper GI x-ray following a barium swallow or by fiberoptic endoscopy. If this disease is in an active phase, an ulcer crater will show up on the x-ray film. In the healed stage, only a deformity caused by scar tissue will show up on the x-ray. Endoscopy provides a method of direct visualization of the ulcer crater, and it may be used if the x-ray findings are normal or questionable even though the patient complains of persistent dyspepsia. Endoscopy also is useful for obtaining a piece of affected tissue for cytologic examination and biopsy.

Peptic ulcers generally are medically treatable by antacids, drugs that inhibit acid secretion, and, in some cases, antibiotics. Ulcer patients should discontinue the use of tobacco, aspirin, NSAIDs, and alcohol. These patients should also limit their caffeine intake, but are not required to adopt a bland diet. Most ulcer patients respond to medical treatment, but a small number of individuals develop intractable pain or hemorrhage, perforation, or obstruction, and thus require surgery. The objectives of surgery for duodenal ulcer are (1) to eliminate the disease in a manner that leaves the gastrointestinal digestive apparatus as normal as possible and (2) to achieve this goal with very low patient morbidity and mortality.

One of the most commonly performed surgical procedures to correct a peptic ulcer is a *vagotomy*, which involves cutting the vagus nerve pathways to the stomach and duodenum. Cutting the nerve relieves spasm in this area, assists in the emptying of the stomach, and reduces excessive gastric acid secretion. A vagotomy is performed in association with an *antrectomy*, which is the removal of part of the pylorus. A surgeon may choose to combine a vagotomy with a *pyloroplasty*, which is an incision into the pylorus in order to facilitate gastric drainage. Complications of surgery are recurrent ulceration, bile reflux gastritis, post-vagotomy diarrhea, anemia from the malabsorption of vitamin B_{12}, and *dumping syndrome*, which is characterized by symptoms including palpitations, light-headedness, and extreme perspiration after eating.

The mortality rate from peptic ulcers is decreasing, and the mortality risk in uncomplicated cases is negligible. Patients who are older than 40 and who have chronic ulcers or complications, however, present a higher mortality risk than do other peptic ulcer patients.

Tumors

Benign tumors sometimes arise in the stomach and duodenum. *Leiomyomas*, which are benign tumors of smooth muscle tissue, develop in the gastrointestinal tract more often than in any other part of the body except the uterus. The most common location for gastrointestinal tract leiomyomas is the stomach. Occasionally, leiomyomas ulcerate, causing hematemesis or melena. Polyps infrequently arise in the stomach and rarely arise in the duodenum.

Worldwide, gastric carcinoma is one of the most common fatal malignancies, but it is less common in the United States than in other countries. This cancer occurs twice as often in men than women. In North America, gastric carcinoma patients have a mean age of 60, and less than five percent of these patients are younger than 40. Individuals who are at greatest risk of developing gastric carcinoma have pernicious anemia, atrophic gastritis, and a family history of stomach cancer. Benign gastric ulcer is not a precursor of gastric cancer. Gastric carcinoma typically begins as a small growth that later ulcerates. The early phase of the growth of this tumor is often symptomless, and, unfortunately, when symptoms do present, direct extension of the malignancy to surrounding tissues may already have taken place. The most frequent manifestations of gastric carcinoma are indigestion, upper abdominal pain, weight loss, anemia, and loss of appetite. The diagnosis is made by x-ray, gastroscopy, and biopsy. Surgical removal of the portion of the stomach that contains the malignancy is the most effective surgical procedure for treating this cancer. However, a gastric malignancy is often metastatic at the time of diagnosis, and so complete removal of the tumor is not possible. The overall five-year survival rate for gastric cancer patients is approximately 10 to 15 percent.

Disorders of the Intestines

The most common disorders of the intestines are inflammatory diseases, such as duodenitis, acute enteritis, regional enteritis, and various forms of colitis. Other disorders of the intestines include irritable bowel syndrome, diverticulosis, and megacolon. The intestines may also be the site of obstruction and malignant tumors.

Duodenitis

Duodenitis is a general, nonspecific term that describes any inflammation of the duodenum. Duodenitis causes symptoms that are similar to those of gastritis and peptic ulcer. An x-ray will show duodenal spasm and irritability even in the absence of a demonstrable ulcer.

Acute Enteritis

Acute enteritis is an inflammation of the lining of the small intestine. This disorder usually has a sudden onset and is of short duration. If the stomach is involved in the inflammatory process, as it often is, the condition is known as *gastroenteritis*. If the entire gastrointestinal tract is inflamed, the disorder is called *gastroenterocolitis*. Acute enteritis is characterized by nausea, vomiting, abdominal cramps, and diarrhea. The condition may follow the ingestion of food contaminated by certain bacteria, especially salmonella organisms, or by staphylococcus toxin. Although most cases of acute gastroenteritis are caused by a virus, the disorder may arise from an allergy to certain foods, overindulgence in alcohol, and the use of certain drugs. It may also be a manifestation of a specific systemic infection, such as typhoid fever.

Regional Enteritis

Regional enteritis, which is also known as *Crohn's disease*, is a chronic, nonspecific inflammatory disease that is characterized by abdominal cramps and the passage of loose stools several times daily. The bowel movements of regional enteritis patients usually are not black or grossly bloody, but may contain minute amounts of blood. Low-grade fever, fatigue, abdominal pain, and unexplained weight loss may also be present in affected individuals. Regional enteritis most commonly affects the terminal portion of the ileum but may involve other segments of the intestine. Diseased segments of the patient's intestine may be interspersed with segments of healthy tissue throughout the intestinal tract. If the process extends from the terminal ileum to the large intestine, the condition is known as *ileocolitis* or *Crohn's disease of the colon*. The cause of regional enteritis is unknown, and most patients experience the onset of this disease between the ages of 25 and 35. If a partial obstruction of the intestine develops, the affected individual may have abdominal distention and vomiting. Inflammation and swelling of the bowel wall may lead to (1) ulceration with hemorrhage, (2) perforation, (3) abscess, (4) extensive scarring associated with narrowing or obstruction of the bowel channel, and (5) multiple abnormal passages, called fistulae, between the intestines and adjacent structures. A *fistula* is an abnormal passage between an internal organ and the exterior of the body or between two internal organs.

Acute regional enteritis is treatable with steroids. Patients who are very ill or who have complications, such as partial or complete small bowel obstruction, are hospitalized to receive intravenous fluids and steroids. Such a patient may require the injection of nutrients through a catheter inserted into the superior vena cava in order to bypass the gastrointestinal tract. Surgery may be necessary to treat persistent obstruction, abscesses, or fistulae. The disease may persist for years and feature periods of exacerbations and remissions, with each recurrence associated with progressive involvement. The prognosis for regional enteritis patients depends on the extent of bowel involvement, the duration of the disease, the condition's response to treatment, the length of periods of disease remission, and the extent of complications. Fatal complications of regional enteritis are rare, but these patients do experience an increased incidence of cancer.

Colitis

Colitis is an inflammation of the large intestine. The inflammation may arise from a wide variety of causes. The manifestations, treatment, and prognosis of a case of colitis depend on the specific cause of the condition. Two types of colitis are granulomatous colitis and ulcerative colitis. Figure 9–7 outlines some of the important differences between these two forms of colitis.

Granulomatous colitis, which is also called *Crohn's colitis*, is a regional enteritis that affects the colon. Although granulomatous colitis displays the clinical manifestations of regional enteritis, some of the features of granulomatous colitis are similar to those of ulcerative colitis, which is discussed below. For example, the symptoms of diarrhea and abdominal pain and the signs of fever, weight

Figure 9–7.
Features of Ulcerative and Granulomatous Colitis.

	Ulcerative Colitis	Granulomatous Colitis
Bleeding	Common	Unusual
Abdominal pain	Unusual	Common
Proctitis	Usual	Occasional
Strictures with obstruction	Rare	Common
Bowel distribution	Continuous	Often segmented
Risk of colonic cancer	Significantly increased	Moderately increased
Colectomy	Usually curative	Often palliative

loss, arthritis, and anemia are common to both ulcerative and granulomatous colitis. Colonoscopy is useful in locating the deep ulcerations, swelling, and fissuring of the mucosa and the narrowed sections of the bowel that occur with granulomatous colitis. *Fissuring* is the development of an ulcerated, narrow, deep crevice. Often, affected areas are interspersed between areas of normal colon. Biopsy will confirm the diagnosis of granulomatous colitis.

Ulcerative colitis is characterized by the frequent passage of stools that contain blood, pus, and mucus. In this form of inflammatory bowel disease, the inflammation consists of ulcerations confined to the innermost lining of the colon. The small intestine remains healthy. The medical treatment of ulcerative colitis is similar to that for granulomatous colitis and consists of corticosteroids, antibiotics, and drugs that lessen abdominal cramps and reduce stool frequency. Blood transfusions are sometimes necessary, and long-term drug therapy may suppress low-grade chronic inflammation. If the individual fails to respond to medical management, surgery is indicated. Surgical treatment of ulcerative colitis involves a total *colectomy*, which is the removal of the colon, and the establishment of a permanent ileostomy. An *ileostomy* is a surgically created opening from the ileum through the patient's abdominal wall. A bag is then taped to the patient's skin to collect liquid stool. Because of the ileum's contents, an individual who has an ileostomy must take meticulous care of the skin around the bowel opening to avoid skin irritations and infection. Other possible surgical procedures include making a distal pouch or connecting the ileum to the anal passage.

The recovery rate from a patient's first attack of ulcerative colitis is very good. A mortality rate of five percent occurs in those patients who have severe disease involving the entire colon. Better medical therapy and earlier colectomy for patients who do not respond to medical therapy have improved the overall prognosis for patients who have the acute form of ulcerative colitis. After an acute attack, 10 percent of patients will have a remission that lasts 15 years or more, 10 percent will have chronic symptoms, and the remaining 80 percent will have remissions and exacerbations of the disease over the years. Another reason for undergoing a colectomy is the increasing incidence of colon cancer in patients who have had ulcerative colitis for ten or more years.

Dysentery is another type of colitis, and it is characterized by abdominal cramps and pain, and frequent, watery stools containing pus, mucus, or blood. Two specific varieties of this condition are amebic and bacillary dysentery. *Amebic dysentery*, which is primarily a disease of tropical or subtropical climates, is an infectious colitis caused by the protozoan Entamoeba histolytica. The major site of involvement of this infectious colitis is the large intestine, but abscesses may occur in the liver, lung, and, rarely, the brain. ***Bacillary dysentery*** is an acute bacterial infection that is characterized by fever and bloody diarrhea. Bacillary dysentery is often spread through contaminated food and water or is carried by flies. Epidemics of this type of dysentery are most likely to occur in overcrowded populations that have inadequate sanitation. Preventing an epidemic of this disease, therefore, requires proper sanitation, including (1) thorough hand-washing, particularly before handling food, (2) immersing the dirty garments and bedding of dysentery patients in covered buckets of soap and water until the garments and bedding can be boiled, (3) using mosquito netting and screens on doors and windows to exclude disease-carrying flies, and (4) isolating infected patients. Bacteria that cause bacillary dysentery include salmonella, campylobacter, and shigella. Adults are more resistant to these infections than are children and usually have less severe attacks of this disorder than do children. Generally, bacillary dysenteries are self-limited and carry a good prognosis, but in isolated instances they may be fatal.

Irritable Bowel Syndrome

Irritable bowel syndrome is a chronic functional disorder of the colon that is characterized by chronic abdominal pain and intermittent and recurrent constipation and/or diarrhea. Additional symptoms include dyspepsia, bloating, headache, flatulence, nausea, and vomiting. Irritable bowel syndrome, which is also incorrectly known as *spastic colitis* or *mucous colitis*, is the most common disorder of the gastrointestinal tract and affects women more often than men. Patients who have irritable bowel syndrome and are tense and anxious, or are under sustained emotional stress, typically experience more symptoms than do those patients who are more calm and are not under stress. Abnormal colon neuromuscular function causes bowel spasm, which is detectable by an x-ray following a barium enema. No inflammation or infection is present with irritable bowel syndrome. The irritable bowel syndrome patient's stool may contain an excessive quantity of mucus, but blood usually is absent. Initial therapy for this disorder includes education about the disorder and dietary bulk. Anti-diarrhea medications are necessary for some patients who have irritable bowel syndrome.

Diverticulosis

A ***diverticulum*** is a mucous membrane-lined pouch or sac that protrudes outward through the wall of a tubular organ. Diverticula may occur in the esophagus, stomach, and the intestines. The presence of several diverticula, particularly in the intestines, is known as *diverticulosis*, a condition that occurs most commonly in the sigmoid colon. *Uncomplicated diverticulosis* is asymptomatic and is diagnosed by a barium enema x-ray study or colonoscopy. If diverticula become infected, *diverticulitis*, or inflammation of diverticula, results. The latter disorder causes fever, abdominal pain, and other manifestations that, except for their location, are similar to those produced by appendicitis. The complications of diverticulitis are (1) hemorrhage, (2) spasm or fibrosis of the sigmoid with narrowing of the passage, leading to obstruction, and (3) perforation, abscess formation, and peritonitis.

Typically, acute diverticulitis is treatable with antibiotics and other medical measures, but surgery may be necessary if complications occur. Repeated attacks of diverticulitis may call for the removal of part of the sigmoid. A *colostomy*, which is a surgically created opening between the colon and the surface of the patient's body, may be necessary in patients who develop intestinal obstruction, perforation, or abscess formation. A colostomy may be temporary or permanent. A temporary colostomy usually is constructed to divert the colonic flow so that a diseased segment of the colon can heal. Diverticulitis is rarely treated with a temporary colostomy.

Megacolon

Megacolon is a condition in which the patient's colon is abnormally enlarged. Congenital megacolon is known as *Hirschsprung's disease* and is a disorder of the intrinsic nervous system in the wall of the rectosigmoid area. The intrinsic nerve abnormality is responsible for a constriction of the bowel that results in massive dilation of the colon from the accumulation of feces near the diseased area. Surgical removal of the contracted segment and attachment of the descending colon to the lower rectum is the usual surgical treatment, but removing part of the colon during a partial colectomy may be necessary for patients who have extensive colon disease. Acquired megacolon may develop in any individual who has inadequate evacuation of fecal matter regardless of the cause of the condition.

Intestinal Obstruction

An *intestinal obstruction* is a major interference with the passage of intestinal contents. Intestinal obstruction may result from mechanical or nonmechanical causes. Mechanical causes of intestinal obstruction include (1) extrinsic lesions, such as adhesive bands and internal and external hernias, (2) intrinsic lesions, such as diverticulitis, carcinoma, and regional enteritis, and (3) direct obstructions, such as intestinal prolapse and a twisted intestine. Nonmechanical causes of intestinal obstruction, on the other hand, result from neuromuscular disturbances which produce either adynamic or dynamic ileus. **Adynamic ileus** is the loss of normal activity of the ileum. It is the most common cause of intestinal obstruction. **Dynamic ileus** is an overly active ileum. This condition is rare and results from intestinal spasm.

The symptoms and signs of intestinal obstruction vary, depending on the location and extent of the obstruction. Most patients who have a bowel obstruction experience intermittent abdominal pain and cramping, distention, and vomiting, and they pass little or no gas or feces through the rectum. Adhesions and strangulated hernias are the most frequent causes of obstruction of the small intestine. **Adhesions** may be thin, narrow, thread-like bands or they may be broad folds of tissue. In either case, adhesions can cause occlusion in many sites in the body, including the bowel. Adhesions may be congenital, inflammatory, traumatic, or neoplastic. They frequently develop after abdominal surgery. A **strangulated hernia** is a nonreducible hernia that is trapped so tightly that the blood supply to the protruding tissue is obstructed and is a surgical emergency. A **nonreducible hernia**, which is also called an *incarcerated hernia*, is one in which the protrusion remains in an unnatural location and cannot return to the customary location. If the protrusion can slip back easily into the abdominal cavity, the hernia is **reducible**. If the relief of the strangulation is not prompt, gangrene will occur in the trapped tissue. Furthermore, other nonreducible hernias may cause either incomplete or complete obstruction, but strangulated hernias always cause complete obstruction.

Intrinsic lesions may result from either inflammatory or neoplastic strictures. Inflammatory lesions, such as those that result from regional enteritis, produce a ring-shaped narrowing that includes scarring and stenosis of the intestinal channel. However, most cases of colonic obstruction result from a ring-shaped constriction that is produced by a cancer.

Two examples of direct obstructions of the intestines are intussusception and a twisted bowel. **Intussusception** is an infolding or telescoping of one segment of bowel into another segment. Most intussusceptions occur in the ileocecal area where the terminal ileum telescopes into the cecum. The largest number of intussusception patients are infants and young children. An obstruction resulting from a twisting of the intestine is called a **volvulus**, and it occurs most frequently in the sigmoid. A twisted bowel has a blocked channel. Furthermore, the twisting may cut off the blood supply to the bowel, thus causing an infarction of the involved segment. Surgery is necessary to correct this condition and to prevent the bowel from becoming gangrenous, although volvuli can frequently be reduced by colonoscopy.

Tumors

Tumors of the small intestine are rare. The most common primary neoplasm of the small intestine is the *carcinoid*, which can occur throughout the gastrointestinal tract, but most commonly occurs in the appendix. Carcinoid tumors of the gastrointestinal tract have endocrine activity. The manifestations of the carcinoid syndrome, which are seen intermittently in about five percent of patients who have carcinoids, include redness, cyanosis, diarrhea, peripheral edema, asthma, and evidence of right heart valvular lesions.

The frequency of metastases from carcinoid tumors varies with the location of the primary tumor. Carcinoids of the appendix metastasize very infrequently, whereas over 50 percent of carcinoids of the colon develop metastatic spread. The cancer can spread to any organ by metastasis, but the liver is the most common target organ. The proper treatment of a carcinoid is wide surgical excision unless the tumor has metastasized. Radiation therapy has little effect and chemotherapy provides pain relief, but not cure.

Polyps of the colon usually are asymptomatic, but in rare cases produce intestinal cramping, bleeding, or obstruction. Two types of polyps of the colon are hyperplastic polyps and adenomas. A **hyperplastic polyp** is an overgrowth of tissue and is not considered to be a neoplasm. Hyperplastic polyps account for 25 percent of all polyps of the colon and most of the polyps of the rectum, and rarely become malignant. Most neoplastic polyps start as adenomas. Therefore, these adenomas are considered to be premalignant. Up to ten percent of all polyps that are removed during colonoscopy show carcinoma-in-situ or early invasion at the tip of the polyp. Generally, the larger the polyp, the more likely that it is malignant.

Carcinoma of the colon has an unknown origin, but dietary factors may play a role in the development of the cancer. The risk of colon cancer is increased in patients who have a personal or family history of colon cancer and polyps of the colon. Ulcerative colitis and multiple polyposis are predisposing conditions for colon cancer, which affects males more frequently than females. **Multiple polyposis** is an uncommon, familial disease in which multiple polyps are scattered throughout the patient's large intestine. Most colonic malignancies are adenocarcinomas. Symptoms of colon cancer, which depend somewhat upon the location of the tumor in the colon, include bloody bowel movements, changes in bowel habits, distention in the abdominal area, and abdominal cramps. Abdominal pain will occur if any significant degree of intestinal obstruction is present. The diagnosis of colonic carcinoma is made following a patient's barium enema and proctosigmoidoscopy or colonoscopy and is confirmed by biopsy. Colostomy is an effective method of relieving the symptoms of obstruction, but complete removal of the lesion, if possible, is the preferable treatment.

Surgical Procedures Used for Treating Intestinal Disorders

Colectomy, ileostomy, and colostomy have already been discussed in this chapter as effective treatments for certain disorders of the intestines. Other types of surgery, such as ileotransverse colostomy and ileoileostomy, are also effective in treating certain intestinal disorders. An *ileotransverse colostomy* is a procedure in which the surgeon removes a diseased portion of cecum or ascending colon and then joins the ileum and the transverse colon. This type of surgery does not require an opening from the intestine to the skin. An *ileoileostomy* is the surgical joining of two segments of ileum and does not require an opening to be created on the surface of the abdomen.

Disorders of the Rectum and Anus

Many disorders of the rectum and anus are extremely painful but are medically and surgically treatable. The rectal and anal disorders that we will discuss in this section include hemorrhoids; fissures, abscesses, and fistulae; proctitis; and cancer.

Internal hemorrhoids, which are also called *piles*, are dilated veins in the lower rectum. *External hemorrhoids* are varicose veins in the skin and subcutaneous area surrounding the anus. Hemorrhoids are a common cause of rectal discomfort and itching and are the most common cause of rectal bleeding. A *thrombosed hemorrhoid* is a condition in which the blood within a dilated rectal vein clots. Although pain arising from hemorrhoids may be quite severe, corrective surgery is rarely necessary.

Rectal fissures are open, ulcerated crevices in the mucosa of a patient's lower rectum. *Anal fissures*, which are also known as *fissures-in-ano*, are open, ulcerated crevices in the mucosa of the anus. Both types of fissures often result from the passage of hard stools. Because of the constant presence of bacteria in this area, the fissures do not heal readily. Fissures can cause severe distress during defecation. An *anorectal abscess*, which is also called a *perirectal abscess* or *perianal abscess*, begins as an infection in the rectal glands that later invades the surrounding tissue. These abscesses cause rectal discomfort and pain upon defecation. A chronically infected fistula may lead from an abscess to the anorectal canal or to the skin near the anus and may be the source of an annoying, constant discharge. Anorectal abscesses and fistulas will not heal spontaneously, making surgical excision necessary.

Proctitis is a general term for an inflammation of the rectal mucosa and has many different causes. Proctitis that occurs in association with ulcerative colitis is called **ulcerative proctitis**. The presenting symptom of ulcerative proctitis is almost always rectal bleeding. In fact, minor bleeding may be the only symptom if the involvement is limited to the rectum. Ulcerative proctitis generally responds to therapy, but often recurs several times a year. This condition may worsen from time to time, but systemic symptoms and disability rarely occur. Other causes of proctitis include trauma, radiation, venereal disease, tuberculosis, intestinal infections, ischemia, and antibiotic therapy. Manifestations of proctitis include rectal discomfort, painful diarrhea, and rectal bleeding. The cause of the proctitis is determined by sigmoidoscopy, biopsy of the rectal mucosa, and laboratory examinations of the stools. Most cases of proctitis respond well to medical treatment.

The rectum is a common site for gastrointestinal tract malignancies. Carcinomas of the rectum usually are adenocarcinomas, but malignancies of the anal canal generally are squamous cell carcinomas. Rectal bleeding, irregularity of bowel movements, anemia, and pain, none of which is specific for malignancy, are common manifestations of rectal cancer. Creation of a permanent colostomy and the removal of a large part of the rectum are the recommended approaches to managing rectal malignancies. The removal of benign rectal polyps and precancerous rectal adenomas has sharply reduced the incidence of rectal cancer.

Disorders of the Liver

Nearly all disorders of the liver can have serious consequences. This section will define and describe some of the most common liver disorders, including jaundice, hepatitis, fatty infiltration of the liver, cirrhosis, and liver tumors.

Jaundice

Jaundice is a condition in which the affected individual's sclera, skin, and other tissues are stained yellow by bile pigments present in excessive amounts in the patient's circulation. Jaundice is one of the common signs that the liver is involved in a disease process, and a yellow tint in the normally white sclera of the patient's eye often is the first sign of this disorder. In healthy individuals, the liver filters *bilirubin*, which is an end-product of the destruction of aged red blood cells, from the bloodstream. The presence of increased levels of bilirubin is usually the result of disease.

Diseases that produce increased levels of bilirubin, and, therefore, jaundice, can be classified into the following categories:

- *Hemolytic diseases*, in which the increased destruction of red blood cells exceeds the capacity of the normal liver to remove the increased levels of bilirubin from the serum
- *Obstructive diseases*, in which the normal pathway from the liver through the cystic and common bile duct into the duodenum for the excretion of bilirubin is blocked, causing a back-up of bilirubin in the bloodstream
- *Hepatocellular diseases*, in which either the diseased liver cells cannot adequately filter bilirubin from the bloodstream or the amount of bilirubin that is excreted into the bile is reduced

Figure 9–8 lists examples of specific diseases that cause jaundice.

Two benign causes of persistent but mild and nonprogressive hepatocellular jaundice are Gilbert's disease and the Dubin-Johnson syndrome. Gilbert's disease results from a decrease in the ability of the liver to excrete bilirubin, resulting in elevated levels of bilirubin in the patient's blood. Patients who have the Dubin-Johnson syndrome have a congenital defect in their ability to excrete bilirubin.

Hepatitis

Hepatitis is an inflammation of the liver, and it can produce fever, malaise, loss of appetite, nausea, vomiting, abdominal pain, jaundice,

Figure 9–8.
Classifications of Jaundice.

Type of Jaundice	Example of Disease
Hemolytic	Congenital hemolytic anemia
Obstructive	Gallstone, cancer of the pancreas
Hepatocellular	Acute hepatitis, cirrhosis, Gilbert's disease, Dubin-Johnson syndrome

and **hepatomegaly**, which is an enlarged liver. The cause of the inflammation can be a viral infection or the abuse of alcohol or other drugs over time. Hepatitis can be acute or chronic. An acute attack of hepatitis is likely to progress to chronic active hepatitis and hepatic necrosis if (1) the patient's serum aminotransferase[1] levels are abnormally high for more than six months and show little sign of return to normal values, (2) tests indicate the continued presence in the patient's bloodstream of hepatitis B antigens, (3) the patient experiences continued symptoms of the disease, and (4) a biopsy of the patient's liver reveals hepatic inflammation that may progress to cirrhosis.

The three most common forms of viral hepatitis are hepatitis A, which is also known as infectious hepatitis; hepatitis B, which was formerly known as serum hepatitis; and hepatitis C, which was formerly known as non A, non B hepatitis. Immunological blood tests are necessary for distinguishing among the types of hepatitis. Hepatitis A, which is caused by the hepatitis A virus (HAV), is transmitted by close person-to-person contact and the contamination of water and food by infected feces. Immune serum globulin, an immunoglobulin, gives effective protection against the clinical manifestations of hepatitis A if the globulin is administered before or within two weeks after exposure to the virus. Hepatitis A is an acute infection and does not lead to chronic hepatitis.

Hepatitis B, which is caused by the hepatitis B virus (HBV), is spread by close person-to-person contact, injection using inadequately sterilized needles and syringes, and transfusion of contaminated blood. Individuals may continue to harbor the HBV long after the clinical infection has subsided, becoming hepatitis carriers who can transmit the disease to others. Vaccination against this disease is advisable for health care workers and other individuals who are at risk for exposure to hepatitis B. Hepatitis B progresses to chronic hepatitis in five to ten percent of affected individuals. Chronic viral hepatitis progresses to cirrhosis in one to three percent of these patients. The progression to cirrhosis may take a few months or a few years.

Hepatitis C, which is caused by the hepatitis C virus (HCV), resembles hepatitis B in its clinical course and complications. Hepatitis C can be transmitted by (1) unclean needles and syringes, (2)

---

[1]*Aminotransferases*, which are also called *transaminases*, are enzymes that are normally present in the blood serum and various body tissues, especially the heart and liver. Aminotransferase is released into the serum as a result of tissue injury. Thus, an increased concentration of an aminotransferase in the serum may indicate myocardial infarction, acute damage to liver cells, or muscle injury.

blood and blood products, and (3) sexual contact. Furthermore, some people may be carriers of the hepatitis C virus.

Most patients who develop an acute viral hepatitis recover completely within eight weeks. Fewer than one percent of these patients have a sudden, intense form of hepatitis that terminates fatally. Morbidity and mortality rates from viral hepatitis increase with patients' ages. Recovery from an attack of acute viral hepatitis can take a patient three to four months, and marked fatigue may be present during the recovery process.

Alcoholic hepatitis is characterized by fever, jaundice, hepatomegaly, and fluid accumulation in the patient's abdomen. Gastritis, pancreatitis, and hematemesis may occur in association with alcoholic hepatitis. Laboratory studies show that patients who have alcoholic hepatitis have abnormalities that are similar to those associated with viral hepatitis. Some alcoholic hepatitis patients who abstain from using alcohol recover completely, but others develop cirrhosis.

Fatty Infiltration of the Liver

Fatty infiltration of the liver most commonly occurs from excessive alcohol intake, but it may also result from excessive fat in the diet, chronic infections, metabolic disorders, or diabetes. In some patients, the cause of this condition is unknown. A fatty liver is enlarged, and tests of its function may or may not be abnormal. If alcohol consumption is the cause of the fatty liver, abstinence often reverses the condition. Acute fatty liver may also be a complication of pregnancy that results in high maternal and fetal mortality. The cause of fatty liver during pregnancy is not known, but is not related to alcohol use.

Cirrhosis

Cirrhosis is a chronic degenerative liver disease that involves the progressive destruction of liver cells. Areas of fibrosis and scar tissue that obstruct drainage through the portal vein of the liver replace the destroyed cells. *Postnecrotic cirrhosis* is a type of degenerative liver disease that results from the death of liver tissue following an attack of viral or toxic hepatitis that did not progress to complete healing. In this type of cirrhosis, the liver is shrunken, and the patient complains of weakness, loss of appetite, and jaundice.

Alcoholic cirrhosis involves the progressive destruction of liver cells resulting from long-term abuse of alcohol, which has a direct toxic effect on liver cells. The abuse of alcohol is the most common cause of cirrhosis. The nutritional deficiency state that commonly is present in chronic alcoholics may exaggerate the detrimental effects of the alcohol abuse itself. Ten to fifteen percent of alcoholics develop cirrhosis. Signs of alcoholic cirrhosis, which is also called *Laennec's cirrhosis* or *portal cirrhosis*, are moderate hepatomegaly, splenomegaly, fluid accumulation in the abdomen, small dilated blood vessels in the skin, redness of the palms, edema in the lower extremities, and, in male patients, testicular atrophy. In the early stages of alcoholic cirrhosis, the patient's liver is firm and nodular, but in the late stage, the liver becomes small and shrunken. The diagnosis of alcoholic cirrhosis is suspected from a history of alcohol intake and the presence of liver enlargement and is confirmed by a liver biopsy. Abstinence from alcohol improves the condition of some patients' livers.

Symptoms of all types of cirrhosis develop slowly and progressively over a period of years. These symptoms may include loss of appetite, vomiting, weakness, and abdominal discomfort. However, the development of jaundice, esophageal varices, and ascites are very poor prognostic signs. **Ascites** is a condition in which the patient accumulates fluid in the abdomen. This condition occurs when the patient's kidney retains sodium and water. Ascites occurs in association with heart failure and certain malignancies, as well as with the late stages of cirrhosis.

The major complications of cirrhosis that contribute to death are gastrointestinal hemorrhage, kidney failure, and brain degeneration, which is called encephalopathy. Uncontrolled gastrointestinal bleeding may result from (1) a decrease in the presence of clotting factors that a healthy liver manufactures in adequate amounts and (2) the rupture of a distended esophageal vein. The death rate attributed to cirrhosis has been increasing gradually but steadily over the past several years. An explanation for the rise in declared cirrhosis-caused deaths may be the increasing use of liver biopsy which leads to greater recognition of the disease. Death rates associated with cirrhosis are substantially higher among men than women and are higher in nonwhites than whites.

Tumors

Hepatomas are the most common primary malignant tumors of the liver, and they are characterized by (1) abdominal discomfort, resulting from an enlargement in the liver, stretching its outer lining; (2) fever; (3) jaundice; and (4) ascites. Sixty to seventy-five percent of hepatomas develop in association with cirrhosis. Although primary cancers of the liver are rare, metastases to the liver are common. The primary sites for these metastatic cancers are often the stomach, intestines, pancreas, lung, gallbladder, reproductive organs, and breast. Manifestations of secondary liver cancers depend on the type and location of the primary lesion. The prognosis for hepatic malignancy patients is grave, because neither surgery nor radiotherapy is an effective treatment for liver cancer. The life expectancy for most patients who have malignant liver tumors is four to six months after the discovery of the tumor.

Procedures Used in Diagnosing Liver Disorders

Specialized examinations are useful in the investigation of liver disease. For example, radionuclide imaging can show diffuse or focal liver enlargement resulting from hepatitis, cirrhosis, abscess, and primary and metastatic tumors. If an abscess or a tumor is present, the scan will show a well-defined area of decreased isotope uptake. In the presence of cirrhosis, the liver generally will be enlarged, but the radionuclide uptake on the scan will be decreased and will lack uniformity. This diagnostic method is also useful in evaluating jaundice. Liver scanning is most often performed on patients who have (1) primary cancers that often metastasize to the liver; (2) persistently abnormal liver function tests; or (3) suspected primary liver cancer. The presence of a discrete filling defect on the scan is an indication that a liver tumor may be present. Ultrasound, CT scanning, and MRI are also used to assess structural changes in the liver.

Arteriography of the hepatic arteries is useful in demonstrating the effect of a cirrhotic liver on the hepatic arterial circulation. Abnormal hepatic circulation may indicate the presence of primary or secondary liver tumors and portal hypertension. However, arteriography cannot distinguish between the various types of hepatic tumors and may not differentiate benign from malignant solitary tumors.

Another useful diagnostic technique for liver disease is a percutaneous liver biopsy, which usually is helpful in diagnosing most forms of liver disease.

Disorders of the Gallbladder

The gallbladder is the site of two relatively common disorders: cholecystitis and cholelithiasis.

Cholecystitis

Cholecystitis is an inflammation of the gallbladder. The disease may be seen as a complication of infections, and in most cases, is associated with gallstones. A cholecystitic gallbladder becomes inflamed and distended. In long-term cases, the gallbladder may become thickened and shrunken. Complications of cholecystitis include (1) *gangrene*, which is tissue death and decomposition, (2) perforation of the gallbladder, and (3) the accumulation of pus.

The pain of cholecystitis occurs in the patient's upper abdomen, particularly the right upper quadrant. The pain may be mild and incorrectly identified as indigestion, or it may be severe and incorrectly identified as a heart attack. Vomiting, fever, and abdominal tenderness are other common manifestations of cholecystitis. Some cholecystitis patients develop *cholangitis*, which is the inflammation of the bile ducts. Cholangitis impairs the ability of the liver cells to excrete bilirubin, thus causing jaundice.

Cholelithiasis

Cholelithiasis is a condition characterized by the formation or presence of gallstones. Gallstones are composed primarily of cholesterol and small amounts of calcium, bilirubin, and bile pigments. Usually more than one stone is present at a time. Stones vary in size from minute calculi resembling grains of sand to solitary stones that are greater than one inch in diameter. "Silent" gallstones produce no symptoms, but many gallstones cause cholecystitis and that condition's characteristic symptoms. When a stone passes from the gallbladder, where it may have remained silent for many years, into the common bile duct, the patient experiences severe biliary colic. This colic develops suddenly over the right upper quadrant, is spasmodic, and is very painful. If a stone blocks the passage of bile through the common bile duct, jaundice will occur. Patients who develop gallstones are likely to be older than 40, female, and/or obese. Women who regularly use oral contraceptives or estrogen, and people who experience malabsorption of bile salts are also more likely than the normal population to develop gallstones.

The management of "silent" gallstones is controversial even though the medical risk for developing complications is low. Symptomatic gallstones, on the other hand, require surgery. A *cholecystectomy*, which is the removal of the patient's gallbladder, is the principal surgical procedure for the treatment of gallbladder disease. Removal of the patient's gallbladder, however, may interfere with the patient's digestion because the large supply of bile normally retained in the gallbladder for the breakdown of ingested fats is no longer available. Individuals who have had a cholecystectomy should, therefore, limit their intake of fats.

Traditionally, the treatment for symptomatic gallstones was a cholecystectomy through an open abdominal incision. The recovery course generally was a five-day hospital stay with three to six weeks' convalescence. However, laparoscopic cholecystectomy is now available also. A laparoscopy, as defined in Chapter 3, *Specialized Diagnostic Techniques*, is a surgical procedure in which the surgeon can examine the interior of the abdomen by means of a fiberoptic laparoscope. The surgeon makes three or four small incisions on the patient's abdomen. Each incision is typically no more than one inch long. The surgeon inserts a fiberoptic light source in one incision and inserts a fiberoptic scope that is attached to a small camera in another incision. During the procedure, the surgeon views the patient's internal organs on a television-like monitor that is connected to the camera. The third incision is the location the surgeon uses to insert long, very thin cutting instruments during a laparoscopic cholecystectomy. **Laparoscopic cholecystectomy** is the surgical removal of the gallbladder during a laparoscopy. It requires general anesthesia and has the same risks and complications as open cholecystectomy, but patients who have undergone the laparoscopic surgery experience less postoperative pain, hospitalization of only one or two days, and a convalescence of only one or two weeks.

Furthermore, laparoscopy can be used in conjunction with laser technology to remove a patient's gallbladder. The surgeon removes the gallbladder by "zapping" it with the laser. The laser technique is like a laparoscopic cholecystectomy in that it typically requires that the patient receive general anesthesia, and most patients experience only a small amount of postoperative pain and do not take long to recuperate from the procedure.

Another method of treating gallbladder disease is the use of pills to dissolve gallstones. Drug therapy has resulted in complete or partial dissolution of stones in 50 percent of gallstone patients. In more than half of the patients, the oral administration of certain drugs will reduce the concentration of cholesterol in the patient's bile. A very high rate of stone reformation will occur after drug therapy is stopped unless stone-producing factors in the patient's diet are altered in the interim.

Still another way to treat patients who have gallstones is with a procedure called a lithotripsy. **Lithotripsy** is a noninvasive technique that involves the use of soundwaves to break down solid masses, in this case gallstones, into small pieces. The patient can easily pass the broken down gallstone out of his or her body. Sometimes lithotripsy is used in conjunction with drug therapy.

Procedures Used in Diagnosing Gallbladder Disorders

Oral cholecystography is a simple method of x-ray visualization of the gallbladder that follows the patient's ingestion of tablets containing a contrast agent. Upon reaching the small intestine, the contrast agent is absorbed into the patient's bloodstream. The liver removes this substance from the patient's blood and excretes it into the bile, which is collected by and concentrated in the gallbladder. An x-ray of the gallbladder, called a *cholecystogram*, detects the concentrated radiopaque dye. Oral cholecystography is highly reliable, having an overall accuracy rate of 97 percent in diagnosing gallstones and other abnormalities of the gallbladder. Interpretation of the test becomes difficult, however, when visualization of the gallbladder is poor or nonexistent. Failure of visualization may result from (1) an obstruction of the cystic duct by a gallstone or inflammation and swelling, (2) an inability of the gallbladder to concentrate the dye, (3) some interference with the normal absorption of the agent from the bloodstream, (4) or from unexplained causes. In general, a gallbladder that cannot be visualized by oral cholecystography is considered to be a diseased organ, because only about five percent of nonvisualized gallbladders prove to be normal.

Although oral cholecystography is the mainstay of test procedures for diagnosing gallstones, radionuclide imaging, ultrasonography, and cholangiography are also useful diagnostic techniques in selected instances. Radionuclide imaging may be used to demonstrate gallbladder, cystic duct, and common duct pathology if oral cholecystography produces poor visualization. Furthermore, radionuclide imaging is often used to diagnose suspected acute cholecystitis. Scanning with radioactive technetium allows the physician to visualize the patient's liver, bile ducts, and bladder. The radionuclide enters the patient's bile in the liver. Only small amounts of the nuclide are necessary for the identification of the gallbladder and bile flow pathways. The presence of the nuclide in the gallbladder implies that the cystic duct is open and effectively rules out acute cholecystitis because, in most cases, the cause of acute cholecystitis is obstruction of the cystic duct. If the gallbladder is unable to collect the radionuclide and, hence, cannot be visualized, acute or chronic cholecystitis is probably present.

Ultrasonography is another investigative technique used when oral cholecystography poorly visualizes the gallbladder. Indications for the use of ultrasonography in the diagnosis of gallstone disease are acute cholecystitis, allergy to cholecystographic contrast agents, jaundice, and nonvisualization of the gallbladder by other methods.

Ultrasonography is a particularly useful diagnostic technique for pregnant women, because this procedure does not expose the women to potentially hazardous radiation.

Endoscopic retrograde cholangiography and percutaneous transhepatic cholangiography are two additional procedures used to evaluate biliary structures. These procedures require special skills on the part of the physician and carry a slight risk of harm to the patient. Investigation using these techniques is useful when jaundice may be resulting from an obstruction in the common bile duct. **Endoscopic retrograde cholangiography**, which is sometimes called *endoscopic retrograde cholangiopancreatography* (ERCP), allows medical personnel to directly visualize the patient's common bile duct and pancreatic duct through a flexible fiberoptic endoscope passed down the patient's esophagus, through the stomach, and into the duodenum. As used here, the term "retrograde" refers to the injection of a radiopaque substance in a direction opposite to the normal flow of bile. X-rays follow the passage of the dye, which was introduced directly into the patient's common bile duct, and will indicate if an obstruction is present in the duct. Furthermore, if the patient has a gallstone, an ERCP may perform both diagnostic and treatment functions. Sometimes the endoscopy will dislodge a gallstone from the patient's duodenal papilla. Under these circumstances, the physician may then be able to remove the stone. Endoscopy can also enlarge the opening of the duodenal papilla to help with the passage of stones. Enlarging the opening of the duodenal papilla during an endoscopy is called a papillotomy.

Percutaneous transhepatic cholangiography is a diagnostic procedure that allows the physician to introduce a contrast agent directly into the patient's liver through a long, thin needle inserted through the patient's skin. This technique permits x-ray visualization of the bile ducts.

Disorders of the Pancreas

The pancreas is subject to inflammation, cystic fibrosis, and benign and malignant tumors.

Pancreatitis

Pancreatitis is an inflammation of the pancreas. Many cases of pancreatitis occur in association with gallbladder or biliary tract disease, alcohol abuse, or hyperlipidemia. **Hyperlipidemia** is a condition characterized by elevated serum cholesterol and/or triglyceride levels. Manifestations of pancreatitis include severe abdominal pain, vomiting, and marked abdominal tenderness. Repeated attacks of pancreatitis cause extensive damage to enzyme- and insulin-producing cells, sometimes resulting in the development of malabsorption syndrome and diabetes mellitus.

One complication of acute pancreatitis is the formation of a pseudocyst or abscess. A few patients have recurrent acute attacks of pancreatitis. Some patients develop chronic pancreatitis, a disease that occurs more commonly in men than in women. Gallbladder disease, peptic ulcer, and chronic alcoholism are predisposing conditions for chronic pancreatitis.

Cystic Fibrosis

Cystic fibrosis, which is also known as *mucoviscidosis* or *fibrocystic disease of the pancreas*, is an inherited disease in which the patient's pancreas develops obstruction of its ducts, resulting from fibrosis and degeneration of the exocrine cells. This disease, which usually first presents in the patient's early childhood, causes a disorder of the mucus-producing exocrine glands in the bronchi, pancreas, liver, and intestines. The resultant deficiency of digestive enzymes results in **steatorrhea**, a condition characterized by large, bulky, fatty, foul-smelling stools. Malnutrition, resulting from malabsorption, may occur despite an apparently adequate caloric and vitamin intake. Repeated pulmonary infections, primarily bronchitis and bronchiectasis, lead to fibrosis, lung abscess, and chronic pulmonary insufficiency.

An increase in the chlorides and sodium excreted by the cystic fibrosis patient's sweat glands forms the basis for the "sweat test" used in diagnosing this disease. Elevated values for these electrolytes in children are diagnostic for cystic fibrosis. The long-term outlook for affected children remains poor, although the prognosis for these patients has improved with the development of more effective methods of treatment. Many of these patients live to early adulthood.

Tumors

Benign tumors of the pancreas include cysts and islet cell adenomas. An abnormal glucose tolerance is registered in over one-half of individuals who have pancreatic cysts. Cysts that are expanding or that are complicated by hemorrhage, ruptures, or abscess require surgical treatment. Islet cell adenomas are relatively rare tumors that produce large amounts of insulin, creating a condition of hyperinsulinism that is characterized by sweating, trembling, flushing of the face, weakness, and mental confusion.

Adenocarcinoma is the most common pancreatic malignancy. The early symptoms arising from this cancer include jaundice, loss of appetite, indigestion, weight loss, and constant upper abdominal midline pain, which may radiate through to the back. Small cancers adjacent to the duodenum may require surgical intervention called *pancreatoduodenectomy*, which involves the removal of the connection between the pancreas and the duodenum, followed by the surgical joining of the pancreatic duct to the jejunum. Cancers elsewhere in the pancreas may not be surgically removable. A small operative mortality is associated with extensive pancreatic cancer surgery, and the long-term prognosis for pancreatic cancer patients is very poor.

Procedures Used in Diagnosing Pancreatic Disorders

Computerized tomography produces the best visual image of the pancreas and surrounding structures, but it cannot detect tumors within the pancreas unless the tumors alter the contour of the gland. Angiography is necessary to detect small tumors located within the gland. ERCP is diagnostic in 75 percent of pancreatic tumor cases and can also identify pancreatic narrowing or obstruction. Percutaneous needle aspiration biopsy of the pancreas under ultrasound or CT guidance is a procedure that can give a definitive diagnosis of pancreatic cancer and can eliminate the need for exploratory surgery.

Other Digestive System Disorders

Numerous other disorders of the digestive system besides those described above exist. This section will discuss a few disorders of the digestive system that do not easily fit into the previous categories. This section will address bleeding from the gastrointestinal tract, appendicitis, peritonitis, the malabsorption syndrome, and morbid obesity.

Bleeding from the Gastrointestinal Tract

Gastrointestinal tract bleeding may manifest as (1) hematemesis, (2) melena, or (3) *hematochezia*, which is the passage of bloody stools. Vomited blood usually is red, but if the blood has been in contact with gastric acids for several hours, the acids will alter the color of the blood to a "coffee grounds" appearance. Furthermore, blood that has been altered in color by the action of intestinal digestive juices gives the patient's stool a black color. Hematemesis and melena may occur as a result of the same episode of bleeding, or either may occur alone. Upper gastrointestinal tract bleeding is likely to produce melena, and bleeding from the lower colon or rectum is likely to produce hematochezia. Figure 9–9 lists some common causes of gastrointestinal tract bleeding.

Hemorrhoids are the most common cause of gastrointestinal tract bleeding. Causes of bleeding from the upper gastrointestinal tract include gastritis, peptic ulcer, and rupture of an esophageal varix. Causes of bleeding from the lower gastrointestinal tract, other than bleeding hemorrhoids, include diverticulitis, polyps, cancer, and ulcerative colitis. Bleeding disorders—both those affecting the platelets, such as thrombocytopenia, and those affecting coagulation, such as hemophilia—are responsible for bleeding from both upper and lower gastrointestinal sites.

Gastrointestinal bleeding is one of the more serious clinical events that can be induced by drugs. Because the bleeding may occur spontaneously as a complication of certain illnesses, physicians may not be certain if the bleeding is a result of the disease or is drug-induced. Anticoagulants, steroids, drugs containing aspirin, and NSAIDs are commonly associated with gastrointestinal bleeding. The most severe gastrointestinal bleeding associated with drug use originates from upper GI tract locations, often from the stomach, and occurs most frequently in elderly patients and in patients who experience impaired kidney function.

The Hemoccult slide test and other similar tests are useful diagnostic methods for detecting blood in the patient's stool. The Hemoccult test is very sensitive and can reveal the presence of very minute amounts of blood originating from any gastrointestinal site.

Figure 9–9.
Common Causes of Gastrointestinal Bleeding.

Location of Bleeding	Common Causes
Mouth, nose, pharynx	Nosebleed
Esophagus	Esophagitis, ruptured esophageal varices
Stomach	Gastritis, ulcer, cancer, hiatus hernia
Duodenum	Ulcer, duodenitis
Intestine	Diverticulosis, ulcerative colitis, regional enteritis, polyp, diverticulitis, cancer
Rectum, anus	Hemorrhoids, polyp, cancer

Barium-contrast upper and lower gastrointestinal x-rays, commonly called an upper GI series and a barium enema, respectively, are generally available diagnostic studies that detect the location of GI bleeding and that produce low morbidity. However, an upper GI series is inferior to properly conducted fiberoptic endoscopy, which can provide a direct visualization of the bleeding site. Endoscopy can detect with high accuracy the presence of bleeding from gastritis, esophageal varices, tears at the gastrointestinal junction, and peptic ulcers. Colonoscopy is a valuable fiberoptic method of identifying the causes of bleeding in the large intestine.

Appendicitis

Appendicitis is an inflammation of the appendix. Typically pain begins in the area around the patient's navel and gradually shifts to the right lower quadrant. Vomiting, constipation, and fever are common manifestations of appendicitis. The major complication of an attack of acute appendicitis is rupture with peritonitis and abscess formation. Adhesions, which form at the site of the inflamed peritoneum, may later cause obstruction of a loop of bowel. The treatment of an acute appendicitis is surgical removal of the organ during an *appendectomy*.

Peritonitis

Peritonitis is an inflammation of the peritoneum, the membrane that lines the abdominal cavity and covers the abdominal organs. The inflammation may result from bacterial or nonbacterial causes. Bacterial causes of peritonitis include (1) rupture of an inflamed appendix, diverticulum, or peptic ulcer, (2) the spread of an inflammation of the fallopian tube, or (3) tuberculosis. Substances such as bile from a ruptured gallbladder, urine from a perforated bladder, or blood from a ruptured tubal pregnancy in women may cause a nonbacterial peritonitis. Abdominal pain is a cardinal feature of peritonitis but manifestations vary, depending on the extent, the location, and the underlying cause of the inflammation. Treatment is directed toward the removal of the source of the contamination.

Malabsorption Syndrome

The *malabsorption syndrome* is a symptom-complex associated with impaired gastrointestinal absorption of nutrients. Many conditions, such as pancreatic insufficiency, gastrectomy, chronic liver disease, biliary tract obstruction, extensive small intestine resection, and certain endocrine and parasitic diseases are associated with malabsorption. Steatorrhea is a common feature in most of these disorders. Other manifestations of the malabsorption syndrome are loss of appetite, weakness, weight loss, anemia, low-grade fever, and joint pain. The prognosis for control of the malabsorption syndrome is fair to good, depending on the cause of the condition and provided that the affected individual follows a proper diet with vitamin supplements. Sometimes steroids and antibiotics are added to the treatment program. Long-term, if not life-long, adherence to a strict medical regimen of treatment is necessary to control malabsorption syndrome.

Morbid Obesity

Morbid obesity is defined as body weight of 100 percent or more above the standard. This disorder causes an accelerated degeneration of important organ systems, such as the circulatory system, the respiratory system, the musculoskeletal system, the digestive system, and the urinary system. Conditions associated with morbid obesity include heart disease, hypertension, respiratory dysfunction, thromboembolic disease, diabetes mellitus, osteoarthritis, hepatobiliary disease, and kidney disease. In addition, morbid obesity causes increased susceptibility to infection and increased operative risk. Morbidly obese individuals experience higher mortality than that of the normal population. The excess mortality principally results from coronary heart disease, stroke, and diabetes mellitus. Morbid obesity is treated with physician supervised dietary restriction, behavior modification, and exercise. If these measures fail, surgery may be necessary. Gastroplasty or gastric bypass procedures limit food intake by reducing the size of the patient's stomach and delaying emptying of food from the stomach, making the patient feel fuller for a longer amount of time. However, studies show little long-term weight reduction in patients who have had these procedures, which currently are rarely medically recommended.

10

The Urinary System

The **urinary system**, which is also called the *urinary tract*, is the group of organs that produce and excrete urine. The most important function of the urinary system is to remove soluble wastes from the body. However, this system also helps to maintain proper water balance and blood pressure. This chapter begins with an introduction to the components of the urinary system and then discusses the investigative techniques available for detecting disorders of this system. Next, common manifestations of these disorders are presented. The final section of this chapter describes disorders that can affect the components of the system.

ANATOMY AND PHYSIOLOGY

The organs that comprise the urinary system are the kidneys, the ureters, the urinary bladder, and the urethra. Figure 10–1 illustrates the organs in a male's urinary system.

The Kidneys

The **kidneys** are organs that filter the blood and concentrate the fluid that will be excreted as urine. Normally, a person has two kidneys that are shaped like large lima beans and that measure about five to

Figure 10–1.
The Organs in a Male's Urinary System.

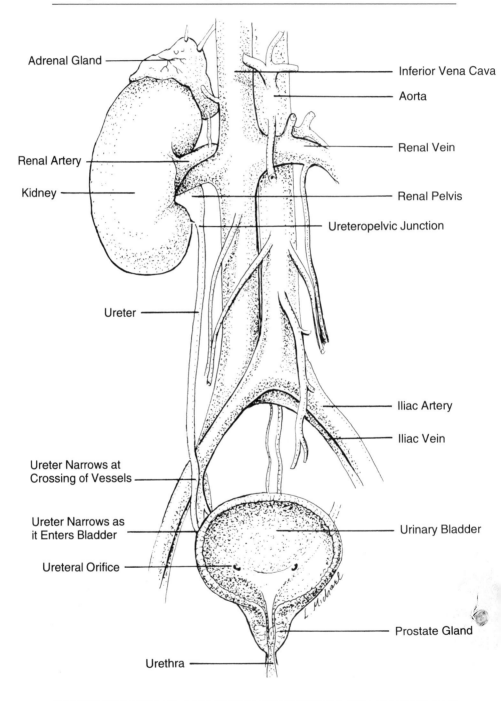

Adrenal Gland

Inferior Vena Cava

Aorta

Renal Vein

Renal Artery

Kidney

Renal Pelvis

Ureteropelvic Junction

Ureter

Iliac Artery

Iliac Vein

Ureter Narrows at
Crossing of Vessels

Ureter Narrows as
it Enters Bladder

Urinary Bladder

Ureteral Orifice

Prostate Gland

Urethra

six inches in length. The kidneys are located in the back of the abdomen, one on either side of the spine. The right kidney is often slightly lower than the left, possibly because of downward pressure on the right kidney from the liver. The kidneys are surrounded by fat that aids in their support and cushions them against trauma.

"*Renal*" means "pertaining to the kidney." The blood supply to each kidney is furnished by a renal artery that is a large branch of the abdominal aorta. The renal artery enters the kidney at an indentation, called the *hilum*, and then divides into successively smaller branches. The branches eventually terminate in a tuft or looped coil of capillaries known as a *glomerulus*. The renal arteries have counterparts in the venous system. These small branching veins unite to form larger vessels that eventually join to form the renal vein. The renal vein carries blood from each kidney to the inferior vena cava.

The outer zone of the kidney is called the cortex, and the inner portion is called the medulla. In the cortex are located one to two million nephrons. A *nephron* consists of a glomerulus, surrounded by its capsule, and a tubule. A kidney tubule pursues a very circuitous course through the cortex and into the medulla and then joins with other tubules to form a straight collecting duct. Figure 10–2 illustrates the parts of a nephron unit. The collecting ducts drain into the *renal calyces*, which are cup-shaped cavities that empty into the kidney pelvis. Fluid and other substances removed from the blood travel from the glomerulus to the renal pelvis through this system of tubules and collecting ducts. Figure 10–3 provides a cross-sectional view of a healthy kidney.

The kidneys respond to changes in the body's internal environment in order to maintain this environment in a steady state. This consistency is accomplished in the following ways:

- Excretion—The kidneys remove waste materials from the blood. The waste is removed by filtration in the glomerulus and by secretion, as well as absorption, in the tubules. These waste materials and other substances would be harmful to the body if they were not removed.
- Regulation of blood volume and osmolarity—Osmolarity is a technical term that refers to the movement of oxygen and other substances in a solution through a membrane. By varying the amount of water and solutes reabsorbed by the tubules, the kidneys assist in the control of body fluids and blood osmolarity. A *solute* is any substance that can be dissolved. The kidneys may reabsorb greater or lesser amounts of water and solutes at any given time to meet the body's needs.
- Maintenance of the normal acid-base equilibrium of body fluids—

Figure 10–2.
The Parts of a Nephron Unit.

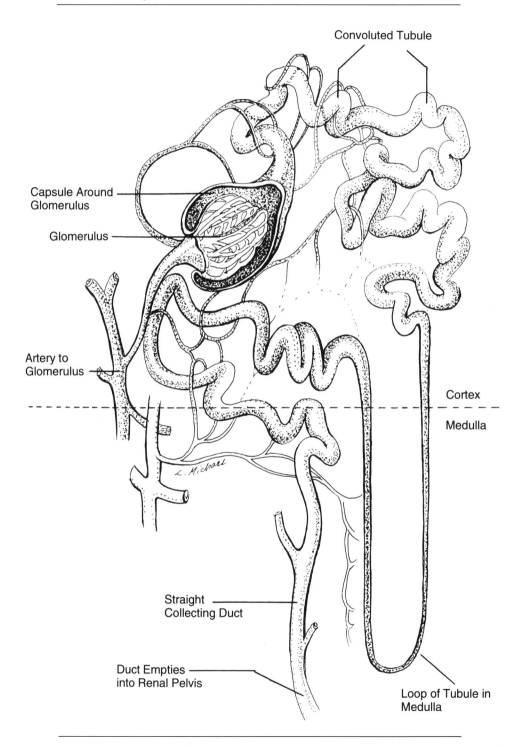

Convoluted Tubule

Capsule Around
Glomerulus

Glomerulus

Artery to
Glomerulus

Cortex

Medulla

Straight
Collecting Duct

Duct Empties
into Renal Pelvis

Loop of Tubule in
Medulla

Figure 10–3.
A Cross-Sectional View of a Kidney.

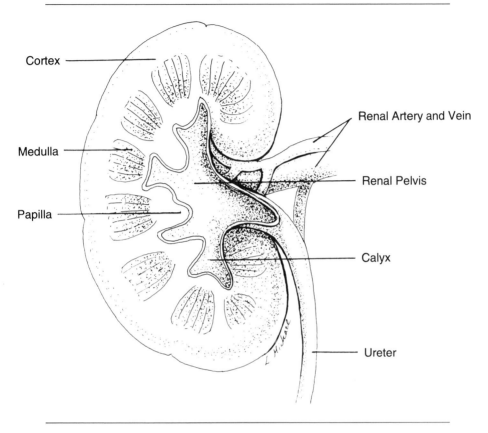

The kidneys remove the acid end-products of metabolism and vary the secretion of both **anions**, which are negatively charged ions, and **cations**, which are positively charged ions.

- Regulation of blood pressure—The kidneys influence blood pressure in several ways. After loss of blood from the body, the renal blood vessels constrict, shunting blood that normally would go to the kidneys into the general circulation where the immediate need for blood is greater. Furthermore, in their role as regulators of blood fluid volume, the kidneys help to maintain blood pressure. When blood pressure drops for any reason, the kidneys release an enzyme, renin, that raises blood pressure by causing the production of other hormones that constrict the arteries and cause salt and water retention.
- Preservation and concentration of important substances—The

kidneys' excretion and reabsorption abilities help to maintain the proper concentration of sodium, potassium, glucose, vitamins, amino acids, hormones, enzymes, and other essential substances in the body.

- Control of red blood cell mass—The secretion of the hormone erythropoietin by the kidneys regulates the production of red blood cells.

The kidneys have a rich blood supply that enables them to filter a large quantity of blood in a short amount of time. Water, glucose, minerals, and some small proteins pass through the thin-walled glomerular capillaries as a *filtrate*, which is a liquid that has passed through a filter. This renal filtrate is collected in the proximal tubule of the nephron. Normally, blood corpuscles remain in the capillaries and do not become part of the filtrate. The glomerular filtrate then passes down the tubules where secretion or reabsorption of various substances occurs. A large portion of the blood liquid passes into the capsule as a filtrate. Much of the liquid must be reabsorbed or the amount of water lost as urine would be enormous and the body quickly would become dehydrated. Thus, the tubules reabsorb sodium, chloride, other substances, and most of the water from the glomerular filtrate. The waste matter and the water that is not reabsorbed become urine.

Usually, glucose is completely reabsorbed by the tubules and does not appear in the urine. However, if a patient's blood glucose concentration is high, glucose may appear in the urine. Some individuals' glucose levels rise to high diabetic levels in the blood before any glucose appears in their urine. Other people have a "low renal threshold" for glucose, a condition called *renal glycosuria*, in which glucose appears in their urine even if they have a normal blood glucose level. Renal glycosuria is very rare and is usually of no medical significance.

The Ureters

A *ureter* is a tube that carries urine from a kidney to the bladder. Normally, people have two ureters, one leading from each kidney to the bladder. In the wall of the ureter are muscle fibers. Alternating contractions and relaxations of these fibers provide the necessary peristaltic activity for propelling urine downward from the kidney into the bladder. A ureter does not retain a uniform size throughout its length. It has three narrowed areas: (1) at the ureteropelvic junction where the ureter leaves the kidney, (2) at the point at which the ureter crosses the iliac blood vessels that go to the leg, and (3) at the entrance of the ureter into the bladder. Problems arise when kidney stones become lodged in these narrowed locations.

The Urinary Bladder

The *urinary bladder* is a hollow, musculomembranous organ that collects and stores urine prior to excretion. In males, the bladder is located in front of the rectum, and in females it is located in front of the vagina and uterus, both of which lie in front of the rectum. The bladder's size and specific position vary according to the amount of urine it contains. At the lower part of the bladder, around the opening of the urethra, is a sphincter composed of circular muscle fibers. Muscles in the wall of the bladder contract in association with relaxation of the sphincter, and urine is discharged into the urethra. The bladder can distend considerably to hold large quantities of urine, but ultimately distention will trigger a desire for urination.

The Urethra

The *urethra* is the excretory duct through which urine, which has been temporarily stored in the bladder, is removed from the body. The excretion of urine from the body is called *urination*, or *micturition*, and is generally under the voluntary control of healthy individuals. In males, the urethra, which also carries semen, extends from the bladder through the length of the penis. The first and widest portion of the male urethra is surrounded by the prostate gland. A woman's urethral external opening is located directly in front of the vaginal opening.

PROCEDURES USED FOR DIAGNOSING URINARY SYSTEM DISORDERS

Physicians can use several methods to detect and diagnose disorders of a patient's urinary system. This section will discuss urinalysis, blood tests, cystoscopy, pyelogram, renal arteriography, ultrasonography, and biopsy.

Urinalysis

The first step in the investigation of urinary system disease is a *urinalysis*, which is the laboratory examination of a patient's urine specimen. Routine tests performed during a urinalysis typically determine (1) the urine's specific gravity, which is its weight compared to water, (2) the urine's pH level, which indicates the acid-alkaline balance, (3) the presence of protein and glucose in the urine, and (4) the presence of red blood cells, white blood cells, or casts. *Casts* are cylindrical structures found in the urine that are composed of protein, red blood cells, white blood cells, or fat, in varying proportions. A routine urinalysis is a screening test. A normal urinalysis does not rule out urinary system disease, nor does the finding of one or more abnormalities in the urine clearly indicate the presence of disease. For example, the finding of red blood cells in the urine is generally an indication of disease somewhere in the urinary tract. In rare instances, the presence of red blood cells in the urine is caused by a disease that affects the body as a whole as well as the kidney. In some cases, red blood cells from the vagina or skin can be found in a urine specimen that was not obtained properly. Further testing is necessary to determine the cause of the presence of the red cells and to identify the point at which the blood is entering the urinary system.

A *dip-stick test* is a diagnostic procedure in which a narrow plastic strip, onto which one or more small test pads are affixed, is dipped into a patient's urine specimen and then removed from the specimen. Alternatively, drops of the urine specimen may be placed on the pads. The test pads contain chemicals that react only to the presence of specific substances, such as protein, glucose, red blood cells, white blood cells, bacteria, or bilirubin. The changes in the colors of the chemicals on the test pads indicate the presence or absence of the specific substances in the patient's urine.

A physician who suspects the presence of a bacterial urinary tract infection usually will request a culture of the patient's urine in order to identify the type of bacteria responsible for the infection. Identification of the specific organism is necessary in order to select the appropriate antibiotic to be used in treatment. A *culture* is the intentional growth of microorganisms in special substances that provide good environments for the microorganisms' growth. A urine culture is generally considered positive, or abnormal, if greater than 100,000 bacteria are grown per cubic millimeter of urine, although sometimes a smaller number may be considered abnormal.

The measurement of the urine's specific gravity provides additional information about kidney function. When oral fluids are withheld, a normal kidney produces a very concentrated urine that has a high specific gravity. After forced hydration, the same kidney will try to get rid of the excess water by producing a very dilute urine that has a low specific gravity. A diseased kidney may excrete urine that has a specific gravity constantly in the mid-range, regardless of the amount of fluids the person has taken in.

Blood Tests

Tests performed on blood samples are useful in the recognition and evaluation of kidney diseases and as a means of following their progress. Two tests commonly used to evaluate kidney function are measurements of blood urea nitrogen and serum creatinine. However, as screening devices for renal disease, these tests may be misleading, because their results remain within normal limits until the kidney has lost more than 50 percent of its function. *Urea* is a substance produced by the liver as the chief nitrogenous end-product of the metabolism of protein. The *urea nitrogen* is the nitrogen component of urea, and it is actually measured in the test. The concentration of urea nitrogen in the blood, which is called *blood urea nitrogen (BUN),* can be an indication of kidney function. For example, abnormally elevated BUN levels indicate the inability of the kidney to excrete urea in normal amounts. Although the BUN level is a widely used measure of renal function, it has several limitations. One limitation is that a person's BUN level may be elevated in the presence of gastrointestinal bleeding—because of the absorption of extra protein—even though the person's kidney function remains normal. Furthermore, a combination of a low protein diet and increased fluid intake may reduce the patient's BUN in the absence of altered kidney function. Furthermore, a person who has a moderate BUN elevation is likely to be symptom-free even if the person's kidney function is poor. The BUN test is useful when the levels are high because its value correlates with symptoms. Patients who have a high BUN are likely to have symptoms of uremia (which is discussed later in this chapter).

    Creatinine is a metabolic end-product that is derived primarily from muscle metabolism, and, to a lesser degree, dietary intake. Its rate of excretion is relatively constant, and its concentration in the blood serum is minimally affected by physical activity. Serum creatinine is thus a better indicator of renal function than BUN is. The creatinine clearance test is an even more precise assay of renal function than the BUN or creatinine tests alone are. The creatinine clearance is the volume of plasma that is completely "cleared" of creatinine by the kidneys each minute. As opposed to the BUN and serum creatinine levels, which rise with renal failure, the creatinine clearance level falls in renal failure.

Cystoscopy

Cystoscopy is a procedure that permits the surgeon to view the interior of the patient's bladder through a fiberoptic instrument known as a *cystoscope*. Working with instruments passed through the cystoscope, the surgeon can crush and remove small stones in the bladder, remove tissue samples for biopsy, and destroy small bladder tumors using electric current. The surgeon can introduce catheters through the cystoscope and pass them into the patient's ureters and the pelvis of each kidney.

Pyelogram

Catheters are passed into the kidney pelvis for the purpose of performing an x-ray study known as a *retrograde pyelogram*. A small amount of a radiopaque dye passes through the catheter into the kidney pelvis, and then a series of x-rays is obtained. A similar procedure performed on the bladder is called a *cystogram*. When it is performed on the urethra, it is called a *urethrogram*. An *intravenous pyelogram (IVP)* is an x-ray study of the kidney and ureters following an intravenous injection of a radiopaque dye. The intravenous study, as opposed to the retrograde pyelogram, furnishes greater information on the kidney's ability to concentrate urine and on the size and general outline of the kidney. The retrograde pyelogram, however, reveals more clearly the size and shape of the renal calyces, renal pelvis, and ureter.

Renal Arteriography

Findings from an intravenous pyelogram of changes compatible with renal artery stenosis will indicate the need for renal arteriography for clarification of the disease. As described in Chapter 3, *Specialized Diagnostic Techniques*, arteriography is the x-ray study of a patient's artery after the injection of a radiopaque dye into the artery. The renal arteriogram can establish the existence of a renal arterial lesion and can aid in determining the cause of the lesion, but cannot prove that the presence of a partial constriction of a renal artery is the cause of hypertension. Nor does a renal arteriogram indicate that the surgical correction of such a constriction would result in a lowering of the patient's blood pressure. However, renal arteriography can detect kidney lesions of small size and can differentiate benign lesions from malignant lesions in a very high percentage of cases.

Ultrasonography

Another useful test in diagnosing kidney disease is an ultrasound examination. The diagnostic accuracy of this technique in evaluating kidney lesions that are larger than 3 centimeters approaches 95 percent. Smaller masses of about one centimeter can also be evaluated by ultrasonography, but with less diagnostic accuracy. Ultrasonography is very helpful in diagnosing renal failure, especially when urinary tract obstruction is suspected.

Biopsy

A biopsy, as described in Chapter 3, is the removal of a small amount of tissue from a living body for microscopic examination. A renal biopsy is especially valuable in determining the extent of kidney damage in glomerulonephritis, the nephrotic syndrome, asymptomatic proteinuria, and renal failure. An open biopsy of kidney tissue may be performed by a surgeon during an operation, and a closed biopsy may be accomplished by inserting a biopsy needle through the skin of the patient's back into a kidney. Possible complications of biopsy include prolonged hematuria, hemorrhage, and infection. Kidney removal and/or death have followed about 0.1 percent of reported closed biopsies. A biopsy may also be performed during a cystoscopy on lesions of the bladder, ureter, or urethra.

DISORDERS OF THE URINARY SYSTEM

Disorders of the urinary system result from congenital malformations, infections, malignant changes within the patient's urinary organs, and diseases of other parts of the patient's body. Most disorders of the urinary system are of minor consequence and respond well to treatment. Other disorders, however, are more serious and may become chronic and difficult to treat. These latter disorders occasionally lead to renal failure and even death. This section will first identify several common manifestations of urinary disease and then will discuss some urinary tract pathology.

Manifestations of Urinary Disease

Diseases that affect the urinary system show themselves in several ways. Some of the more common urinary tract manifestations that are associated with various disorders include uremia, hematuria, pyuria, and proteinuria.

Uremia

As defined in Chapter 7, *The Circulatory System,* uremia is a toxic condition that is characterized by the retention of large amounts of the by-products of protein metabolism in the blood. Urea is often present in large amounts in the blood of uremic patients. Uremic patients typically experience nausea, vomiting, headache, vertigo, dimness of vision, coma, and convulsions.

Hematuria

Hematuria is a condition in which red blood cells are present in the patient's urine. When the urine is not contaminated by uterine or vaginal secretions, hematuria is pathologic and is a sign of a urinary tract abnormality. Although not all instances of hematuria result from serious disease, each case needs thorough investigation. *Microscopic hematuria* is a condition in which very small amounts of blood that can be detected only on microscopic examination are present in the patient's urine. *Gross hematuria* is a condition in which blood is readily apparent in the patient's urine. Gross hematuria usually results from an infection, kidney stone, or tumor. Microscopic hematuria may be more serious than gross hematuria. Systemic causes of hematuria may arise from damage to any part of the urinary system, but the mechanism depends on the nature of the disease. Hemorrhagic diseases, such as hemophilia, may cause hematuria, as can sickle cell disease, lupus erythematosus, and polyarteritis nodosa. Furthermore, hematuria can be a complication of anticoagulant drug therapy or may even result from long-distance running. The sites and major causes of bleeding into the urinary tract are shown in Figure 10–4.

Pyuria

Pyuria is a condition in which white blood cells are present in the urine. A few white cells may be present normally, but, when the urine has not been contaminated by a vaginal discharge, white cells are numerous only in association with a pathologic process. White cells escape into the urine at the same sites that red blood cells escape into the urine—the kidney, ureter, bladder, prostate and accessory structures, and urethra. In general, the causes of pyuria are acute infections, primarily pyelonephritis, cystitis, prostatitis, epididymitis, and urethritis. Chronic pyelonephritis, a persistent urinary tract stone, and obstructive urinary tract disease also may produce constant or intermittent pyuria.

Proteinuria

Proteinuria is a condition in which protein is present in the urine. Urine from healthy individuals may contain small amounts of protein,

Figure 10–4.
The Sites and Major Causes of Bleeding into the Urinary Tract.

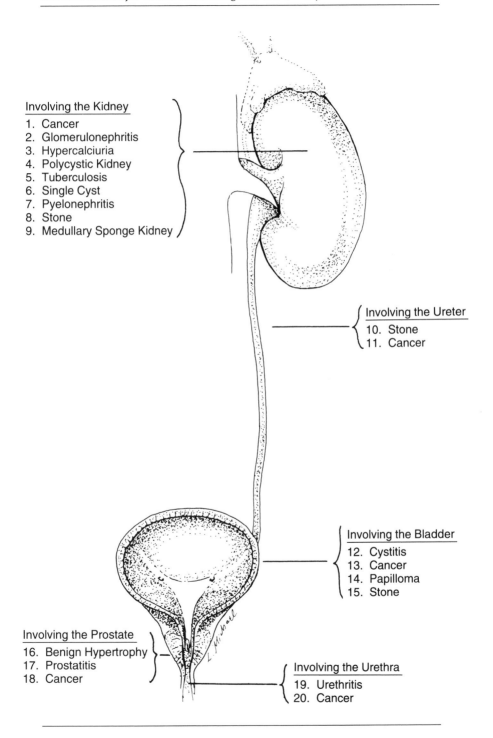

Involving the Kidney
1. Cancer
2. Glomerulonephritis
3. Hypercalciuria
4. Polycystic Kidney
5. Tuberculosis
6. Single Cyst
7. Pyelonephritis
8. Stone
9. Medullary Sponge Kidney

Involving the Ureter
10. Stone
11. Cancer

Involving the Bladder
12. Cystitis
13. Cancer
14. Papilloma
15. Stone

Involving the Prostate
16. Benign Hypertrophy
17. Prostatitis
18. Cancer

Involving the Urethra
19. Urethritis
20. Cancer

including albumin and many other renal cell proteins. Proteinuria and albuminuria are generally considered to be synonymous terms. Proteinuria is classified into three main types: (1) false proteinuria, (2) non-renal proteinuria, and (3) renal proteinuria. *False proteinuria* is a condition in which protein is present in the urine as a result of contamination. For example, the urine may become accidentally mixed with fluids, such as blood and pus, that originated outside the urinary tract. *Non-renal proteinuria* is a condition in which protein is present in the urine as a result of a disorder outside the organs of the urinary system. This type of proteinuria can be caused by fever, strenuous exercise, certain medications, cardiac disease, or endocrine diseases. *Renal proteinuria* is a condition in which protein is present in the urine as a result of abnormalities in the glomeruli, or, in rare cases, in the tubules. Proteinuria exceeding 75 milligrams per 100 milliliters of urine usually indicates the presence of renal proteinuria. If the proteinuria is associated with erythrocyte or hemoglobin casts, intrinsic kidney disease is even more likely. Significant proteinuria in the presence of hypertension is a poor prognostic sign, indicating advanced kidney disease that may progress into chronic renal failure.

Another type of proteinuria is *orthostatic proteinuria*, which is a condition in which protein is increased in the urine only when the patient is upright. This condition is not uncommon in teenagers and usually has no morbidity or mortality significance.

Congenital Abnormalities

Congenital abnormalities are more common in the urinary system than in any other organ system. The kidneys, ureters, bladder, urethra, and renal blood vessels can be the sites of congenital urinary system disorders.

Congenital abnormalities may include the absence of one kidney, the presence of an extra kidney, or an abnormally shaped kidney. The absence of one kidney is rare, but when it occurs, the patient's solitary kidney usually will be normal. This normal kidney is capable of carrying on the function of two kidneys, but a serious problem may arise if the solitary kidney becomes infected or develops stones or other pathologic conditions. A supernumerary, or extra, kidney may develop near one or both kidneys. The extra kidney may lie free from, or may be fused to, another kidney. A relatively common kidney abnormality is the horseshoe kidney, which usually involves fusion of the two kidneys across the midline of the body at the lower poles to form a horseshoe-shaped structure. Horseshoe kidneys may not produce any symptoms, but may be subject to hydronephrosis, pyelonephritis, or stone formation.

Another congenital disorder that can affect the kidneys is cystic disease. Renal cystic disease is a condition that is characterized by the replacement of functioning kidney tissue with fluid-filled cysts. The cysts may be either solitary or multiple and may affect one or both kidneys. Polycystic disease is an inherited condition that causes a slow deterioration of kidney function and often results in renal failure. Medullary sponge kidney is a condition that is characterized by cystic dilation of the collecting ducts in the renal medulla. It rarely causes renal failure. Sponge kidney often is complicated by hematuria, recurrent infection, and calculi formation. The medullary sponge kidney patient's prognosis is related to the degree of development of these complications. Many people have a few benign isolated kidney cysts, some of which may measure up to several centimeters in diameter, that never cause problems.

Duplications of the ureters and/or renal pelvis are common anomalies and generally are of no medical significance. However, if one of the extra ureters drains a rudimentary, supernumerary kidney, the latter could become infected. Furthermore, if a ureter is congenitally narrowed or obstructed, the abnormality must be surgically corrected by dilating the narrowed area.

A fairly common urinary tract disorder that occurs in some children is vesicoureteral reflux. *Vesicoureteral reflux* is a condition in which urine flows back up the ureters when the bladder contracts during urination. This backward flow causes pressure on the kidneys which may lead to kidney damage or may cause pyelonephritis.

Congenital abnormalities of the bladder include exstrophy, diverticula, double bladder, and obstructing valves or strictures at the bladder neck. *Exstrophy* is a rare, but treatable urinary tract malformation in which the front wall of the bladder is absent. If the overlying abdominal wall is also absent, the exstrophic bladder opens directly to the exterior of the body. Failure of the pubic bone to fuse, difficulties with gait, and abnormalities of the urethra also may be associated with exstrophy. Exstrophy typically is surgically corrected at birth. A diverticulum, as defined in Chapter 9, *The Digestive System*, is a pouch or sac of mucous-membrane-lined tissue that protrudes outward through the weakened wall of a tubular organ. The bladder can be the site of diverticulae. In addition, the bladder neck can be the location of congenital narrowing or obstruction.

Urethral abnormalities may include an absent or abnormally

closed urethra. Other urethral abnormalities involve abnormally opened urethras. For example, **epispadias** is a condition affecting some males in which the urethra opens on the upper, or dorsal, surface of the penis. Similarly, **hypospadias** is a condition in which the urethra opens on the underneath, or ventral, surface of the penis. The treatment of hypospadias and minor degrees of epispadias is surgical, and normal function typically follows the surgery. Extensive abnormalities of the urethra can only be partially corrected by surgery.

The most common congenital abnormality of the renal blood vessels is an aberrant renal artery. An aberrant vessel is one that is not located in the normal site for that vessel. An aberrant artery may cross and obstruct the ureter, giving rise to symptoms. Surgery relieves the obstruction.

Figure 10–5 presents some common congenital abnormalities that affect urinary system organs.

Obstructive Diseases

Obstruction to the flow of urine may occur at any point in the urinary tract. Locations and common causes of urinary tract obstruction are shown in Figure 10–6. The most common cause of urinary tract obstruction in males is an enlarged prostate. Another common cause of urinary obstruction is the presence of stones, or calculi, that may develop in the kidney or bladder. Although the cause of the stone formation is frequently unknown, chronic urinary infections, increased urinary calcium, increased urinary uric acid, and medullary sponge kidney are the most common causes of kidney stones.

Figure 10–5.
Congenital Abnormalities of the Urinary Tract.

Organ	Abnormalities
Kidney	Absence of one kidney, presence of an extra kidney, fusion of two kidneys
Ureter	Presence of an extra ureter, narrowing of a ureter, vesicoureteral reflux
Bladder	Exstrophy, diverticulum, narrowing of the bladder neck
Urethra	Epispadias, hypospadias
Renal blood vessels	Aberrant renal artery

Figure 10–6.
Locations and Common Causes of Urinary Tract Obstruction.

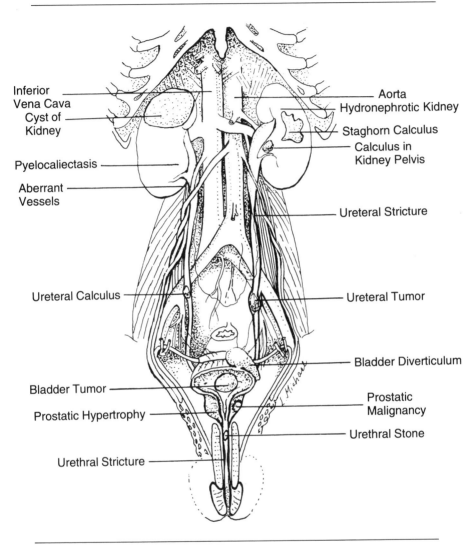

Inferior Vena Cava

Cyst of Kidney

Pyelocaliectasis

Aberrant Vessels

Ureteral Calculus

Bladder Tumor

Prostatic Hypertrophy

Urethral Stricture

Aorta

Hydronephrotic Kidney

Staghorn Calculus

Calculus in Kidney Pelvis

Ureteral Stricture

Ureteral Tumor

Bladder Diverticulum

Prostatic Malignancy

Urethral Stone

Strictures and kinks of the ureter may also cause obstructions. A stricture is a narrowing which may be congenital or acquired. A congenital stricture may result from faulty development of a segment of a ureter or may be produced by an aberrant blood vessel. Acquired strictures are more common than congenital strictures and may result from

- infection originating in the urinary tract
- injury from the passage of a stone, with infection and residual scarring
- scarring from surgical removal of a stone
- benign or malignant tumors of the ureter
- scarring from radium treatments given for a malignancy of the bladder or uterus
- extrinsic pressure on the ureter by a benign or malignant tumor located in an adjacent structure
- infection of an adjacent organ with involvement of the ureter

Patients who have malignant tumors that cause urinary tract obstruction have a poor prognosis. For other causes of stricture, the patient's prognosis depends on (1) the duration of the stricture, (2) the degree of distention of the kidney resulting from the stricture, and (3) the feasibility of operative correction.

Disorders of the Kidney

The most serious diseases of the urinary system are those that affect the kidneys. *Nephropathy* is a general term for kidney disease. Acute and chronic infections, inflammatory diseases, kidney stones, and tumors can impair kidney function. In addition, disorders of other parts of the body, such as hypertension, diabetes mellitus, and some connective tissue diseases, can damage the kidneys.

Pyelonephritis

Pyelonephritis is a bacterial infection that causes inflammation of the kidney and its pelvis. Microscopic evidence of inflammation is seen in the glomerulus and collecting tubules. Pyelitis refers to a bacterial infection that is limited to the renal pelvis. However, infection of the kidney pelvis usually does not occur without involvement of at least part of the kidney. For this reason, *pyelonephritis* is the more accurate term. Pyelonephritis occurs in acute and chronic forms.

Acute Pyelonephritis. Acute pyelonephritis is a bacterial infection of the kidney that appears suddenly and is characterized by high fever, chills, rapid pulse, flank pain, frequency of urination, and *dysuria*, which is pain upon urinating. The infecting organisms usually ascend to the kidney from the lower urinary tract, but in rare cases the kidney becomes infected via the bloodstream or lymphatic system. Predisposing conditions for acute pyelonephritis include ureteral strictures, ureteral reflux, tumors of the urinary tract, stones, and neurogenic bladder, among others. The urine sediment of a person who has pyelonephritis is loaded with white blood cells and bacteria and also may contain numerous red blood cells and casts. Urine sediment is obtained by spinning a urine sample in a machine called a centrifuge.

A urine culture is included in any thorough investigation of an attack of pyelonephritis. An initial culture identifies the specific offending organism, and further testing shows the sensitivity of the offending organism to various antibiotics. The prognosis for full recovery from one acute attack of pyelonephritis is excellent. After more than one attack, the prognosis is still good. Each recurrence, however, increases the likelihood of permanent kidney damage and progression to chronic pyelonephritis. Nonetheless, most patients who have acute pyelonephritis do not develop chronic pyelonephritis.

Chronic Pyelonephritis. Chronic pyelonephritis is a slowly progressive infection that usually affects both kidneys. This condition may be associated with the persistence of a kidney stone or obstruction or may follow as the consequence of repeated acute attacks of pyelonephritis. Chronic pyelonephritis may run a protracted course over many years and the individual may be relatively symptom-free. Proteinuria and pyuria generally are present, but may be intermittent. Recurrent attacks are characterized by fever, headache, fatigue, loss of appetite, weight loss, excessive thirst, backache, dysuria, and pyuria. In advanced stages, the disease may lead to renal failure and/or hypertension. The terminal stage of chronic pyelonephritis cannot be clinically distinguished from the corresponding end-stage of chronic glomerulonephritis.

Nephrolithiasis

Nephrolithiasis is a condition marked by the presence of kidney stones. The size of the kidney stones varies from tiny particles to large staghorn calculi that fill the patient's renal pelvis. Initially, calcium separates from the patient's urine to form microscopic crystals, which become attached to the mucous membrane of the kidney pelvis. In time, these deposits enlarge as more calcium separates and collects. Finally the deposit is large enough to be considered a stone. Very small stones, usually smaller than five millimeters, may be passed in the urine with minimal or no difficulty. On the other hand, large stones may remain silent within the kidney for many years. If a stone passes into the ureter, the patient will experience renal colic, flank tenderness, and hematuria. *Renal colic* is acute abdominal pain produced by the passage of a stone within the urinary tract. Pain resulting from the presence of a kidney stone is usually caused by the strong peristaltic contractions of the ureter attempting to move the stone down into the bladder. Renal colic may be excruciating if the stone obstructs the ureter.

If the stone is not passed promptly or removed surgically, hydronephrosis develops. ***Hydronephrosis*** is a pathologic condition characterized by distention of the renal pelvis and calyces with urine, as a result of obstruction of the ureter from any cause. Initially the renal pelvis distends, then kidney tissue is progressively compressed by the pressure of the unexcreted urine. Functioning kidney cells die from the constant pressure of this retained urine. In advanced cases, only a thin-walled, functionless sac remains of the previously healthy kidney. Kidney damage is proportional to the degree and duration of the obstruction. Complications of hydronephrosis are stone formation, infection, and hypertension. In the absence of these complications, the outlook is good if the obstruction involves only one kidney, is discovered early, and is corrected promptly, provided that the kidney is not too badly damaged. Considerable function will return when adequate drainage returns, even after weeks of obstruction. Persistent or repeated intermittent obstruction leads to infection, which, in turn, increases kidney damage. If the obstruction has affected both kidneys and has resulted in substantial kidney damage, the patient's life may be significantly shortened.

For many patients, the cause of the stone formation is unknown. However, chronic dehydration probably is responsible for the higher incidence of stone formation in tropical climates. For these nephrolithiasis patients in particular, and for others whose stones have an unknown origin, drinking additional fluids to maintain a dilute urine is the primary treatment for preventing urinary calculi formation. The long-term administration of thiazide diuretics, which increase tubular reabsorption of calcium out of the urine by 30 to 50 percent, reduces the recurrence rate of stone formation. Furthermore, repeated urinary tract infection, medullary sponge kidney, and Crohn's disease are conditions that predispose patients to stone formation. Hypercalciuria, which is characterized by the presence of large amounts of calcium in the urine, is common in patients who have kidney stones. Twenty-five percent of all patients who have kidney stones experience only one episode of symptomatic stone passage.

Patients usually spontaneously pass obstructing stones that are located in lower levels of the ureter, but they may require surgical removal of some of these stones via cystoscopy. Physicians can surgically remove large stones in the renal pelvis or can treat the stones with lithotripsy. Lithotripsy, as discussed in the treatment of gallstones in Chapter 9, *The Digestive System*, is a noninvasive technique that uses soundwaves to break up stones so that they can be easily passed from the patient's body in the urine. Lithotripsy is the most common treatment for kidney stones that do not pass spontaneously.

Glomerulonephritis

Glomerulonephritis is a fairly common inflammatory disease of the kidney, and it is characterized by pathologic changes in the glomeruli and smaller arterioles of the kidney. A main distinction between glomerulonephritis and pyelonephritis is that no bacterial invasion of the kidney occurs in glomerulonephritis, whereas bacterial invasion does occur in pyelonephritis. Glomerulonephritis typically is characterized as being either immunologic or nonimmunologic in origin. Glomerular disease resulting from immunologic reactions may follow some infections, such as streptococcal infection of the upper respiratory tract, scarlet fever, or pneumonia. Nonimmunologic glomerular disease is less common and may be caused by metabolic, infiltrative, toxic, or hemodynamic processes.

Acute Diffuse Glomerulonephritis. Acute diffuse glomerulonephritis is an acute form of glomerulonephritis that typically is characterized by massive proteinuria, hematuria, anemia, hypertension, decreased urinary output, and generalized retention of tissue fluids. Many cases of acute diffuse glomerulonephritis follow tonsillitis or pharyngitis and are called *post-streptococcal glomerulonephritis*. The fatality rate for acute diffuse glomerulonephritis patients is about five percent, usually resulting from congestive heart failure, recurrent convulsions, or uremia. Most patients who have acute diffuse glomerulonephritis recover completely, although the amount of time required for recovery varies from a few days to one year. A small percentage of patients do not recover fully, and they continue to suffer from chronic glomerulonephritis or later develop high blood pressure.

Chronic Diffuse Glomerulonephritis. Chronic diffuse glomerulonephritis is a progressive disease that may take years to run its full course and is characterized by irreversible damage to the renal glomeruli and tubules. Patients may initially complain only of mild swelling, headache, and shortness of breath, but renal function often deteriorates over time. Ultimately, kidney or heart failure will develop as terminal events. Chronic diffuse glomerulonephritis may appear as a primary disease, as a disorder that is secondary to a systemic disease, or as a sequel to the acute form of glomerulonephritis. The chronic form of the disease may occur with or without the loss of large amounts of protein in the urine. The manifestations of chronic glomerulonephritis vary with the stage of the condition. In the latent stage, the patient often has no symptoms and may appear to be in good health. The only evidence of the disease is proteinuria and/or hematuria, and, occasionally, hypertension. The nephrotic stage is characterized by generalized edema, recurrent headache, hypertension, shortness of breath, fatigue, and heavy proteinuria. The symptoms may subside to the latent stage with treatment, but the nephrotic stage usually leads to kidney failure. Nephrotic symptoms may develop one or more times during the course of chronic glomerulonephritis.

Focal Glomerulonephritis. Focal glomerulonephritis is a kidney condition in which only some glomeruli show inflammatory changes and other glomeruli appear to be normal. Focal glomerulonephritis is characterized by recurrent attacks of hematuria and mild proteinuria. Microscopic hematuria may persist between attacks. Although focal glomerulonephritis generally runs a benign course, hypertension and renal failure occur as complications in rare instances.

Nephrotic Syndrome

The **nephrotic syndrome** is a condition that is characterized by low serum albumin, elevated cholesterol, massive proteinuria, and generalized edema and is seen as part of many diseases affecting the kidney. The syndrome may occur in association with glomerulonephritis, diabetic kidney disease, lupus erythematosus, allergic reactions, syphilis, and other disorders. The prognosis of nephrotic syndrome is better for children than for adults. About 80 percent of children progress to eventual cure, but only 25 percent of adults with this syndrome do so.

Hypertension and Kidney Disease

Severe and persistent hypertension causes damage to many organs, especially the heart, kidneys, and the brain. As discussed in Chapter 7, *The Circulatory System*, hypertension may be primary or secondary. Secondary hypertension results from some known systemic disorder. One cause of secondary hypertension is renal artery disease resulting from obstruction of renal bloodflow. The obstruction typically arises from an arteriosclerotic plaque or an abnormality in the renal blood vessels. When the kidney senses a drop in blood pressure caused by arterial stenosis, the organ responds by producing renin, an enzyme that indirectly raises blood pressure. Renin produced under conditions of shock serves a very useful purpose of assisting in the maintenance of a level of blood pressure sufficient to protect vital organs. Conversely, in the absence of shock, a rise in blood pressure to elevated levels has a negative effect—to an already failing kidney, the renin-produced hypertension causes still further deterioration. Renal arteriography is useful in identifying obstructed renal vessels. This procedure involves the injection of a radiopaque dye through a catheter into each renal artery so that the location and degree of narrowing of each renal artery can be identified.

Signs of kidney damage arising from hypertension include proteinuria, hematuria, and cylindruria. The effects of hypertension on the kidney parallel the severity of the disorder. Unless severe hypertension is lowered by medication, renal failure may occur. Over 90 percent of untreated renal patients die within two years of the onset of hypertensive nephropathy. Hypertension caused by renal disease that affects only one kidney is occasionally treated surgically and may arrest the progression of this potentially life-shortening condition.

Renal Failure

Renal failure is a condition in which the kidney is unable to normally excrete the substances produced by metabolism. It is characterized by (1) a decrease in the rate of filtration by the glomerulus, manifested by **oliguria**, which is the reduced excretion of urine, and (2) a rise in the blood urea nitrogen and serum creatinine concentrations. Uremia is the end-stage of renal failure.

If signs of renal failure develop suddenly, the condition is referred to as *acute renal failure*. A common cause of acute renal failure is a disorder known as **acute tubular necrosis**, which is the sudden death of the cells of the renal tubules. This condition can follow exposure to toxic drugs or chemicals, severe hemorrhage, septicemia, crushing injuries, and incompatible blood transfusions. It rarely occurs without any predisposing illness. A patient experiencing acute renal failure has the potential for full recovery, but the nature and severity of any associated illness or injury influences his or her clinical course of treatment.

Chronic renal failure is a progressive condition that is characterized by disorders in all aspects of renal function. The period over which chronic renal failure develops can range from months to years. The condition can be caused by a wide variety of kidney diseases. Figure 10–7 lists the most common of these kidney disorders. The symptoms of renal failure affect the whole body. These symptoms include hypertension, heart failure, edema, anemia, diarrhea, vomiting, fatigue, neuropathy, severe itching, bone changes, and many

Figure 10–7.
Causes of Chronic Renal Failure.

Category of Disorder	Example of Illness
Disease of the glomerulus	Chronic glomerulonephritis
Congenital kidney disease	Polycystic kidney disease
Infectious kidney disease	Chronic pyelonephritis
Obstructive disease	Stones, prostatic hypertrophy
Disease of the kidney tubules	Acute tubular necrosis
Vascular disease of the kidney	Hypertensive nephropathy, renal arterial stenosis
Systemic disease	Systemic lupus erythematosus, diabetes mellitus

other conditions. The treatment for renal failure involves aggressive treatment of the underlying disease, if possible. Control of blood pressure is essential, and certain diets, especially low protein ones, may slow the progression of renal failure. End-stage renal failure is treated with hemodialysis, peritoneal dialysis, or renal transplantation. These treatment procedures are discussed later in this chapter.

Cancer of the Kidney

Renal cancer represents slightly more than two percent of cancers in males and somewhat less than two percent in females. Adenocarcinomas account for slightly more than 80 percent of the renal malignancies in adults. *Embryonal nephroma*, which is also called *Wilms tumor*, is a malignant tumor of the kidney and is the most common kidney cancer occurring in patients younger than five. Manifestations of kidney malignancies are nonspecific and include hematuria, abdominal and flank pain, weight loss, and fever. The treatment of renal cancers is surgical, sometimes combined with postoperative radiation therapy and postoperative chemotherapy. The outlook for these patients is poor, because symptoms generally occur only after the tumors have grown to a large size.

Renal Manifestations of Systemic Disorders

The kidneys are often affected by disorders that develop in other parts of the body. Among these systemic diseases that commonly affect the kidneys are diabetes mellitus, hypertension, polyarteritis nodosa, systemic lupus erythematosus, and diffuse scleroderma. Diabetes mellitus is discussed in Chapter 12, *The Endocrine System*, hypertension and polyarteritis nodosa are discussed in Chapter 7, *The Circulatory System*, and systemic lupus erythematosus and diffuse scleroderma are discussed in Chapter 5, *The Skin*.

Polyarteritis nodosa is a multisystem disorder that is characterized by widespread inflammation of arteries in many organ systems. This disorder affects the kidneys in 75 percent of all cases, and is more common in men than in women. Systemic lupus erythematosus is a generalized connective tissue disorder that mainly affects women. Glomerulonephritis that is associated with systemic lupus erythematosus is known as *lupus nephritis*. Lupus nephritis develops in approximately half of the cases of systemic lupus erythematosus. Proteinuria is a constant finding in lupus nephritis and at times may be severe. Diffuse scleroderma is a systemic disorder that is characterized by the hardening and shrinking of the connective tissues of any part of the body and that occurs most often in women between the ages of 30 and 50. In most diffuse scleroderma patients who have kidney involvement, proteinuria may be present for many years without evidence of progressive renal disease. However, rapidly progressive kidney failure associated with severe hypertension may develop at any time during the course of diffuse scleroderma. Kidney failure usually leads to early death from uremia unless the patient receives dialysis. The kidney disease associated with connective tissue disorders is often progressive, but is sometimes effectively treatable with corticosteroids.

Procedures Used for Treating Renal Disorders

Renal disorders can be treated using a variety of surgical and other procedures. This section will define and describe a few of the more common treatments for kidney disease, including dialysis, transplantation, and percutaneous transluminal angioplasty.

Dialysis. Dialysis is the process of separating substances that are dissolved in a solution by diffusing the substances through a semipermeable membrane. *Hemodialysis* utilizes the process of diffusion across a membrane to remove toxic substances from the patient's blood while adding desirable components. Blood from the arterial side of the patient's circulatory system passes in a constant flow on one side of the membrane, and a cleansing solution passes on the other side. This procedure allows removal of waste products in a manner that is similar to glomerular filtration in the kidney. The blood then returns to the venous system of the patient. Hemodialysis requires access to the patient's vascular system and is generally performed in a hospital inpatient or outpatient setting. ***Continuous ambulatory peritoneal dialysis (CAPD)*** involves an indwelling abdominal catheter that permits the addition of dialysis fluid to the peritoneal cavity followed by drainage of fluid containing nitrogenous wastes three to four times daily. Because CAPD can be performed at home and is less costly than hemodialysis, CAPD offers the patient greater freedom and self-reliance than does hemodialysis. Some patients use dialysis until a suitable, matched donor kidney becomes available.

Many dialysis patients are able to continue their predialysis lifestyles, and most can resume a functional, but less strenuous, lifestyle. Other patients have limited stamina, but are able to care for themselves. Patients who are involved in chronic dialysis programs have mortality rates of five to ten percent per year. Age is an important factor in determining mortality rates, because patients who are younger than 35 have a 74 percent 5-year survival rate, whereas patients who are older than 64 have a 16 percent 5-year survival rate. Less than half the patients who start dialysis over age 55 live 5 years.

Transplantation. Transplantation is a surgical procedure in which tissues or organs taken from one individual are implanted in another individual to replace diseased or nonfunctioning tissues or organs. Tissues or organs that come from donors who are alive typically work better and for a longer time than do tissues and organs that come from cadavers, provided that the donor tissues and organs are well-matched to the recipient. About 95 percent of renal transplants obtained from living parents or siblings function adequately for longer than a year. However, living donors supply only a small percentage of needed kidneys. By contrast, about 80 percent of well-matched cadaver kidneys function successfully for longer than a year. Immunosuppressive drugs help prevent immunological rejection of the donor kidney, but often make the patient more susceptible than usual to infection. Other possible complications of renal transplantation include acute renal failure; acute and chronic transplant rejection; surgical problems, such as urinary fistulas and wound infections; duodenal ulcer with bleeding and perforation; hypertension; and liver disease.

Percutaneous Transluminal Angioplasty. Percutaneous transluminal angioplasty (PTA) is a procedure that involves the dilation of a blood vessel by means of a balloon-tipped catheter that is inserted through the patient's skin and into the chosen vessel and then passed to the site of the obstruction. The balloon is then inflated in order to open the channel of the artery. PTA is sometimes used to treat obstructions of the renal arteries. A successful PTA to clear these renal obstructions often promptly leads to a reduction of hypertension. If the PTA is unsuccessful, however, a surgical bypass of the obstructed renal artery may be necessary. Compared with surgical treatment of the renal obstructions, PTA has several advantages. Some of these advantages are that (1) PTA patients need only a local anesthetic, whereas patients who undergo surgery require a general anesthetic, (2) the period of hospitalization for PTA patients is shorter than that for patients who undergo surgery, (3) PTA costs less to perform than surgery does, and (4) PTA causes less morbidity and mortality than surgery does. Complications of PTA rarely occur; however, catheter-induced trauma may necessitate urgent surgical intervention.

Disorders of the Urinary Bladder and Urethra

The urinary bladder and urethra may be the sites of infections, malignant tumors, or mechanical problems resulting from nerve damage. Although they are not immediately serious, bladder and urethral infections must be treated aggressively, because they present some danger of spreading first to the kidney and then throughout the body.

Cystitis and Urethritis

Cystitis is an inflammation of the bladder epithelium that is usually acute and is characterized by frequency of urination, fever, and dysuria. Red and white blood cells are present in the urinary sediment of a cystitis patient. *Urethritis* is an inflammation of the urethra. Urethritis may result from infection by common urinary bacteria or may be secondary to gonorrhea or chlamydia. Cystitis and urethritis are treated with antibiotics or sulfa drugs. For some individuals, treatment may be prolonged, because these conditions have a strong tendency to persist and/or recur.

Neurogenic Bladder

Neurogenic bladder is any condition of urinary bladder dysfunction resulting from a lesion of the central or peripheral nervous system. Diabetes, trauma, tumors, infections, and degenerative diseases involving the brain, spinal cord, and sacral nerve roots are the most common causes of neurogenic bladder. The presence of residual urine leads to calculus formation and infection, the two most common complications of neurogenic bladder. Neurogenic bladder may occur in one of two forms. In one type, the bladder has no muscle tone and is flaccid. Sensation of filling disappears, and the bladder becomes greatly distended. The quantity of residual urine is large and overflow dribbling is constant. The other type of neurogenic bladder is the hypertonic type, which is also known as the spastic bladder. The capacity of a spastic bladder is variable but generally is considerably less than normal. When the bladder's reduced maximum capacity is reached, it empties itself spontaneously and without warning.

Tumors of the Bladder

Malignant tumors of the bladder rarely develop in individuals who are younger than 40. Moreover, smokers and certain workers in the leather and rubber industries have an increased risk of developing these malignancies. These tumors have a tendency to recur following removal and may become more invasive with each recurrence. Malignant tumors of the bladder are staged on the basis of the degree of their invasion into the bladder wall. The greater the depth of infiltration, the higher the tumor stage and the poorer the prognosis. The most common malignant tumor of the urinary tract develops in the epithelium lining the bladder. If the urinary bladder tumor is confined to the epithelial layer, it can be removed through a cystoscope. The prognosis for survival following tumor removal from the epithelial layer is good, having an 85 to 90 percent 5-year survival rate. Treatment of invasive bladder cancers may include chemotherapy, radiation treatment, and/or the surgical removal of the bladder in a procedure called a *cystectomy*. If the tumor has gone through the bladder wall, in about half the cases the tumor cells will have also spread into the patient's pelvic lymph nodes. Long-term survival for invasive tumor patients is rare, even if only one pelvic node is involved.

11

The Reproductive System

Reproduction is the process by which a species creates a new generation of its own kind. In humans, the process is a sexual one, requiring the fusion of an ovum from a female and a sperm from a male. In this chapter, the anatomy and physiology of the male reproductive system and the disorders affecting it will be described first, followed by the anatomy and physiology of the female system and the disorders affecting it. The chapter will then discuss the physiology and disorders of pregnancy and childbirth, nonsurgical and surgical forms of contraception, and the anatomy of, and diseases that affect, the breasts. This chapter concludes with a section on sexually transmitted diseases.

ANATOMY AND PHYSIOLOGY OF THE MALE REPRODUCTIVE ORGANS

The reproductive organs of the male are the penis, testes, epididymis, and accessory glands. Figure 11–1 illustrates the male reproductive organs.

Figure 11–1.
Cross-Sectional Views of the Male Reproductive Organs.

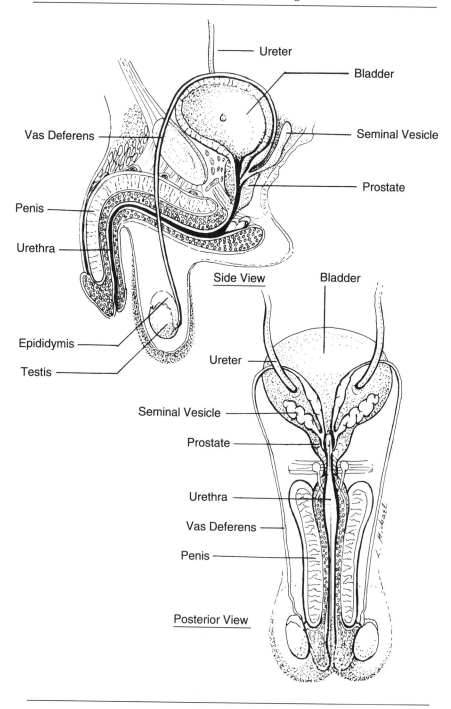

Ureter

Bladder

Vas Deferens

Seminal Vesicle

Prostate

Penis

Urethra

Side View   Bladder

Epididymis

Ureter

Testis

Seminal Vesicle

Prostate

Urethra

Vas Deferens

Penis

Posterior View

The Penis

The **penis** is the primary male reproductive and urinary excretion organ, and it contains the major portion of the urethra through which semen and urine are discharged from the male's body. This chapter will focus upon the penis in its function as an organ of reproduction. (Chapter 10, *The Urinary System*, focuses upon the excretion function of this organ.) The penis has a rich supply of blood. Sexual stimulation increases the supply of blood to the penis, resulting in penile erection.

The Testes

The **testes**, or *testicles*, are two egg-shaped glands that produce sperm cells. Sperm cells, which are also called **spermatozoa**, are the mature male cells that fertilize the female's eggs during reproduction. Sperm cells are contained in **semen**, which is a thick, whitish fluid that is composed of spermatozoa and secretions from the testes and other organs of the male reproductive system. In a normal adult male, the testes are situated in the **scrotum**, which is an elastic, external pouch that lies just below the penis and contains the testes and their accessory organs. Because the scrotum lies outside the body, the intrascrotal temperature is slightly lower than that in the abdominal cavity. This lower temperature is necessary for sperm cell production, which is called **spermatogenesis**. Spermatogenesis does not occur satisfactorily in undescended testicles, and so, if both testes remain in the male's abdomen, sterility will result.

In addition to manufacturing sperm, the testes also produce hormones called androgens. An **androgen** is any substance that possesses masculinizing activities. One androgen is **testosterone**, which is responsible for growth of hair in a male distribution pattern and other masculine characteristics. Testosterone affects bone growth, protein metabolism, and normal male sexual responses.

Epididymis and Vas Deferens

Positioned along an edge of each testis is a long, narrow, highly coiled duct, called the **epididymis**. Sperm cells and fluids produced in the testis pass into the epididymis and then into the vas deferens. The **vas deferens**, which is also called the *vas* or *spermatic cord*, is a continuation of the epididymis, extending into the pelvis and around the bladder and emptying into the urethra.

Accessory Glands of Reproduction

The accessory glands of reproduction in males are the seminal vesicles and the prostate gland. The *seminal vesicles* are two membranous sacs that join with the vas deferens as it opens into the urethra. These vesicles produce a large part of the seminal fluid, as well as the glucose necessary for sperm cell survival. The *prostate gland* is a structure that surrounds the neck of the bladder and the urethra. It adds an alkaline secretion to the seminal fluid.

DISORDERS OF THE MALE REPRODUCTIVE SYSTEM

Disorders of the male reproductive system may result from congenital abnormalities, infection, or tumors. This section will discuss some of the more common disorders that affect the male reproductive system. However, sexually transmitted diseases, which include some of the most serious infections of the male reproductive system, are discussed in a separate section at the end of the chapter. Furthermore, most disorders of the penis involve the urethra and are discussed in Chapter 10, *The Urinary System*. Therefore, disorders of the penis are not addressed here. This section will discuss disorders of the testes, scrotum, and accessory glands.

Disorders of the Testes and Scrotum

Disorders affecting the testes and the contents of the scrotum include congenital abnormalities, infections, and tumors.

Congenital Abnormalities

Congenital anomalies of the testes are rare. For example, absence of a testis rarely occurs, although imperfect descent of a testis from the abdominal cavity into the scrotum is fairly common. *Cryptorchidism*, which is also called *cryptorchism*, is a condition in which a male has an undescended testis. It is the most common congenital anomaly of the male reproductive system. In early fetal life, the testes are contained in the abdominal cavity, but prior to birth the testes normally descend into the scrotum. However, up to ten percent of male infants are born with an undescended testis. In most of these cases, the testis descends into the scrotum spontaneously within the first year of life, but in about 1 of every 500 males, the condition persists beyond that first year. The cause of cryptorchidism, which usually affects only one testis, is not known.

An undescended testis is relatively immobile and unprotected, and so is more subject to damage from trauma than is a descended testis. In addition, an undescended testis is usually sterile and frequently undergoes varying degrees of atrophy. However, the primary medical significance of cryptorchidism is the increased risk of cancer in both the descended and undescended testes. Cryptorchidism can be corrected by an operation called an **orchiopexy**, in which the surgeon anchors the patient's undescended testis in the scrotum. Although anchoring the testis in its normal location is desirable, the operation does not necessarily protect the testis from later malignant change.

Torsion of the Spermatic Cord

Torsion is an act of twisting. Torsion of the spermatic cord, which has an unknown cause, results in the sudden onset of acute pain in the scrotum and occurs most often in adolescents. A twisting of the spermatic cord interferes with the blood supply to the testis, resulting in swelling in the area of the torsion and obstruction of the cord. Surgery is necessary to correct the condition. If the torsion is not surgically corrected, the affected testis will have to be surgically removed.

Epididymitis

Epididymitis is an inflammation of the epididymis and can exist alone or in combination with an inflammation of the testes. If both the epididymis and the testes are involved, the condition is called **epididymo-orchitis**. Epididymitis may (1) occur as a complication of infections of the prostate, urethra, or bladder, (2) follow prostatic surgery, or (3) result from the use of a catheter. Manifestations of epididymitis include pain and swelling in the scrotum, painful urination, and urethral discharge. Physicians use diagnostic techniques, such as radionuclide scanning of the testes, to differentiate acute epididymitis from torsion of the spermatic cord. Antibiotics will cure most cases of epididymitis, although total resolution of the disease process may take several weeks.

Tumors

Some testicular tumors are benign, and others are malignant. Three of the more common types of benign tumors are spermatoceles, varicoceles, and hydroceles. A **spermatocele** is a cyst originating in the cells that connect the testis to the epididymis. These cysts vary in size and contain varying numbers of spermatozoa. They usually exist as solitary cysts but can be present as a cystic mass. A small or moderately sized spermatocele may cause no symptoms, but a large cyst will produce symptoms of pain in the area of the growth. The treatment for a spermatocele, if necessary, is surgical removal. A *varicocele* is a dilated, elongated, tortuous network of veins that usually occur on the left scrotum. Varicoceles may be asymptomatic or may cause a dragging, weighty sensation, and most do not require surgical intervention. They vary in size and are found in some men who are evaluated for sterility. However, the extent to which a varicocele contributes to sterility, if at all, is not known. A *hydrocele* is an abnormal accumulation of fluid within the sac that envelops the testis as it lies within the scrotum. Normally, this sac contains only a few drops of fluid. A hydrocele can be congenital or acquired, and may be associated with hernia. Treatment of a hydrocele may consist of needle aspiration to drain the excess accumulated fluid. If fluid reaccumulates, as it often does following needle drainage, surgical excision of the hydrocele may be necessary.

Most testicular tumors are malignant and are often curable. Malignant tumors of the testicles most often develop in males in the 15 to 44 age group. Physicians classify these tumors as being either seminomas or nonseminomas. Seminomas are malignant tumors of the testis that derive from abnormal, sperm cell precursors. Nonseminomas contain several types of abnormal cells. The first sign of a testicular tumor is a mass in the scrotum that is usually painless. Treatment typically involves the surgical removal of the tumor and of the testis. The pathologist then examines the tumor and determines whether it is a seminoma or a nonseminoma. CT scanning of the patient's abdomen and chest is used to stage the invasiveness of the disease and can also be used to monitor treated patients.

Under the TNM staging system, stage I disease is localized to the testes, stage II disease has spread to the abdominal lymph nodes, and stage III disease has spread to other abdominal structures or has metastasized above the diaphragm. Treatment for testicular cancers is evolving. Presently, *orchiectomy,* which is the surgical removal of a testis, and abdominal radiation are the usual treatments for stage I and early stage II seminomas. More advanced seminomas are treated with orchiectomy and chemotherapy, possibly followed by further surgery and/or radiation. Nonseminoma tumors are treated very much the same as seminomas at the various stages. Present day cure rates for seminomas and nonseminomas are greater than 95 percent for those patients who have stage I disease, 85 to 90 percent for patients whose disease is in early stage II, and 80 to 85 percent for patients whose disease is in more advanced stage II or stage III.

Disorders of the Accessory Glands

The three main disorders associated with the prostate gland and seminal vesicles are infection, hypertrophy, and cancer.

Infection

Acute prostatitis is a bacterial infection of the prostate characterized by (1) an abrupt onset of fever, (2) pain at the base of the penis, (3) rectal aching, (4) frequent, urgent, and painful urination, and (5) an uncontrolled discharge of cloudy fluid from the urethra. Rectal examination of a patient who has prostatitis will reveal a tender, hot, swollen prostate gland, and urinalysis will show the presence of white blood cells, bacteria, and, in some cases, blood. Complications of prostatitis include prostatic abscess, urinary obstruction from a swollen gland, pyelonephritis, and epididymitis. Antibiotic therapy usually is effective in treating prostatitis, although the infection tends to be recurrent. The disease frequently is mild, and only the complications, when they occur, are of serious medical concern. *Chronic prostatitis* is a recurrent, low-grade infection or inflammation of the prostate that is difficult to treat because often no bacterium can be identified as the cause of the disorder. In older men, chronic prostate infections may be associated with enlargement of the prostate gland.

Most infections of the prostate also involve the seminal vesicles. The symptoms and treatment of seminal vesicle infections do not differ from those of prostatitis.

Hypertrophy

Benign prostatic hypertrophy (BPH) is a condition that involves the noncancerous enlargement of the prostate gland and occurs with greatest frequency in males over age 50. By age 60, almost all men have some degree of prostatic enlargement, which may be related to hormonal changes associated with aging. Symptoms of BPH include difficulty in starting the flow of urine, decreased force of the urinary stream, dribbling of urine after voiding, urinary frequency, and waking from sleep to urinate. Benign prostatic hypertrophy can cause serious health problems if the enlarged prostate gland presses on the urethra, thus obstructing the flow of urine. In this situation, the patient's bladder may not empty completely, leaving some urine remaining in the bladder after each act of voiding. In time, the residual urine may become infected, which sometimes leads to an ascending pyelonephritis, a condition in which bacteria ascend from the bladder to the kidney through the ureters. The increasing residual urine and pressure required to excrete the urine may thin the bladder's muscular wall, thus permitting a diverticulum to form in the bladder. Sooner or later the ureters will dilate and eventually the kidney tissue will atrophy.

The surgical procedure generally used to correct the obstruction resulting from an enlarged prostate is called a transurethral resection. During a ***transurethral resection (TURP),*** the surgeon removes the obstructing prostatic tissue through the patient's urethra by means of a specially designed cystoscope and an electrical cutting device. Following the TURP, the individual may experience blood in his urine until the cut surfaces heal. Another surgical procedure for treating BPH is prostatic angioplasty, which involves the dilation of the prostatic urethra with a balloon-tipped catheter. Although prostatic angioplasty has successfully managed some cases of BPH, this procedure is not considered to be standard therapy. Furthermore, drug therapy may eventually be useful in treating BPH.

Cancer

In males, carcinoma of the prostate is the third leading cause of cancer death and the second most common cancer in men. Prostate cancer rarely affects males younger than age 50 and often is discovered at an early stage as an incidental finding at TURP, as an abnormal lump during a rectal exam, or at the time the condition produces symptoms, such as hematuria, urinary obstruction, and bone pain. A relatively new blood test, called a prostatic specific antigen (PSA) test, shows promise for the early detection of prostatic cancer. A PSA is typically used in conjunction with ultrasonography and biopsy. A biopsy of a tissue sample is necessary to confirm the diagnosis of prostate cancer. A tumor that is classified as low grade has a much better prognosis than one that is classified as high grade. Physicians usually stage prostate cancers by either the TMN system or the A to D system. In this latter system, A means that the cancer is localized and D means that the cancer has metastasized to distant tissues. The seminal vesicles are often the site of prostate cancer metastasis. B and C refer to intermediate stages of prostate cancer invasion.

Treatment of carcinoma of the prostate generally involves surgical removal of the lesion and/or radiation therapy. A patient whose cancer is localized can expect a long-term cure, and a five-year survival rate of 58 percent is possible even for those patients who have stage D disease. Easing the patient's level of discomfort can be accomplished by radiation, chemotherapy, or antiandrogen treatment.

ANATOMY AND PHYSIOLOGY OF THE FEMALE REPRODUCTIVE ORGANS

The female reproductive organs are the uterus, ovaries, fallopian tubes, vagina, vulva, associated accessory glands, supporting structures, and external genital organs. Figure 11–2 illustrates the female reproductive organs.

The Uterus, Ovaries, and Fallopian Tubes

The *uterus* is a hollow, thick-walled, pear-shaped muscular organ that performs functions that are primarily related to childbearing. It is situated between a woman's bladder and her rectum. The *ovaries* are two solid, oval sexual glands in which ova, or eggs, are formed. The ovaries are located behind and on either side of the uterus and are suspended below and close to the outer end of the fallopian tubes. The *fallopian tubes*, which are also known as *oviducts*, lie on either side of the uterus and are open passageways that function to move ova from the surface of the ovary into the uterus.

The larger, upper part of the uterus is called the *corpus*, or body, and it contains a small triangular space known as the *endometrial cavity*. The wall of the corpus is composed of two layers of tissue. The inner, thin layer, which lines the cavity of the uterine corpus, is called the *endometrium*. The outer, thicker layer of the corpus is muscular and is called the *myometrium*. A very thin layer of peritoneum covers the myometrium.

The body of the uterus is loosely supported in its position by various ligaments and can move with considerable freedom. The part of the uterus that lies above the fallopian tubes' points of entrance is called the *fundus*. The *cervix* is the lower constricted neck of the uterus. The cervical canal communicates with the endometrial cavity above and, through its external opening, with the vagina below. During pregnancy, the cervix enlarges and softens and, with labor contractions, dilates to permit passage of the fetus. The cervix does not change position readily, because it has strong ligamentous attachments. The uterus is said to be in a "normal" position when the uterine body is anterior to and slightly bent forward on the cervix.

The inner end of a fallopian tube opens into the endometrial cavity, and the outer opening communicates with the peritoneal cavity. Each fallopian tube has fringed ends called *fimbriae* that drape down over the ovary.

The size of different individuals' ovaries varies considerably and may even vary in a given individual at different times during her life. At birth, a female's ovary contains hundreds of thousands of micro-

Figure 11–2.
Cross-Sectional Views of the Female Reproductive Organs.

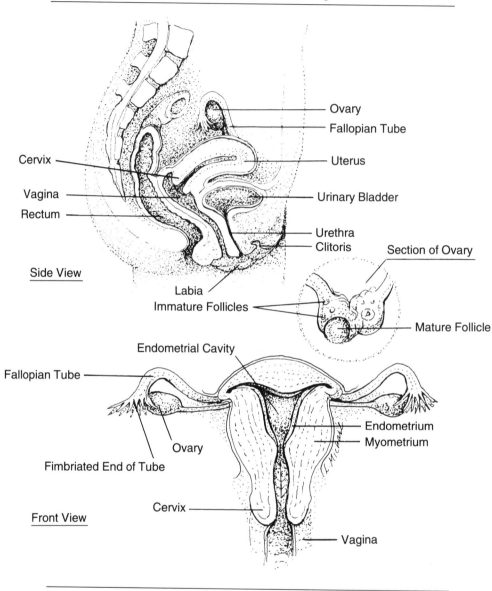

Ovary
Fallopian Tube
Cervix
Uterus
Vagina
Urinary Bladder
Rectum
Urethra
Clitoris
Section of Ovary
Side View
Labia
Immature Follicles
Mature Follicle
Endometrial Cavity
Fallopian Tube
Endometrium
Myometrium
Ovary
Fimbriated End of Tube
Cervix
Front View
Vagina

scopic ova. Each ovum is surrounded by fluid and is contained in a
sac or follicle. As the woman approaches her childbearing years,
these primitive ova begin to enlarge and mature. The ripening of an
ovum and bursting of the follicle with the release of a mature ovum

occurs in the process called ***ovulation***, usually about 14 days before the woman's next expected menstrual period. Generally, only one ovum develops fully and is released during any one menstrual cycle. Occasionally ovulation will not occur at all or will occur only infrequently, a situation that is more common during the very early and very late years of a woman's menstrual life. Sometimes ovulation occurs twice during the same menstrual cycle. Although the maturation of an ovum is not believed to occur in each ovary on an alternating basis, over a period of time both ovaries take part in this process. During an average woman's reproductive life, about 400 eggs will reach maturity and be released by the ovary.

In addition to the manufacture of ova, the ovaries produce estrogens. ***Estrogens*** are female hormones that stimulate growth of the endometrium and myometrium, cervix, vaginal mucosa, and the ducts and glands of the breasts. Estrogens may affect hair and fat distribution and may slow the aging processes that are manifested by wrinkles, arteriosclerosis, and loss of bone calcium.

The Vagina and Vulva

The ***vagina*** is a hollow, elastic, muscular tube that functions as a birth canal, the passageway for the escape of menstrual fluid, and a receptacle for semen during intercourse. The vagina extends from a woman's external genitalia to her cervix, around which it is attached. The vagina lies behind the bladder and in front of the rectum. A significant characteristic of the muscular and elastic fibers in the vaginal walls is that they are capable of great distention, which is important during passage of the fetus at delivery. The area that contains the external genital organs of a female is called the ***vulva***. The external female genitalia are the labia, clitoris, and hymen. The ***labia*** are elongated skin folds that extend down and back on either side around the vaginal opening. The ***clitoris*** is a small, cylindrical erectile structure that is located above the urethral opening at the most forward position of the vulva and is partly concealed by the labia. A circular fold of tissue known as the ***hymen*** surrounds the vaginal opening and partially closes it in virginal females.

DISORDERS OF THE FEMALE REPRODUCTIVE SYSTEM

Many disorders of the female reproductive system affect more than one component of the system. This section will first introduce some of the more common procedures that physicians use to diagnose female reproductive system disorders. Then this section will address some of the more common of these disorders, including disturbances in the menstrual cycle, disorders associated with menopause, infections, endometriosis, uterine tumors, and ovarian tumors.

Gynecology is the branch of medicine that treats diseases of the genital tract in females. Many specialized diagnostic procedures are used in the investigation of gynecologic disorders. We will discuss several of these diagnostic techniques, including pelvic exams, Pap smears, ultrasonography, colposcopy, hysterosalpingography, dilation and curettage, conization, hysteroscopy, and laparoscopy.

A *pelvic exam* is an office procedure for (1) directly visualizing a female's external genitalia, vagina, and cervix and (2) palpating her ovaries, uterus, fallopian tubes, uterine ligaments, and rectal area for abnormalities or tenderness. A Pap smear or samples for culture or biopsy may also be taken during a pelvic exam. A *Pap smear* is a screening test for cervical cancer in which the physician gently scrapes the surface of the female patient's cervix and posterior vagina and places the obtained mucus on a glass slide. A pathologist then stains and examines the cells contained in the mucus on the slide. Some pathologists use a system that classifies the appearance of the patient's cervical and vaginal cells by describing the cells as being normal, dysplastic, inflamed, cancerous, and so on. *Dysplastic cells* are adult cells that display an alteration in their size, shape, or organization, and *dysplasia* is the condition in which the size, shape, and organization of adult cells is altered. Another classification system some pathologists use labels the classes of cervical and vaginal cells from I to V:

- Class I—normal cells
- Class II—slightly abnormal cells with either mild dysplasia or inflammation
- Class III—greater degree of dysplasia
- Class IV—severe dysplasia or carcinoma-in-situ
- Class V—malignant cells

Conization is a procedure that is used for both the diagnosis and treatment of cervical dysplasia. In a *conization* procedure, the surgeon removes a cone of tissue from the patient's cervical canal. The sample tissue can be microscopically evaluated by a pathologist for the presence of dysplasia or cancer. Conization is now used more for treatment than for diagnosis alone. Laser surgery, which is typically performed on an outpatient basis, may be used instead of conization to eliminate dysplastic cervical cells.

Another diagnostic technique that sometimes accompanies a pelvic exam is colposcopy. *Colposcopy* is an office procedure that involves the insertion of an instrument called a colposcope into the patient's vagina for the examination of the cervical and vaginal tissues. A colposcope does not utilize fiberoptic technology, but instead contains a magnifying lens that aids in the identification of premalignant cells and areas for biopsy.

Ultrasonography, which was defined and described in Chapter 3, *Specialized Diagnostic Techniques*, is a valuable noninvasive tool for evaluating the female genital tract and for diagnosing abnormalities of the ovaries, tubes, uterus, and uterine ligaments. For example, ultrasound technology can reveal problems, such as ectopic pregnancy, ovarian cysts, or certain tumors, that will be discussed later in this chapter. Ultrasonography can also provide information during pregnancy about the developing fetus. Moreover, ultrasonography can be performed in conjunction with fine needle aspiration biopsy in the diagnosis of reproductive tract malignancy.

Hysterosalpingography, which is also known as *uterosalpingography*, is a diagnostic procedure involving an x-ray study of the patient's uterine cavity and the canal of the fallopian tubes after the injection of a radiopaque substance or gas into the patient's uterus. The x-ray record from this study is called a ***hysterosalpingogram*** or *uterosalpingogram*. Hysterosalpingography is performed on infertile women to see if an obstruction is blocking the fallopian tubes and to determine the possible role that any existing uterine disorder plays in causing infertility.

Dilation and curettage, which is commonly called *D&C*, is an operative procedure in which the physician dilates the canal of the patient's cervix with a series of graduated dilators. The dilation is followed by a scraping, which is called a ***curettage***, of the patient's uterine cavity. In some patients, the scraping removes the endometrial lining of the uterus for microscopic examination and is performed to examine the causes of infertility, menstrual irregularities, postmenopausal bleeding, and painful menstruation. Dilation and curettage is also commonly performed on women who have had a miscarriage in order to remove all remaining placental tissue.

Although fiberoptic endoscopy was discussed in Chapter 3, at least two specialized applications, hysteroscopy and abdominal laparoscopy, are often used in diagnosing gynecologic disorders. ***Hysteroscopy*** involves the insertion into the patient's uterus of a modified fiberoptic scope, known as a hysteroscope, for visual examination of the cervical canal and endometrial cavity. Typically, the physician fills the patient's uterus with gas in order to create bigger spaces among the organs and structures in the endometrial cavity so that the hysteroscopic inspection can be more effective.

The hysteroscope is a valuable instrument for diagnosing the cause of infertility. Through the hysteroscope the physician can observe intrauterine adhesions, tumors, and abnormalities of the uterus. ***Abdominal laparoscopy*** is the inspection of the patient's abdominal and pelvic organs using a fiberoptic scope, known as a laparoscope, that the surgeon inserts through a small incision in the front wall of the patient's abdomen. Laparoscopy is a common procedure for diagnosing and treating gynecologic conditions such as endometriosis, tumors, pelvic pain, and ectopic pregnancy.

Disturbances in the Menstrual Cycle

Many of the reproductive system disorders affecting women are the result of disturbances in the menstrual cycle. During a menstrual cycle, an ovum is liberated from its follicle onto the surface of an ovary and then moves into the fallopian tube. The mechanism by which an ovum moves from ovary to tube is not understood, but the fimbriae may play a role in this process. Once in a tube, the ovum moves toward the uterus by peristaltic contractions of the tubal muscles. If the ovum is not fertilized, the ovum, part of the endometrium, and blood are discharged from the woman's body through the vagina. The cycle is under hormonal control and normally recurs approximately every four weeks, in the absence of pregnancy. ***Menstruation***, which is the discharge of the blood and tissues from the uterus through the vagina, generally lasts three to five days.

Premenstrual Tension Syndrome

Premenstrual tension syndrome is a monthly disorder of unknown cause that usually occurs during the seven to ten days prior to menstruation. An estimated 10 to 12 million women experience some symptoms of this disorder. Symptoms of premenstrual tension syndrome include irritability, fluid retention, insomnia, fatigue, emotional instability, craving for sweets, depression, and acne. The extent of the symptoms ranges from minimal to severe, and treatment is variably successful. Oral contraceptives, diuretics, vitamin B_6, tranquilizers, and, on rare occasions, psychiatric consultation for severe mood symptoms have all been used. For most affected women, the symptoms of the syndrome are unpleasant but not impairing.

Dysmenorrhea

Dysmenorrhea is painful and difficult menstruation and is commonly associated with lower abdominal cramps. A significant number of menstruating women have menstrual pain that is severe enough to miss work for one to three days each month. In instances in which the painful menstruation has no demonstrable cause, the disorder is known as *primary dysmenorrhea*. If the painful menstruation results from a known condition, the disorder is known as *secondary dysmenorrhea*. Primary dysmenorrhea may result from abnormal prostaglandin[1] production. Medications, such as birth control pills or ibuprofen, that decrease prostaglandin secretion are often very effective treatments for the pain. Vaginal delivery of a child also helps relieve the mother's symptoms of dysmenorrhea, perhaps by dilating the cervix. Patients who do not respond to the normal treatments need further evaluation.

Amenorrhea

Amenorrhea is the absence of menstruation. Most causes of amenorrhea do not indicate serious disease. For example, pregnancy, lactation, and the lack of adequate ovarian hormonal stimulation at menopause are three common causes of this condition. Nutritional deficiencies, stress, and disorders of the uterus, ovaries, or the pituitary, thyroid, or adrenal glands are other causes of amenorrhea. Furthermore, amenorrhea is associated with an abnormally low level of body fat. Excessive exercise, such as marathon running or ballet, or an eating disorder may lead to amenorrhea. Treatment of this condition depends on its cause.

Menorrhagia and Metrorrhagia

Menorrhagia is an excessive menstrual flow, and *metrorrhagia* is uterine bleeding between normal menstrual periods. Uterine hemorrhage, as manifested by menorrhagia and metrorrhagia, may result from many causes. The control of menstruation is supported by a very delicately controlled hormone balance, and in some women this balance is disturbed. Some other causes of uterine hemorrhage not directly related to hormone imbalance are infections of the pelvic organs, disease of the ovaries, tumors of the uterus, and certain systemic diseases, such as anemias, bleeding disorders, and leukemia. However, for many uterine hemorrhage patients, the cause of the disorder is not demonstrable. These patients are said to have functional, or dysfunctional, uterine bleeding.

---

[1]*Prostaglandin* is a group of fatty acids that stimulate contractions of uterine and other smooth muscle tissues and perform other functions in the human body.

In women older than 40, a D&C procedure often will establish a diagnosis of the cause of the abnormal bleeding. In many instances, the D&C also has a therapeutic benefit because a normal menstrual pattern returns after the procedure, although the reason this occurs is not clear. Younger women who experience uterine hemorrhage may be treated with oral contraceptives or other hormones if a pelvic exam produces no evidence of disease and an evaluation for pregnancy is negative.

Infections

The organs of the female reproductive system can be infected by bacteria, fungi, protozoa, or viruses. Some of these organisms are transmitted mainly through sexual contact, and some are often transmitted by other methods. This section will address infections that often are **not** obtained through sexual contact with an infected partner. These infections, which may affect any organ of the system, include vaginitis and Bartholin's gland abscess. Infections that are primarily transmitted by sexual contact are discussed in a separate section at the end of this chapter.

Vaginitis

A *vaginitis* is any infection or inflammation of the mucous membrane of the vagina and is characterized by itching and a vaginal discharge that is usually heavy, pus-filled, and foul-smelling. The vaginitis may be noninfectious or infectious. A chemical irritation of the vagina resulting from the use of feminine hygiene products is an example of a noninfectious vaginitis. An infectious vaginitis may arise from a fungus, bacterium, or a protozoa. In about 15 percent of vaginitis cases, a combination of infectious organisms is present. Treatment with oral and topical drugs is usually successful, but the specific drug depends on the cause of the infection.

Bartholin's Gland Abscess

Bartholin's glands, which are two small glands that are situated on either side of the vaginal opening, may be the seat of infection. A *Bartholin's gland abscess* occurs when an infection involves the entire gland and a collection of pus distends the gland, forming an abscess. Symptoms and signs of an abscess are localized pain, swelling, and painful sexual intercourse. The oral administration of antibiotics and a surgical incision into the gland in order to drain the collected pus are the customary forms of treatment for an abscessed Bartholin's gland.

Endometriosis

Endometriosis is a condition in which very small pieces of endometrial tissue become implanted and grow in areas outside their normal location in the lining of the uterine cavity. These endometrial implants are known as *endometriomas*. How endometrial tissue escapes from the uterine cavity to grow elsewhere is the subject of many theories, but no single theory fully explains the phenomenon. The theory that has received the widest medical acceptance states that menstrual blood containing endometrial cells flows backward through the fallopian tubes and that the viable endometrial cells implant wherever they land after escape from the fimbriated ends of the tubes.

Endometriomas grow on the surfaces of the fallopian tubes, ovaries, uterus, bladder, vagina, rectum, uterine ligaments, and other pelvic and abdominal structures. Under the influence of the female hormones, these endometriomas undergo the cyclic changes of menstruation that affect normal endometrium tissue. Endometriomas on the surface of the ovary hemorrhage with each menstrual period. Each successive menstrual period adds more blood within a thin-walled cyst until finally a large structure called a "chocolate cyst," so called because old blood has a dark brown color, is formed. *Adenomyosis* is a condition in which the endometrial implants are located in the myometrium.

The signs and symptoms of endometriosis depend on the location and number of the implants. Common manifestations of endometriosis include dysmenorrhea, sterility, pelvic pain, rectal discomfort, painful sexual intercourse, and abnormal menstruation. Endometrial implants on peritoneal surfaces may produce dense adhesions, which can cause intestinal obstruction if a loop of bowel is involved. The activity of the endometrial implants subsides as ovarian activity wanes at menopause, but during the active phase, endometriosis may be the cause of considerable impairment.

Removal of endometrial implants or scar tissue through laparoscopic surgery may successfully treat endometriosis, but sometimes multiple surgical procedures are necessary to effect a complete cure. Hormone treatment will suppress normal ovarian activity during the menstrual cycle, but occasionally the endometrial problems are of such magnitude that the surgical removal of the uterus in a *hysterectomy* and/or the surgical removal of both ovaries in a *bilateral oophorectomy* are necessary. Drug therapy with Danocrine has been quite successful in relieving endometrial symptoms and improving fertility. Furthermore, although endometriosis can impair a woman's ability to become pregnant, pregnancy often improves the condition.

Disorders Associated with Menopause

Strictly speaking, *menopause* refers to the specific biologic event of the last menstrual period, and *climacteric* encompasses those years beginning when the ovarian function starts to wane and ending after the cessation of menses, when the hormone output from the ovaries has stabilized at a lower level. However, this text will follow the common use of **menopause** to mean both the last menstrual period and the years of declining ovarian activity. Most women experience menopause in their late 40s or early 50s. Some evidence indicates that menopause begins at a slightly later age now than it did several generations ago. Preceding the cessation of menstruation, a woman may experience irregular menstrual flow that is either more frequent or less frequent than she usually experiences and that may be heavier or more scanty than she usually experiences. The primary symptoms of menopause are hot flashes, sweating, irritability, headaches, and fatigue. Some women also experience mild depression during menopause. Many women experience these symptoms to at least some degree. Only severe symptoms should be any cause for concern. However, some women experience no symptoms related to menopause. Few reliable statistics about the incidence of serious menopausal pathology are available. This section will describe a few of the more common problems associated with menopause.

Dysfunctional Uterine Bleeding

In the years immediately preceding menopause, decreased progesterone secretion often produces irregular uterine bleeding. Oral doses of progesterone are usually the most satisfactory treatment for irregular menstrual periods. Lack of a satisfactory response to progesterone suggests that the bleeding may arise from causes such as uterine polyps, fibroid tumors, or cancer, which are discussed in a later section.

Postmenopausal Bleeding

Vaginal bleeding that occurs six months or more after the cessation of menses is always a sign for concern and must be investigated promptly. A D&C and Pap smear are performed to rule out carcinoma of the cervix and endometrium as a cause of this bleeding. Other causes of postmenopausal bleeding include the improper use of estrogen medication, atrophic vaginitis, ulcers of the cervix, estrogen-secreting ovarian tumors, blood disorders, and uterine polyps.

Atrophic Vaginitis

Atrophic vaginitis, which is also called *senile vaginitis*, is a form of vaginitis that occurs in postmenopausal women and is associated with an estrogen deficiency. The vaginal mucous membrane in postmenopausal women is prone to superficial ulceration and infection. Vaginal burning, itching, and bleeding are common symptoms of atrophic vaginitis, and treatment with low-dose estrogens often is helpful. The major significance of this condition is that the bleeding may raise a suspicion of cancer or of other serious causes of postmenopausal bleeding. Atrophic vaginitis typically responds to topical or oral estrogen treatment.

Tumors of the Uterus

The uterus is a common site of tumors, many of which are benign. However, the uterus, especially the cervix, is also subject to malignant tumors. Widespread use of the Pap smear in recent years has greatly contributed to the early identification of cervical malignancy in a treatable stage. This section will first look at benign uterine tumors and then will address malignant uterine tumors.

Benign Tumors

The most common types of benign uterine tumors are polyps and leiomyomas. Uterine polyps typically arise from the mucosa of the endocervical canal and the endometrium, and are soft, red, fleshy, structures that bleed readily and may be responsible for a discharge. The surgical removal of a polyp is a minor procedure.

Fibroids, which are also called *myomas* or *leiomyomas*, are benign tumors that are composed primarily of uterine muscle that has undergone excessive growth. These tumors rarely become malignant. Fibroids, which are the most common tumors of the uterus, generally develop during a woman's active menstrual years and stop growing at menopause. About 40 percent of adult women have fibroids, but most of these tumors are too small to be medically significant or clinically recognized. The manifestations of fibroids may include menorrhagia, prolongation of the menstrual period, dysmenorrhea, failure to conceive, increased incidence of miscarriage, difficult labor, and pelvic discomfort caused by large fibroids that place pressure on the woman's bladder and rectum. The choice of treatment for fibroids is influenced by many factors, including the age of the patient, the location and size of the fibroid, and the nature of the patient's symptoms. Small tumors generally require no treatment, but large growths or those growths that cause symptoms often are treated by the removal of the fibroid in an operative procedure called a **myomectomy**, which can be performed using traditional surgical or fiberoptic and laser techniques. A hysterectomy is performed only in extreme cases.

Malignant Tumors

Uterine malignancies arise either from the cervix or from the body of the uterus. A Class IV or V Pap smear strongly suggests cervical cancer, which is confirmed by biopsy. The most common cervical malignancy arises from squamous epithelium and is, therefore, a squamous cell carcinoma. Carcinoma of the cervix often produces no symptoms, but will show up on an abnormal Pap smear. However, abnormal bleeding or symptoms of metastatic disease may occur in more advanced cases of cervical cancer. Treatment of this cancer is by hysterectomy, radiation therapy, or laser surgery to remove the affected area, depending on the stage of the malignancy. Five-year survival rates depend primarily on the stage of the lesion at the time of initial treatment, as well as on the grade of the tumor. For example, surgery to remove carcinoma-in-situ has a cure rate greater than 98 percent. Cone biopsy may also be curative in very localized cervical cancer.

The most common carcinoma of the body of the uterus arises from the glandular endometrium and is known as an adenocarcinoma. The most common symptom of an adenocarcinoma is bleeding that is irregular, between menstrual cycles, or postmenopausal. In addition, the patient's uterus may enlarge slightly because of the presence of the growing tumor. The adenocarcinoma patient's prognosis depends on the stage of the disease and the grade of tumor at the time of the initial treatment. Cancers of the uterus cannot be staged based on clinical examination. Instead, they are staged in association with surgery. Hysterectomy is the traditional method of treating these cancers. Typically, the surgery will also include the removal of the fallopian tubes, the ovaries, and the pelvic and para-aortic lymph nodes, in order to look for malignant cells. The surgery is often preceded or followed by radiation. The 5-year survival rate for patients who have tumors that are limited to the endometrium is 90 to 95 percent. If the tumor has invaded the uterine wall through less than half of the wall's thickness, the 5-year survival rate is approximately 80 percent. Invasion of the uterine wall by more than half of the wall's thickness provides a 5-year survival rate of approximately 70 percent. Patients whose endometrial malignancy has invaded either the glands that line the cervix or the cervix itself face a 5-year survival rate of up to 60 percent. If the malignancy (1) involves the uterine surface, the tubes, and/or the ovaries, (2) appears in the abdominal fluid, or (3) has metastasized to the pelvic and/or para-aortic lymph nodes, the associated 5-year survival rate is approximately 30 percent. The 5-year survival rate for patients whose tumor has invaded the bladder or rectum is approximately 5 percent.

Tumors of the Ovaries

The medical community recognizes many different benign and malignant ovarian tumors. Unlike cancerous tumors of the uterus, ovarian malignancies usually are asymptomatic in the early stages and are often fast-growing.

Benign Tumors

Cysts constitute the most common type of benign ovarian tumor. As defined in Chapter 5, *The Skin*, a cyst is any closed cavity or sac, normal or abnormal, that is lined by epithelium. Cysts may be single or multiple, and they may develop on one ovary or on both simultaneously. One type of simple cyst develops from an ovarian follicle if the follicle fails to rupture and release an ovum during ovulation. Follicle cysts usually are single and vary in size, but are seldom larger than a lemon. Their size may change during different stages of the woman's menstrual cycle. After several menstrual cycles, the fluid within the cyst may be reabsorbed, thus allowing for the complete disappearance of the cyst.

Another type of cystic disorder of the ovaries is polycystic ovary syndrome. **Polycystic ovary syndrome**, which is also called *Stein-Leventhal syndrome*, is a symptom-complex that is characterized by menstrual irregularities, obesity, sterility, and, occasionally, a male type of body hair distribution. Sterility from the polycystic process is the result of hormonally induced **anovulation**, which is the absence of ovulation, in both ovaries. Treatment of the Stein-Leventhal syndrome typically consists of hormone therapy or the surgical removal of a wedge of tissue from the ovaries.

Some types of benign cysts are considered to be precancerous.

For example, cystadenomas and dermoid cysts are common neoplastic cysts that usually are benign, but may undergo malignant transformation. Cystadenomas were discussed in Chapter 4, *Tumors*. A **dermoid cyst** is a tumor that is composed of several different types of tissue, none of which is native to the location of the growth, and that results from abnormal cell development in the embryo.

Malignant Tumors

The most common ovarian cancers are primary growths. However, the ovary may also be the seat of metastatic spread from carcinomas that have their primary growth in other organs. Treatment of all ovarian cancers includes the full spectrum of methods used in the treatment of any malignant disease: surgical excision, radiation, and chemotherapy. The five-year survival rates for patients who have ovarian malignancies depend on the cell type, grade, and stage of the cancer. Because most ovarian tumors do not produce symptoms in the initial phase of their growth, a malignant neoplasm may not be detected at an early point in its growth. The benefits of early diagnosis, such as the best opportunity for complete removal of the tumor, are often obtained by patients who have regular physical examinations. Symptoms that occur later in the growth of ovarian malignancies include pelvic discomfort, cramps or steady dull pelvic pain, and menstrual disturbances. Symptoms that are produced by ovarian cancers that have spread to other locations depend on the location of the metastatic lesions.

Hormone-Secreting Tumors

Certain ovarian tumors, some of which are malignant and some of which are benign, manufacture sex hormones. For example, **granulosa cell tumors**, which are malignant neoplasms that arise out of the cells that surround the ovarian follicles, secrete estrogen. These tumors are low grade, and affected patients can expect a 50 to 60 percent survival rate after 20 years. Symptoms produced by granulosal cell tumors are related to its estrogen production and include irregular menstrual bleeding. Another sex hormone-producing ovarian tumor is the **Sertoli-Leydig cell tumor**, which arises from the supporting tissue of an ovary and secretes a male sex hormone. Symptoms of Sertoli-Leydig cell tumors include defeminizing phenomena, such as amenorrhea and diminished breast size, and signs of virilism, such as a heavy growth of facial hair.

PHYSIOLOGY AND DISORDERS OF PREGNANCY AND CHILDBIRTH

Obstetrics is the branch of medicine that deals with the management of pregnancy from fertilization through labor and childbirth. *Fertilization*, which is the union of an ovum and a spermatozoa and includes the fusion of male and female chromosomes, usually occurs in a woman's fallopian tube. Sensitive blood pregnancy tests may be positive as soon as seven to ten days after fertilization, and urine tests may be positive in two to three weeks. Repeated cell division of the fertilized ovum takes place as it moves down the tube and implants in the endometrium. The endometrium provides a healthy environment for the implantation and growth of the fertilized ovum. After an ovum leaves an ovarian follicle, the empty follicle becomes known as the *corpus luteum*, which manufactures progesterone. Progesterone performs two important functions related to pregnancy: (1) it helps prepare the endometrium for the implantation and growth of a fertilized ovum and (2) it helps develop the system of the breast that allows the woman to produce and secrete milk. If the woman becomes pregnant, the corpus luteum lasts until the end of the third month of pregnancy. During pregnancy, the corpus luteum maintains the implanted ovum until the placental hormones can assume this responsibility. If conception does not occur, the levels of progesterone and estrogen decrease, causing the endometrium to collapse and be discharged in the menstrual flow. This process repeats itself approximately every 28 days from a woman's puberty to menopause unless pregnancy or disease, including emotional illness, supervenes.

During the first two weeks of pregnancy, the product of conception is called a *conceptus* or *zygote*. From the third to the fifth week of pregnancy, during which time the fertilized ovum develops into a recognizable form, the product of conception is called an *embryo*, and after the fifth week, it is called a *fetus*. Soon after the fertilized ovum implants in the endometrium, the development of the placenta begins. The *placenta* is an organ that is found only in mammals, and it provides nutrition to the conceptus throughout the pregnancy. The placenta also manufactures hormones that are required in order for the pregnancy to last for the full term. Blood vessels that communicate with the maternal and fetal circulatory systems develop within the placenta, but these two circulatory systems remain separate. Although maternal blood cells do not enter the fetal circulation and fetal blood cells do not enter the maternal circulation, glucose, oxygen, and other vital substances pass through placental tissues from mother to fetus. In addition, waste products of fetal metabolism pass into the maternal circulation for elimination by the mother.

By the end of the third month of pregnancy, the mother's uterine cavity is filled with amniotic fluid, which surrounds, supports, and protects the growing fetus. The uterus undergoes great enlargement during pregnancy, so that by the time the fetus reaches full term, the mother's uterine capacity has increased over 500 times. This enlargement results in the displacement of the mother's stomach and intestines and considerable stretching of the mother's abdominal wall.

The normal pregnancy lasts about 40 weeks and is typically divided into "trimesters" of approximately 13 weeks each. The expected date of confinement (EDC), which is also called the "due date," is calculated by adding 280 days to the first day of the mother's last normal menstrual period (LNMP). Although the EDC is only an approximation, about 90 percent of all pregnancies will terminate within two weeks of the calculated delivery date. A *premature infant* is a baby that is delivered before its organs have completed normal intrauterine development. The infant's length, weight, and "age"—as measured from the mother's LNMP—are frequently used to define the limits of prematurity. However, some authorities think that birth weight is the single most important criterion for determining prematurity and consider any baby that weighs 2,500 grams or less at birth to be premature.

Labor is the series of events that results in the delivery of the baby. During labor, the strong uterine muscles contract to assist in the descent of the fetus through the birth canal. The onset of labor occurs as the result of several factors, all working toward the same goal. Labor begins with "labor pains," which are intermittent, involuntary contractions of the muscles in the body of the uterus. These contractions increase in intensity and duration as labor progresses. Thinning, relaxation, and dilation of the cervix are also associated with these contractions. At some point in this process, the membrane that contains the amniotic fluid and the fetus bursts. When the dilation of the cervix is complete, the baby begins its descent into the vagina and, with the bearing down efforts of the mother, is delivered from the mother's body. Several minutes after the baby's delivery, continuing contractions of the uterus expel the placenta. In the weeks following childbirth, the mother's pelvic organs, which were so markedly stretched during pregnancy and delivery, gradually return to their normal size.

Complications of Pregnancy

A normal pregnancy, labor, and vaginal delivery usually offer no threat to the life of the mother or the child and only insignificant morbidity for either. Even a *cesarean section*, which is an incision through the mother's abdominal and uterine walls in order to deliver a fetus, by skilled physicians utilizing modern methods of anesthesia, properly matched blood, and well-trained postoperative care, has an exceedingly favorable outlook for mother and child. A cesarean section may be performed if the mother has a pelvic deformity or active genital herpes or if her body fails to make normal progress during labor. A cesarean section may also be indicated if (1) the fetus is in distress during or prior to labor or has not moved into the normal position for delivery or (2) if the placenta is in an abnormal position or is not functioning properly. Once a woman has given birth by cesarean section, she may or may not need to have a cesarean section for each subsequent child.

Abortion

An *abortion* is the termination of pregnancy before the conceptus, embryo, or fetus is capable of living outside the uterus. Abortions are classified as spontaneous, therapeutic, or voluntary. A *spontaneous abortion*, or *miscarriage*, is a termination of pregnancy that occurs naturally. Up to 50 percent of conceptions end in miscarriage, which most often occur in the first trimester of pregnancy. Typical causes of spontaneous abortions are abnormalities in the fetus or in the mother's uterus, placenta, or ovary. A systemic illness in the mother may also cause a spontaneous abortion. Most women do not repetitively miscarry. A *therapeutic abortion* is the deliberate interruption of pregnancy for medical reasons that usually pertain to the health of the mother or fetus. A *voluntary abortion* is the deliberate interruption of pregnancy that is performed in the absence of a medical need.

Bleeding during Pregnancy

Vaginal bleeding during pregnancy may have many causes. In the first trimester of pregnancy, vaginal bleeding may result from a *threatened spontaneous abortion*, a condition in early pregnancy that is characterized by bleeding, menstrual-like cramps, and abdominal pain. In many cases, these signs disappear, and the pregnancy continues to full term. At other times, the bleeding and cramps become more severe, and placental tissue is expelled from the woman's vagina. Curettage may be required to stop the bleeding and remove all remaining fetal and placental tissue.

A second cause of bleeding and pain in the first trimester of pregnancy is an ectopic pregnancy. An ***ectopic pregnancy***, which is also called a *tubal pregnancy*, is a condition in which the fertilized ovum implants and develops outside the mother's uterine cavity. The most common location for an extrauterine pregnancy is the fallopian tube. The reason the fertilized ovum stops in the tube and does not implant in the uterus is not known, but pelvic adhesions, endometriosis, and prior infections of the tube may contribute to an ectopic pregnancy. Ectopic pregnancies do not develop to full term, and many spontaneously abort into the mother's abdominal cavity through the tube's fimbriated end, causing few symptoms and minimal intra-abdominal bleeding. On the other hand, some ectopic pregnancies cause tubal rupture and massive intra-abdominal hemorrhage that endanger the life of the mother and require immediate surgical intervention. However, most ectopic pregnancies are diagnosed before rupture and are removed surgically.

Another cause of uterine bleeding in the first trimester of pregnancy is hydatidiform mole, which occurs slightly more often among women over the age of 40 than among women at younger ages. ***Hydatidiform mole*** is a disease in which placental cells proliferate and form small, grape-like cysts. Usually fetal tissue is absent from the cystic growth. Treatment for hydatidiform mole involves emptying the uterus promptly after the diagnosis has been established, usually by a suction evacuation procedure followed by curettage. Fifteen to twenty percent of hydatidiform patients have persistent cases of the disease. Chemotherapy cures persistent molar disease in many women. A malignant form of hydatidiform mole, called the chorio carcinoma, is also effectively treated with chemotherapy.

Two common causes of bleeding in the third trimester of pregnancy involve placental disorders that may be life-threatening for both the mother and the child. One of these conditions is ***placenta previa***, in which the placenta lies partially or completely over the internal opening of the uterus. Abnormal bleeding occurs when this internal opening begins to thin and dilate in preparation for the passage of the baby. The other common cause of bleeding in the third trimester of pregnancy is abruptio placenta. ***Abruptio placenta*** is a condition in which the placenta begins to separate from its implanted position in the mother's uterus before the birth of the baby. Under normal circumstances, the placenta does not separate until after the delivery of the baby. Abruptio placenta is associated with considerable hemorrhage from the mother's uterus. In many instances of placenta previa or abruptio placenta, a cesarean section is necessary to preserve the life of the mother and her child.

Preeclampsia and Eclampsia

Preeclampsia is a disorder that affects women in late pregnancy, results from a metabolic disturbance, and is characterized by hypertension, swelling, and proteinuria. Symptoms of preeclampsia include headache, dizziness, nervous irritability, and visual disturbances. Preeclampsia most often affects young women who are pregnant for the first time, but its cause is not known. The objectives of treatment for preeclampsia are (1) to prevent eclampsia from developing and (2) to induce delivery of the baby by the quickest means available that will do the least harm to the mother and her child. Preeclampsia that is not stabilized by treatment nor interrupted by delivery may develop into eclampsia. *Eclampsia* is a condition that has the same symptoms and signs as preeclampsia, except that the former is also associated with convulsions and coma. Eclampsia is potentially fatal and is an obstetric emergency that requires the prompt lowering of the mother's blood pressure and the control of her convulsions. Immediate termination of the pregnancy by induction of labor and either vaginal delivery or cesarean section is essential for treating eclampsia.

The medical significance of preeclampsia and eclampsia, apart from the immediate prognosis for the mother, is the long-term effect of these disorders on the mother's blood pressure and kidney function. Within ten days after delivery, the majority of women who have preeclampsia or eclampsia experience a full recovery, but some of these patients develop residual hypertension. The severity of the preeclamptic or eclamptic attack influences the patient's ultimate prognosis. For example, the higher the mother's blood pressure during the attack, the greater the likelihood that she will later have hypertension. Similarly, many women who have severe preeclampsia or eclampsia will experience some permanent kidney damage later in life.

Chronic Hypertensive and Renal Disease

Closely related to preeclampsia and eclampsia are chronic hypertensive disease and chronic renal disease. Although chronic hypertension and chronic renal disease are not directly related to pregnancy, pregnancy can cause marked exacerbations of these disorders. Women who have chronic hypertension will become more hypertensive as pregnancy progresses. Similarly, women who have chronic renal disease often will show increasing proteinuria as pregnancy advances. Furthermore, women who have these chronic diseases are very prone to develop preeclampsia, which, in turn, increases the severity of the underlying chronic disease process.

Complications of Labor and the Postpartum Period

Abnormal labor or childbirth is called **dystocia**. Dystocia may result from any one of many factors, such as a large baby, a small pelvis, and/or weak, ineffectual uterine contractions. The condition in which the mother's pelvis is too small for the size of the baby is called **cephalopelvic disproportion**. The causes of weak uterine contractions are not known, although (1) heavy sedation during labor, (2) extreme apprehension, fatigue, malnutrition, and anemia, and (3) weakened and stretched uterine muscles from repeated childbirth may contribute to this disorder. The babies of women who have dystocia are often delivered with the help of forceps or by cesarean section.

The **postpartum period** is the period of time following childbirth. Two potentially serious physical postpartum complications that may affect the mother are postpartum hemorrhage and postpartum infection, both of which require prompt diagnosis and vigorous treatment. **Postpartum hemorrhage** is the loss of excessive amounts of blood from the blood vessels soon after childbirth. This condition may arise from

- tears in the birth canal
- uterine rupture
- retention of a piece of placenta, preventing the uterus from contracting to its normal size
- blood clotting disorders caused by or unrelated to the pregnancy
- **uterine atony**, a condition in which the uterine muscles lack their normal tone or strength as a result of a long labor, heavy sedation, anesthesia, multiple pregnancies, or excessive fluid within the uterus
- a large baby

Postpartum infections commonly involve the mother's genital tract, particularly the vagina or uterus. Renal and breast infections are other common postpartum disorders. Postpartum infection is not the major problem today that it used to be before the development and widespread use of germ-free delivery techniques. However, the condition does occur occasionally and is attended by significant morbidity. Postpartum infections are typically responsive to antibiotics.

Childbirth causes a stretching of the supporting structures around the mother's uterus, vagina, perineum, and rectum. The *perineum* is the region in males and females that lies between the urogenital area and the rectum. In females, it specifically lies between the vagina and rectum. In some patients, these supporting structures are so weakened and torn by childbirth that other organs sag into the patient's vagina. The sagging of the urethra and its supporting structures is known as a *urethrocele*, and the sagging of the bladder is called a *cystocele*. A *cystourethrocele* is a sagging urethra and bladder. The stretching and relaxation of the structures in the wall between the vagina and rectum may permit a *rectocele*, or sagging of the rectum, to protrude into the vagina. Stretching of the uterine supports may allow the uterus to descend into the vagina, which is often accompanied by a cystourethrocele. Frequently, women who have one of these displacements experience some loss of urinary and bowel control, a condition called *incontinence*, and difficulty in completely emptying the bladder. Failure to completely empty the bladder is a cause of both bladder infection and urinary obstruction. In its severe form, urinary obstruction will lead to hydronephrosis, a condition that is discussed in Chapter 10. If the structures and organs around the vagina are severely weakened or displaced, or if the weaknesses and displacements are associated with recurrent bladder infections, vaginal plastic surgery is probably indicated.

Furthermore, some women have a uterus that is tipped out of its normal position as a result of childbirth or from some other cause. This condition is often asymptomatic, but may be associated with a backache. Occasionally, a tipped uterus causes dysmenorrhea or infertility, and in these circumstances, surgery to return the uterus to its normal position is the suggested treatment.

CONTRACEPTION

Contraception is the intentional prevention of pregnancy. Methods for the prevention of pregnancy may be nonsurgical or surgical. Nonsurgical contraceptive techniques are usually temporary and can be abandoned at will. Some surgical contraceptive techniques are permanent; others can be abandoned only after another surgery.

Nonsurgical Methods

Nonsurgical methods of contraception include (1) methods that do not involve any outside physical mechanism, (2) vaginal insertion methods, and (3) birth control pills. The two most common types of contraceptive methods that do not involve an outside mechanism are coitus interruptus and the rhythm method. ***Coitus interruptus***, which is commonly called "withdrawal method," is a contraceptive method that involves the male's removal of his penis from the woman's vagina just prior to ejaculation. The ***rhythm method*** of contraception involves timing sexual intercourse around the days during each month when the woman is fertile. Coitus interruptus and the rhythm method provide pregnancy rates that are much higher than the rates provided by other forms of contraception.

Vaginal insertion methods of contraception include spermicidal jelly or foam, the diaphragm, the cervical cap, the spermicidal sponge, and condoms. These contraceptives are sometimes called "barrier" methods of contraception because they are intended to prevent sperm cells that are in the woman's vagina from entering her uterus. Spermicidal jelly and spermicidal foam are contraceptive methods that involve the insertion of a sperm-killing substance inside the woman's vagina at the cervix. Spermicidal jelly is also used in conjunction with other contraceptives, such as the diaphragm and cervical cap. A ***diaphragm*** is a contraceptive device that is made of molded rubber or soft plastic and that has a metal spring rim. A properly placed diaphragm covers the back wall of the vagina, including the cervix. Cervical caps are very similar to diaphragms, but typically are smaller and cover only the cervix, rather than a larger section of the back of the vagina. Cervical caps should also be coated with spermicidal jelly prior to vaginal insertion. A spermicidal sponge is a contraceptive device that involves the vaginal insertion of a small sponge that is coated with a sperm-killing substance. If inserted properly, the sponge sits directly on the cervix. There are two main types of condoms: the female condom and the male condom. The female condom is a plastic sheath that, when properly inserted, lines the entire vagina. A spermicide coats the interior of the female condom. The male condom is the only common nonsurgical contraceptive method that directly affects the male sexual intercourse partner. The male condom is a latex, rubber, or plastic sheath that covers the man's penis during sexual intercourse. The male condom should be put on prior to penile insertion into the woman's vagina. Vaginal insertion contraceptives have two main drawbacks: (1) they must be used prior to each sexual intercourse exposure and (2) they may lead to vaginal infection. Furthermore, although the use of these methods typically results in lower pregnancy rates than does the use of coitus interruptus and the rhythm method, the use of vaginal insertion contraceptives results in higher pregnancy rates than do the use of birth control pills and surgical methods of contraception. An advantage of vaginal insertion contraceptives, particularly condoms worn by males, is that they provide some protection against sexually transmitted diseases.

Birth control pills, or *oral contraceptives*, are hormonal compounds that women take orally in order to block ovulation and thus prevent pregnancy. Most types of birth control pills contain some level of estrogen. The advantages of oral contraceptives, when used properly, include (1) almost 100 percent effectiveness in preventing pregnancy, and (2) spontaneity of sexual intercourse without fear of pregnancy. Other benefits of birth control pills are that they can regulate a woman's menstrual cycle and often lessen menstrual discomfort from cramps. Minor side effects of oral contraceptives, such as weight gain, acne, and small patches of discoloration on the skin, are common, but these side affects often disappear with continued use. Major side effects from the use of oral contraceptives occur very infrequently. However, a woman who has or has had phlebitis, hypertension, or abnormal glucose tolerance, or who uses tobacco products, should not use birth control pills.

Surgical Methods

Surgical methods of contraception generally provide longer term, more permanent protection against the possibility of pregnancy than do nonsurgical methods. This section will discuss hysterectomy, tubal ligation, vasectomy, intrauterine devices, and subcutaneous progesterone implants.

Although in the past hysterectomies were used as a form of contraception, today the surgical removal of a woman's uterus is rarely performed for primarily contraceptive purposes. Typically, a hysterectomy is performed only if the woman exhibits evidence of uterine disease. A far more common contraceptive method than hysterectomy is tubal ligation. A **tubal ligation** is a surgical procedure in which a woman's fallopian tubes are constricted, severed, or crushed, to prohibit the passage of sperm. A tubal ligation, which is a fairly simple procedure that is associated with a short recovery period, is often performed in conjunction with a laparoscopy and can be performed on an outpatient basis. The male equivalent of a tubal ligation is a vasectomy. A **vasectomy** is the surgical removal of a portion of a man's vas deferens to prohibit the passage of sperm. Both tubal ligations and vasectomies are nearly 100 percent effective in preventing pregnancy. Furthermore, these procedures are sometimes reversible with follow-up surgery.

Another type of contraception involves an intrauterine device. An *intrauterine device (IUD)* is a small object that is implanted into a woman's uterus for the purpose of preventing pregnancy. The exact method by which IUDs prevent pregnancy is not known. IUDs come in a variety of different materials, such as steel, other metals, and plastic, as well as a variety of designs, such as spirals, double coils, loops, bows, rings, and shields. The pregnancy rate associated with IUDs is slightly higher than the rate associated with oral contraceptives. Side effects that may accompany the use of an IUD are pelvic pain and abnormal bleeding. Complications of this contraceptive method include uterine perforation that leads to pelvic infection, uterine infection, and unrecognized expulsion of the device. In addition, women who become pregnant while wearing an IUD are more likely to have abnormal pregnancies than are women who do not use an IUD. A woman who becomes pregnant while wearing an IUD should have the device surgically removed as soon as possible in order to avoid complications.

Subcutaneous implants of progesterone are relatively new contraceptives. These implants require minor surgery in which hormones are inserted under the skin of a woman's arm. The implants are effective in preventing pregnancy for approximately five years, at which time they should be replaced. Progesterone implants prevent pregnancy by preventing ovulation in a manner that is similar to the way in which birth control pills prevent ovulation. Moreover, these implants produce side effects that are similar to those produced by birth control pills. Although progesterone implants can be removed in a relatively minor surgical procedure, women who intend to become pregnant within two or three years are typically encouraged to use another contraceptive method.

ANATOMY, PHYSIOLOGY, AND DISEASES OF THE BREASTS

The breasts are discussed here in a separate section because, although they are not true organs of reproduction, breast development in females is closely associated with the beginning of menstruation and pregnancy. The female breast, which is more developed than the male breast, develops during the same time period in which the organs of the female reproductive system also begin to mature. Furthermore, the hormones that prepare other parts of the female body for pregnancy also affect the breasts.

The breasts, which are also called mammary glands, physiologically are closely related to the skin. Female breasts increase in size at puberty as the result of hormone stimulation and typically reach their full development in the early childbearing period, although they generally become even larger during milk production. Milk production is called *lactation* and is normally associated with childbirth. The breast contains 15 to 20 lobes, each of which has its own excretory duct, which terminates in multiple alveoli. These lobes are arranged around a central conical projection, which is called the nipple. A variable amount of fatty tissue fills out the breast between the lobes. During pregnancy the alveoli enlarge in preparation for lactation. The breast may be the site of benign and malignant tumors.

Benign Tumors

This section will discuss some of the benign tumors or growths, including abscesses and cysts, that may affect the breast.

Occasionally the breast may be the site of an abscess, which is a localized pocket of pus. Breast abscesses are typically bacterial infections, and the staphylococcus bacterium is the most common cause of these growths. An infected breast will be swollen, and the skin overlying the abscess will be hot, red, and tender. Abscesses of the female breast most often develop after the delivery of a baby. Although antibiotics may keep the infection under control, usually incision and drainage of the abscessed area are required to eliminate the infection.

The breast is a common site for cysts. Small solitary cysts and benign solid tumors often develop in the female breast and are typically asymptomatic. Cysts and benign tumors are of medical significance primarily because many benign growths are indistinguishable from malignant ones upon initial examination of the patient's breast. Biopsy will establish the diagnosis with certainty. A pathologist evaluates a cyst's fluid following needle aspiration of the fluid. Documentation of the cyst's disappearance confirms its benign nature. *Fibrocystic disease of the breast* is a condition that usually affects both breasts and is characterized by the formation of multiple, benign, painful lumps that become increasingly tender just prior to and during menstruation. On palpation, fibrocystic breasts have a lumpy or "B-B shot" consistency. The cause of fibrocystic disease is unknown, but may be related to the use of caffeine or chocolate, or it may arise from a hormonal effect. After menopause, the condition often becomes asymptomatic. Fibrocystic breast disease does not predispose the patient to breast cancer. However, certain arrangements of normal cells as indicated upon biopsy may carry a higher risk of later developing into cancer.

Malignant Tumors

A woman has a one in nine chance of developing breast cancer during her lifetime. Of the women who develop breast cancer, about one in three will die from the malignancy. The cause of breast cancer is unknown, but the risk of developing the disease is greater in women who have a family or personal history of breast cancer than in the general population. This disease has few manifestations in its early stage, but a palpable solitary hard lump in the breast and/or a bloody discharge from the nipple are suggestive of cancer. Early diagnosis before the cancer can spread is important in the control of the disease. Asymptomatic women are encouraged to perform monthly breast self-exams and to have periodic exams performed by their doctors. The appropriate frequency of screening for breast cancer with an x-ray technique called mammography depends on the woman's age and risk factors. However, mammography misses approximately ten percent of breast tumors. If a woman discovers a lump in her breast, her doctor should have the lump biopsied or followed very closely until a clear diagnosis is made.

The TNM system relating tumor size, spread to nodes, and distant metastases is a commonly used method of describing breast cancer. A small tumor size and the absence of spread to local nodes are favorable factors in determining the patient's prognosis. Noninfiltrating carcinoma-in-situ of the lobes is an increased risk factor for infiltrating carcinoma. Women who have lobular carcinoma-in-situ should be examined carefully for evidence of infiltrating cancer. Some of these patients might elect to have both breasts surgically removed before the cancer can spread. The surgical removal of a breast is called a *simple mastectomy*.

Noninfiltrating carcinomas that are limited to the mammary duct system typically are curable. Intraductal carcinoma-in-situ has not spread from the initial site of development. Although a simple mastectomy for ductal carcinoma-in-situ provides a 98 to 99 percent cure rate, other less extensive procedures may also be curative. Unfortunately, most breast cancers are not discovered until after invasion of the surrounding breast tissue has occurred. Infiltrating ductal carcinoma is by far the most common form of mammary cancer. The patient's prognosis depends on the clinical stage of the lesion. Primary breast cancer that is strictly confined to this organ has about a 75 percent disease-free 10-year survival rate. Significantly lower survival rates are associated with breast cancer that has infiltrated the lymph nodes or metastasized to other organs.

The basic treatment for all forms of breast cancer is surgical removal of the tumor and, sometimes, the entire breast. The surgical removal of a tumor or lump is called a *lumpectomy*. A *modified*

radical mastectomy is the surgical removal of the entire breast and the associated lymph nodes in the armpit area. Some surgeons remove the lymph nodes that lie above the collarbone and behind the mammary glands also, because nodes in these locations are common sites for the spread of the cancer. A modified radical mastectomy preserves the underlying chest muscles that were removed in the older standard radical mastectomy procedure. Any surgery to remove a malignancy in the breast may or may not be supplemented with radiation therapy, chemotherapy, or hormonal therapy. The patient's age, the number of cancerous nodes that are present, and the presence or absence of distant metastases are some of the factors that help the physician determine the best treatment for an individual breast cancer patient.

Breast Reconstruction and Augmentation

Breast implants are an integral part of breast reconstruction and augmentation. **Breast reconstruction** is the surgical reformation of a breast, typically following any type of mastectomy, and **breast augmentation** is the surgical enlargement of a breast. Both reconstructive and augmentative procedures are usually cosmetic in nature. Breast implants traditionally have been made of either a silicon or salt solution inner filling and an outer containment shell. Concern over complications of silicon implants led to the 1992 Federal Drug Administration (FDA) decision to limit the use of these implants to controlled clinical studies. The FDA assured women who want the implants following breast cancer surgery that they would have access to the studies. Complications of any type of breast implants include rupture, infection, scar formation, and poor cosmetic results. Furthermore, some implants are suspected of inducing autoimmune diseases. Implants also make checking for breast cancer more difficult.

SEXUALLY TRANSMITTED DISEASES

Sexually transmitted diseases (STDs), which are also called *venereal diseases*, are disorders that one person passes to another primarily through intimate sexual contact. Because most sexually transmitted diseases affect both males and females, these disorders warrant a separate discussion in this text. This section will define and describe some common STDs, including gonorrhea, nongonococcal urethritis, syphilis, genital herpes, and genital warts. Although AIDS is often spread by intimate sexual contact, it is also spread by other methods. Moreover, unlike the other STDs, AIDS is a disorder of the immune system, and so is discussed in Chapter 2, *Scientific Background for the Study of Disease*. Hepatitis B is also commonly spread by intimate sexual contact, but is discussed in association with other forms of hepatitis in Chapter 9, *The Digestive System*.

The genital manifestations of STDs in men are often trivial compared to the severe complications these diseases can cause in women. The most severe of these complications is ***pelvic inflammatory disease*** (PID), which is any inflammatory infection that affects the reproductive organs in the pelvis. PID is caused by microorganisms that initially multiply in the vagina and then later ascend through the endometrial cavity to the uterine tubes and adjacent structures. Any of the pathogens which cause STDs in males can cause PID, although gonococcal and chlamydial bacteria cause most of these infections. Often, a female who has a PID will also have an infection caused by bacteria which are normally present in the gastrointestinal or urinary tract, but which cause infection if they appear in other locations.

Symptoms of PID include pain and tenderness in the pelvis, fever, vaginal discharge, backache, painful urination, and menstrual disturbance. The long-term complications of PID result from both the initial infection and the healing process. For example, as inflamed fallopian tubes heal, they frequently become blocked by scar tissue and adhesions. Totally blocked tubes cause sterility. Partial tubal obstruction predisposes the individual to ectopic pregnancies. Adhesions that occur during the healing of an acute PID result in chronic pelvic pain. Hospitalization and intravenous antibiotic therapy are often necessary to cure a PID. Furthermore, abscesses of the fallopian tubes or ovaries, adhesions, and other complications of a PID may require surgical treatment.

Gonorrheal Infections

Gonorrhea is an infection that is caused by the *Neisseria gonorrhoeae*, which is commonly called the gonococcus bacteria. In males, gonorrhea occurs primarily as urethritis and is characterized by a thick yellow penile discharge and painful urination. In females, the gonococcus bacteria cause inflammation of the urethra and cervix, characterized by frequent and painful urination, urethral discharge, vaginal and vulval redness and burning, and a heavy, thick, yellow, foul-smelling vaginal discharge. Gonococcal infection can also involve the anal canal and pharynx. Complications of gonorrhea include prostatitis, epididymitis, cystitis, inflammation of the fallopian tubes, urethral stricture, and arthritis. The treatment of gonorrhea traditionally involved penicillin. However, the recent emergence of penicillin-resistant strains of gonococcus has shifted treatment toward a group of antibiotics called cephalosporins.

Nongonococcal Urethritis

Nongonococcal urethritis (NGU), which is also called *nonspecific urethritis*, is an inflammation of the urethra that is caused by a microorganism other than the gonococcus bacterium. The discharge produced by nongonococcal urethritis is less profuse than that produced by gonorrhea, but other symptoms of NGU are the same as those for gonorrhea. In many cases, NGU is caused by chlamydia bacteria, but other microorganisms may also be responsible for the disease. Chlamydial infection often occurs in association with gonorrhea, and so most patients receive treatment for both types of bacteria. Complications of chlamydial genital tract infections include epididymitis, prostatitis, urethritis, cervicitis, conjunctivitis, and arthritis. Treatment of NGU depends on the infecting organism, but most cases of NGU respond to antibiotic therapy.

Syphilis

Syphilis, which is also called *lues*, is a venereal disease that is caused by the spirochete *Treponema pallidum*. Although syphilis can be a congenital disease, this text will consider only the acquired, venereal form. Syphilis can involve any organ in the body. The primary lesion, which is known as a chancre, appears in males on the penis two to four weeks after exposure. In females, the chancre appears on the vulva, labia, or cervix three to four weeks after exposure. Menstrual disturbances and vaginal discharge may be present in syphilitic females, but many of these patients have no symptoms other than the chancre for a period of time. Antibiotic treatment at the beginning stage of syphilis will generally provide a complete cure. On the other hand, untreated syphilis will proceed through a latent stage following the slow healing process of the chancre, and then will progress to secondary syphilis. This second stage of syphilis is characterized by fatigue, slight anemia, headaches, and a rash that comes and goes. Antibiotic treatment at this stage typically effects a cure and prevents late complications of the disease. Syphilis often goes through another latent stage following the clearing of the rash that accompanies secondary syphilis. If still untreated, the syphilis will enter into a third stage that is called tertiary syphilis. Tertiary syphilis may involve any organ, the most important of which are the brain and heart. Slow, continuous destruction of brain tissue may lead to

Figure 11–3.
Sexually Transmitted Diseases.

Disease	Pathogen	Common Genital Manifestations
Gonorrhea	Neisseria gonorrhoeae	PID, urethritis
Syphilis	Treponema pallidum	Chancre
Nongonococcal urethritis	Chlamydia	PID, urethritis
Genital herpes	Herpes simplex virus	Vulvovaginitis, balanitis
Genital warts	Human papilloma virus	Warts
HIV infection	Human immuno-deficiency virus	None
Hepatitis B infection	Hepatitis B virus	None

disorders of sensation, mental function, vision, and coordination. Ultimately, uncontrolled tertiary syphilis leads to paralysis, dementia, aortic insufficiency, and/or aortic aneurysm. Proper medical treatment during the third stage of this disease will arrest the progression of the disorder, but cannot restore destroyed tissue.

Genital Herpes

Genital herpes is an inflammatory skin disease affecting the genitals that is caused by the herpes simplex virus and is characterized by the formation of small, clustered vesicles and an enlargement of the glands in the groin. The most common manifestations of genital herpes are extremely painful sores that are surrounded by areas of inflammation on the penis in affected males and on the vagina, labia, clitoris, or cervix in affected females. The affected areas quickly form ulcers and become covered with a gray-white film. Spontaneous healing of the lesions typically occurs within several weeks of their initial appearance, but recurrences of the lesions are common. Oral antiviral therapy will treat the primary herpes infection or will prevent genital herpes infection. A woman who has genital herpes can transfer the virus to her child at the time of vaginal delivery. Although such a transfer is uncommon, the illness in an infant can be severe, and so delivery by cesarean section may be recommended to prevent this complication.

Genital Warts

Genital warts are caused by the human papilloma virus (HPV). The warts appear in either the genital area or the area around the anus in males or females. In females, genital warts often cause mildly abnormal Pap smears, and a few subtypes of these warts are associated with cervical cancer. Genital warts are difficult to treat and tend to be persistent. Common treatments for removing genital warts are "freezing" them or "burning" them with chemicals or heat.

Figure 11–3 outlines some STDs, their causes, and their manifestations.

12

The Endocrine System

The human body contains two types of glands: (1) exocrine glands and (2) endocrine glands. As explained in Chapter 9, *The Digestive System*, exocrine glands have ducts and endocrine glands do not have ducts. Each endocrine gland manufactures one or more hormones and releases them directly into the bloodstream or lymph channels. A **hormone** is a chemical substance that is produced and secreted by an organ or the cells of an organ and that travels through the circulatory system to a target organ where the hormone elicits a response. The nature of the target organ's response to a hormone depends on the target organ. The **endocrine system** is the group of glands and other structures in the body that create hormones and release the hormones directly into the circulatory system.

Hormones serve many useful purposes, including the regulation of

- the balance of salt and water in the body
- blood pressure
- metabolism
- reproduction
- blood sugar
- nerve impulse transmission
- digestion

This chapter will first address the primary components of the endocrine system, except for the ovary and testis, which are discussed in Chapter 11, *The Reproductive System*. The text will then discuss some of the disorders that affect endocrine glands.

ANATOMY AND PHYSIOLOGY

The primary components of the endocrine system include the pituitary gland, hypothalamus, thyroid gland, parathyroid glands, adrenal glands, pancreas, and the ovary and testis. Figure 12–1 illustrates the male endocrine system and Figure 12–2 illustrates the female endocrine system.

The Pituitary Gland

The *pituitary gland*, which is also called the *hypophysis*, is the master gland, so named because it is involved in most endocrine activities. The pituitary gland rests at the base of the brain in a small bony cavity, called the *sella turcica*, within the floor of the cranium. The pituitary gland is divided into an anterior lobe and a posterior lobe. Most pituitary hormones affect the action of peripheral endocrine target tissues and organs, causing these tissues and organs to produce additional hormones.

The anterior lobe of the pituitary secretes the following six hormones:

- *adrenocorticotropic hormone (ACTH)* stimulates the production of hormones from the adrenal cortex
- *follicle-stimulating hormone (FSH)* causes maturation of the ovum and induces estrogen production in the female and the production of sperm in the male
- *human growth hormone (HGH)* exerts a major influence on the growth of all tissues
- *thyroid-stimulating hormone (TSH),* also called *thyrotropin,* stimulates the thyroid gland to manufacture and release thyroid hormones
- *luteinizing hormone (LH),* in females initiates ovulation and stimulates the ovary to produce progesterone and in males causes the testis to secrete testosterone
- *prolactin (PRL)* stimulates the development of ducts and glands in breast tissue and is responsible for the secretion of milk

Figure 12–1.
The Organs in a Male's Endocrine System.

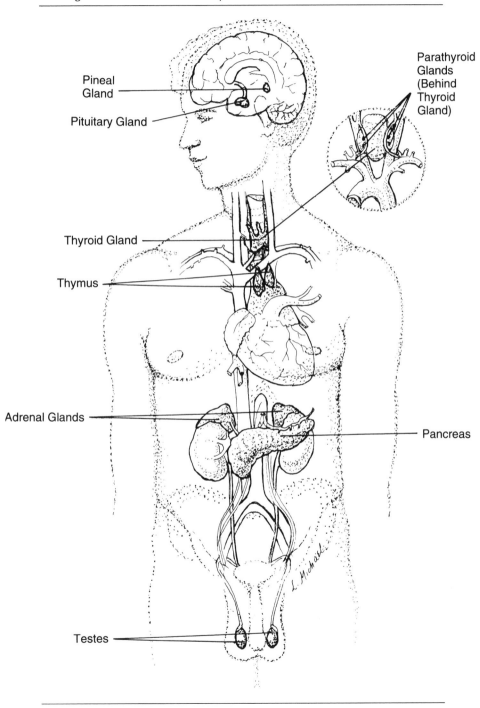

Figure 12–2.
The Organs in a Female's Endocrine System.

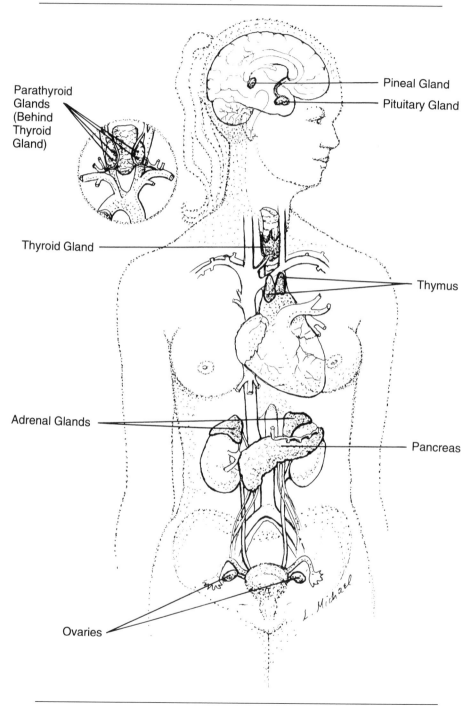

The Hypothalamus

The *hypothalamus* is an area at the base of the brain that is adjacent to, and interconnected with, the pituitary gland. A narrow stalk consisting of nerve fibers and blood vessels connects the hypothalamus with the pituitary. In addition to this close *anatomic* relationship, a close *functional* relationship between the hypothalamus and the pituitary exists. The hypothalamus produces several **releasing factors**, which are hormones that act on the pituitary gland to affect the release of pituitary hormones. These releasing factors are

- *thyrotropin-releasing hormone (TRH),* which causes the release of TSH
- *growth hormone-releasing hormone (GRH),* which causes the release of HGH
- *corticotropin-releasing hormone (CRH),* which causes the release of ACTH
- *luteinizing-releasing hormone (LHRH),* which causes the release of LH

In addition, the hypothalamus produces the following two hormones:

- *antidiuretic hormone (ADH),* which causes the kidney tubules to increase their reabsorption of water, thus leading to decreased urine output, and causes the constriction of the smooth muscle found in the walls of blood vessels
- *oxytocin,* which causes contraction of the smooth muscle of the uterus, and so is of primary importance during labor and after the delivery of the child

After their manufacture, ADH and oxytocin are stored in the posterior pituitary gland and are secreted in response to appropriate stimuli.

The Thyroid Gland

The *thyroid gland*, which is located in front of the trachea below the Adam's apple, consists of right and left lobes that are connected by a narrow mid-portion, which is called the *isthmus*. The thyroid is made up of many microscopic follicles that contain the thyroid hormones. The thyroid—under the control of the pituitary gland's TSH—secretes two principal hormones, triiodothyronine (T3) and thyroxin (T4), into the circulation. The thyroid hormones may enter the bloodstream directly for immediate use or they may be stored in the follicles for later use.

Only small amounts of T3 and T4 travel in the circulation unbound. Instead, most T3 and T4 hormones bind to serum proteins, such as thyroxin-binding-globulins (TBGs). However, only unbound T3 and T4 hormones are able to enter cells. T3 is three times as active as T4, and in turn affects most of the metabolic functions of the thyroid hormones. Thyroid hormones are involved in tissue and organ growth, metabolism, and the formation of bones. These hormones stimulate many target organs, including the adrenal glands, reproductive organs, and the organs of the nervous system. Because the thyroid gland uses iodine to produce T3 and T4, an adequate dietary supply of iodine is necessary for the manufacture of thyroid hormones and the proper functioning of the gland.

Measurements of thyroid hormone levels provide diagnostic information regarding the state of the gland's activity. However, test values may be normal despite clinical evidence of thyroid disease, or values may be abnormal in a patient who appears to have clinically normal thyroid function. The clinical condition of normal thyroid function is called *euthyroidism*. The most common tests used to detect disturbances of thyroid function are radioimmunoassay (RIA) techniques and the thyroid scan. RIA techniques measure total serum T3 and T4, which include the unbound hormones plus the hormones bound to the protein carriers. Changes in serum concentrations of these hormones reflect not only changes in the free active hormone but also changes in the concentration of the thyroid-binding proteins. Conditions in which TBG increases, not necessarily with a corresponding increase in the free hormone, are pregnancy, estrogen or tamoxifen citrate[1] use, hepatitis, and primary biliary cirrhosis. TBG decreases with androgen or high-dose corticosteroid use, severe systemic illness, cirrhosis, and acromegaly. In patients who do not have underlying systemic illnesses or conditions known to alter the level of thyroid-binding proteins, total serum T4 is a sensitive and specific index of both *hyperthyroidism*, which is the overproduction by the thyroid gland of thyroid hormones, and *hypothyroidism*, which is the inadequate production by the thyroid of thyroid hormones. T3 is not a sensitive indicator of *hypo*thyroidism, but is a highly sensitive indicator of *hyper*thyroidism. Typically, T4 decreases in *hypo*thyroidism and increases in *hyper*thyroidism. TSH is also easily measurable, and normally it increases in *hypothy-*

---

[1]*Tamoxifen citrate* is an oral antiestrogen medication that is used to treat breast cancer patients.

roidism and decreases in *hyper*thyroidism if the disorder is within the thyroid gland.

Another important test in the diagnosis of thyroid disease is thyroid scanning following administration of radioactive iodine that then concentrates in the thyroid gland. After the patient receives the radioactive iodine, the amount of iodine the thyroid removes from the circulation can be measured by scanning devices during radioactive iodine uptake tests. Thyroid scanning is useful in confirming the diagnosis of hyperthyroidism and in establishing the diagnosis of subacute and chronic thyroiditis. Certain scans will show thyroid anatomy, nodules, goiter, and so on. Because the test involves a small dose of a radioactive substance, thyroid scanning generally should not be administered to children or pregnant women and should not be used as a screening procedure for thyroid disease in apparently healthy people.

The Parathyroid Glands

The four *parathyroid glands* are tiny, flattened, oval discs that are located on the back of the thyroid gland. The principal cells of these glands secrete the parathyroid hormone, which is necessary for the regulation of blood calcium and phosphorus and for the utilization of these substances by the bones. The parathyroid hormone also contributes to the normal functioning of nerves and muscles, because the blood level of calcium affects the functioning of these tissues.

The Adrenal Glands

The *adrenal glands* are small, flattened, cup-shaped structures that lie immediately above and in front of the upper end of each kidney. Because of their location, these two glands are sometimes referred to as *suprarenal glands*. Each adrenal gland has an outer cortex and an inner medulla. Each of these zones produces hormones that are essential to life and health. The cortex produces two steroids: (1) *glucosteroids*, which are also called *glucocorticoids*, are steroids that assist in regulating the body's sugar metabolism and numerous other functions, and (2) *mineralocorticoids* are steroids that aid in maintaining the body's sodium and potassium levels. In addition, the adrenal cortex is the source of small amounts of estrogen and androgens, such as testosterone. The adrenal medulla secretes *epinephrine*, which is also called *adrenalin*, a hormone that causes acceleration of the individual's heart rate, relaxation of the smooth muscle of the bronchial tubes, and constriction of the peripheral blood vessels, but not of vessels furnishing blood to the heart, brain, and active muscles. Epinephrine is liberated in response to stress, excitement, and hypoglycemia.

The Pancreas

The pancreas, which was first discussed in Chapter 9, *The Digestive System*, is both an exocrine gland and an endocrine gland. The *exocrine* secretion of the pancreas, which is called pancreatic juice, is discussed in Chapter 9. This section will focus upon insulin, which is the *endocrine* secretion of the pancreas. Insulin is the hormone that regulates sugar metabolism. It is produced in collections of cells, known as the *islets of Langerhans*, that are scattered throughout the pancreas.

Other Hormone-Secreting Structures

The limits of endocrinology are not easy to define because the brain, liver, stomach, and kidney manufacture substances that regulate various functions in the body. These substances qualify as hormones although they are not traditionally included under the endocrine system. Moreover, other tissues manufacture substances that are considered to be endocrine hormones. For example, the placenta manufactures three hormones. Very early in a woman's pregnancy, her placenta secretes a hormone called *chorionic gonadotrophin* that stimulates the ovaries and prevents the degeneration of the corpus luteum. After the third month of the pregnancy, the placenta secretes both estrogen and progesterone in quantities sufficient to maintain the pregnancy.

Another structure that secretes a hormone is the pineal body. The *pineal body* is a small gland in the brain that is located behind the medulla and above the cerebellum and that is connected to the substance of the brain by a small stalk. The pineal body secretes many biologically active substances, but only *melatonin*, which suppresses the menstrual cycle, is classified as a hormone. Although the pineal body may become filled with calcium as the individual grows older, calcification has no apparent effect on pineal function. Pineal tumors are rare, but they may cause precocious puberty in males and may also cause diabetes insipidus.

Interactions

Considerable interaction occurs among the endocrine glands. Hormones secreted by one gland may affect not only a target organ or organs, but also other endocrine glands. For example, the pituitary gland secretes hormones that stimulate the ovary to produce estrogen. Estrogen affects the uterus, vagina, and breast. In a process called negative feedback, estrogen will also slow or inhibit the manufacture of the pituitary hormones that initially stimulated the ovary to produce the estrogen. The body maintains these hormones in a very delicate balance. The pituitary gland releases just enough pituitary hormone to affect the secretion of adequate quantities of estrogen. An excess of estrogen will suppress pituitary activity temporarily until the levels of circulating hormones are brought back into balance.

The endocrine system also closely interacts with the nervous system. One function of some hormones and of certain components of the nervous system is to affect communication between cells. The nervous system can also stimulate or interrupt the release of hormones by sending stimuli from the nervous system to a gland. For example, the hypothalamus receives stimuli from the nervous system. In response to these nervous system stimuli, the hypothalamus then stimulates or interrupts the release of certain pituitary hormones by releasing its own hormones to the pituitary.

Furthermore, other organs besides those of the nervous system and the endocrine system regulate the body. For instance, the liver modifies the action of certain hormones by detoxifying the hormones into less active forms. In certain diseases, the liver may fail to carry out this role with the result that excessive amounts of one or more hormones circulate throughout the body, adversely affecting several organ systems.

DISORDERS OF THE ENDOCRINE GLANDS

Most disorders of the endocrine glands, except for certain tumors, result in either an over- or underproduction of hormones. Figure 12–3 provides a list of endocrine disorders arising from hormone production abnormalities.

Disorders of the Pituitary Gland and Hypothalamus

The anterior and posterior lobes of the pituitary gland and the adjoining hypothalamus can be the seat of endocrine disorders. Some of the more common disorders of the pituitary gland and hypothalamus include diabetes insipidus, inappropriate secretion of ADH, hypofunction of the pituitary, and tumors.

Figure 12–3.
Disorders of the Endocrine Glands Resulting from Alterations in Hormone Production.

Endocrine Gland	Diseases Caused by Overproduction	Diseases Caused by Underproduction
Pituitary	Acromegaly	Dwarfism
Thyroid	Hyperthyroidism	Hypothyroidism
Parathyroid	Hyperparathyroidism	Hypoparathyroidism
Adrenal	Cushing's syndrome	Addison's disease
Pancreas	Hypoglycemia	Diabetes mellitus

Diabetes Insipidus

Diabetes insipidus is a condition that results from a deficiency of ADH, which is an important regulator of water balance. Lacking the stimulus for the reabsorption of water by the kidney tubules, the diabetes insipidus patient excretes an excessive amount of very dilute urine, a condition called *polyuria.* Many diseases and conditions cause diabetes insipidus, but some cases of this disorder have no known cause. Among the known causes of diabetes insipidus are head trauma, neurosurgical procedures on the pituitary gland, tumors and infections involving the pituitary gland, and cerebrovascular accidents. Diabetes insipidus that results from kidney disease is called *nephrogenic diabetes insipidus*. Manifestations of diabetes insipidus are polyuria, excessive thirst, dry skin, dehydration, headache, dizziness, fatigue, and irritability. Treatment of diabetes insipidus depends, in part, on the origin of the condition, but most patients benefit from life-long administration of a vasopressin compound that has an antidiuretic action. Desmopressin, a drug that has great antidiuretic potency and is self-administered as a nasal spray, is the safest and most convenient therapeutic agent for diabetes insipidus patients.

Inappropriate Secretion of Antidiuretic Hormone

Inappropriate secretion of antidiuretic hormone is a syndrome that results from the overproduction of ADH. Although water retention is a common occurrence associated with this syndrome, the majority of the manifestations of inappropriate secretion of ADH result from a low serum sodium level. Manifestations of low sodium levels include mental confusion, fatigue, muscle weakness, headache, nausea, vomiting, and loss of appetite. Progression of the disease may result in convulsions and coma. An increase in the secretion of ADH may occur in association with malignancies, endocrine disorders, diseases of the lungs and central nervous system, and the use of certain drugs. Restriction of fluid intake is an effective treatment in most cases of inappropriate secretion of ADH.

Hypofunction

Hypofunction means diminished activity. Hypofunction of the anterior pituitary gland may result from tumors, congenital defects, infections, infarctions, or aneurysms. If target glands do not get stimulating pituitary hormones, these glands, in turn, may show reduced output. *Panhypopituitarism* is a generalized decrease in pituitary function resulting from the reduced production of all anterior lobe hormones, and is characterized by weakness, sensitivity to cold, drowsiness, premature aging, facial and generalized swelling, intolerance to stress, amenorrhea, and genital atrophy. The treatment of this condition involves the administration of thyroid hormone and hydrocortisone. A child whose pituitary gland fails to produce sufficient levels of hormones may need treatment with growth hormone to attain adequate height. In addition, hypofunction of the testes is often treated with testosterone and the hypofunction of the ovaries is often treated with estrogen.

Tumors

Pituitary tumors typically present in one of three ways: (1) the expanding mass puts pressure on adjacent structures, thus causing symptoms, such as visual disturbances and headaches, (2) the excess or deficiency of hormones associated with these tumors causes disorders, such as Cushing's disease, acromegaly, and amenorrhea, and (3) the tumor appears on a patient's x-ray film, CT scan, or MRI study that was taken to investigate some unrelated condition. Although some pituitary tumors produce symptoms before they can be visualized, many of these tumors are large before they cause symptoms. Pituitary tumors generally grow slowly, and many patients who have pituitary tumors do not seek medical attention until their vague symptoms have been present for a number of years. The most common lesion involving the sella turcica is the pituitary adenoma. Functionally, these adenomas are divided into hormone-secreting tumors and non-hormone-secreting tumors. The hormone-secreting tumors produce an excess of prolactin, growth hormone, or ACTH.

Acromegaly is a chronic, often disabling disorder caused by an adenoma of the anterior pituitary lobe that produces an excessive amount of growth hormone. Symptoms of acromegaly are headache, visual disturbances, a broadened face, and enlarged head, hands, and feet. Hypertension, heart disease, arthritis, and amenorrhea may also be present in acromegaly patients. Pituitary adenomas, which usually are benign, can be removed by means of a very delicate microsurgery, called a *transseptal, transsphenoidal hypophysectomy*, in which the surgeon approaches the gland through the patient's nose. Drug therapy and radiotherapy to the pituitary gland also are used to treat some acromegaly patients. Adenomas of the pituitary can also produce an excessive amount of ACTH. The overproduction of ACTH results in Cushing's disease, a condition that is similar to Cushing's syndrome, which will be discussed later in this chapter in the section on diseases of the adrenal gland.

Benign prolactin-secreting adenomas, which are the most common pituitary tumors, are noncancerous and are characterized by elevated blood levels of prolactin. Microadenomas are those tumors that are smaller than one centimeter, and macroadenomas are those that are larger than one centimeter. Common symptoms of prolactin-secreting adenomas are (1) *galactorrhea*, which is an abnormal discharge of milk from the breast, (2) impotence, (3) menstrual irregularity, and (4) fertility problems. A CT scan or MRI study of the patient's head defines the size of the tumor. Oral drug treatment with bromocriptine, which lowers elevated prolactin levels, is often effective in treating microadenomas, but macroadenomas may require surgical removal or radiation therapy.

Figure 12–4 outlines the hormonal bases for several hypothalamic-pituitary syndromes.

Disorders of the Thyroid Gland

The most common symptoms associated with disorders of the thyroid gland are thyrotoxicosis and hypothyroidism. *Thyrotoxicosis* is a general term for any condition that is characterized by the presence of excessive amounts of circulating thyroid hormones, regardless of the cause. Some common symptoms of thyrotoxicosis are (1) nervousness, (2) sweating, (3) hypersensitivity to heat, (4) fatigue, (5) palpitations, and (6) weight loss. Some common signs of this disorder are (1) goiter, (2) tachycardia, (3) tremors, and (4) *exophthalmos*, a condition in which the patient has abnormally protruding eyeballs. *Thyroid storm* is a sudden severe attack of thyrotoxicosis and may be fatal. Thyroid storm, which may be precipitated by surgery, emotional stress, or severe infections, is

Figure 12–4.
Hormonal Bases for Hypothalamic-Pituitary Syndromes.

Hormone	Syndromes Caused by Overproduction	Syndromes Caused by Underproduction
ACTH	Cushing's disease	Adrenal insufficiency
TSH	Hyperthyroidism	Hypothyroidism
FSH, LH	Sexual precocity	Infertility, amenorrhea
HGH	Acromegaly	Dwarfism, hypoglycemia
PRL	Amenorrhea, galactorrhea	(None)
ADH	Inappropriate ADH production	Diabetes insipidus

characterized by hyperthyroidism, high fever, cardiac arrhythmias, and, occasionally, congestive heart failure. Hyperthyroidism is a type of thyrotoxicosis. The treatment of thyrotoxicosis depends upon the cause of the disorder.

Hypothyroidism is a graded phenomenon, although no precise point of separation exists between the mild deficiency state of hypothyroidism and more advanced states. *Cretinism* is fully developed and advanced hypothyroidism in infants and small children, and *myxedema* is advanced hypothyroidism in adults. Mild deficiency states of hypothyroidism are much more common than the advanced states, which are relatively rare. Clinical abnormalities associated with hypothyroidism include decreased T4 and increased TSH. Hypothyroidism often occurs as the result of treatment by a physician for other disorders. For example, the majority of patients who receive radioactive iodine treatments for hyperthyroidism will eventually become hypothyroid. In addition, a substantial number of patients who undergo a *subtotal thyroidectomy*, which is the surgical removal of part of the thyroid, eventually develop hypothyroidism. Another common cause of hypothyroidism is thyroiditis, which is discussed later in this section. Some typical manifestations of adult hypothyroidism include (1) dry, coarse, cold, puffy skin, (2) fatigue and lethargy, (3) thin hair and scant eyebrows, (4) swelling of the hands, face, and eyelids, (5) intolerance to cold, (6) mental and physical slowness, and (7) hoarseness. Some patients who have severe cases of hypothyroidism experience cardiac enlargement, coma, and psychotic symptoms. Treatment by synthetic thyroid hormones often achieves a dramatic response and returns many patients to normal. Hypothyroidism is one of the easier diseases to treat.

The rest of this section will discuss a few specific thyroid disorders, including Graves' disease, goiter, thyroiditis, and tumors.

Graves' Disease

Graves' disease is an autoimmune disease of unknown cause that is characterized by hyperthyroidism, exophthalmos, and characteristic skin changes. Graves' disease is one of the most common endocrine disorders, appearing most often in women between the ages of 20 and 40. Several methods, such as drugs, surgery, and radioactive iodine, may be used in treating Graves' disease. These drugs may be used on a continuous basis as the sole therapy for Graves' disease or may be given to the patient for several weeks prior to thyroid surgery. Surgical treatment, which is rarely performed on Graves' patients, is a permanent form of therapy. However, complications occur in about ten percent of surgically treated patients. Complications of thyroid surgery include the development of hypothyroidism if the surgeon removes too much functioning thyroid tissue, recurrence of hyperthyroidism if the surgeon does not remove enough tissue, and damage to nerves or the parathyroid glands that lie adjacent to the thyroid gland. Radioactive iodine is also used as a method of destroying thyroid tissue, thereby reducing the amount of hormone manufactured. The long-term complication of radioactive iodine therapy is hypothyroidism. However, radioactive treatment generally is administered only to patients who are at least 30 years old, and it is usually not considered to be appropriate therapy for women of childbearing age.

Goiter

An enlargement of the thyroid gland is known as a *goiter*. If the enlargement results from a relative or absolute deficiency in iodine, which is needed for the manufacture of thyroid hormones, and if the patient has no symptoms, the thyroid enlargement is referred to as a *simple goiter*, or a *nontoxic goiter*. A simple goiter is the result of the thyroid gland's attempt to maximize the capture and utilization of iodine. A simple goiter may occur during those periods, such as puberty, pregnancy, and prolonged infections, when the patient experiences a temporary increased demand for thyroid hormones. When the patient's body's demand for thyroid hormones returns to normal, the enlargement usually disappears. Simple goiter may also be secondary to other mechanisms. The thyroid enlargement of a simple goiter may be smooth and symmetrical, or it may be slightly nodular or cystic. A simple goiter's enlargement generally is sufficient to maintain normal thyroid hormone levels in the patient's blood, but occasionally the patient will develop hypothyroidism. Fortunately, the widespread use of iodized salt, which compensates for diets deficient in iodine, has sharply reduced the number of simple goiters. Simple goiters may also improve with oral drug therapy to replace T4.

If the thyroid gland enlargement results in the excessive manufacture of thyroid hormones, thus leading to the manifestations of hyperthyroidism, the enlarged thyroid is known as a *toxic goiter*. A toxic goiter may occur in association with a number of causes of hyperthyroidism. The thyroid gland of a patient who has toxic goiter may show a smooth, generalized enlargement, which is called a *diffuse toxic goiter*. However, if the toxic goiter patient's gland consists of one or several nodules, the enlargement is called a *nodular toxic goiter*.

Thyroiditis

Thyroiditis is an inflammation of the thyroid gland. The medical community recognizes several forms of thyroiditis. The most common of type of thyroid inflammation is *Hashimoto's thyroiditis*, which is an autoimmune disease of unknown cause that may be associated with other autoimmune diseases, such as pernicious anemia and systemic lupus erythematosus. Hashimoto's thyroiditis most commonly affects middle-aged women and is characterized by the presence of a firm, painless, rubbery goiter. The Hashimoto's patient initially may be euthyroid, but as the disease progresses, hypothyroidism often will occur and require treatment.

Tumors

A common type of thyroid tumor is the thyroid nodule. *Thyroid nodules* are localized areas of enlargement in the thyroid gland and are usually painless and benign. Thyroid nodules commonly occur, especially in women who are middle-aged or older. The chief clinical concern of the physician is to differentiate benign nodules from those that are malignant so that he or she can determine which nodules are most likely to require surgical removal. Two common procedures that are used to diagnose thyroid nodules are radioisotope scanning and fine needle biopsy. However, few thyroid nodules require excision because thyroid carcinoma is a relatively rare condition. Many patients who have thyroid cancer, which occurs twice as often in women as in men, have a medical history that includes irradiation to the neck. The initial manifestation of thyroid cancer is a painless thyroid swelling, which is easily noticed during palpation. Thyroid cancers are relatively slow growing, even if the carcinoma has metastasized to another location in the patient's body. A thyroid cancer patient's prognosis depends on factors such as the (1) size of the tumor at the time of discovery, (2) tumor's cell type, and (3) presence or absence of metastatic spread.

Disorders of the Parathyroid Glands

The parathyroid hormone controls the levels of calcium and phosphorus in the blood and bone. An increase in the level of the parathyroid hormone causes (1) a decrease in the patient's serum phosphorus level and (2) an increase in the patient's serum calcium level, a condition called *hypercalcemia*. Other causes of hypercalcemia include certain cancers, sarcoidosis, vitamin D overdose, and thiazide or lithium use. Routine blood screening often detects asymptomatic or mildly symptomatic hypercalcemia. Symptoms of hypercalcemia include kidney stones, abdominal pain, loss of appetite and weight, vomiting, bone pain, fatigue, weakness, depression, and personality changes. A decrease in the level of the parathyroid hormone results in (1) an increase in the patient's serum phosphorous level and (2) a decrease in the patient's serum calcium level, a condition called *hypocalcemia*.

Hyperparathyroidism is a condition characterized by an excessive amount of the parathyroid hormone. *Primary hyperparathyroidism* is hyperparathyroidism that results from increased parathyroid hormone production by one or more of the four parathyroid glands. This condition occurs twice as often in women as in men, and most cases result from a parathyroid adenoma. A few cases of primary hyperparathyroidism occur as the result of *idiopathic parathyroid hyperplasia*, which is a condition in which an abnormal increase in the number of parathyroid cells occurs for no known reason. Moreover, only about five percent of primary hyperparathyroidism cases arise from parathyroid carcinoma. The treatment of primary hyperparathyroidism is surgical.

Hypoparathyroidism is a condition that is characterized by a lack of parathyroid hormone. The most common cause of hypoparathyroidism is the accidental removal of or damage to the parathyroid glands in the course of an operation on the thyroid gland. The symptoms of hypoparathyroidism include paresthesia, restlessness, depression, fatigue, and muscle cramps as a result of hypocalcemia. Some patients also experience symptoms of tetany, such as spasms in certain muscle groups. Treatment with vitamin D and calcium is effective in raising the patient's blood calcium level, thus minimizing the symptoms of hypoparathyroidism.

Disorders of the Adrenal Glands

The adrenal cortex produces several hormones, each of which has a different effect. The excess or deficiency of one or more adrenal hormones will produce well-defined syndromes, such as aldosteronism, Cushing's syndrome, and Addison's disease.

Aldosteronism

Aldosterone is an adrenal hormone that regulates the body's water and salt balance. *Aldosteronism* is the secretion of aldosterone in excessive amounts. *Secondary aldosteronism* is a condition in which the secretion of aldosterone in excessive amounts is stimulated by agents outside the adrenal gland. Secondary aldosteronism is often associated with the nephrotic syndrome, cirrhosis of the liver, and heart failure. Primary aldosteronism, as defined in Chapter 7, *The Circulatory System,* is a condition in which the secretion of aldosterone in excessive amounts is stimulated by agents within the adrenal gland. Primary aldosteronism is characterized by hypertension and low serum potassium. Low serum potassium causes muscle weakness, fatigue, and polyuria. The most frequent cause of primary aldosteronism is an aldosterone-producing adenoma in the adrenal cortex. Less common causes of primary aldosteronism are (1) *bilateral adrenocortical hyperplasia*, a condition in which the cortexes of both adrenal glands are the sites of the abnormal multiplication of cells in a normal arrangement, and (2) adrenal carcinoma. Hyperplasia is typically treated with an oral aldosterone antagonist. On the other hand, adrenal carcinoma generally requires the surgical removal of the tumor.

Cushing's Syndrome

Cushing's syndrome is a condition in which hormones—corticosteroids—that affect metabolism exist in excessive amounts for a sustained period of time. This condition results from either overproduction or oral administration of the hormones. The overproduction of these hormones can arise from a benign adrenal adenoma, adrenal cancer, or spontaneous adrenal hyperplasia. Oral administration of these hormones often involves taking cortisone, prednisone, or other drug. The manifestations of Cushing's syndrome include obesity, hypertension, decreased glucose tolerance, weakness and fatigue, osteoporosis, personality changes, and menstrual and sexual dysfunction. If the Cushing's disease results in the overproduction of adrenal cortical androgen, the condition is called ***adrenal virilism***. (Adrenal virilism can also result from the overproduction of adrenal cortical androgen arising from an adenoma.) Adrenal virilism produces manifestations that are more noticeable in women than in men. Some of the signs of adrenal virilism in women include a male-type pattern of hair distribution, deepening of the voice, acne, amenorrhea, and decreased breast size. Treatment of Cushing's syndrome depends on the site of the underlying problem and is usually surgical, but may involve low doses of steroids.

Addison's Disease

Addison's disease is a condition in which the adrenal glands underproduce corticosteroids and mineralocorticoids and is characterized by progressive weakness, brownish pigmentation of the skin, low blood pressure, dizziness, fainting spells, diarrhea, and weight loss. The inability of the adrenal cortex to maintain an adequate hormonal output most often results from atrophy of the adrenal gland for unknown reasons or from an immunologic reaction. Other causes of adrenal cortex failure include adrenal hemorrhage, adrenal tumors, bilateral adrenal tuberculosis or other infection, and disease of the pituitary gland that is associated with decreased ACTH production. Adrenal failure may also result when oral steroids are withdrawn too quickly from a chronic user of the steroids. The treatment of Addison's disease patients by the daily administration of drugs to replace the hormones that are underproduced has increased the life expectancy of most of those patients to a normal duration.

Disorders of the Pancreas

Endocrine disorders of the pancreas are characterized by either (1) the overproduction of insulin, (2) the underproduction of insulin, or (3) the reduced ability of the body to utilize insulin properly. The overproduction of insulin results in ***hypoglycemia***, which is a blood sugar level that is too low for the body's needs. The underproduction of insulin or the inability of the body to utilize the amount of insulin that is produced results in ***hyperglycemia***, which is a blood sugar level that is too high.

Hypoglycemia

Some hypoglycemic individuals report no symptoms, even when their blood sugar levels are quite low, but others report symptoms of palpitations, sweating, weakness, tachycardia, trembling, headache, hunger, dizziness, and anxiety, even when their blood sugar levels are in the normal range. However, these symptoms are not specific for hypoglycemia, and other diseases can cause similar manifestations. Therefore, establishing a diagnosis of hypoglycemia is difficult. Nonetheless, most authorities agree that blood sugar levels below 50 milligrams percent, the simultaneous presence of symptoms, and the relief of these symptoms by the ingestion of carbohydrates indicate the presence of hypoglycemia.

Hypoglycemia may arise from any one of several causes. For example, *fasting hypoglycemia*, which is hypoglycemia that occurs after abstinence from eating so that all glucose contents of the intestines have been absorbed, occasionally arises in individuals who have taken an overdose of oral antidiabetic agents or insulin. Fasting hypoglycemia can also result from an adenoma of the pancreatic islet cells, adrenal insufficiency, hepatic insufficiency, or the underproduction of some pituitary hormones. *Reactive hypoglycemia*, which is also called *postprandial hypoglycemia,* is a temporary condition that occurs two to four hours after the ingestion of carbohydrates and is associated with an excessive release of insulin and, in turn, a decrease in blood sugar. *Idiopathic hypoglycemias* are those hypoglycemias that have no known cause. *Pseudohypoglycemia* is a condition in which a patient experiences the symptoms of hypoglycemia, but has normal blood sugar levels. The treatment of hypoglycemia depends on the cause of the condition. Generally, mild cases of hypoglycemia do not require treatment unless the patient's symptoms occur often. Smaller and more frequent meals that are high in protein and relatively free of simple sugars is the usual treatment for reactive hypoglycemia.

Hyperglycemia

Glucose is the form in which complex sugar appears in the blood, is the end-product of carbohydrate metabolism, and is a major source of energy in living organisms. People who have hyperglycemia are said to be glucose intolerant because they do not metabolize glucose properly. The body's ability, or inability, to metabolize glucose is shown by the oral glucose tolerance test (OGTT). The test involves the oral ingestion of a solution containing 75 grams of glucose after a 10- to 16-hour overnight fast. Blood samples are drawn before the patient drinks the solution and at one and two-hour intervals afterwards. The plasma glucose levels at these times are then compared to normal values. Figure 12–5 presents the plasma glucose concentration levels that indicate health, impaired glucose tolerance, and

Figure 12–5.
Venous Plasma Glucose Levels Diagnostic for Various Conditions.

Condition	Fasting	Level on Oral Glucose Tolerance Test (mg%)	
		1-hour Sample	2-hour Sample
Normal	< 115	< 200	< 140
Impaired glucose tolerance	< 140	> 200	< 200
Diabetes mellitus	> 140	> 200	> 200

diabetes mellitus. (Impaired glucose tolerance and diabetes mellitus are discussed later in this chapter.) However, the medical community is not in universal agreement about these categories. Some authorities feel that the levels required for the diagnosis of diabetes mellitus are too high.

The measurement of glycosylated hemoglobin, which is designated hemoglobin A1c, is an important test used for monitoring a patient's average blood glucose levels over a period of time. Unlike blood glucose levels, which vary widely during a 24-hour period, glycosylated hemoglobin concentrations rise and fall slowly and are unaffected by recent glucose ingestion. The level of a patient's hemoglobin A1c is a reflection of that patient's average blood glucose level over the prior two to three months. A random blood sugar determination indicates the patient's glucose control at any given time, but hemoglobin A1c represents a check on the degree of control of diabetes over a longer period. Patients whose diabetes is either uncontrolled or poorly controlled may possess levels of glycosylated hemoglobin that are twice as high as those levels in nondiabetics and some diabetics who have their disease under excellent control.

Glucose intolerance typically is classified into three categories: diabetes mellitus, gestational diabetes mellitus, and impaired glucose tolerance, each of which is discussed below.

Diabetes Mellitus. Diabetes mellitus (DM) is a heterogeneous group of disorders that, because of the body's inability to metabolize glucose properly, are characterized by hyperglycemia. Another indication of DM is glycosuria, which was defined in Chapter 2 as a condition in which an excessive amount of glucose is present in the patient's urine. DM can be classified into three main types: (1) insulin-dependent diabetes mellitus (IDDM), which is sometimes called Type 1 diabetes or juvenile diabetes, (2) non-insulin-dependent diabetes mellitus (NIDDM), which is sometimes called Type 2 diabetes or adult onset diabetes, and (3) diabetes associated with other disorders. Genetic factors probably are involved in the development of DM. NIDDM appears to have a genetic origin, because a family history of diabetes is extremely common in these patients. A family history of DM is less common in IDDM patients than in NIDDM patients. In fact, if one identical twin has IDDM, the chance that the other twin will be diabetic does not exceed 50 percent.

In many people who have IDDM, the disorder first manifests in childhood. Furthermore, the symptoms of IDDM, such as polyuria, excessive thirst, hunger, weakness, and weight loss, typically occur abruptly and are often precipitated by illness or stress. On the other hand, NIDDM tends to develop in people who are older than 40 and may be asymptomatic. If symptoms do occur, they usually develop gradually. Patients who have IDDM usually are not overweight and may even be thin, but many NIDDM patients are overweight or morbidly obese. IDDM patients require more careful management of their disease than do NIDDM patients.

Treatment of all types of DM lower the patient's blood sugar levels and relieve the patient of annoying symptoms. Lower blood sugar levels can be achieved through diet, exercise, the use of oral antidiabetic drugs, the regular injection of insulin, or a combination of these methods. The management of NIDDM is easier than the management of IDDM, because the former causes narrower fluctuations in the patient's blood glucose level than does the latter. A nutritionally adequate diet with calorie restriction is the mainstay of treatment for all overweight DM patients. Many NIDDM patients can control their diabetes very well on a proper diet alone without medication. However, some individuals will also need to take antidiabetic drugs for control. These drugs, taken orally, act by stimulating the pancreas to release its own insulin. A few patients who meet most of the criteria for NIDDM achieve better control of their disease if they take small daily doses of insulin, because their pancreases do not produce enough insulin to maintain proper levels of blood sugar.

Generally, as soon as a patient is diagnosed as having DM, the patient begins a specialized diet and may require either insulin injection or oral antidiabetic drug therapy. Usually, the endocrinologist and patient work together during a trial period to determine the smallest dose of insulin or antidiabetic drug that will control the patient's diabetes. Patients typically take oral antidiabetic drugs one or two times a day, depending on the patient's response to the drugs. Insulin is administered by injection. Several different types of insulin are available, and they vary considerably in the speed and duration of their activity. Regular insulin acts rapidly to produce a sudden and dramatic lowering of the patient's blood sugar level, but lasts for only a short amount of time. Ultralente and protamine zinc insulin are two types of insulin that are very long-acting and have a slower, sustained blood sugar-lowering effect for 24 hours or more. NPH and lente insulin are types of insulin that are intermediate in rapidity of action and duration of effect between regular insulin and ultralente or protamine zinc insulin. Insulin used for injection therapy may have been obtained from cattle or swine or may have been genetically engineered from human cells. The conventional insulin regimen includes one or two doses, which often are a combination of regular insulin and a longer-acting type each day. A second treatment regimen employs multiple doses of insulin, typically containing only regular insulin before meals followed by a longer-acting preparation later in the day. A third insulin regimen involves the patient's use of a programmable insulin pump, which allows for a nearly continuous, low-dose, subcutaneous injection of insulin throughout the day. The latter two regimens require the patient to take frequent blood sugar measurements, but provide the best control over the patient's blood sugar levels.

The acute complications of DM include hypoglycemic reactions and insulin deficiency states. Hypoglycemic reactions, which are the most common complication of insulin therapy, may result from an excess of insulin or of oral antidiabetic drug, from delay in eating a meal, or from unusual physical exertion. Manifestations of hypoglycemic reactions include tachycardia, palpitations, sweating, confusion, or mental changes. If untreated, a hypoglycemic reaction may progress to coma and seizures. If the reaction lasts long enough, it may also cause permanent brain cell damage. All manifestations of hypoglycemia are relieved by glucose administration.

On the other hand, hyperglycemic coma is associated with insulin deficiency and is often precipitated by another illness or by stress. This type of coma is preceded by several days of polyuria, polydipsia, fatigue, nausea, vomiting, and mental stupor. In addition, the patient's breath will have a fruity odor. If the hyperglycemia is left untreated, the condition will progress to coma and death. Hyperglycemic coma occurs more often in patients who have IDDM than in patients who have other types of DM.

The chronic complications of DM include severe, premature atherosclerosis leading to coronary artery disease, stroke, aortic aneurysms, and peripheral vascular disease. DM is also a leading cause of blindness, even though most diabetics do not become blind. Furthermore, many cases of end-stage renal disease result from DM. In fact, the major causes of death of diabetic patients are ischemic heart disease, hypertension, and renal failure. Most of the increased mortality and morbidity associated with DM occurs in patients who have had the disease for 15 to 20 years. However, improper or inadequate treatment of low or high blood sugar can lead to significantly increased morbidity or mortality at any stage of the illness.

Gestational Diabetes Mellitus. Gestational diabetes mellitus (GDM) is DM that develops during a woman's pregnancy. When the GDM patient is no longer pregnant, her glucose tolerance typically returns to normal. Congenital anomalies, large size for gestational age, and fetal death are the most significant health risks of GDM to the fetus. Complications, such as low blood sugar and calcium levels, infection, and high bilirubin levels soon after delivery may occur in the infant. Meticulous care in maintaining the mother's blood sugar at proper levels during pregnancy will alleviate many of these conditions.

Impaired Glucose Tolerance. Impaired glucose tolerance (IGT) is a group of conditions that fall in the borderline zone between normal glucose tolerance and DM. Several terms, including subclinical diabetes, borderline diabetes, and latent diabetes, were formerly used to describe disorders that are now called IGT. The results of repeated glucose tolerance tests for the same person will vary over time. Over the long term, individuals who have IGT may develop full-blown DM, may revert to normal glucose tolerance, or may remain in the IGT range. Individuals who have IGT are more likely to develop atherosclerotic disease than are individuals who have normal glucose tolerance. However, most IGT patients do not develop clinically significant eye or renal disease, as many DM patients do. Overweight individuals who have IGT can improve their glucose tolerance by losing weight. A small percentage of IGT patients will develop full-blown DM despite adequate treatment during the IGT phase.

Figure 12–6 outlines the types of glucose intolerance.

Figure 12–6.
Classification of Glucose Intolerance.

- Diabetes mellitus (DM)
  - Insulin-dependent (IDDM)
  - Non-insulin-dependent (NIDDM)
- Gestational diabetes mellitus (GDM)
- Impaired glucose tolerance (IGT)

13

The Musculoskeletal System

The *musculoskeletal system* consists of the body's bones, joints, muscles, cartilage, ligaments, and tendons. Bones, muscles, cartilage, ligaments, and tendons are connective tissues and are defined and described in Chapter 2, *Scientific Background for the Study of Disease*. Scientific investigation of the musculoskeletal system involves the study of the anatomy of the connective tissues, as well as the study of the function of these tissues and their contribution to the normal working of the body. Specifically, the scientific study of bones is called *osteology*, and the scientific study of muscles is called *myology*. This chapter will discuss the components of the musculoskeletal system and then will detail the primary disorders of that system.

ANATOMY AND PHYSIOLOGY

In the fetus, most of the temporary skeleton consists of cartilage, which forms a model from which most bones develop. Gradually, most of the fetal cartilage is absorbed and replaced by permanent bone. Some cartilage remains at the ends of long bones, at joints, in the areas surrounding the trachea and bronchi, in the external ear and nose, and in other locations in the body. The purpose of cartilage is to furnish elastic support and protection and to provide greater flexibility than bone. Bones come together at joints. A *joint*, which is also known as an *articulation*, is the place of union or junction between two or more bones, especially a junction that permits motion of one or more of the bones. An **articular capsule** is a sac-like envelope that encloses the cavity of a joint. Ligaments extend between bones at joints to give the joints strength. Skeletal muscles, by their contractions, move bones and are responsible for all voluntary motion. Tendons attach the ends of muscles to bones. In many locations in the body, tendons are subject to injury from stress and strain.

Bones

An infant is born with about 350 bones, but during its growth many of these bones fuse, leaving the adult with approximately 206 bones. Bone is one of the hardest structures in the body. The outside layer of a bone is composed of very dense tissue, commonly called **compact bone**, and the central core of the bone consists of a spongy latticework-like tissue, called **cancellous bone**. Coating the compact bone is a protective fibrous membrane, the **periosteum**, which contains the blood vessels that supply nourishment to the bone. Marrow fills the cavities in cancellous bone tissue. Red marrow, which is responsible for the production of red and white blood cells, is found in flat and short bones, at the ends of long bones, and in the vertebrae, breastbone, and ribs. Yellow marrow is found exclusively in the cancellous tissue of long bones. Yellow marrow consists of fatty tissue, and, in healthy adults, is not actively engaged in the manufacture of blood cells. Bone tissue performs the following important functions:

- Bones move in response to muscle contractions to put the body in motion and maintain its upright position.
- Bones provide support for, and shape to, the body and protect vital structures, such as the brain, spinal cord, heart, and lungs, from injury.
- Red bone marrow in certain bones is the site of manufacture of blood cells.
- Bone contains the body's reservoir of calcium.

Calcium is needed to give the bones their hardness and strength and is also necessary to prevent paresthesia, muscle cramps, and tetany. Furthermore, calcium insures normal heart contractions and the proper functioning of the blood-clotting mechanism.

The Spine

The *spine*, which is also called the *vertebral column*, the *spinal column*, or the *backbone*, consists of a flexible series of bones called vertebrae and provides the primary support for the body's structures. A *vertebra* is any one of the bones of the spine, which are labeled according to their location along the column.

- *Cervical vertebrae* lie at the top end of the spine, supporting the head and neck.
- *Thoracic vertebrae* attach to the ribs and form part of the back wall of the chest cage.
- *Lumbar vertebrae* lie at the small of the back, between the chest cage and the pelvis.
- *Sacral vertebrae* lie behind the pelvis.
- *Coccygeal vertebrae* form the lowest segments of the spine.

Normally, at birth a person has 33 vertebrae, but an adult has fewer because the five sacral vertebrae unite to form the *sacrum*, which is the triangular bone that is wedged between the two hipbones. Furthermore, the four coccygeal vertebrae fuse to form the *coccyx*, which is the bone at the very base of the adult spine. Because the lower vertebrae are responsible for supporting greater weight, they are significantly larger than the upper vertebrae. The thoracic vertebrae are intermediate in size between the cervical and lumbar vertebrae, and the lower thoracic vertebrae are larger than the upper ones.

An infant's vertebral column is more or less straight, but gradually curves develop, and by adulthood, the vertebral column has four curves—cervical, thoracic, lumbar, and sacral—that are named for the four major sections of the spine. Figure 13–1 outlines the major

Figure 13–1.
The Vertebral Column.

Major Sections	Number of Vertebrae	Designation of Vertebrae
Cervical	7	C1–C7
Thoracic, or dorsal	12	T1–T12, or D1–D12
Lumbar	5	L1–L5
Sacral (5 fused)	1	S1
Coccyx (4 fused)	1	C1

sections of the vertebral column and the number of vertebrae in each section.

A typical vertebra consists of two major segments: an anterior body and a posterior vertebral arch. A vertebral body and arch enclose an opening, called the ***vertebral foramen***, that contains the spinal cord. A ***vertebral body*** is a solid, flat, oval structure and is the largest part of the vertebra. Within the vertebral body is cancellous tissue containing red bone marrow. Each vertebral body is separated from the bodies of adjacent vertebrae by a flat plate of tissue called an ***intervertebral disc***. The outer margin of this disc is a tough ***fibrocartilage***, which is a type of connective tissue that consists of typical cartilage cells and parallel thick, compact collagenous bundles. The fibrocartilage that surrounds the intervertebral disc is called the ***anulus fibrosus***, and it surrounds a soft, gelatinous central section of tissue, called the ***nucleus pulposus***. The vertebral arch forms the posterior portion of the vertebra. On its surface are several projections and recesses into which ribs and muscles attach. Each vertebra is bound to adjacent vertebrae by several strong ligaments. The connection of a vertebral body above to a vertebral body below provides the spine with the ability to perform its major function of supporting body structures. Figure 13–2 illustrates the connections between vertebrae by providing two views of the thoracic vertebrae.

The Skull

The ***skull***, which is the bony framework of the head, is composed of a series of flattened, irregular bones and lies on the top of the vertebral column. Eight cranial bones house and protect the brain. The skull has openings for blood vessels, cranial nerves, the spinal cord, and other vital structures. The skull also has many cavities, including (1) the nasal cavity, (2) the ear canals and cavities, (3) the ***orbits***, which shelter the eyeballs, and (4) the paranasal sinuses, which lie within the skull bones adjacent to the nasal cavity. The ***maxilla***, which is the upper jaw, holds the upper teeth. The ***mandible***, which is the lower jaw, holds the lower teeth and is the largest and strongest bone of the face. The mandible is hinged at the temporomandibular joint to permit chewing. With the exception of the mandible and the three tiny ossicles within each middle ear, the skull bones are immovably fused together.

Figure 13–3 provides side views of the vertebral column and the skull.

Figure 13–2.
Two Views of the Thoracic Vertebrae.

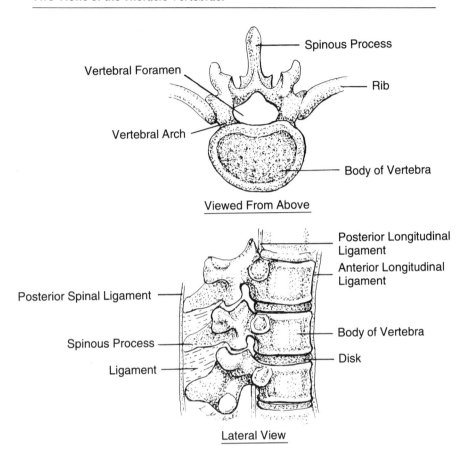

Viewed From Above

Lateral View

The Thorax

The **thorax**, or chest cage, contains the principal organs of circulation and respiration. The back of the thorax is formed by the 12 thoracic vertebrae and the posterior parts of the 12 ribs. The front of the thorax is formed by the elongated, flattened breastbone. The ribs form the sides of the thorax. Each rib articulates directly and individually on the back with a corresponding vertebra. Each of the first seven ribs terminates in a separate cartilaginous extension that joins the breastbone, or sternum, directly. The eighth, ninth, and

Figure 13–3.
Side Views of the Vertebral Column and Skull.

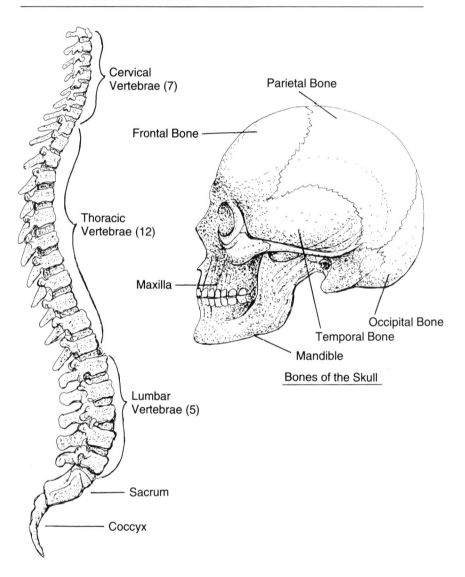

Cervical
Vertebrae (7)

Parietal Bone

Frontal Bone

Thoracic
Vertebrae (12)

Maxilla

Occipital Bone

Temporal Bone

Mandible

Bones of the Skull

Lumbar
Vertebrae (5)

Sacrum

Coccyx

tenth ribs terminate in cartilage that fuse as they communicate with the sternum. The eleventh and twelfth ribs are not attached to the sternum and end in muscle and soft tissue.

The Shoulder Girdle and Upper Extremities

The front of the shoulder girdle is formed by the **clavicle**, or collarbone. The **scapula**, or shoulder blade, is an irregular, flat, triangular bone that forms the rear part of the shoulder girdle. The **humerus**, the longest and largest bone of the upper extremity, is the bone of the upper arm. The head of the humerus, together with the bones of the shoulder girdle, form the shoulder joint. The **radius** is the forearm bone that lies on the same side as the thumb. The radius lies beside the **ulna**, which is the longer of the two forearm bones. The wrist bones are known as **carpal bones**, the small bones of the hand are the **metacarpal bones**, and the bones of the fingers are the **phalanges**. Knuckles are the **metacarpal phalangeal** joints.

The Hipbone and Lower Extremities

The **innominate bone**, or hipbone, in adults results from a fusion during growth and maturity of three separate bones: the ilium, ischium, and pubis. The **ilium** becomes the wide, top portion of the innominate bone; the **ischium** becomes the lower, back portion of the innominate; and the **pubis** becomes the lower, front part of the innominate. The union of these three bones occurs in and around a cup-shaped socket, called the **acetabulum**. (Figure 13–4 provides an illustration of the hip joint.) The **pelvis** is a strong, bony ring composed of the two hipbones on the sides and front and the sacrum and coccyx in the rear. The **femur**, the strongest and longest bone in the body, is the long bone in the upper leg. The rounded head of the femur fits into the acetabulum to form a ball and socket joint. The flat, triangular bone located in front of the knee joint is the **patella**, or knee cap. The **tibia**, or shin bone, and the **fibula,** or calf bone, are the two bones of the lower leg. The tibia is the longer of these two bones and is second only to the femur as the longest bone of the body. The bones of the ankle are the **tarsal bones**, the small bones of the foot are known as **metatarsal bones**, and the bones of the toes are called **phalanges**, as are the bones of the fingers.

Figure 13–5 provides an anterior view of the bones in the human skeleton.

Figure 13–4.
The Hip Joint.

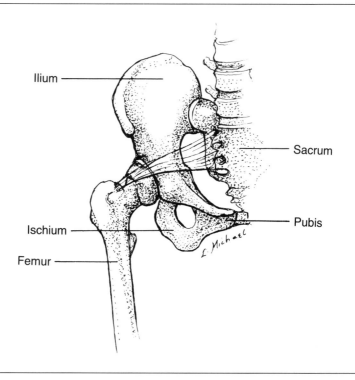

Joints, Ligaments, and Bursae

Many joints are protected and supported by strong ligaments that bind the joints together. Some joints, such as the connections between most of the skull bones, permit no movement at all, and some other joints, such as those between the vertebral bodies, allow slight movement. However, most joints in the body are freely movable. The surfaces in these movable joints are covered with cartilage and are connected by strong ligaments. The joint space is lined by a thin membrane, called the synovial membrane, which secretes a small amount of lubricating fluid. Freely movable joints may be classified as follows:

- *Hinge joints* permit only forward and backward motion.
- *Rotary joints* permit only rotation.
- *Ball and socket joints* permit motion in an indefinite number of axes.

Figure 13–5.
An Anterior View of the Bones in the Human Skeleton.

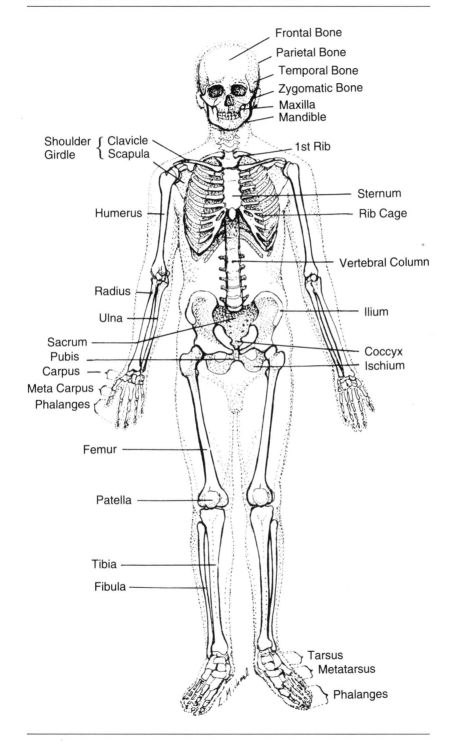

Figure 13–6.
Classification of Freely Movable Joints.

Type of Joint	Example of Joint
Hinge	Between humerus and ulna
Rotary	Between radius and ulna
Ball and socket	Between femur and innominate
Gliding	Between vertebrae
Saddle	Between carpal and metacarpal bones

- *Gliding joints* permit only gliding movements.
- *Saddle joints* permit flexion, extension, abduction, and circumduction[1].

Figure 13–6 provides an example for each of these types of joints and Figure 13–7 illustrates a few of these examples.

Many freely movable joints are surrounded by one or more two-layered sacs, called **bursae**, which are filled with fluid. The function of a bursa is to permit ligaments and muscles to move freely about a bone or joint without friction and with a minimum of irritation. Approximately 80 bursae lie on each side of the body. Certain bursae are recognized with proper names. For example, the bursa located between the lower end of the femur and the tendons of the patella is known as the **suprapatellar bursa**, and the bursa located between the **deltoid muscle**, which is the triangular muscle at the shoulder joint, and the shoulder joint capsule is known as the **subdeltoid bursa**. Figure 13–8 illustrates the shoulder joint and subdeltoid bursa.

Muscles

Because Chapter 2, *Scientific Background for the Study of Disease*, contains a full discussion of the three types of muscle tissue, this section will provide a short summary and recap. Smooth muscle tissue is located in the walls of blood vessels and in the digestive tract. Cardiac muscle tissue appears only in the myocardium. Skele-

---

[1]*Flexion* is the act of bending; *extension* is the movement by which the two ends of a joint are drawn away from each other; *abduction* is movement away from the midline; and *circumduction* is movement in a circle.

Figure 13–7.
Examples of Rotary, Ball and Socket, and Hinge Joints.

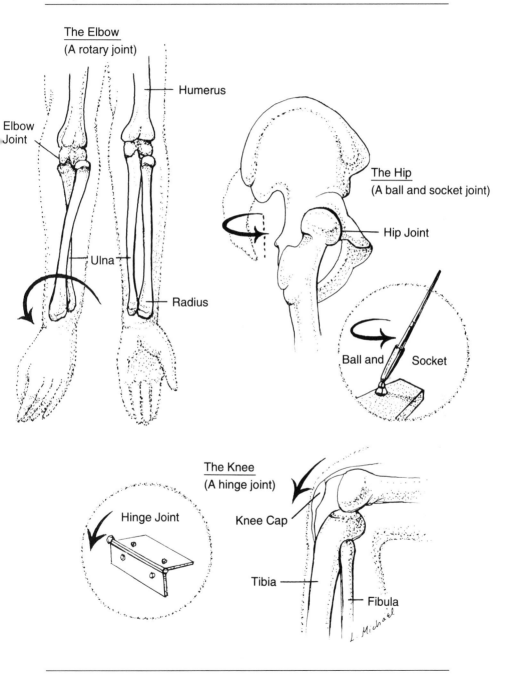

Figure 13–8.
The Shoulder Joint and Subdeltoid Bursa.

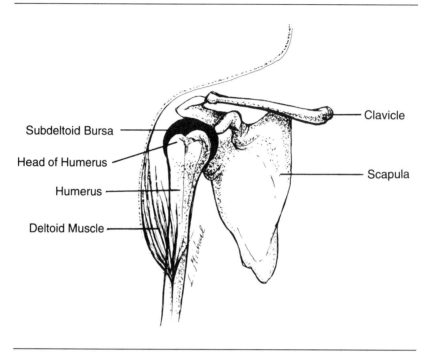

tal muscles, which are also known as *striated muscles*, are located in organs of voluntary motion. Most skeletal muscles are attached to bones by means of tendons. However, a few facial muscles do not have bone attachments.

This chapter will focus upon skeletal muscles. Skeletal muscles, which can contract rapidly and powerfully, but fatigue easily and need rest, are under voluntary control. However, a person cannot make an individual skeletal muscle contract, because these muscles work in groups to produce motion. Most muscles are opposed by other muscles that have an opposite action. In order to flex the arm, for example, flexor muscles must contract and extensor muscles must relax simultaneously. The nervous system coordinates the actions of the muscle groups.

DISORDERS OF THE MUSCULOSKELETAL SYSTEM

Disorders of the musculoskeletal system may involve the bones, muscles, ligaments, or all three, especially at joints. Musculoskeletal disorders may result from trauma, mechanical displacement, or pathologic conditions, such as inflammation, degeneration, immune disorders, infection, defects in metabolic processes, or tumors. This section will first discuss some common general disorders of the musculoskeletal system. Then, it will address a few of the many disorders that may affect specific joints.

General Disorders

This section will discuss diseases and conditions that can affect almost any component of the musculoskeletal system. We will define and discuss fractures, dislocations, sprains and strains, bursitis, and arthritis.

Fractures

A *fracture* is a break in the surface of a bone. Fractures are classified in three ways: (1) by the integrity of the overlying tissue, (2) by the specific location in the bone, and (3) by the degree of displacement.

The classification of a fracture by the integrity of the overlying tissue is subdivided into closed fractures and open fractures. In a *closed fracture*, the overlying skin and soft tissues remain intact after the bone surface has been broken. On the other hand, in an *open fracture*, the overlying skin and soft tissues are disrupted and part of the broken bone surfaces penetrate to the outside of the body.

Fractures may occur in the bone shaft, which is called the *diaphysis*, in the end of the bone, which is called the *metaphysis*, or in the articular surfaces. The site of the break is important because the type of bone tissue harmed determines the mode and speed of healing. The outer layer of bone heals by a process, called *external bridging*, in which new bone tissue grows over the area of the break. Metaphyseal bone, however, heals by the growth of new bone tissue next to the damaged *trabeculae*, which are tiny, sharp projections in cancellous bone that form a mesh of intercommunicating spaces that are filled with bone marrow. The new bone tissue that is formed during the healing process is called *callus bone*. Fractures in metaphyseal bone tissue heal more quickly than do fractures in diaphyseal tissue.

Displacement is a change from a normal position or relationship. It can occur in many structures in the body. Classification of a fracture by the degree of displacement describes the resultant position of bone fragments after the fracture. The degree of displacement may vary from "nondisplaced," which means that the bone fragments remain next to each other and in proper alignment, to a variety of deformities produced by the displacement. These deformities will reflect (1) **angulation**, which means that the bone no longer lies in a straight line, (2) **rotation**, which means that the bone has turned, without any side-to-side or up-and-down movement, (3) a change in the bone's length, (4) or **translation**, which means that the bone fragments lie in totally different planes. Fracture patterns on x-rays are further described as being transverse, oblique, or spiral. A **transverse fracture** is one that occurs at a right angle to the long axis of the bone, an **oblique fracture** occurs at a slant to the long axis of the bone, and a **spiral fracture** winds around the short axis of the bone.

The medical community uses many other terms to describe fractures. For example, a **comminuted fracture** is a break that involves more than two bone fragments, an **impacted fracture** is a break that involves two bone fragments that are firmly driven into each other, and a **multiple fracture** is a break that involves two or more lines of fracture that are not physically connected to each other in the same bone. Some descriptive terms relate to the origin of the fracture: a **pathologic fracture** occurs when a bone, weakened by tumor or disease, breaks during normal daily activities or minor trauma, and an **avulsion fracture** occurs as the result of a sudden, severe muscle pull that tears the ligaments and muscles from the bone.

Fractures may be **reduced**—that is, brought into proper alignment—by closed or open methods. Closed methods of reduction are noninvasive and include manipulation and traction, which uses the exertion of a pulling force to align the bone fragments. Open reduction is accomplished by surgery. Typically, the surgeon makes an incision in the skin over the fracture and exposes the bone in order to achieve proper bone fragment alignment. Once the fracture is reduced, the bone must be kept in perfect alignment. External fixation with casts and internal fixation with screws, rods, pins, wires, and plates are methods used to maintain proper alignment.

The proper healing of fractures depends upon several factors, including:

- the accuracy of the initial realignment
- the level of immobilization of the fracture and the length of time of immobilization
- the blood supply the fractured bone receives
- the type of bone involved
- the type of fracture involved
- the location of the fracture on the bone
- the age and general physical health of the patient
- the presence or absence of infection at the site of the fracture

Problems associated with any of these factors may arise and result in the delay or the incompletion of the healing process. A delay in the healing process of fractures is called *delayed union*, and the failure of the process is called *nonunion*. Figure 13–9 outlines some of the problems that may be associated with each of the factors involved with healing. Other recognized potential complications of fractures are (1) neurovascular injuries, (2) adult respiratory distress syndrome, (3) chronic **osteomyelitis**, which is an inflammation of bone tissue resulting from a pus-forming organism, (4) deformity of new bone growth, (5) posttraumatic arthritis, (6) **osteonecrosis**, which is the death of bone tissue, and (7) **reflex sympathetic dystrophy**, which is a disturbance in the sympathetic nervous system marked by pain, pallor, sweating, swelling, or atrophy of the skin.

The treatment of delayed union or nonunion may involve **bone grafting**, which is the implanting or transplanting of bone tissue from one site to another. Bone chips from the tibia, fibula, and ilium are most frequently used in bone grafts. The bone chips provide a

Figure 13–9.
Healing of Fractures.

Factors Involved with Healing	Problems Encountered
Realignment	Faulty reduction will result in delayed union
Immobilization	Movement will delay the healing process; nonunion may result
Blood supply	Inadequate nourishment delays healing; some bones have a characteristic limited blood supply, and fractures in these bones heal slowly
Bone involved	The larger the bone, the longer the time required for healing
Type of fracture	Transverse fractures heal more slowly than oblique and spiral fractures
Location of fracture	Location affects the rate of healing; for example, a fracture in the lower third of the tibia takes longer to heal than a fracture in the upper third
Age and condition of the patient	Fractures in elderly people take longer to heal than fractures in young people; fractures in sick patients heal more slowly than fractures in healthy patients
Infection	Infection at the fracture site causes delayed union or nonunion

building-block for joining the pieces of the fracture, and they usually are put into place with some type of internal fixation method, such as a pin or wire. A recent development in promoting the healing of fractures is the use of electrical stimulation. The electrical stimulation technique involves placing wires on the surface of the body directly above the break in the bone and sending an electric current through the wires. This technique has shown excellent results in treating the nonunion of fractures. Electrical stimulation can achieve a rate of union comparable to that of bone graft operations, with less risk of harm and infection to the patient.

Dislocations

A bone **dislocation**, which is also known as a *luxation*, is a total displacement of one or more bones that comprise a joint, causing a complete change in the normal relationship between these bony surfaces. A **subluxation** is a partial change in the customary alignment of these surfaces, which still retain some contact with each other. Acute dislocations usually result from external trauma and only rarely result from unbalanced muscular action. In individuals who have abnormally relaxed muscles and ligaments, the dislocation may be recurrent. Furthermore, some dislocations are congenital, and others are spontaneous. Complications of dislocations frequently occur and include impairment of circulation to local tissues or to an extremity; injury to nerves; injury to other important, surrounding structures; associated chip fractures; traumatic arthritis; and death of bone tissue. Specific treatment of dislocations depends on the joint affected and the nature of associated injuries. Generally the patient is placed under anesthesia while a dislocation is reduced. Then, the joint must be immobilized by sling, splint, or cast to give the surrounding tissues an opportunity to heal. Surgical repair of torn ligaments is often necessary to prevent recurrent dislocations.

Sprains and Strains

A **sprain** is a condition that results from an overstretching or tearing of supporting ligaments at a joint and generally occurs whenever movement in the joint extends beyond the normal range. Sprains occur in the ankle, knee, finger, wrist, elbow, and spine. A **strain** results from the overstretching or tearing of muscles or tendons. The distinction between sprains and strains is more academic than practical, because these injuries often occur simultaneously, and clinically differentiating between the two is difficult. Both disorders cause pain and disability. The diagnosis of these musculoligamentous disorders is often made by excluding other causes of pathology, such as fracture, upon clinical and x-ray examination. Usually, resting the painful area is sufficient to effect a cure for a sprain or strain, but physiotherapy and external support may be helpful in selected cases.

Bursitis

Bursitis is an inflammation of a bursa. It may exist in an acute or chronic form, and in either case is secondary to mechanical irritation or bacterial infection. Acute bursitis is marked by a swelling of a bursa arising from an outpouring of synovial fluid. The swelling results in localized tenderness and limitation of joint movement, either by mechanical abnormality or pain. Motion at the neighboring joint irritates the bursa, producing or aggravating the pain. The effusion of fluid associated with acute bursitis generally is absorbed within a week or two, and recovery is usually complete. In the chronic form of bursitis, the bursal wall becomes thickened by a chronic inflammatory reaction, which results in the degeneration of the bursa. If the condition does not respond to rest, heat, needle aspiration, local corticosteroid or anesthetic injection, and analgesics, surgery may be necessary to remove the bursa itself. Such surgery may result in permanent limitation of joint motion.

Trauma is a common cause of bursitis, which may be induced by a single traumatic episode or by repeated episodes of trauma. The trauma itself may be external, such as a blow to a joint, or internal, such as irritation of a calcific deposit or from excessive pressure or friction. Although infectious bursitis is uncommon, acute infectious bursitis typically results from infection by a pus-producing agent, and chronic infectious bursitis most often results from tuberculosis.

Arthritis

Arthritis is a general term for several disorders in which anatomic change produces pain and stiffness in joints. Many people who have arthritis also have restricted motion in the affected joints. Two fundamental pathologic processes, inflammation and degeneration, coexist in arthritis patients, and both processes can exist in acute or chronic forms. In certain arthritic disorders, such as rheumatoid arthritis, inflammation is the predominant process, and in other conditions, such as osteoarthritis, degeneration is the more important process. Arthritis may also accompany, or be the major manifestation of, many other disease states. Figure 13–10 provides a classification of arthritis and an example of each class.

Figure 13–10.
Classification of Arthritis.

Manifestation	Example of Disease
Synovitis, which is the inflammation of a synovial membrane	Rheumatoid arthritis
Disease in the transition region where ligament attaches to the bone	Ankylosing spondylitis
Cartilage degeneration	Osteoarthritis
Crystal-induced synovitis	Gout
Joint infection	Staphylococcal and gonococcal infection

Rheumatoid Arthritis. Rheumatoid arthritis is a chronic, systemic disease characterized by inflammation in and around many joints. The cause of rheumatoid arthritis is unknown, although autoimmunologic, infectious, metabolic, endocrine, or allergic influences may be involved. The course of the disease, which is marked by periods of improvement and worsening, is slowly progressive and highly variable. The chief complaints of most rheumatoid arthritis patients are pain and tenderness, swelling, stiffness, and unpredictable periods of restricted motion in the affected joints. In addition, many patients express specific systemic complaints of malaise, fatigue, and, occasionally, low-grade fever. Typically, discomfort and stiffness are severe early in the morning and lessen with the day's activity.

In adults, rheumatoid arthritis may have a gradual or an abrupt onset. More than 80 percent of adult rheumatoid arthritis cases arise in patients who are younger than age 40, and 75 percent of affected persons are women. Joint manifestations consist of redness, swelling with joint fluid, and tenderness. Adult rheumatoid arthritis may affect any joint, but the disease principally involves the joints of the fingers, wrists, elbows, and knees. In the hands, the joints on the back of the hand and the joints of the fingers are the most likely to be affected. Symmetrical joint involvement is a common finding and helps to distinguish rheumatoid arthritis from other forms of the disorder. Subcutaneous fibrous nodules occur only in the rheumatoid form of arthritis, but are found in only 15 to 20 percent of rheumatoid arthritis patients.

Laboratory studies of rheumatoid arthritis patients frequently indicate a mild anemia and the presence of an autoantibody known as the rheumatoid factor (RF). RF is an immunoglobulin M (IgM) antibody that is directed against normal human immunoglobulin G (IgG). Immunoglobulins are discussed in more detail in the Immunology section of Chapter 2. The characteristic clinical course of adult rheumatoid arthritis is one of remissions and recurrences, with the tendency to become gradually more disabling with each recurrence. However, in some patients the disease may be present for years without change and may cause only minimal disability. Chronic joint changes associated with adult rheumatoid arthritis, including calcification of the joint space and destruction of surrounding cartilage, "freeze" the joint, rendering it incapable of movement. Once joints become frozen and deformed by chronic disease, the chance of a return to full function is extremely poor.

In children, rheumatoid arthritis typically has its onset before the patient is 16 years old. This type of rheumatoid arthritis, called juvenile chronic arthritis or juvenile rheumatoid arthritis, is more common in girls than in boys, and most often presents between ages two and four, although it has a secondary peak of onset between the ages of ten and twelve. A subset of juvenile chronic arthritis is called *Still's disease*, which is characterized by high spiking daily fevers, body rash, and other manifestations of systemic disease. In many respects, the juvenile chronic arthritis is similar to adult rheumatoid arthritis. However, the systemic symptoms, such as fever, rash, splenomegaly, and generalized lymphadenopathy, are likely to be more severe in children than in adults. Furthermore, cardiac involvement and pleural effusion are more common in juvenile patients than in adult patients. The juvenile form of this disorder affects large joints, and a juvenile patient may develop a bird-like face from impaired growth of the mandible. The RF in juvenile arthritis patients is usually negative. When the disease occurs in growing joints, some changes in growth and development may occur. The prognosis for a juvenile chronic arthritis patient, therefore, depends on the age of onset, as well as the severity of joint involvement. The chronic changes, such as freezing of joints, seen frequently in the adult variety are not common in the juvenile form. Complete remission can be anticipated in 75 percent of children who have juvenile chronic arthritis.

Spondylarthropathy. The *seronegative spondylarthropathies* are forms of arthritis that are characterized by the absence of RF, an involvement of the spine and related bones, and at least some degree of peripheral inflammatory joint disease. Pathologic changes associated with these spondylarthropathies are found in the *enthesis*, which is the site of ligamentous attachment to bone. By comparison, pathologic changes associated with rheumatoid arthritis are found in the synovial membranes. Moreover, spondylarthropathies show a significant hereditary pattern. ***Ankylosing spondylitis***, which is also known as *Marie Strumpell disease*, is a chronic, slowly progressive form of arthritis, which primarily involves the spine and sacroiliac joints. This condition is the most common spondylarthropathy and has a peak onset in males between the ages of 15 and 35. Ankylosing spondylitis is one of the most common causes of back complaints in young men. Early in the course of the disease, an acute attack is characterized by pain or stiffness in the lumbosacral region. This symptom is worse in the morning and is relieved somewhat by modest activity. About one-third of ankylosing spondylitis patients have symptoms related to pain and/or stiffness in the hips, knees, and ankles. Up to 30 percent of affected people suffer from complications, such as aortic insufficiency, cardiac enlargement, or inflammation of the aorta or iris, which are not directly related to bones. The sacroiliac joints and the joints between the lower lumbar vertebrae in ankylosing spondylitis patients show bilateral destruction and fusion as early manifestations of the disease. Exacerbations and remissions occur, and the disease progresses up the patient's spine with each recurrence. Eventually, the entire thoracic and lumbar spine becomes straight and rigid. As the thoracic spine and the rib-vertebral joints become involved, chest expansion diminishes. A "hunchback" invariably results as a late manifestation. Morbidity from ankylosing spondylitis is substantial, and patients who have this disorder experience a higher mortality rate than that of the general population. This increased mortality rate is attributable to conditions, such as ulcerative colitis, nephritis, cardiovascular disease, and respiratory disease, that often accompany this form of arthritis.

Psoriatic arthritis is a spondylarthropathy that is characterized by the presence of psoriatic skin and nail lesions. About 20 percent of patients who have psoriasis develop this inflammatory joint disease that often initially resembles rheumatoid arthritis. In addition, psoriatic arthritis is seen in people of all ages and with equal frequency in both males and females. Most frequently, the psoriasis presents prior to the arthritis. Often psoriatic arthritis runs a benign, intermittent course, but occasionally untreated psoriatic arthritis may cripple as severely as does rheumatoid arthritis.

Reiter's syndrome is a spondylarthropathy that is characterized by urethritis, conjunctivitis, and arthritis. This disorder is predominately genetic in origin. Although peripheral joints are more commonly involved in the arthritic process of Reiter's syndrome, at least 20 percent of affected patients show evidence of sacroiliitis and ascending spinal disease. Reiter's syndrome sometimes results from a venereal or intestinal infection. In the past, Reiter's syndrome was thought to affect only males, but the medical community now recognizes that women may also be affected. Although the initial manifesta-tions of peripheral arthritis and systemic illness may be mild, the disease is no longer thought to be self-limited, and researchers have found that approximately 80 percent of patients examined five years after the initial episode of Reiter's have some evidence that the disease is still active. No specific treatment for this arthritis exists, and research has proved that the use of antibiotics, despite the infectious origin of the disease, is ineffective.

   Osteoarthritis. *Osteoarthritis*, which is also known as *degenera-tive arthritis, degenerative joint disease*, and *hypertrophic arthritis*, is generally a chronic, noninflammatory, degenerative disease that usually affects several joints, particularly those, such as the knees, hips, and spine, that involve weight-bearing and daily wear-and-tear. Joints of the hand, most often the joints nearest the fingernails, are also commonly affected. Joints affected by osteoarthritis become distorted and damaged, but, except for the spine, do not become frozen. The joint changes result from a combination of bone degener-ation and the proliferation of new bone, tendon, cartilage, and synovial membrane tissue. The cause of osteoarthritis is unknown, but aging, heredity, obesity, and prior joint disease, including joint trauma, are predisposing factors. Osteoarthritis is the most common variety of arthritis and is about twice as common in women as in men. After the age of 55, most persons have some x-ray evi-dence of osteoarthritis, although in only one-third of the popula-tion does the presence of arthritis cause symptoms. Symptoms of osteoarthritis, which are nonsystemic, rarely manifest before age 40, and they typically include pain and swelling in one or several joints. Generally, the pain associated with osteoarthritis is worse at the end of the day and is aggravated by strenuous exercise. How-ever, light exercise, which "loosens up" the joint, may relieve the pain.

   Osteoarthritis is a slowly progressive disease, which in many cases never reaches the stage at which specific treatment is required. Graded exercises, heat, mild analgesics, and rest are often sufficient to control the symptoms. Even if surgery is required, osteoarthritis presents a less severe prognosis than does rheumatoid arthritis because the former is more amenable to surgical correction of joint distortion. Surgical replacement of the hip joint has revolutionized the treatment of osteoarthritis in that location and, to a lesser extent, knee replacement has assumed the same role. The development of other artificial joints is progressing rapidly.

   Arthritis Associated with Systemic Disease. Arthritis, in which anatomic change in a joint produces pain, and ***arthralgia***, in which pain occurs in a joint without anatomic change, are commonly associated with systemic disease and may herald or mask the underlying clinical problem. For example, almost all patients who have sickle cell disease experience some musculoskeletal symptoms. In fact, the onset of arthralgia is often the first sign of a sickle cell crisis, and the death of bone tissue in the head of the femur is frequently one of the late manifestations of sickle cell disease. Moreover, many blood-clotting disorders, such as hemophilia, have musculoskeletal manifestations, because repeated bleeding episodes within joint spaces eventually lead to synovial changes and destruction of joints. These manifestations mimic those of rheumatoid arthritis. Virtually all patients who have severe forms of clotting disorders show some form of chronic joint impairment by the age of 15. Furthermore, some endocrine diseases, particularly hypothyroidism and acromegaly, are associated with arthritis and arthralgia.

Infectious arthritis, as its name implies, is joint disease that results from a bacterial, viral, or other infection. Bacterial arthritis usually results from a blood-borne infection. Acute bacterial infections are usually divided into gonococcal and nongonococcal classifications. Gonococcal arthritis usually presents with skin changes, as well as pain and swelling in several joints at a time. Typically, the pain and swelling associated with this disorder *migrate*, which means that they spontaneously move to other locations in the body. Staphylococcus is the most common infectious agent of nongonococcal arthritis, which usually presents in a person who is either very young or very old and has a compromised immunologic system. Staphylococcal arthritis typically presents with symptoms of fever and malaise and usually affects a single joint, which is swollen, painful, and reddened. Neither gonococcal nor nongonococcal arthritis results in permanent joint damage if treated quickly and appropriately.

Tuberculous arthritis, as its name implies, is a joint disorder resulting from tubercular infection. This disorder is characterized by chronic inflammation of, and effusion of fluid in, a single joint. This type of arthritis also causes destruction of the neighboring bones. Children who have tuberculous arthritis typically experience the collapse of the lower spine, leading to a misshapened back.

Viral arthritis is a relatively common problem and is associated with a wide spectrum of viral illnesses, including hepatitis B and measles. The arthritis arising from hepatitis B occurs in 10 to 30 percent of all hepatitis B patients and frequently precedes the recognition of the underlying infection. On the other hand, arthritis arising from measles usually follows the appearance of the rash characteristic of the underlying disease by several days.

Gout. Gout is a hereditary form of arthritis that is characterized by an excess of uric acid in the blood, a condition called *hyperurice-*

mia, and by recurrent acute attacks of arthritis in the peripheral joints. Contributing to hyperuricemia are a protein-rich diet, the use of thiazide diuretics, and the intake of alcohol. A protein-rich diet increases the urates in the body, while thiazides and alcohol decrease uric acid excretion from the body. Although hyperuricemia predisposes a person to gout, an elevated blood uric acid level is not diagnostic of gout in an asymptomatic person. Conversely, an acute gouty arthritis may occur in a person who has normal blood uric acid levels. However, the higher the blood level of uric acid, the greater the likelihood that symptoms of gout will appear. Gout most often affects men over age 40, especially those who are overweight or hypertensive. The classic acute attack of gout occurs in an obese, sedentary man who suddenly develops severe joint pain. The affected joint becomes swollen, hot, tender, and red-purplish in color. The most common initial site of involvement of gout is the first joint of the big toe. The instep, ankle, and knee are other common locations for attacks of gout. In about eight percent of patients who have gout, the first sign of the disorder is the passage of a uric acid kidney stone. Initial mild attacks of gout last only a few days, but subsequent attacks may persist for several weeks.

The chronic phase of gout is characterized by *tophi*, which are deposits of uric acid, or urate, crystals in the tissues. Tophi occur most often in and around joints, in cartilage, bone, bursae, and in subcutaneous tissues. A frequent site of tophi is the external ear. Permanent deformity from these deposits results only after numerous attacks of gout over a period of years. Movement in a gouty joint may be limited, or the joint may be frozen. Renal disease is the most serious complication of gout. Urate crystals precipitate to form urinary tract calculi, which impair renal function and, in severe cases, may lead to renal failure. In the past, about ten percent of patients who had gout died from uremia, but newer antihyperuricemic drugs minimize the complications of the disease.

Disorders of Specific Joints

This section will discuss musculoskeletal disorders that affect specific joints. We will look at disorders of the temporomandibular joints, shoulders, wrists, hips, and knees.

The Temporomandibular Joint

The *temporomandibular joints (TMJs)* are the hinge joints that connect the lower jawbone with the side of the skull. The lower jawbone, or mandible, fits into a hollow depression in the temporal bone of the skull. As the mouth opens, the mandible glides forward slightly under the temporal bone at the same time that the jaw opens with the hinge-like action of the joint. A cartilage within the joint acts as a cushion facilitating the gliding motion of the mandible. The TMJ may be the site of several musculoskeletal and other diseases.

Symptoms of TMJ disease are pain in or around the ear, which is often increased by chewing or by opening the mouth, and headache. Physical findings in TMJ disease are localized tenderness over the temporomandibular joint, clicking when the mouth is opened, and restriction or limitation of jaw motion. Some causative factors in the origin of TMJ disease are congenital abnormalities, trauma, infection, irradiation, and arthritis. However, the most common disorder involving the TMJ area is the *myofascial pain-dysfunction syndrome (MPD),* which is a nonarticular condition that mimics true TMJ disorders by producing pain, limitation of jaw movement, or a combination of both. MPD occurs more frequently in women than in men, and most cases are psychophysiologic in origin, produced by jaw clenching and/or tooth grinding secondary to emotional stress. Although MPD is not initially accompanied by anatomic alteration within the joint, repeated microtrauma may result in damage to the cartilage and the joint, which in turn may lead to malocclusion. *Malocclusion* is the improper meeting of the teeth when the jaw is closed.

Most patients who have a TMJ disease or MPD will achieve complete relief of symptoms with conservative therapy consisting of jaw rest, heat, and muscle-relaxing or pain-relieving medications. A few patients will be helped by the elimination of dental occlusion problems. Psychologic counseling may also be helpful in treating patients who have persistent MPD. Only a very small number of patients who have TMJ disorders or MPD will require surgery on the joint itself. In these few cases, arthroscopic surgery is particularly useful for correcting cartilage deformities or actually removing the cartilage and replacing it with an artificial one. *Arthroscopy* is a procedure that permits direct visualization of a joint through fiberoptic imaging that is visualized on a monitoring cathode-ray tube screen. The instrument allows not only the direct visualization of the joint anatomy, but also tissue biopsy, the removal of damaged tissue, and a variety of corrective surgical procedures. Arthroscopy is usually performed on patients who have received a local anesthesia, and it has resulted in marked reduction of postoperative recovery and impairment time. Magnetic resonance imaging, which is defined and discussed in Chapter 3, *Specialized Diagnostic Techniques*, is very useful in evaluating anatomic changes in the TMJ and other joints.

The Shoulder

The shoulder joints and the shoulder area may be the sites of musculoskeletal problems. The causes of shoulder joint disease include rheumatoid arthritis, gout, infection, and degenerative arthritis, often resulting from acute or chronic trauma. The causes of pain and impairment in the shoulder area other than the joint typically originate in the rotator cuff. The **rotator cuff** is a musculotendinous structure that surrounds the capsule of the shoulder joint, providing it with mobility and strength. The rotator cuff is subject to **calcific tendinitis**, which is an inflammation and calcification of the bursa in a joint, resulting in pain, tenderness, and limitation of motion in the joint. The cuff is also subject to complete and incomplete tears. Another problem of the tissue in the shoulder area other than the joint is **adhesive capsulitis**, which involves an adhesive inflammation between a joint capsule and the peripheral cartilage of the joint. Adhesive capsulitis is characterized by the gradual onset of pain, leading to increasing pain, stiffness, and limitation of motion. Adhesive capsulitis occurs more often in middle-aged females than any other group and is of unknown origin. Diagnosis of shoulder joint disorders typically is based on the patient's medical history, a physical exam, x-ray, MRI tests, and/or arthroscopy. Arthroscopy can also be used as a therapeutic tool in correcting problems with the rotator cuff by restoring the shoulder's function.

The Wrist

Each wrist consists of multiple joints of the radius and ulna with the carpal bones. The multiple articulations within this area are subject to systemic arthritis, particularly rheumatoid arthritis and osteoarthritis, which is usually secondary to previous injury of the articular surfaces. The wrist area is also subject to other disorders, including: (1) fractures, such as **Colles'**, which is a fracture of the distal end of the radius, (2) **ganglions**, which are benign cysts on the back of the wrist, (3) **DeQuervain's disease**, which is a painful inflammation of the abductor and extensor muscles of the thumb, and (4) **carpal tunnel syndrome**, which is a condition that arises when the median nerve that crosses the carpal tunnel is entrapped as a result of repetitive motion, injury, pregnancy, or endocrine diseases such as diabetes mellitus or thyroid disease. The treatment for disorders of the wrist typically restores painless function of the joints through the use of splints, rest, corticosteroid injection, or, in rare cases, surgery. Diagnosis and therapy by arthroscopy are very common for the small wrist joints.

The Hip

Chronic hip disorders in adults may result from (1) osteoarthritis, (2) rheumatoid arthritis, (3) ankylosing spondylitis, (4) injuries, (5) tumors, (6) infection, and (7) osteonecrosis. Osteonecrosis typically follows fracture or dislocation and has become increasingly common following renal transplantation, corticosteroid therapy for systemic disease, alcoholism, diabetes mellitus, and sickle cell disease. Bone tissue death can often be identified by bone scans and MRI studies before it is apparent on an x-ray.

Virtually all cases of chronic hip disease in adults lead to progressive functional loss. In these cases, surgical reconstruction may be indicated. Operative procedures for chronic hip disease include arthrodesis, total hip replacement with an artificial joint, and bone grafting. **Arthrodesis**, which is also known as *artificial ankylosis*, is the surgical fixation of a joint through a procedure that causes the joint surfaces to fuse by promoting the proliferation of bone cells. Arthrodesis is sometimes used to treat young patients who have disease in only one hip, although even in this situation, total hip replacements are being utilized more frequently. Some of the disadvantages of total hip replacement include problems, such as infection at the site of the incision, phlebitis, and pulmonary embolism, that are associated with any type of surgery. Problems that are specific to joint replacement surgery include the possibility of the dislocation or loosening of the artificial joint and the deterioration of the artificial joint resulting from normal use. After artificial joints have been in place ten years, mechanical failure of the device is a significant problem. Bone grafting is infrequently used, but can be employed to treat nonunion of fractures of the hip.

The Knee

Each knee is a hinge joint controlled by the quadriceps muscle, which lies on the front of the thigh, and four ligaments: the medial and lateral collateral ligaments, the anterior cruciate, and the posterior cruciate. The **anterior cruciate** lies on the front of the knee joint and the **posterior cruciate** lies behind the knee joint. Each knee also has two menisci. A **meniscus** is a crescent-shaped fibrocartilage disk that is located in a joint. The **medial meniscus** lies in the middle line of the knee, and the **lateral meniscus** lies on the side of the knee joint. The knee is the most frequently injured joint, and many knee injuries result from the person's participation in contact sports. Furthermore, of all joints in the body, the knee is the most likely to show primary degenerative arthritis or osteoarthritis. Injuries of the knee region include fracture of the kneecap, distal femur, proximal tibia, and proximal fibula; dislocation of the kneecap and knee joint; tears of the tendons and kneecap ligaments; and a variety of internal disorders. Some common internal disorders of the knee include the accumulation of blood, fluid, or pus and chips of bone or cartilage in the joint space; arthritis; infection; and injury to a meniscus.

The diagnosis of knee disorders can be difficult, but typically begins with a physical examination that tests for stability and internal derangement of the ligaments and/or cartilage. The physical examination is supplemented by x-ray and/or MRI examination and arthroscopic diagnostic study. Arthroscopy has become a primary therapeutic method and has resulted in marked advances in the ability to reconstruct and/or compensate for internal structural derangements. Arthroscopy has also reduced the length of a patient's postoperative impairment. Other diagnostic measures include arthrocentesis and arthrograms. **Arthrocentesis** is the needle puncture of a joint for the removal of joint fluid. Arthrocentesis relieves joint pain caused by the presence of fluid that distends the joint capsule. In many cases, analysis of the joint fluid will assist in the establishment of a diagnosis. The knee is the joint in which arthrocentesis is performed most commonly. An **arthrogram** is an x-ray of a joint taken after a dye has been injected into the joint. The dye outlines the joint space and helps to distinguish joint pathology. An **arthrotomy** is a procedure in which a surgeon makes an incision through the patient's skin and into the joint for direct visualization and manipulation of the structure. Arthrotomy is now performed only when arthroscopy is not feasible. Total knee replacement with an artificial joint is another available therapy, but thus far it is not as widely used nor as well-established as hip replacement surgery.

Disorders of the Back and Neck

Chronic back pain is an exceedingly common problem. Most episodes of chronic back pain are related to localized regional mechanical problems that subside with or without therapy, usually within two months. The medical community recognizes at least 60 relatively common causes of back pain, some of which are categorized in Figure 13–11.

Successful treatment for many of these back problems remains elusive, because precise diagnosis is often difficult to obtain. Even in the presence of anatomic evidence of a back disorder by x-ray

Figure 13–11.
Classification of Back and Neck Disorders.

Category of Disorder	Examples of Disorder
Rheumatologic	Rheumatoid arthritis, ankylosing spondylitis, psoriatic arthritis, Reiter's syndrome
Mechanical	Back strain/sprain, herniated intervertebral disk, cervical rib, osteoarthritis, spondylolisthesis/spondylolysis, scoliosis
Metabolic-endocrine	Osteoporosis, osteomalacia, parathyroid disease, pituitary disease
Infectious	Osteomyelitis, intervertebral disk space infection, tuberculosis
Benign tumors	Osteoid osteoma, giant cell tumor, osteochondroma
Primary malignancies	Multiple myeloma, chondrosarcoma
Metastatic malignancies	Breast, prostate, kidney, rectum, thyroid cancers

examination, some patients are symptom-free. On the other hand, some patients complain of considerable pain and disability, even though only minimal objective evidence of back disease can be found. Much chronic back pain can be attributed to bone and joint diseases that were previously discussed in this chapter, and so the remainder of this section will discuss other disorders of the back and neck that have not yet been addressed.

Ruptured Disk

The rupture of an intervertebral disk involves an abnormality in the disk's fibrous outer ring, the anulus fibrosus, allowing the extrusion of the soft central portion of the disk, the nucleus pulposus, which then compresses the spinal cord and spinal nerves, causing pain. This protrusion of the nucleus pulposus is called a ***herniation of an intervertebral disk***. A disk may rupture and herniate following a tear resulting from injury or from the spontaneous degeneration associated with age. The most common location for rupture and herniation of a disk is the lumbar area of the back. Patients who have disk injuries often say that "something gave way" in their backs during exercise or exertion. This injury will produce back pain and stiffness. If the herniation is in the lumbar area, it will produce pressure on the sciatic nerve roots, and pain called ***sciatica*** will radiate down the back of the patient's leg on the affected side beyond the knee. Pain from a disk is aggravated by exercise and relieved by rest. Coughing or sneezing usually accentuates the pain.

The physician first suspects a rupture of an intervertebral disk has occurred upon the patient's complaints of characteristic symptoms, and x-ray evidence confirms the diagnosis. Myelography, which was defined in Chapter 3, is performed by injecting an oily, radiopaque dye into the patient's spinal canal, and then making an x-ray study of the movement of the dye through the canal. The dye travels freely up the spinal canal until it meets an area of constriction or obstruction. A protruding disk distorts or blocks the flow of dye, and the x-ray identifies the exact location of the lesion. Many physicians now consider MRI to be as effective as myelography in diagnosing a ruptured disk and prefer MRI because it is noninvasive. Another objective measure of sciatic nerve involvement is an ***electromyography (EMG),*** which utilizes the natural electrical properties of skeletal muscle by recording the electrical activity evoked in a muscle by the electrical stimulation of its nerve.

Treatment consisting of bed rest alone, or in combination with traction or a corrective cast, is helpful in relieving the symptoms of most patients who have a ruptured disk. Natural healing frequently occurs as the extruding disk shrinks. Surgery is indicated when severe sciatic pain is not relieved by normal therapy or occurs on a frequent, recurrent basis causing repeated periods of impairment. Surgery is also performed to prevent neurologic damage from the compression of the spinal cord or spinal nerve. The surgeon exposes the herniated disk by removing part of the bony vertebral arch, which is called the ***lamina***, in an operation known as a ***laminectomy***. The surgeon then removes the nucleus pulposus, and in some cases, performs a bone graft to create a bridge over the involved area in order to give greater support to the spinal column. Bone for this spinal fusion graft usually is obtained from the ilium. However, five years or more after surgery, the functional and symptomatic status of a patient who has undergone an operation is statistically no different than the comparable status of the patient who has not undergone surgery.

Peripheral Nerve Compression

One condition in which an individual may experience peripheral nerve compression is called cervical rib syndrome. A ***cervical rib*** is an extra rib resulting from a congenital overdevelopment of the seventh cervical vertebra. This condition, which is rare, may be unilateral or bilateral. A cervical rib usually causes no symptoms, but, if the extra rib impinges on blood vessels and nerves that serve the upper arm, it may cause numbness, tingling, and weakness of the hand and fingers. These symptoms are more pronounced when the individual's arm is raised. However, numbness, tingling, and weakness of the hand and fingers occasionally occur in the absence of x-ray evidence of a bone abnormality. If the symptoms are confined to the hand, two conditions are suspect: (1) a tight muscle in the neck, which creates pressure on the nerves that serve the arm, or (2) a constriction of the median nerve as it passes through the wrist, creating carpal tunnel syndrome. These conditions are fully correctable by surgical procedures that relieve the pressure on the affected nerve.

Spondylolisthesis

Spondylolisthesis is a displacement of a vertebral body over the vertebra below it. The displacement usually is forward and occurs most frequently in the lumbar area. Spondylolisthesis may be symptomless or may produce chronic backache, with or without sciatica. However, severe symptoms occur infrequently. The displacement associated with this condition may arise from a congenital or acquired defect and is measured in degree of slippage as determined by x-ray. Spondylolisthesis is a common cause of back pain in patients younger than 25, but is rarely the sole cause of back pain in patients older than 40. Treatment for this condition varies, depending on the degree of the patient's vertebral displacement. In some cases, rest, analgesics, exercise, and/or a back brace are sufficient to correct the problem, but in other cases, surgery is necessary.

Tuberculosis of the Spine

Tuberculosis of the spine, which is also known as *tuberculous spondylitis* or *Pott's disease*, is a chronic destructive lesion of one or more vertebrae and is secondary to tuberculosis elsewhere in the body. Collapse of the affected vertebrae may produce abnormal curvature and compression of the spinal cord. Other bones, especially the hips, knees, and hands, may be attacked by the tubercle bacillus. Symptoms depend on the particular bone involved. In addition to requiring treatment for the pulmonary symptoms of tuberculosis, patients who have spinal tuberculosis may require prolonged immobilization or spinal fusion. Chemotherapy is the mainstay treatment for the underlying tuberculosis.

Spinal Curvature

Curvature of the spine is a common disorder. Many mild degrees of spinal curvature produce no symptoms or functional impairment and either are discovered accidentally by x-rays taken for some other purpose or are noticed during a physical examination. Three types of spinal curvature are scoliosis, lordosis, and kyphosis.

Scoliosis, which is the most common of the three types, is defined as one or more lateral curvatures of the spine. The abnormal spinal curve may occur on only one side of the midline, or it may occur on both sides. The deformity may be a permanent, structural anatomic change, or it may be a temporary alteration produced by reflex spasm of the muscles around the spine. Females, particularly adolescent girls, are more commonly affected than are males. Usually, the younger the child when the structural abnormality develops, the more serious the prognosis. Scoliosis may also occur on a congenital basis because of defects in vertebral formation. In addition, genetic problems may cause scoliosis. Scoliosis may also develop after trauma and certain diseases, such as poliomyelitis, rheumatoid arthritis, cerebral palsy, muscular dystrophy, neurofibromatosis, and tuberculosis of the spine. The most common structural form of scoliosis is idiopathic and begins in childhood or adolescence.

Walking may be a problem for individuals who have severe scoliosis, and certain activities may be performed awkwardly. Abnormal stress may be placed on certain muscle groups and bones because of a shift in the individual's center of gravity. Scoliosis patients may experience injuries because they lack agility and flexibility. The most serious sequela of scoliosis is decreased room for lung expansion, resulting from a narrowing of the chest cavity. Severe deformities that interfere with full respiratory motion predisposes scoliosis patients to frequent episodes of pneumonia. Narrowing of the chest cavity can also interfere with the ability of the heart to function. Mild cases of scoliosis cause no problems and require no treatment. Early recognition and prompt treatment of severe cases of this condition have lessened the incidence of the many severe deformities that were formerly associated with scoliosis and have greatly improved the prognosis. Treatment typically involves the use of a well-fitting brace or cast, and, for severe cases, surgery may be necessary.

Lordosis is a condition characterized by excessive forward convexity in the lumbar and cervical region of the spine. *Kyphosis*, or a hunchback, is an excessive posterior curvature of the cervical and thoracic sections of the spinal column. Lordosis and kyphosis are caused by many of the same conditions that cause scoliosis. In addition, a senile type of kyphosis affects the elderly, usually reflecting bone loss through osteoporosis, which is discussed later in this chapter. Severe lordosis and kyphosis cause orthopedic and medical problems similar to those caused by scoliosis. In particular, marked kyphosis causes a significant loss of lung capacity.

Low Back Strain and Sprain

Low back strains are an ill-defined group of disorders that are characterized by a persistent backache that is believed to arise from stresses on the muscles and ligaments that surround and support the vertebral column. Strains of this nature, which comprise the largest category of back pain problems seen in clinical practice, occur when vertebral muscles fail to protect the deep ligaments that maintain posture. Strain in the sacroiliac and lumbosacral areas occurs more often in women than in men. Typically, twisting the trunk, stooping, or bending aggravates the pain associated with these back problems. Most strains and sprains recover completely with rest, but some patients also require a surgical corset. Physiotherapy is generally prescribed to strengthen the patient's back muscles. Nevertheless, some patients experience backaches for many years despite treatment, although the pain they experience is usually a nagging discomfort rather than a serious handicap.

Torticollis

Torticollis, or wryneck, is caused by a spasm or contraction of the neck muscles that results in a rotation of the neck and an unnatural position of the head. A common form of wryneck is *infantile torticollis*, a condition which results from an injury during birth to the muscles on one side of the infant's neck. Other forms of torticollis include myogenic torticollis and psychogenic torticollis. *Myogenic torticollis* is transient and results from a muscle spasm caused by localized inflammation of a neck muscle. Torticollis may also arise from structural deformities, inflammatory lesions, or arthritis of the cervical spine. The treatment of the torticollis depends on treating the underlying cause of the disorder.

Whiplash

The term *whiplash* describes a heterogeneous collection of pathological conditions of the neck, typically an acute sprain or strain, involving the muscles and ligaments of the cervical spine. In fact, the simple musculoligamentous neck sprain/strain is the most common of all neck injuries. This type of injury is characterized by neck pain and limitation of movement of the neck and back and usually results when a patient is in a car that is hit from behind. Results of physical and x-ray examination usually are normal, except for a certain degree of lordosis resulting from spasm of the muscles around the cervical spine. The duration of the symptoms depends on the severity of the injury, emotional factors, and, in a few patients, the status of litigation proceedings related to the injury. Treatment for whiplash typically consists of a neck brace to immobilize the damaged muscles and ligaments, physical therapy to return the muscles and ligaments to proper functioning, and, in some cases, drug therapy.

Metabolic Bone Disease

The main types of metabolic bone disease are characterized by osteopenia. *Osteopenia* is a metabolic disease that is associated with a decrease in the patient's bone mass. A variety of diseases, including parathyroid gland dysfunction, nutritional deficiencies, estrogen deficiency, and liver, gastrointestinal, or renal disease, present as osteopenia. Two forms of osteopenia are osteomalacia and osteoporosis.

Osteomalacia is the abnormal mineralization of bone and cartilage in adults, whose bones have, for the most part, stopped growing. *Rickets* is the abnormal mineralization of bone and cartilage in children, whose bones are still growing. Rickets usually results from vitamin D deficiency. In either disorder, the bone is softened, making it subject to deformities in growth and fracture. Prompt recognition of the bone problem and appropriate treatment of the underlying cause can forestall or minimize the bone abnormality.

Osteoporosis is an absolute decrease in bone mass and is a major health problem. The causes of osteoporosis are many and varied and may include endocrine, gastrointestinal, bone marrow, and connective tissue disorders. The most common type of osteoporosis is post-menopausal osteoporosis, which usually occurs in females 15 to 20 years after menopause, although both sexes may show age-related decrease in bone mass at age 70 or older. Postmenopausal osteoporosis frequently manifests as fractures of the wrist and vertebrae, and general age-related osteoporosis often leads to hip and vertebral fractures. The fractures occur either spontaneously in the weight-bearing bones or in any bone after minor trauma. Even without fractures, vertebral changes in the thoracic region of the spine commonly lead to a kyphosis, or the "dorsal hump" of the post-menopausal female. The treatment of osteoporosis relates to the underlying cause. Calcium and bone-promoting agents, such as estrogen, fluoride, vitamin D, and *calcitonin*, which is a hormone secreted by cells within the thyroid gland, have all been used with limited success in treating patients who have post-menopausal osteoporosis. To be of greatest benefit, these agents must be administered to the patient before the patient has lost much bone density, because they retard the rate of bone loss but do not increase bone density. The most common cause of secondary osteoporosis is the use of corticosteroids. The most effective means of preventing this type of osteoporosis are simply reducing the prescribed dosage of the drug, limiting the duration of the drug therapy, or using alternate-day dosage of the corticosteroid.

Osteomyelitis is a pus-producing infection of bone, usually resulting from staphylococcus or streptococcus bacteria. This disease may exist in either an acute or a chronic form. The acute process may occur in the course of a bacterial invasion of the bloodstream that develops either from infection elsewhere in the body or from organisms that reach the bone directly through open fractures, wounds, and orthopedic procedures. The infection, which usually affects only one bone, causes a fever and results in tenderness over the involved tissue. Satisfactory treatment of acute osteomyelitis depends upon an accurate bacteriologic diagnosis and prompt, specific antibiotic therapy. Surgical drainage of pus may also be necessary. Antibiotics control many osteomyelitis infections. Several serious complications can result from inadequate or delayed treatment of an acute attack of osteomyelitis. Pus, as it develops, tends to spread to other parts of the involved bone, surrounding soft tissues, and the skin. This spreading infection results in extensive death of bone and other tissues. Extension of the infection to a neighboring joint produces an arthritis. Occasionally, infected bone will serve as a focus for the spread of microorganisms through the bloodstream to distant organs.

Chronic osteomyelitis develops as a sequel to the acute process. The chronic form may cause few symptoms as it smolders for many years, with intermittent drainage of pus from a deep-seated infection around dead bone tissue. From time to time, the lesion may appear to heal, only to increase in activity with external drainage later on. Frequently, chronic osteomyelitis manifests some or all of the complications of the acute form of the disease. Chronic osteomyelitis may become progressive, resulting in continuing bone loss and eventually debilitation. It may also be associated with the accumulation of abnormal complex proteins known as *amyloids*. *Amyloidosis* is a condition in which amyloids infiltrate multiple organs such as the liver, the heart, the stomach, and the kidney. When the disease process is advanced, the amyloids surround and destroy the organs' cells, injuring the affected organs. Frequently, amyloidosis is fatal.

Tumors

Although most tumors that arise from the various connective tissues remain noncancerous, benign tumors have some medical signifi-cance because they can destroy bone tissue, thus leading to frac-tures. Furthermore, some benign tumors undergo malignant change. The physician diagnoses bone lesions by x-ray, aided by knowing the patient's age, the duration of the patient's symptoms, the number of bones involved, and the location of the tumor within the bone. For example, multiple bone tumors usually are benign in children and malignant in adults.

Three of the many primary bone cancers are (1) osteogenic sarcoma, (2) Ewing's tumor, and (3) multiple myeloma. **Osteogenic sarcoma**, which is also known as *osteosarcoma,* is a malignant primary tumor of the bone that consists of cancerous connective tissue. **Ewing's tumor** is a malignant tumor of the bone that always arises in bone marrow. **Multiple myeloma**, which is a malignant tumor made of plasma cells, usually arises in the bone marrow. Multiple myeloma is the most common primary bone tumor, and osteosarcoma is the second most common. However, most bone tumors in adults are metastatic, not primary. In males, most meta-static bone tumors arise from prostate and lung malignancies, and in females, metastatic bone tumors arise from breast and lung cancers. Other common origins of metastatic bone tumors are thyroid, renal, and gastrointestinal cancers. Figure 13–12 provides a list of benign and malignant tumors of bone and other connective tissues.

Noninvasive investigative techniques, such as radionuclide and CT scanning, can be used to diagnose bone tumors. Bone scans are usually positive long before changes on x-ray are visible. Biopsy of the tumor typically establishes a specific diagnosis. Small, benign tumors producing no symptoms often are not removed unless for cosmetic reasons. However, a benign tumor that causes symptoms or interferes with function will usually be surgically removed. Bone grafts and joint replacement using artificial joints are two common types of bone surgery. Furthermore, improvements in bone "bank-ing" have made transplantation feasible. Because primary bone cancers metastasize quickly and widely, early recognition of the lesion and, often, prompt radical surgery, including amputation, are necessary. Even with the use of chemotherapy and radiation, the

Figure 13–12.
Classification of Connective Tissue Tumors.

Tissue of Origin	Benign	Malignant
Fibrous tissue	Fibroma	Fibrosarcoma
Cartilage	Chondroma	Chondrosarcoma
Bone	Osteoma	Osteogenic sarcoma
Blood cell-producing tissue	(None)	Multiple myeloma, reticulum cell sarcoma, leukemia, lymphoma
Unknown origin	Giant cell tumor	Malignant giant cell tumor, Ewing's sarcoma

five-year survival rate from bone malignancies remains low. The prognosis for osteosarcoma and Ewing's tumor patients is particularly poor because of the high rate of distant metastases these tumors produce. Treatment of one of these tumors depends upon the nature of the growth, its location, and its manifestations.

The Nervous System

The nervous system is the group of organs and structures that work with the endocrine system (1) to keep the body in communication with both its own organs and tissues and the external environment and (2) to produce, control, and coordinate appropriate responses to internal and external conditions. This chapter first will discuss the components of the human nervous system. It then will address many disorders that affect the nervous system and will present several procedures used to diagnose nervous system disorders.

ANATOMY AND PHYSIOLOGY

The human **nervous system** consists of the central nervous system and the peripheral nervous system. The **central nervous system (CNS)** is highly developed and specialized and includes the brain and the spinal cord. The **peripheral nervous system** includes the cranial and spinal nerves and the **autonomic nervous system**, which regulates the activities of cardiac muscle, smooth muscle, and glands. The CNS is the control center of the body. The peripheral nerves carry nerve impulses, which are messages, to the brain and spinal cord from the various muscles and organs of the body. In response to these messages, the brain and spinal cord send controlling impulses to the tissues and organs of the body.

This section will discuss the components of the nervous system, including the brain, the meninges and the cerebrospinal fluid, the spinal cord, and the components of the peripheral nervous system.

The Brain

The **brain** is the organ of the CNS that is contained within the **cranium**, which is the skull, and rests upon the floor of the cranial cavity. The brain contains four hollow chambers that are called **ventricles of the brain**. The brain is divided into several sections, including the cerebrum, the cerebellum, and three smaller structures called the midbrain, the pons, and the medulla.

Cerebrum

The **cerebrum** is the upper part of the brain and is the largest part of the human CNS. The **cerebral cortex**, which is the surface of the cerebrum, is arranged in a large number of folds called **convolutions** or *gyri*. The cerebrum is divided into two cerebral hemispheres. The hemispheres are further subdivided into four main lobes. The **frontal lobe** lies at the forward part of the cerebrum and is the origin for most voluntary motor activity. In addition, a large part of the frontal lobe governs an individual's personality, judgment, and social adaptation. A smaller area of this lobe functions as the speech control center. The **parietal lobe** lies at the top and on the side of the cerebrum and is the area of the brain that receives, interprets, correlates, and stores most sensations, such as temperature, pressure, position, and pain. Control over hearing, smell, and understanding speech occurs in the **temporal lobe**, which sits near the bottom and to the side of the cerebral hemisphere. The **occipital lobe**, which sits at the back of the cerebrum, controls visual sensations. In addition, the cerebral cortex consists of other areas that are concerned with memory, learning, emotional reactions, and judgment.

Cerebellum

The **cerebellum** is the second largest division of the brain, and it lies beneath the cerebral hemispheres in the back of the cranial cavity. The cerebellum coordinates movement of muscles, especially to maintain posture, and provides muscle contractions to control equilibrium.

Midbrain, Pons, and Medulla

The midbrain, pons, and medulla are located in front of the cerebellum and beneath the cerebral hemispheres. The *midbrain* contains the nuclei of important cranial nerves and assists in the regulation of posture and equilibrium. The *pons* contains the nuclei of other important cranial nerves and provides a pathway for nerve impulses. The pons is located beneath the midbrain. The *medulla* is an extension of the spinal cord and contains the nuclei of the cranial nerves that are not in the midbrain or pons. The medulla, which is located below the pons, also contains nerve centers for regulating heartbeat and respiration rate.

The Spinal Cord

The spinal column, which was defined and described in Chapter 13, *The Musculoskeletal System*, contains the *spinal cord*, which is a cylindrical mass of nerve tissue that occupies the vertebral canal. The spinal cord extends from the medulla to the level of the first or second lumbar vertebra and is the main cable for nerve-impulse transmission, which is vital to all types of sensation and movement. Ascending nerve tracts conduct impulses up the spinal cord to the brain, and descending tracts conduct impulses from the brain to the lower end of the spinal cord. The tracts have specialized functions— some conduct impulses for temperature or pain, others conduct impulses for touch, and still others conduct impulses for sense of balance or muscle tone. Anesthesiologists can use the nerve-impulse transmission properties of the spinal cord to inhibit the conduction of pain stimuli to the brain.

The Meninges and the Cerebrospinal Fluid

The brain and spinal cord are protected by three membranes, which are collectively called the *meninges*. The three meninges are (1) the dura, (2) the arachnoid, and (3) the pia. The *dura*, which is the outermost of the membranes, is thick and tough. Nerve impluse inhibition that takes place in the area outside the dura is called *epidural anesthesia*. The *arachnoid*, which lies beneath the dura, is very delicate. The arachnoid and dura are separated from each other by a tiny space that is called the *subdural space*. The *pia*, which is the innermost membrane, consists of elastic and collagenous fibers. (Figure 14–1 provides side views of the brain and the meninges.) Separating the arachnoid and the pia is a tiny space that is called the *subarachnoid space*. The subarachnoid space contains

Figure 14–1.
Side Views of the Brain and Meninges.

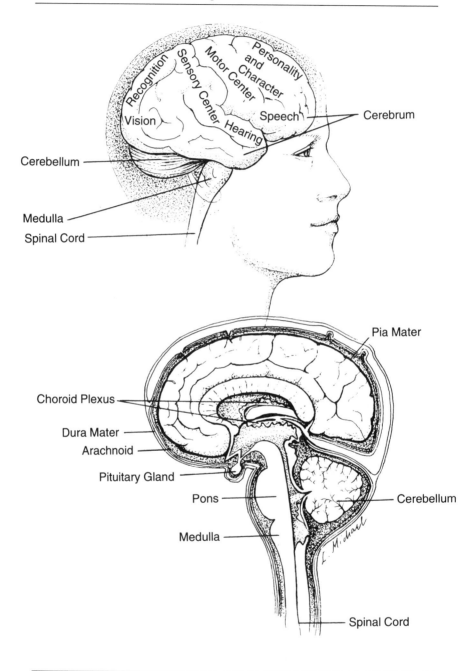

cerebrospinal fluid. *Cerebrospinal fluid* is a clear, watery liquid that is produced in the ventricles of the brain and the meninges. It cushions the brain and spinal cord against mechanical jolts and sudden changes in pressure.

The Peripheral Nervous System

The peripheral nervous system consists of the nerves outside the brain and spinal cord. Its function is to conduct nerve impulses between the CNS and the body. The peripheral nervous system includes the cranial nerves, the spinal nerves, and the autonomic nervous system.

The Cranial Nerves

The *cranial nerves* are the twelve pairs of nerves that originate in nuclei found in the brain. Each nerve is designated by a roman numeral in addition to a specific name, and each has a specific function. For example, the *olfactory nerve*, I, is responsible for transmitting nerve impulses related to the sense of smell, and the *optic nerve*, II, is responsible for transmitting nerve impulses related to the sense of sight. The *acoustic nerve*, VIII, is responsible for transmitting nerve impulses related to the sense of balance and hearing. The *vagus nerve*, X, which is the largest of the cranial nerves, transmits nerve impulses arising from the pharynx, larynx, trachea, bronchi, lungs, aorta, stomach, and other internal organs. The vagus assists in the act of swallowing and helps to control the actions of the internal organs. It transmits sensations of hunger and pain from these organs and is involved with respiratory reflexes. The Appendix contains a complete list of the cranial nerves.

The Spinal Nerves

The spinal nerves are arranged in 31 pairs and are named for the area of the spinal cord from which they arise. One nerve from each pair lies on one side of the spinal cord, and the other nerve from each pair lies on the other side of the cord. The spinal nerves and their branches travel to the skin and muscles of the entire body except for the part of the head that is served by the cranial nerves. The spinal nerves consist of eight pairs of cervical nerves, twelve pairs of thoracic nerves, five pairs of lumbar nerves, five pairs of sacral nerves, and one pair of coccygeal nerves. In the thoracic region of the spine, these nerves run independently of each other, but in other areas they unite to form networks that are called cervical, brachial, lumbar, sacral, and coccygeal plexuses, respectively. The *sciatic nerve* arises from the lumbo-sacral plexus and is the largest nerve in the body, serving nearly all of the skin of the leg, the muscles of the back of the thigh, and the muscles of the leg and foot. Figure 14–2 provides a side view of the sciatic nerve.

The Autonomic Nervous System

The autonomic nervous system serves the vital organ systems, such as the digestive, cardiac, circulatory, respiratory, urinary, reproductive, and endocrine systems, and functions independently of conscious control. The main nerve complexes in this system are two cords, called the *sympathetic trunks*, that extend vertically through the neck, thorax, and abdomen, one trunk on either side of the vertebral column. Loose networks of nerves extend from the sympathetic trunks. The autonomic nervous system also prepares an individual for "fight or flight." Working in conjunction with the adrenal gland in response to stress, this system causes a rapid heart rate, an increase in blood pressure, increase in cardiac output, dilated pupils, dry mouth, and dilation of the blood vessels to the skeletal muscles.

Blood Supply to the Brain and Spinal Cord

The principal blood vessels that carry blood to the head are called the common carotid arteries. Each common carotid divides into two branches: the internal carotid artery, which supplies the front of the brain, the eye, and parts of the forehead and nose, and the external carotid artery, which is the major source of blood for the head, face, and the greater part of the neck. The vertebral arteries arise from the subclavian blood vessels, and supply blood to the back of the brain. The arterial blood supply to the spinal cord is furnished by branches of the vertebral, intercostal, and lumbar arteries. Blood travels away from the brain primarily through the internal jugular vein, and, to a lesser extent, through the vertebral vein.

Transmission of Sensory and Motor Stimuli

Afferent nerves convey sensations from peripheral nerve endings over afferent pathways, which are also called sensory pathways, to the brain and spinal cord. A peripheral nerve ending is a highly

Figure 14–2.
A Side View of the Sciatic Nerve.

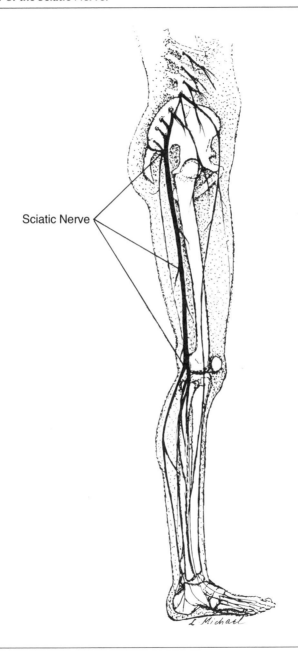

Sciatic Nerve

specialized receptor for a specific stimulus—a nerve ending that receives pain does not receive touch, temperature, or other sensation. The specific sensation is carried over separate nerve fibers, either directly to the brain through sensory cranial nerves or to the brain through specific sensory tracts in the spinal cord. When the brain receives afferent nerve sensations, it interprets the sensations and, often, transmits impulses to efferent nerves. **Efferent nerves** convey impulses from the CNS over efferent pathways, which are also called motor pathways, to the peripheral nervous system. In turn, the cranial and spinal nerves stimulate skeletal muscles, other smooth and striated muscles, glands, and the internal organs of the thorax and abdomen. In this fashion, a sensation can be translated into activity. For example, assume that an individual hears a noise. The individual's external ear picks up the soundwaves generated by the noisy event and transmits the soundwaves through the ossicles of the middle ear to the cochlear division of the eighth cranial nerve. Eventually, the sound impulses reach the auditory cortex of the temporal lobe of the brain, which interprets the impulses. From the auditory cortex, central connecting nerve pathways communicate with other parts of the brain, including the principal motor area in the frontal lobe. In response to the impulse that it receives, the motor area releases motor impulses that travel on efferent pathways to muscles of the skeleton and eyes, other muscles, and glands. The individual's muscles react to the motor impulses, causing the individual to turn to investigate the source of the noise and preparing the individual to take appropriate action. Figure 14–3 illustrates the transmission of motor and sensory stimuli in the body.

However, not all sensory stimuli result in impulses that reach the brain or higher centers. Certain reflex activities, such as the withdrawal of the hand following a painful pinprick to the fingertip, are controlled solely by the spinal cord and the spinal nerves. These reflex activities are controlled by reflex arcs that have several essential parts, including

- a receptor or nerve ending that receives the stimulus and initiates the impulse
- a sensory nerve pathway that carries the sensory information to the spinal cord
- a connecting pathway within the spinal cord that relays the impulse to a motor nerve
- a motor nerve pathway that carries the motor response to the end organ
- a muscle or other end organ that carries out an action

Figure 14–3.
The Transmission of Motor and Sensory Stimuli.

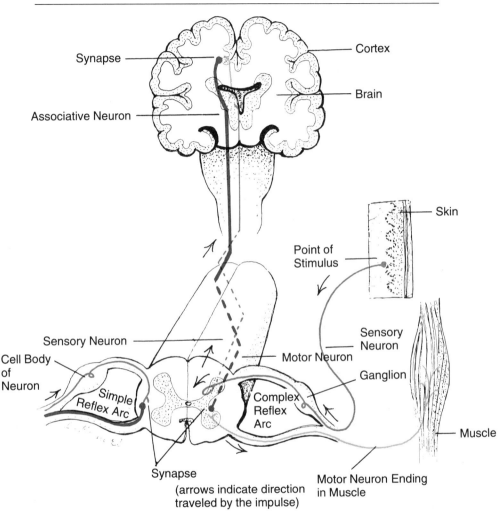

DISORDERS OF THE NERVOUS SYSTEM

Clinical manifestations of nervous system disease depend on the nature of the disorder and its location in the nervous system. Common symptoms and signs of nervous system disorders include headache, defective vision or hearing, abnormal temperature, touch, and pain sensations, abnormal reflexes, paralysis, convulsions, and unconsciousness. These symptoms are nonspecific. The causes of the symptoms are determined from the results of appropriate neurologic examinations. The list of conditions in which headache is a prominent symptom is almost endless, and so headache will be discussed in its own subsection. Then, the remainder of this section will discuss some specific disorders of the nervous system, including trauma, epilepsy, vascular diseases, disorders of the peripheral nerves, infections, hereditary and congenital disorders, diseases of muscle and the neuromuscular junction, tumors, and idiopathic diseases.

Headache

Headache can be a manifestation of serious disease, but usually results from benign, although possibly recurrent, causes. A *vascular headache* results from the distention and dilation of intracranial arteries. The major examples of vascular headaches are migraine and cluster headaches.

A *migraine headache* is a relatively common, intense, paroxysmal, recurrent, vascular type of headache that is often associated with irritability, nausea, and vomiting. The cause of migraines is unknown, although stress, bright sunshine, certain foods, and the administration of nitroglycerine and birth control pills may trigger migraine attacks. The frequency of migraine headaches varies from one or two attacks each year to several times weekly, often increasing during periods of emotional stress. The duration and severity of the headaches are variable. Severe, throbbing attacks may last 6 to 18 hours. Many attacks of migraine headaches are preceded by warning symptoms, such as dizziness, visual sensations, and double vision. Warning symptoms that precede a migraine are called an *aura*. At the height of a migraine attack, the patient may experience nausea and vomiting. Between migraine attacks, the patient typically remains in good health. Migraine headaches are more common in women than in men and in patients who have a family history of migraines than in patients who have no family migraine history. Migraine is a benign condition, which, with very rare exceptions, does not affect the patient's longevity. On rare occasions, a migraine can cause a stroke. Individual episodes may respond to medications that contain ergot, such as Cafergot, or to other pain medications such as aspirin, NSAIDs, or codeine. In addition, some individuals take daily doses of beta-blockers or calcium channel-blockers as preventive therapy. Drug treatment of migraines is typically very successful.

Cluster headaches are vascular headaches that are characterized by severe pain of a short duration, located behind or near one eye. Cluster headaches are generally not preceded by an aura. These headaches typically occur more often in the spring and fall and affect males more often than females. Treatment of a cluster headache often involves some of the medications that are used to treat migraine headaches. Sometimes a short course of prednisone is very effective. Lithium or antidepressants may be used to prevent cluster headache attacks.

Tension headaches, unlike vascular headaches, arise from persistent contractions of the muscles of the head and neck. Tension headaches affect 80 percent of the population at one time or another and affect adult females more than any other population group. Tension headache patients generally describe their discomfort as a steady tightness, often located in the forehead, temples, or back of the head or neck. Analgesics, such as aspirin, acetaminophen, or ibuprofen may effectively treat tension headaches, but some patients need treatment with anti-depressant medications. In addition, headaches may result from pressure on pain-sensitive structures of the head or from distention and inflammation of these structures.

More than one headache mechanism may be responsible for a patient's head pain. Furthermore, although headaches usually result from fairly harmless conditions, persistent headaches can be a manifestation of organic disease. Brain tumors can cause any type of headache. Other illnesses may precipitate headaches resembling typical tension or vascular headaches. Headache arising from disorders of the nervous system is discussed in the context of each of those disorders.

Trauma to the Cranium, Brain, and Spinal Cord

Trauma to the cranium and brain is frequently classified on the basis of the type of skull injury involved. A *closed head injury* is one in which the patient's skull has not received injury or at most has incurred a simple, nondisplaced, linear fracture without scalp laceration. *Open head injuries* involve injury to the skull and include scalp lacerations and linear or depressed fractures of the skull. In a depressed fracture, a fragment of bone is displaced below the level of the skull, pressing upon and injuring the brain, and requiring surgical correction. However, the medical significance of head trauma is related to the nature and severity of brain damage and not to the presence or absence of a fractured skull.

Loss of consciousness with injury to the brain may be brief—from seconds to minutes—or prolonged—from hours to days. Mild injury may produce a *concussion*, which is a brief loss of consciousness without permanent neurologic changes. Moderate injury may produce cerebral swelling and a longer period of unconsciousness. *Cerebral contusion*, which is a bruise of the brain, or laceration may follow severe injury. Both conditions are associated with prolonged unconsciousness and abnormal neurologic signs.

Hemorrhage is a common complication of severe head injury. The bleeding can occur into the subarachnoid space, into the subdural space, into the tissues outside the dura, or into the substance of the brain itself. Bleeding into the subdural space causes a *subdural hematoma*, which is a localized collection of clotted blood lying underneath the dura, usually requiring surgical treatment. Bleeding into the tissues outside the dura may cause an *epidural hematoma*, which is a localized collection of clotted blood around and above the dura and can be fatal if not treated promptly. Other complications of head injury include cranial nerve paralysis, seizures, and post-concussion syndrome. *Post-concussion syndrome* is characterized by amnesia, headache, and nausea for the period immediately following a head injury and for a short period following the patient's recovery of consciousness. Headache, dizziness, easy fatigability, and personality changes may also occur in association with post-concussion syndrome. This syndrome may remain for months after the head injury, or it may be a permanent clinical feature. Atrophy of the brain substance or other organic change in the brain may also occur in association with post-concussion syndrome. Patients may suffer permanent impairment of memory, thought, concentration, or certain sensory or motor functions.

Trauma to the vertebral column is significant because of possible damage to the spinal cord, and spinal cord injuries often produce more permanent impairment than head injuries produce. Injury to the spinal cord results when it is compressed from a fracture-dislocation of a vertebra or damage to the blood supply of the cord. The patient may lose motor and sensory function below the level of the spinal cord injury. If the injury is severe, the loss of function may be complete and permanent. If the spinal cord is injured in the cervical area, paralysis of all upper and lower extremities, which is called *quadriplegia*, may result. Paralysis of the lower extremities only, which is called *paraplegia*, results from injuries that occur at lower levels of the spinal cord. Spinal cord injuries may cause the patient to lose bladder and rectum control, possibly leading to urinary tract infections and obstructions that may be fatal.

Epilepsy

Epilepsy is any one of a group of neurologic disorders resulting from abnormal electrical activity of the patient's brain. This abnormal electrical activity leads to recurrent alterations in the patient's neurologic function. Each episode of neurologic dysfunction is called a *seizure*, and an episode of neurologic dysfunction that involves the patient's motor activity is called a *convulsion*. Epilepsies can be classified in several ways. Epilepsy can be classified as being either acquired or idiopathic. Many causes of acquired epilepsy are listed in Figure 14–4.

Epilepsy is idiopathic if the patient does not exhibit evidence of an organic brain lesion. Because most adults who experience seizures do not exhibit evidence of a brain lesion, "epilepsy" usually refers to idiopathic epilepsy. Idiopathic epilepsy tends to run in families and typically first appears in patients who are between the ages of three and fifteen. Physical stimuli, such as light and sound, may precipitate a seizure in an individual who has idiopathic epilepsy. Alcohol consumption, emotional tension, and lack of sleep may also produce seizures in susceptible individuals. Alterations in the electrical activity of a patient's brain may be detected during an epileptic attack. In addition, epileptics often have abnormal electrical brain activities between attacks.

A severe form of epileptic seizures is a state known as *status epilepticus*, which is characterized by frequent, generalized convulsions and failure to regain consciousness between attacks. Fortunately, status epilepticus is not common because most patients who have epilepsy respond well to anticonvulsant medication. A *febrile seizure* is an episode that occurs in association with a high fever.

Figure 14–4.
Causes of Acquired Epilepsy.

Category	Examples
Genetic and birth factors	Birth trauma, fetal infection, congenital malformations
Infectious disorders	Encephalitis, meningitis, brain abscess
Toxic factors	Alcohol or other drug abuse, abruptly stopping the administration of seizure medication
Trauma	Subdural hematoma
Circulatory disorders	Subarachnoid hemorrhage, aneurysm
Metabolic disorders	Hypoglycemia, hypocalcemia
Tumors	Primary or metastatic intracranial tumor
Degenerative diseases	Huntington's disease

Approximately five percent of young children experience at least one of these episodes. One or two isolated febrile seizures is usually of no medical significance in children under the age of five. However, a convulsion that occurs in association with a fever could be the first epileptic attack, particularly in those children who (1) have family histories of epilepsy, (2) experience the initial seizure after age five, and (3) have a relatively low fever at the time of the attack.

One classification system of epileptic seizure patterns has two major categories: partial seizures and generalized seizures. **Partial seizures**, which are also called *focal seizures,* originate with electrical activity in one area of the brain and may or may not spread to other areas of the brain. **Generalized seizures**, on the other hand, affect several areas of the brain from the beginning of the attack.

Simple Partial Seizures

A **simple partial seizure** is the result of an irritation of a small area of the brain. The convulsive activity typically starts as a focal seizure in one part of the body, such as the patient's face, thumb, arm, or leg. The attack may be limited to the focal seizure, or the convulsion may move to muscle groups in other parts of the patient's body in a process called a **Jacksonian March**. If the convulsion becomes generalized, the individual often loses consciousness. Simple partial seizures may indicate the presence of a brain tumor, but scars resulting from injury may also be responsible for the attacks.

Complex Partial Seizures

Complex partial seizures, which are also called *psychomotor seizures* or *temporal lobe seizures*, are behavioral seizures in which the patient loses consciousness, but experiences involuntary movements during the loss of consciousness. Common movements associated with complex partial seizures are rotation of the head and eyes, smacking of the lips, twisting and writhing motions, walking around, and picking at one's clothes. Episodes of complex partial seizures may be preceded by a sensory aura such as an unusual smell, intensive emotion, or sensory hallucination. Some patients have personality disorders and/or psychiatric disturbances that are associated with their complex partial seizures. Approximately half of all complex partial seizure patients exhibit evidence of a tumor or of scar tissue from trauma or infection in the temporal lobe of the brain. Complex partial seizures differ from absence seizures, which are discussed below, in that the former type of seizure lasts longer and is associated with a deeper clouding of consciousness and a greater range of involuntary muscular movement.

Tonic-Clonic Seizures

Tonic-clonic seizures are generalized convulsions that are characterized by loss of consciousness, as well as tonic-clonic activity. The seizure begins with a *tonic convulsion* in which all of the patient's muscles stay in a continuous state of rigid tension. The tonic convulsion is quickly followed by a *clonic convulsion*, which is characterized by rhythmic, generalized involuntary contractions and relaxations of muscles. During tonic-clonic attacks, affected persons may bite their tongues, fracture bones, or injure themselves in other ways. Often, these patients lose control over bowel and bladder functions during the seizure. Following a tonic-clonic seizure, the patient will enter a *postictal state*, which is a period of sleep and stupor that may last up to several hours. Tonic-clonic seizures are the most common type of seizure pattern and may be preceded by an aura so that the patient may be aware that an attack is imminent.

Absence Seizures

An *absence seizure* is a generalized episode characterized by a brief lapse of consciousness that is often so fleeting that the affected person may be unaware of the seizure, even if several of these seizures occur per day. An absence seizure may present as a sudden, momentary blank expression or a fixed gaze, followed by prompt return to full mental activity. This type of seizure, which mainly affects children four to twelve years of age, is usually not preceded by an aura.

Other Seizure Patterns

Other types of seizure patterns include atonic seizures and myoclonic seizures. *Atonic seizures* are characterized by a transient loss of postural tone, causing the affected person to fall suddenly. *Myoclonic seizures* are characterized by involuntary contractions or jerks of muscles of the patient's extremities, trunk, or face, without loss of consciousness. Myoclonic attacks are more common in the morning or during periods of drowsiness.

Figure 14–5 lists the classifications of several types of epileptic seizures.

Figure 14–5.
Epileptic Seizure Classification.

- Partial seizures
  - Simple partial
  - Complex partial
  - Secondary generalized partial

- Generalized seizures
  - Tonic-clonic
  - Absence
  - Atonic
  - Myoclonic

More than one seizure pattern may be present in the same individual. For example, some people have both generalized tonic-clonic and absence seizures. Furthermore, atonic and myoclonic seizures may be associated with either absence or tonic-clonic attacks.

A number of drugs can control most epileptic convulsions, and many epileptics must take anticonvulsant medication throughout their lives. Of the many anticonvulsants available, all have side effects and some are preferred for the control of particular seizure types. Some patients must take more than one medication in order to control their seizures. If a patient has been seizure-free for a certain amount of time, often four years, the physician and patient may decide to remove the patient from anticonvulsant medication for a trial period. However, the medication dosage should be tapered off very slowly.

Vascular Diseases of the Brain

Any interference with the vascular systems that supply blood to the brain or with the free exchange of oxygen and glucose and the removal of the end-products of cellular metabolism will produce symptoms of anoxia. *Anoxia* is a condition that is characterized by an absence of oxygen to the tissues. The precise nature of the anoxic symptoms will depend on the area of the brain affected by the lack of oxygen. A *cerebral vascular accident (CVA),* which is more commonly called a *stroke,* is any disease of the cerebral vascular system that results in cerebral, cerebellar, or brain stem anoxic damage. Conditions, such as hypertension, diabetes mellitus, elevated blood cholesterol, and certain types of heart disease, that produce or aggravate arterial disease predispose individuals to CVAs. Hypertension is the greatest risk factor in vascular brain diseases, and even mild hypertension dramatically increases the patient's risk of having a stroke.

Treatment of CVAs depends on the particular type of stroke, its severity, and its location and underlying cause. Similarly, the prognosis for stroke patients depends on the cause of the stroke and the location and extent of the brain infarction. The larger the infarct and the greater the degree of the patient's neurologic symptoms as a result of the infarction, the poorer the patient's prognosis. However, mortality trends for stroke patients have been declining for many years. A complete explanation for the declining death rate attributed to CVAs is not known, but more effective drug therapy to control hypertension and improved methods of management of stroke and rehabilitation of the stroke victim may be contributing factors.

The main syndromes produced by vascular disorders of the brain are (1) transient ischemic attack, (2) cerebral thrombosis, (3) cerebral embolism, (4) intracerebral hemorrhage, and (5) subarachnoid hemorrhage.

Transient Ischemic Attack

A *transient ischemic attack (TIA)* is a brief episode in which the vascular system of the brain fails to function properly, but does not produce persistent neurological dysfunction. TIAs, which precede up to 75 percent of all strokes, are characterized by temporary blindness in one eye or other visual disturbance, a speech disorder, vertigo, numbness, weakness, and localized paralysis. All symptoms and signs of a TIA usually disappear within 24 hours, and most manifestations last for less than one hour. The most common cause of a TIA is a microembolism to the brain that develops from atherosclerotic lesions in large blood vessels, particularly the blood vessels of the neck. A TIA also may result from significant narrowing or spasm of any arteriosclerotic blood vessel supplying the brain. Generally, full recovery occurs after the first TIA, but these episodes are warnings of a possible impending full-scale stroke.

Cerebral Thrombosis

A thrombus, as defined in Chapter 8, *The Respiratory System*, is a blood clot. *Cerebral thrombosis* is a condition in which a blood clot develops in a cerebral artery and blocks the flow of blood to the area of the brain served by that artery. Arteriosclerosis is the major underlying cause of cerebral thrombosis, but other diseases producing injury to a blood vessel may also be responsible. The manifestations of cerebral thrombosis include ischemia and infarction, and depend, in large part, on which portion of the brain has been deprived of its oxygen supply. Cerebral thrombosis is the second most common cause of CVAs and occurs most often in patients who are between 50 and 70 years old.

Cerebral Embolism

An embolus, as discussed in Chapter 8, is material that travels through the bloodstream to another location in the body. *Cerebral embolism* is the occlusion of a cerebral vessel by a traveling blood clot, air bubble, tumor, or other piece of material. Emboli generally are not infected. However, an infected embolus that travels to the patient's brain typically will produce a brain abscess. Myocardial infarction and auricular fibrillation are conditions that predispose the individual to the development of cerebral embolism. For example, a thrombus may form in a diseased heart, and a small fragment of this clot may break away and travel to the brain. However, more commonly the embolus originates in the carotid artery. *Air embolism*, which is an air bubble that occludes a blood vessel, may result from an injury to the lung. *Fat embolism*, which is a particle that consists of fat and that occludes a blood vessel, may result from a fracture of a long bone. Emboli, like thrombi, cause cerebral ischemia and infarction, the manifestations of which depend on the part of the brain affected.

Intracerebral Hemorrhage

Intracerebral hemorrhage is bleeding into the substance of the brain and occurs from the rupture of a cerebral blood vessel, usually one that has undergone arteriosclerotic changes in its wall. Most intracerebral hemorrhage patients are hypertensive. The immediate mortality from intracerebral hemorrhage is high, and the residual effects, such as paralysis and the loss of certain body functions, are often severe. Intracerebral hemorrhage rarely occurs in patients who are younger than 40.

Subarachnoid Hemorrhage

Subarachnoid hemorrhage is a condition in which the patient experiences bleeding into the space between the arachnoid and pia membranes. Subarachnoid hemorrhage results from the rupture of an aneurysm in most patients and from rupture of an arterial-venous malformation in other patients. Subarachnoid hemorrhage also may result from an open or closed head injury, a brain tumor, an infectious disease, or a bleeding disorder. Symptoms produced by a ruptured blood vessel include acute severe headache, fainting, vomiting, dizziness, and alterations in the patient's mental status. However, an unruptured aneurysm can also cause symptoms and signs as it dilates and expands, producing pressure on vital adjacent brain structures. Some of the symptoms of an unruptured aneurysm are visual disturbances and facial pain. The mortality rate associated with subarachnoid hemorrhage is high, and survivors of these hemorrhages may experience significant neurologic disorders.

Disorders of the Peripheral Nerves

Neuropathy is a general term for any abnormal function or structure involving a peripheral nerve. The term "neuritis" is often used improperly to describe a disorder of a peripheral nerve from any cause and of any type. However, **neuritis** correctly describes an inflammation of a peripheral nerve, a condition that is associated with pain and tenderness, unusual sensations, lack of sensations, paralysis, and muscular and subcutaneous tissue wasting over the area served by the affected nerve. Because inflammation usually is not present in most instances of structural and functional disorders of the peripheral nerves, neuropathy is the correct term to generally describe these conditions.

Neuralgia

Neuralgia is a condition that is characterized by sudden, intense pain that extends along the course of one or more nerves. The many varieties of neuralgia are distinguished from each other according to the particular nerve involved. For example, the fifth cranial nerve, which is called the ***trigeminal nerve***, serves the side of the face and head. A functional disturbance of the trigeminal nerve is known as ***trigeminal neuralgia***, or *tic douloureux*, a condition of unknown cause that is characterized by sharp pain over one or more branches of this nerve. The painful attacks of trigeminal neuralgia, which is the most common of all the neuralgias, may last only a minute or two or they may be prolonged for 15 minutes or more. The frequency of these attacks range from several each day to one or two a month. Another neuralgia involving a cranial nerve is ***glossopharyngeal neuralgia***, which is a condition of unknown cause that is characterized by sudden intense pain in the area of the tonsils, the back of the pharynx, the back of the tongue, and the middle ear. The areas affected by glossopharyngeal neuralgia are served by the ninth cranial nerve, which is called the **glossopharyngeal nerve**. Treating these neuralgias of the fifth and ninth cranial nerves is difficult. Operations of various types and injections of alcohol into the nerve have been used, but no treatment relieves the pain in every patient. Drug therapy can effectively treat these neuralgias in many patients and may even prevent neuralgic attacks.

Mononeuropathy

Mononeuropathy is a functional or structural disorder affecting a single peripheral nerve. Mononeuropathies are usually secondary to local pressure or trauma. **Ulnar neuropathy** is characterized by numbness in the patient's fourth and fifth fingers and weakness of certain hand muscles. This condition often results from injury or pressure at the point at which the ulnar nerve crosses the elbow at the ulnar notch or "crazy bone." Local care to the area or, occasionally, surgery is necessary for relieving the mononeuropathic symptoms. Carpal tunnel syndrome, which was discussed in Chapter 13, *The Musculoskeletal System*, is a mononeuropathy that is characterized by night pain in the first through fourth fingers, numbness and tingling in these fingers, and weakness of the hand muscles. Simple therapy with splints, steroid injection, and work modification typically will treat carpal tunnel syndrome effectively, although surgery may be necessary for some patients.

Polyneuropathy

A **polyneuropathy** is any syndrome that is produced by the abnormal function or structure of multiple peripheral nerves. The cause of many cases of polyneuropathy is unknown, although usually the neuropathy does not result from infectious agents. Known causes of polyneuropathy include

- toxic agents, such as drugs, including alcohol, and chemicals, such as lead
- metabolic disorders, such as uremia, vitamin deficiencies, and diabetes mellitus
- vascular factors, such as periarteritis nodosa or lupus erythematosus, which interfere with the blood supply to the peripheral nerves

The severity of the signs and symptoms of polyneuropathy, which may include sensory loss, paresthesia, pain, and muscle weakness, depend on the number of nerves involved, their location, and the extent of the nerves' involvement.

Intercostal Neuritis

Intercostal neuritis is an inflammation of the nerves that lie between the ribs that is usually secondary to spinal cord or nerve root irritation, and that is characterized by chest pain. The primary medical importance of intercostal neuritis is that it produces pain that is similar to that associated with coronary artery disease. *Radiculitis* is an irritation of a nerve root at the point at which the root emerges from the spinal cord. *Cervical radiculitis* is an irritation of a nerve root at the point at which the root emerges from the cervical spine. Cervical radiculitis can cause pain over the chest area, and, like intercostal neuritis, can be confused with more serious causes of chest pain.

Guillain-Barré Syndrome

The *Guillain-Barré syndrome*, which is also known as *acute idiopathic polyneuritis*, is a disorder involving both cranial and peripheral nerves and is characterized initially by acute weakness and paralysis of the patient's legs. Within a few days, this weakness spreads to the patient's arms, trunk, and face. The muscular weakness progresses for a week or two, and then the patient gradually recovers over the next several weeks. Guillain-Barré patients rarely experience residual weakness or paralysis, and the mortality rate associated with this disorder is very low. This syndrome most frequently follows an upper respiratory infection or gastroenteritis, but may also follow an immunization and may occur in patients at any age and at any time of the year.

Infections of the Nervous System

Bacteria and viruses are the most common causes of infections of the nervous system. Fungi, protozoa, rickettsiae, and other microorganisms are much less common causes of these infections. Any part of the brain and cranial nerves may be involved in the infectious process. Although these infections often involve more than one anatomical division, nervous system infections usually are classified on the basis of the major site of involvement. This section will discuss only a few major nervous system infections, including meningitis, encephalitis, and poliomyelitis.

Meningitis

A *meningitis* is an inflammation of the membranes covering the brain and spinal cord. *Purulent meningitis* is a bacterial infection of the membranes covering the brain and spinal cord. Symptoms of purulent meningitis include severe headache, stiff neck, elevated temperature, stupor, and delirium. The invading bacteria reach the patient's meninges from primary infections of the heart, lungs, or other organs via the bloodstream. Bacteria may also reach the meninges in the course of a systemic infection or by direct extension from an abscess in an adjacent structure. Although almost any type of bacteria may cause meningitis, H. influenza, pneumococcus, and meningococcus bacteria are the most common. A purulent meningitis patient's prognosis for survival is good if effective antibiotic treatment begins early in the course of the illness. However, these patients may experience residual neurologic deficits, especially loss of hearing.

Meningitis can also result from a viral infection. Viral meningitis, which is also known as aseptic meningitis, typically develops in the summer or early fall. Although the symptoms of viral meningitis are generally the same as those of bacterial meningitis, they usually are not as severe. Essentially all patients who have viral meningitis experience a full recovery.

Encephalitis

Encephalitis is an acute inflammation of the brain that may be caused by many different strains of viruses or other infectious organisms and that is generally characterized by high fever, headache, lethargy, tremors, and delirium. The immediate mortality from an encephalitis is high, reaching over 50 percent of affected individuals in certain forms of the disease. Those patients who recover from encephalitis usually do so without complications, but mild headache, easy fatigability, residual paralysis, mental deterioration, and convulsions may occur as residual effects of the disease. However, a given patient's symptoms, prognosis, and residual effects depend in large measure on the responsible virus. For example, *herpes encephalitis (HSE)* is an inflammation of the brain that is caused by the herpes simplex virus and that is characterized by headaches, fever, personality changes, disorientation, hallucinations, focal neurologic signs, and coma. Without treatment, the mortality rate of HSE patients is high, and few patients return to normal. Drug therapy may be curative for many HSE patients, but they often experience neurologic residual effects.

Poliomyelitis

Poliomyelitis, which is also called *infantile paralysis*, is a disease of the central nervous system that is caused by a virus that destroys the nerve cells responsible for motor activity and that affects skeletal muscles and the muscles involved with swallowing, breathing, and talking. The physician cannot estimate the patient's prognosis for the return to full function of weak or paralyzed muscles until several months after the acute process has subsided, because partially damaged cells may recover completely. Nonetheless, if the patient's paralysis is extensive, the prognosis is poor. Poliomyelitis can, occasionally, lead to death, usually from respiratory failure or other pulmonary complications. However, since the late 1950s, the wide-spread availability of a highly effective vaccine that prevents polio-myelitis infection has resulted in a steady decline in the incidence of the disease.

Some poliomyelitis patients develop a "post-polio syndrome" 20 to 30 years after the original infection. The cause of this syndrome is unclear, and its symptoms include mild to moderate deterioration of motor function, weakness, joint pain, and fatigue. No effective treat-ment for post-polio syndrome exists, and physicians cannot deter-mine in advance which patients will develop the disorder.

Hereditary and Congenital Disorders of the Nervous System

The nervous system is subject to both hereditary and congenital disorders. *Hereditary disorders* are disorders that are genetically transmitted from parent to offspring. Some hereditary disorders manifest at the time of the child's birth, and others appear years later. Some hereditary disorders are also congenital disorders. *Congenital disorders* are disorders that are present at the child's birth and that may result from heredity or from disease or injury to the fetus before delivery. This section will discuss only four of these disorders: cerebral palsy, congenital hydrocephalus, spina bifida, and Huntington's disease.

Cerebral Palsy

Cerebral palsy (CP) is a general term for nonprogressive disorders of the central nervous system resulting from damage sustained by the infant during the mother's pregnancy, at delivery, or shortly after the infant's birth. This damage may result from intrauterine infection, anoxia during pregnancy or delivery, the trauma of labor, and other unclear causes. CP is characterized by spasticity of one or more limbs, speech defects, deafness, and, in about half the cases, mental retardation. *Athetoid movements*, which are ceaseless, slow, involuntary, writhing motions, especially of the hands, are also common in CP patients. The range of CP's clinical features is broad and extends from mild, almost unnoticeable spasticity of one limb to marked, generalized spasticity that is associated with great physical handicap, mental retardation, and convulsions. The prognosis for CP patients depends on the extent of muscular and neurologic involvement. Some CP patients live normal lives. Mildly affected CP patients benefit from physiotherapy, speech training, and orthopedic surgery for the correction of deformities. A patient who has severe CP may be confined to a wheelchair and may require extensive care throughout his or her life.

Congenital Hydrocephalus

Congenital hydrocephalus is an enlargement of the ventricles of the brain that arises from the excess accumulation of cerebrospinal fluid. This condition first appears before birth or shortly thereafter. Congenital hydrocephalus results either from an increased production or a decreased absorption of cerebrospinal fluid or from blockage in the pathways through which this fluid normally flows. Various surgical shunting procedures that divert excess cerebrospinal fluid away from the brain and into the heart or peritoneal cavity may be effective therapies for treating congenital hydrocephalus. A shunting procedure's outcome depends on the cause of the hydrocephalus, the degree of damage before shunting, and the effects of complications—including infection or obstruction of the shunt.

Spina Bifida

Spina bifida is a congenital disorder that results from a defect in the fetal development of a vertebra. The condition can exist as the relatively common asymptomatic spina bifida occulta in which a lumbar or sacral vertebra fails to close, or the condition can be more extensive and exist in association with a defect through which a sac-like herniation occurs. If the sac contains meninges alone, the protruding mass is called a *meningocele*, and a protruding mass that contains meninges and spinal cord tissue is called a *meningomyelocele*. A meningocele or meningomyelocele may be associated with hydrocephalus, neurogenic bladder, and paraplegia. Meningoceles and meningomyeloceles require surgical therapy.

Huntington's Disease

Huntington's disease is a dominantly inherited, progressive disorder characterized by depression, erratic behavior, emotional outbursts, abnormal body movements, and dementia. The Huntington's patient often is disabled by the characteristic depression, erratic behavior, and emotional outbursts before the abnormal body movements and dementia become disabling. Huntington's most often develops in patients who are between the ages of 35 and 40 and can progress for 15 to 20 years. No treatment for this condition, which ends in death, currently exists.

Diseases of Muscle and the Neuromuscular Junction

The *neuromuscular junction* is the interface between a muscle and the nerve that stimulates that muscle. Diseases of muscle and the neuromuscular junction are mostly genetic in origin. The muscular dystrophies and myasthenia gravis are the primary diseases in this group.

Muscular Dystrophies

The *muscular dystrophies* are inherited muscular disorders that show progressive degeneration. Several disorders are classified as muscular dystrophies, but each is a distinctive clinical syndrome. Duchenne's muscular dystrophy is the best known of these disorders and has become synonymous with muscular dystrophy. *Duchenne's muscular dystrophy* is characterized by weakness and the eventual atrophy of affected muscles, and the patient's gait and posture are noticeably abnormal. The prognosis for all muscular dystrophy patients is variable, but for most affected individuals the course is one of progressive deterioration. The most favorable prognoses are for those patients in whom the onset of muscular dystrophy symptoms occurred after the patient had reached age 20. Many muscular dystrophy patients, however, are unable to walk within 10 years after the weakness commences. No treatment for any of the muscular dystrophies has proven to be effective.

Myasthenia Gravis

Myasthenia gravis is an autoimmune disorder that is characterized by muscle weakness and easy muscle fatigability. Early in the course of the disease, the patient may feel well in the morning, but may show gradual loss of strength during the day. Other patients may show weakness only after exercise. The cranial nerves that myasthenia gravis most commonly affects are those which stimulate the facial, laryngeal, pharyngeal, eye, and respiratory muscles. Movements of the eyes, facial expression, mastication, swallowing, and respiration are particularly compromised by this disorder. Most myasthenia gravis patients complain of double vision, drooping of the upper eyelids, and difficulty with chewing, swallowing, and speaking. The course of the disease tends to fluctuate with periods of remission and exacerbation. In late stages of the disease, the weakness is constant and more profound, so that simple tasks, such as combing the hair, present difficulties for the patient. Drug therapy is often used in treating myasthenia gravis patients. The surgical removal of the **thymus**, which is a small gland-like body located in the upper, front chest cavity, has also had a beneficial effect for many patients. Medical treatment programs have improved the prognosis for patients who have this disease, which, in the past, was often fatal.

Tumors of the Nervous System

Primary tumors of the nervous system may arise from the brain, the meninges, cranial nerves, nerve sheaths and supporting tissues, pituitary gland, cranial blood vessels, spinal cord, and peripheral nerve tissues. Cancer of the brain and spinal cord kills an estimated 90,000 people in North America each year. In adults, cancer of the brain and spinal cord accounts for only two percent of the total number of cancer deaths, but in children, tumors of the central nervous system are the second most common cancer, surpassed in incidence only by leukemia. For many brain tumor patients, the average survival period following discovery of the tumor is discouragingly brief. Moreover, metastatic tumors to the nervous system, particularly the brain, may originate in almost any organ in the body, but tumors of the lung and breast account for the majority of metastatic nervous system neoplasms.

Symptoms produced by a nervous system tumor are related to the nature of the tumor and its location. The manifestations of brain tumors—including persistent and unrelenting headaches, nausea, vomiting, mental changes, disturbances of consciousness, progressive neurologic disturbances, behavioral changes, and seizures—result from the local destruction of normal nerve tissue and the effects of increased intracranial pressure. Brain tumors differ from cancers arising in other organs in two important ways: (1) the most common brain cancers do not metastasize, and (2) because of limited room for expansion within the cranial cavity, even a small growth can produce considerable damaging effects. Furthermore, brain tumors are difficult to treat because they are often in inaccessible locations or in locations where complete removal may damage vital structures.

The most important nervous system tumors are gliomas and meningiomas. **Gliomas**, which are tumors of supporting tissues, typically are not well-encapsulated and are difficult to remove completely. Gliomas constitute about 40 percent of all intracranial tumors. The most common type of glioma is the highly malignant glioblastoma, which accounts for almost one-quarter of reported cases of primary brain tumors. **Meningiomas**, which are benign tumors arising from the meninges, typically are slow-growing and are encapsulated. Meningiomas comprise about one-sixth of all intracranial tumors. Because they are encapsulated, meningiomas often can be removed completely. Although these tumors are classified as benign, they may recur even after apparently complete removal. Recurrent meningiomas requiring reoperation may have more malignant characteristics than the original tumor.

Spinal cord tumors are usually benign and may arise from the functional elements of the cord, its roots, and meningeal coverings. These tumors often are similar to the corresponding intracranial tumors. Gliomas, meningiomas, and neurofibromas are the most common spinal tumors. **Neurofibromas** are tumors of the peripheral nerves that contain both nerve and fibrous tissue elements. Neurofibromas may be solitary, but often many of these tumors exist together as part of a syndrome called von Recklinghausen's disease, or neurofibromatosis type I, which was discussed in Chapter 5, *The Skin*. Von Recklinghausen's disease is an inherited disorder characterized by multiple tumors of the CNS or cranial or peripheral nerves, multiple skin tumors, and cutaneous pigmentation. The course of this condition is variable depending on the site of the tumors. Neurofibromatosis type II is a dominantly inherited disorder in which the neurofibromas affect the acoustic nerve exclusively and bilaterally. Gliomas, meningiomas, and neurofibromas cause symptoms—such as localized pain, muscle weakness, abnormal sensations, paralysis, sensory loss, and loss of bowel and bladder control—by compressing the nerve root and spinal cord. The location of the tumor and the degree of compression determine the clinical manifestations.

Treatment of a spinal cord tumor typically consists of its surgical removal. A patient whose tumor has grown deep within the substance of the spinal cord has a poorer prognosis than a patient who has a more superficial tumor. Nonetheless, some spinal tumor patients experience improvement and/or cure following the excision of the affected tissue. Spinal tumor patients can expect little or no improvement, however, if they have experienced paralysis from complete death of spinal cord tissue.

Idiopathic Nervous System Diseases

Many diseases of the nervous system have no known cause. Narcolepsy, Parkinson's disease, multiple sclerosis, Reye's syndrome, amyotrophic lateral sclerosis, and Alzheimer's disease will be discussed in this section as examples of these idiopathic diseases.

Narcolepsy

Narcolepsy is a syndrome that is characterized by recurrent episodes of uncontrollable daytime sleep and abnormal nighttime sleep. Narcolepsy may be associated with muscle weakness and a transient loss of muscle tone, a condition called *cataplexy*. The sleep attacks usually have their onset during the patient's teenage or early adult years. Attacks of sleep may occur several times daily and usually are of short duration. Narcoleptic sleep attacks differ from normal sleep in that narcoleptic attacks often occur in circumstances that are not conducive to, and may be inappropriate for, sleep. Some patients experience drowsiness they cannot suppress, and others fall asleep abruptly, without warning, often in embarrassing or dangerous situations. The diagnosis of narcolepsy is accomplished by a typical medical history and sleep studies. Treatment of the sleep attacks may involve drug therapy or behavioral modification. The associated cataplexy may be treated with antidepressant drugs.

Parkinson's Disease

Parkinson's disease is a chronic disorder of the central nervous system and usually first appears in patients after age 45. Parkinsonism is characterized by three main clinical features: tremor, rigidity, and stiffness and slowness of movement. Tremor at rest is typical of Parkinsonism and is abolished or reduced by voluntary movement. The affected limb frequently shows rigidity, experienced as a resistance to passive movement. A Parkinson's patient may experience difficulty in performing simple tasks, such as buttoning a shirt. As the manifestations of this disease gradually become more severe, the Parkinson's patient tends to assume a stooped position and walks with a slow, shuffling gait, and, in time, will develop a generalized slowness of all body movements. This disease becomes progressively disabling with the passage of years. Parkinsonism may include several syndromes with slightly differing prognoses. The cause of the most common form of Parkinsonism, which is known as primary Parkinsonism or paralysis agitans, is unknown, although a small percentage of cases occur following an attack of encephalitis or in association with cerebral arteriosclerosis or syphilis.

Drug therapy has dramatically altered the pattern of life for patients who have Parkinsonism. Not only is the average patient's life span increased with the use of drug therapy, but in 75 percent of affected individuals, treatment causes an improvement in these patients' signs and symptoms. Unfortunately, drugs used to treat Parkinsonism have significant side effects, and, after several years of treatment, the drugs' effectiveness declines. The long-term course of Parkinsonism is progressively downhill.

Multiple Sclerosis

Multiple sclerosis (MS) is a slowly progressive, chronic, degenerative disease that affects the brain and spinal cord and is one of the most common causes of neurologic disability in adults. MS patients experience alterations in nerve functions resulting from a loss of the myelin sheath covering the nerve. The myelin sheath helps speed the conduction of nerve impulses. Thus, damage to the sheath adversely affects the nerve's ability to function normally. MS affects males and females with about equal frequency, and a patient's initial attack of MS typically occurs before age 30. Symptoms of the initial attack often include double vision and blurred vision resulting from an inflammation of one of the nerves that serve the eye. Inflammation of the optic nerve, which is called *optic neuritis*, is the initial event in 35 percent of men and 75 percent of women who eventually develop multiple sclerosis and may precede the diagnosis of MS by as much as 15 years. Other symptoms and signs of MS include weakness, vertigo, abnormal sensations, tremors, and incoordination. The symptoms and signs of the initial attack of MS may be followed by complete clearing, and many months or years may elapse before the next attack occurs. Although many MS patients experience periods of improvement, up to 30 percent of affected individuals never have a remission and progress steadily downhill after the initial attack. For the majority of MS patients, the course of the disease is unpredictable. Each new attack typically results in a gradual accumulation of neurologic dysfunction. In some patients, these attacks may lead to progressive disability and even death. However, other patients will experience little or no impairment. The diagnosis of MS is difficult to make because no specific test for the disease exists. Generally, the diagnosis is made following (1) a clinical history that is consistent with MS, (2) MRI study, (3) spinal fluid analysis, and (4) evoked potentials study. (Evoked potentials studies are discussed later in this chapter.)

Reye's Syndrome

Reye's syndrome is a relatively rare acute condition that is characterized by an enlarged liver and degenerative brain disease and that follows common viral illness, especially influenza and chickenpox, in children. It develops suddenly and is often accompanied by fever and vomiting. A clouding of consciousness, seizures, and coma are manifestations of the degenerative brain disease. Most affected children recover completely, although some patients develop progressively worsening disease, which ultimately becomes fatal. Specific therapy for Reye's syndrome is unavailable, although supportive therapy is very important for the patient's survival.

Amyotrophic Lateral Sclerosis

Amyotrophic lateral sclerosis (ALS), which is also known as *Lou Gehrig's disease*, is a slowly progressive disease that is characterized by impairment of the patient's motor function, muscle weakness, and wasting of tissues. However, ALS, which affects males twice as often as females, does not impair the patient's intellectual function. ALS has no known cure, and approximately 50 percent of all ALS patients die from extreme debility within three to five years of the onset of the illness.

Alzheimer's Disease

Alzheimer's disease is a slowly progressive disorder that is characterized by loss of memory and intellectual, speech, and motor function that may progress to total helplessness. This disease, which is the most common cause of dementia in the elderly, rarely affects individuals who are younger than 50. Because more people are living longer and the general population contains more people who are over age 65 than ever before, Alzheimer's has enormous economic, social, and personal impact. The onset of Alzheimer's is subtle, and its symptoms typically evolve over ten or more years. However, most Alzheimer's patients die from an incidental illness. No specific treatment for Alzheimer's exists, although the physician can treat coincident diseases, such as depression or thyroid disease.

Procedures for Diagnosing Nervous System Disorders

The diagnosis of a nervous system disorder depends on the results of a neurological examination and any of several tests. A *neurological examination* of a patient begins with a detailed medical history of that patient and includes a general physical exam, as well as a specific neurologic examination. One useful test for diagnosing nervous system disorders is a lumbar puncture. A *lumbar puncture*, which is also called a *spinal tap,* is a procedure in which the physician inserts a long needle between adjacent vertebrae in the patient's lower back and removes some cerebrospinal fluid from the subarachnoid space. An analysis of the fluid removed during a lumbar puncture can determine the fluid's content of sugar, protein, infection, and cell types. The presence of certain diseases of the nervous system, especially infections, will produce abnormal cerebrospinal fluid analysis results.

Biopsy of brain, nerve, or muscle tissue is occasionally necessary to confirm certain diagnoses, such as herpes encephalitis, peripheral neuropathy, or a primary muscle disease. However, advances in other diagnostic techniques, including MRI and CT scans, are making tissue biopsies less necessary.

MRI studies and CT scans often supplement and complement each other as diagnostic techniques. MRIs are particularly effective in visualizing disease of the patient's neck and spinal cord and in helping to diagnose MS. CT scans sometimes provide the best information in evaluating head trauma and in checking for certain tumors. Depending on the clinical situation, an MRI or a CT scan may be the preferred imaging technique, although a CT scan is often performed first.

Myelography, which was discussed in Chapters 3 and 13, is another useful technique for diagnosing disorders of the spinal cord or nerve roots. Myelography involves an x-ray study of the spinal canal following the injection of a contrast medium into the patient's spine. Myelograms are often performed in conjunction with CT scans. However, MRIs provide diagnostic information that is as good as, if not better than, information provided by myelograms, and MRI studies are not as uncomfortable for the patient as myelograms are.

Angiography, which was discussed in Chapter 3, is a diagnostic procedure that involves the injection of a contrast medium into an artery, followed by a series of x-rays of the medium's circulation through the patient. In order to conduct an angiographic study of the brain, the physician typically makes the injection into the patient's internal carotid artery. This procedure is useful in demonstrating aneurysms, vascular malformations, brain tumors, hematomas, and thromboses of cerebral vessels.

Electroencephalography is the study of the electrical activity of the brain. Brain wave patterns, recorded on an electroencephalogram (EEG), provide useful information about organic brain disease, especially seizures. However, electroencephalography has its limitations. For example, a normal EEG does not exclude the diagnosis of epilepsy, and the finding of minor EEG variations does not confirm the diagnosis of epilepsy.

Other useful examinations are evoked potentials, electromyography, and nerve conduction studies. Evoked potential studies are useful for evaluating the integrity of sensory pathways to the brain. Visual evoked potentials check the patient's visual pathway, and auditory evoked potentials check the patient's hearing pathway. Somatosensory evoked potentials evaluate the pathway from a particular peripheral nerve to the brain. Evoked potential tests can help in evaluating diseases such as MS or vitamin B_{12} deficiency. Electromyography helps to differentiate among diseases of a muscle, peripheral nerve, or nerve-muscle junction. Nerve conduction studies aid in the evaluation of peripheral sensory or motor nerve diseases by supplementing clinical findings and other testing results.

15

The Sense Organs

The **senses** are the faculties by which human beings perceive their external and internal environment. The senses include sight, hearing, smell, taste, and touch. The **sense organs** are those structures in the body that contain highly specialized nerve endings, called **receptors**, that receive sensations which are then transmitted to the brain so that the individual can perceive the sensations. Heat, cold, pain, hunger, thirst, balance, well-being, malaise, color, shape, sound, smell, sweet, and sour are among the external and internal sensations that a person can perceive. The primary sense organs are the eyes, ears, nose, tastebuds, and segments of the skin.* However, the senses of smell, taste, and touch typically have little morbidity or mortality significance. Therefore, this chapter will focus upon the senses of sight and hearing and so will discuss the eyes and ears.

ANATOMY AND PHYSIOLOGY OF THE EYE

The orbits or eye sockets, as defined in Chapter 13, *The Musculoskeletal System*, are cavities in the front of the skull that protect the eyeballs from injury. The **eyeballs** are the organs of sight and are spherical in shape. Each eyeball contains three sections: the sclera and cornea, the choroid, and the retina. The **sclera**, which is the external coat of the eye, is made of white, fibrous tissue, and the *cornea* is a transparent convex structure that forms the very front section of the eyeball. A thin mucous membrane called the *conjunctiva* lines the front of the sclera and cornea, as well as the back of the eyelids. The *choroid* is the middle section of the eyeball, and it contains a dense network of blood vessels that serve the structures of the eye. The third section of the eyeball is the *retina*, a thin, delicate membrane that is primarily composed of nerve fibers and that lies at the back of the eyeball. The retinal nerve fibers unite to form the *optic nerve*. At the point at which the optic nerve penetrates the retina lies a small, round, pale yellowish-white, slightly raised area known as the *optic disk*, which contains no receptors that are sensitive to light. Because the optic disk contains no light-sensitive receptors, it produces a "blind spot" in an individual's normal field of vision. The six muscles which attach the orbit to the outer layer of the eyeball are responsible for eye movements.

Covering the outer anterior surface of the eyeball are the upper and lower eyelids. The lids have hairs, called eyelashes, along their outer margins to protect the eyes against dust and other particles. The eyelids protect the eyes from injury and have pain and touch receptors on the lids' front surfaces. A single *lacrimal gland*, which is also called a *tear gland*, lies on the inside of each upper eyelid. Normally, this gland secretes just enough liquid to keep the conjunctiva clean and moist. Increased secretion of tears occurs as a result of physical or emotional stimulation. Decreased secretion of the lacrimal gland fluid produces dry eyes, which may result in damage to the cornea.

Other important structures of the eye are the lens, iris, and pupil. The *lens* is a transparent structure that focuses light rays onto the retina. The *iris* is the pigmented part of the eye and is a circular membrane that lies in front of the lens. The *pupil* is an opening at the center of the iris through which light enters the eye. The chamber between the cornea and the iris is filled with a fluid called the *aqueous humor*. A transparent semifluid, jelly-like substance that is called the *vitreous humor* fills the chamber between the lens and the back of the eye.

Connected to the choroid behind the iris are the ciliary muscle and suspensory ligament of the lens. The *ciliary muscle* joins the sclera and the outer ring of the iris, is continuous with the choroid, and suspends the iris. The ciliary muscle attaches to the *suspensory ligament*, which holds the lens in place. The muscle of the iris contracts or relaxes in response to the amount of light entering the eye through the pupil, thus changing the shape of the iris. The ciliary muscle acts to change the shape of the lens. In adjusting the lens for viewing objects that are near the individual, the ciliary muscle contracts, thereby relaxing the suspensory ligament. In adjusting the lens for viewing objects that are far away from the individual, the ciliary muscle relaxes, thereby contracting the suspensory ligament. Figure 15–1 provides a cross-sectional illustration of the eyeball.

When light enters the eye, it is refracted, which means that it is bent or changed in direction, by the cornea, aqueous humor, lens, and vitreous humor. The lens of the eye, like any lens, actually turns the light waves upside down. The light waves create an image—what we call *sight*—when they strike the retina, where highly specialized light-sensitive cells transform the light into electrical energy that is then transmitted as a nerve impulse to the brain. The two types of these highly specialized light-sensitive cells are called cones and rods. **Cones** contain compounds responsible for color vision, and they require more light for stimulation than do the rods. **Rods**, on the other hand, permit vision in low light, but do not transmit impulses for color vision. Rods are also responsible for the detection of motion. The part of the retina directly behind the center of the lens is the **macula**. At the center of the macula is a small depression known as the **fovea**, which is the location of sharpest vision. The fovea contains only cones. The number of cones in the retina decreases as the distance from the macula increases. No cones lie at the periphery

Figure 15–1.
A Cross-Sectional Side View of the Eyeball.

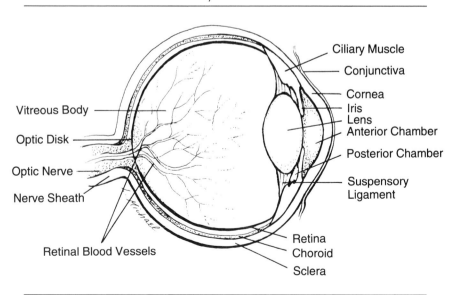

of the retina, and so peripheral vision produces only black and white images. The optic nerve transmits impulses from the rods and cones of the retina to the brain. As part of the process of interpreting electrical impulses as visual images, the brain reverses the received impulses so that the individual perceives viewed objects as being "rightside up," rather than upside down.

DISORDERS OF THE EYE

Many special instruments and procedures are used in the examination of the eye. For example, the *ophthalmoscope* is an instrument that has a special illuminating and lens system that permits an examiner to look into the patient's inner eye and to study the patient's retina. A *tonometer* is an instrument that measures the pressure of the fluids in the eye. Tonometry aids in the diagnosis of glaucoma, which is discussed later in this chapter. *Gonioscopy* is an examination of (1) the angle of the anterior chamber of the eye and (2) the ability of the eye to move normally. Gonioscopy is performed with an instrument, called a gonioscope, that is similar to a microscope and is useful in differentiating between types of glaucoma. In addition, a *slit lamp* is an instrument with which a physician projects a beam of intense light into the patient's eye and examines the eye directly by magnifying lenses. The slit lamp allows for the microscopic study of the patient's conjunctiva, cornea, iris, lens, and vitreous humor.

Some procedures check for the level of the patient's visual acuity, rather than for eye disease. *Visual acuity* is the sharpness of visual perception, or "how well a person sees." Typically, tests of visual acuity measure the sharpness of the person's central vision and the limits of the person's visual fields. A *visual field* is the entire area within which a person can see an object while keeping his or her eye fixed upon a central point. The visual field represents the outer limits of peripheral vision. Peripheral vision is less distinct than is central vision but is important for guidance in the environment and for safety.

Physicians generally test a patient's central visual acuity by means of charts that display block letters, broken rings, or "E"s. If a patient wears corrective lenses—either eyeglasses or contact lenses—the patient's central visual acuity should be measured twice. One test should be performed while the patient is wearing the corrective lenses, and the other test should be performed while the patient is not wearing the corrective lenses. Visual acuity is recorded as a fraction in which the numerator is the distance of the patient from the chart and the denominator is the number assigned to the smallest line on the chart that the patient can read correctly. A patient has normal central vision if his or her visual acuity measurements are 20/20 for distance vision and 14/18 for near vision.

During a test to discover the limits of a patient's visual fields, the patient looks straight ahead. The physician slowly brings a white test object toward the patient in a straight line at 45-degree intervals throughout a complete 360-degree test. The patient signals the physician at the first point at which the patient can see the test object at each 45-degree interval. The physician then records the angle, measured in degrees from the central point of the eye being tested, at which the patient could first see the object. Both of a patient's eyes are tested separately—one eye is covered when the other is being tested—and the fields of vision are plotted for each eye on a special test chart.

Blindness, as defined legally, is a condition in which an individual whose vision has been corrected with glasses or contact lenses has distance vision of 20/200 or worse in the better eye or a visual field restricted to 20 degrees or less in the better eye. A person whose distance visual acuity is 20/200 is able to see clearly 20 feet from the chart what a person who has normal visual acuity can see 200 feet from the chart. Furthermore, a person who has a visual field of 20 degrees has essentially no peripheral vision.

A person who has lost vision in one eye will have a problem with depth perception. The passage of time, however, allows the person to adjust to this impairment so that the person will be able to participate in the normal activities of daily living. Even so, people who have sight in only one eye are not suited for jobs in which full visual fields are necessary for safety.

The eyelids, conjunctiva, cornea, lens, retina, and optic nerve are subject to inflammation, trauma, infections, certain systemic diseases, muscular dysfunction, tumor, degenerative processes, and other conditions. This section will discuss some common eye disorders.

Glaucoma

Glaucoma is a condition in which an increase in the pressure within the patient's eyeball is sufficient to damage the optic nerve and interfere with the patient's vision. The increased pressure in the patient's eye results from an imbalance between the amount of aqueous humor that is manufactured and the amount that is able to drain. Glaucoma often has no symptoms until progressive increased pressure causes visual loss, and it usually affects both eyes. Manifestations of advanced glaucoma include eye pain, decreased visual acuity, and the perception of colored halos around lights. Untreated glaucoma ends in permanent blindness. This eye disease primarily affects people who are middle aged or older, and it is a leading cause of blindness.

Glaucoma is classified as being either open-angle or closed-angle, and as being either primary or secondary. The diagnosis of open-angle or closed-angle glaucoma depends on whether the drainage obstruction is associated with an open or a closed anterior chamber of the patient's eye. Glaucoma is primary if it does not result from some other eye or systemic disorder, and it is secondary if it does result from some other eye or systemic problem. **Developmental glaucoma**, which is also called *congenital glaucoma*, is a type of primary glaucoma that results from an abnormality in the growth of embryonic tissue and that produces an anterior chamber angle defect in the child when it is born.

The most common type of glaucoma is primary open-angle glaucoma, and it accounts for more than 60 percent of all adult glaucoma cases. **Primary open-angle glaucoma** is a chronic, slowly progressive disease that is initially asymptomatic and that typically affects both eyes. People who have a family history of glaucoma are at a higher risk to develop primary open-angle glaucoma than the general population is. Furthermore, individuals who have diabetes mellitus develop primary open-angle glaucoma approximately three times as frequently as do nondiabetics of comparable age. In addition, diabetics develop visual field losses at lower intraocular pressures than do nondiabetics. Nonetheless, the diabetes is not thought to be the cause of the glaucoma. Primary open-angle glaucoma also occurs more often in people who are very nearsighted than in people who have normal eyesight or less severe myopia. **Secondary open-angle glaucoma** is a condition of increased pressure within the patient's eye that results from inflammation, drug use, or mechanical abnormality. Secondary open-angle glaucoma has the same symptoms as primary open-angle glaucoma. People who have an open-angle glaucoma, or who have elevated intraocular pressure without loss of vision, typically receive treatment with beta-blocker eyedrops.

A less common type of primary glaucoma is closed-angle glaucoma, which comprises approximately ten percent of all glaucomas. **Primary closed-angle glaucoma** is characterized by a sudden and acute increase in intraocular tension and, if not treated, will lead to prompt loss of vision. It results from an obstruction of the flow of the aqueous humor. This type of glaucoma typically affects only one eye and develops in patients who are farsighted. It occurs three times more often in females than in males. **Secondary closed-angle glaucoma** is a condition of increased pressure in the eye that most often results from either an intense inflammatory process that causes adhesions to form between the iris and the pupil or from some other condition that causes the lens to come into contact with the iris. Closed-angle glaucoma arising from any cause is an emergency. Emergency medical treatment or a **peripheral iridectomy**, which is the surgical removal of a small piece of the edge of the iris, and the drainage of some of the aqueous humor must be performed promptly in order to avoid permanent damage to the patient's eye.

Disorders of the Eyelids

Eyelid disorders are among the most common eye problems. Examples of eyelid disorders are inflammations of the lids and degenerative disorders of the lids. A **hordeolum**, which is commonly called a *stye*, is a localized, red, tender, swollen abscess of the lid's lacrimal gland. A **chalazion** is a localized enlargement of an eyelid gland that results from blockage of its duct. A chalazion is usually painless, but can become red and painful if infected. **Blepharitis** is an inflammation of the lid edges in which the patient's eyes are red-rimmed and the lid edges are covered with crusts. Tiny, shallow ulcers may also be present in association with blepharitis.

Elderly persons are particularly subject to degenerative disorders of the eyelids, including dermatochalasis, ectropion, entropion, and ptosis. **Dermatochalasis** is a condition characterized by bagginess and loss of elasticity in the skin of the patient's eyelids. **Ectropion** is a condition characterized by the turning outward of part or all of the patient's lid edges. **Entropion** is a condition characterized by the inward relaxation of the patient's lid edges. **Ptosis** is a condition characterized by a drooping of the upper lid and may be secondary to neurological problems. Surgery is seldom necessary for any of these conditions unless the sagging skin obstructs the patient's field of vision or causes significant cosmetic deformity.

Disorders of the Conjunctiva and Cornea

Three of the most common disorders of the conjunctiva and cornea are conjunctivitis, keratitis, and keratoconus. **Conjunctivitis**, which is also called *pinkeye*, is an inflammation of the conjunctiva and is characterized by a watery or mucous discharge. Conjunctivitis may arise from bacterial, viral, fungal, or parasitic infections or from noninfectious agents, such as dust, pollen, smoke, chemicals, and intense light. Infectious conjunctivitis is treated with antibiotic eyedrops and eye rest. Noninfectious conjunctivitis is treated with eye rest and elimination of the irritant. Healing of inflammation of the conjunctiva is usually rapid following appropriate local treatment, and the disorder rarely recurs.

Keratitis is an inflammation of the cornea with or without ulceration. However, ulcerations of the cornea are common and most often result from bacterial infection. Corneal ulcerations may also arise from viruses, fungi, trauma, and vitamin deficiency. The deeper the ulcer, the more severe are the symptoms and complications. Symptoms of corneal ulcers include pain and discharge from the eye, and complications include scarring and perforation, both of which may lead to visual loss.

Keratoconus is a congenital or acquired disease of the cornea that often affects both eyes and is characterized by a cone-shaped protrusion of the center of the cornea. In the early stages of keratoconus, the patient may complain of blurred vision. Treatment of this disorder usually includes the use of hard contact lenses. (Contact lenses are discussed in the section on disorders of the lens later in this chapter.) If a patient's keratoconus is left untreated, the patient may eventually become blind.

Two surgical procedures that are available to treat disorders of the cornea are keratoplasty and radial keratotomy. *Keratoplasty* is a corneal transplant. This procedure greatly improves the visual acuity of those individuals who experience corneal scarring or keratoconus. In a *radial keratotomy*, the surgeon makes a series of bicycle-spoke-like incisions in the patient's cornea from its outer edge toward the center. The series of incisions flatten the cornea and reduce myopia, which is discussed later in the chapter. Although radial keratotomy patients do typically experience much improved visual acuity following the procedure, most must still wear glasses or contact lenses after surgery for optimal vision.

Disorders of the Lens

Disorders of the lens of the eye probably constitute the most common of all eye disorders. Most of these disorders can be corrected with eyeglasses or contact lenses. *Contact lenses* are corrective lenses that, unlike traditional eyeglasses, sit directly on the patient's cornea. Three main types of contact lenses are in use today: hard lenses, soft lenses, and gas-permeable lenses. *Hard contact lenses* are the oldest type of contacts and are made of a rigid plastic. Hard lenses generally are small and durable and offer high visual quality. However, patients often experience difficulty in getting used to wearing hard lenses, and these lenses are more likely than the other two types to "pop out" of the patient's eye. Furthermore, hard lenses can cause corneal swelling if worn for too many hours, because the older types of these lenses do not allow for the flow of oxygen and carbon dioxide across the patient's cornea. However, newer types of hard lenses may allow better flow of gases across the patient's cornea. **Soft contact lenses**, which were developed more recently than the hard lenses, consist of a malleable cover that contains a gelatinous substance. Soft lenses allow for the flow of oxygen and carbon dioxide across the patient's cornea. Soft lenses are larger than hard lenses and are less likely to "pop out" of the patient's eye. Patients generally are able to adjust readily to soft lenses and can wear them for many hours without any swelling of the cornea. However, the vision achieved with soft lenses frequently is not as sharp as that achieved with hard lenses. The third, and newest, type of contact lens is the gas-permeable lens. **Gas-permeable contact lenses**, which are also called *semi-rigid contact lenses*, may be made of any one of several materials, all of which allow oxygen and carbon dioxide to pass across the cornea freely, but also offer high visual quality. Moreover, gas-permeable lenses are about the same size as hard lenses, but provide comfort similar to that of soft lenses.

Most people who wish to wear contact lenses are able to do so. Occasionally, however, contact lenses may cause a chemical irritation, an allergic reaction, or a corneal infection that can progress to ulceration. Contact lenses are not recommended for patients who are prone to develop eye allergies or infections or who, because of a physical or mental handicap, would have difficulty inserting, removing, or maintaining the lenses.

Errors of refraction and cataracts are two types of disorders that can affect the lens.

Errors of Refraction

In order to understand refractive eye disorders, the student must first understand a few properties of light. When a light ray strikes a transparent substance at an angle, the light is bent, or refracted, once as it enters the substance and then again as it passes from the substance to another medium of different density. In a normal eye, light is bent at the cornea and at the lens so that the light focuses on the retina. Focus also depends on the shape of the person's eye. An eye that is too thick or thin, from front to back, will not focus properly. Normally the action of the ciliary muscles can change the shape of the lens, in a process called **accommodation**, to accomplish precise focusing of near and distant objects. **Refractive errors**, therefore, are eye disorders in which rays of light that enter the eye are not brought into proper, precise focus on the retina. Because errors of refraction often involve lens disorders, these abnormalities will be discussed in this section. The common refractive errors are hyperopia, myopia, presbyopia, and astigmatism.

Hyperopia is farsightedness and occurs when rays of light are brought to a focus behind the retina. The result of hyperopia is indistinct vision at all distances up to approximately 20 feet and normal vision beyond this distance. Hyperopia is the most common refractive error. *Myopia*, on the other hand, is nearsightedness, and it occurs when rays of light come to a focus in front of the retina. Myopia produces an inability to clearly distinguish objects that are in the distance. Corrective lenses that bring the rays of light into precise focus on the retina are the most common treatments for hyperopia and myopia. *Presbyopia* is a condition associated with aging in which the patient's ciliary muscles lose their powers of accommodation. A presbyopic lens is flattened, tough, and inelastic. Presbyopia produces difficulty in focusing on near objects and reading fine print. Glasses for reading or for close work will correct the presbyopia, but, because this condition worsens with age, the presbyopic patient may frequently need new prescriptions for stronger lenses. In addition, if the patient has another refractive error, he or she may require bifocal lenses. *Bifocal lenses* consist of two sections—one section corrects for distance vision and the other corrects for near vision.

Astigmatism is a refractive error of the eye in which rays of light are brought to a focus at different points along the retina. This condition usually results from changes or irregularities in the curvature of the cornea. Astigmatism may exist alone or in combination with other refractive errors. In most instances, glasses will correct the astigmatism.

Cataracts

A *cataract* is any opacity or cloudiness in the lens of the eye and is characterized by blurred distance and near vision that cannot be corrected by optical devices. The opacity of the lens interferes with the ability of the lens to focus light rays onto the retina. Cataracts, which typically are painless, can be congenital or acquired. Acquired cataracts may result from eye diseases, toxins, or systemic diseases, but aging is the most common cause of cataracts. Without treatment, a cataract arising from any cause will develop from an early, immature stage, in which the lens is only slightly obscured, through various intermediate stages, until the cataract is mature and the lens is almost totally obscured. An estimated five to ten million individuals are visually impaired by cataracts each year.

The typical treatment of cataracts is surgical and is usually effective, although successful cataract surgery of any type will increase the risk of subsequent retinal detachment. (Detachment of the retina is discussed later in this chapter.) An ***intracapsular cataract extraction*** is the surgical removal of the entire lens. This procedure improves the visual acuity of more than 90 percent of cataract patients and is particularly effective in treating hard cataracts. An ***extracapsular lens extraction*** is the surgical removal of only the front of the lens, followed by the application of sound waves to fragment the center layer of the lens. These fragments are then suctioned out of the patient's lens. The primary advantage of an extracapsular lens extraction, which is particularly effective in treating soft cataracts, is that the patient requires a shorter recovery period than if he or she had undergone an intracapsular lens extraction.

Aphakia is a condition in which the individual does not have a lens in his or her eye, for any reason. The most common reason for aphakia is cataract surgery. Patients who are aphakic as a result of cataract surgery may experience 20/20 vision following the surgery. Cataract surgeries may lead to some minor complications and concerns. For example, many patients complain that the corrective lenses they must wear after cataract surgery magnify objects, and the magnification increases from the center of the patient's visual field to its edges, causing an apparent displacement of the objects. Corrective eyeglasses typically magnify objects 30 percent and contact lenses magnify objects 5 to 10 percent. Many of these patients also note that they experience a reduction of their peripheral vision. In spite of the difficulties cataract patients encounter, most of these patients eventually adjust to the visual and perceptive problems associated with aphakia. With their corrective lenses and improved visual acuity after cataract surgery, they lead normal, useful lives.

Some patients who may not be comfortable with postoperative eyeglasses or contact lenses may benefit from an intraocular lens following cataract surgery. An ***intraocular lens (IOL)*** is a plastic lens that the surgeon permanently inserts in the patient's eye to replace the removed cataractous lens. The IOL provides only one to three percent magnification and allows the patient to have depth perception and full visual fields. However, IOL surgery is technically more difficult to perform and carries a greater risk of complications than routine cataract extraction procedures.

Disorders of the Retina

This section will discuss a few common disorders of the retina, including retinitis, detachment, and retinopathy.

Retinitis

Retinitis is an inflammation of the retina that is characterized by a reduction in the patient's visual acuity, alterations in the patient's perception of the shapes of objects, and eye discomfort. The physician will be able to see retinal hemorrhage, exudate, and edema upon ophthalmoscopic examination of the retinitis patient's eye. Retinitis frequently affects both eyes and is commonly associated with diseases of the choroid and the optic nerve. Retinitis commonly results from the involvement of a systemic disease or from bacterial, viral, fungal, or parasitic infection. Retinitis may also follow direct trauma. A retinitis patient's prognosis depends on the severity of the inflammation and the underlying cause. A patient's vision may return to normal when the lesion is completely healed, but some patients experience a degree of permanent vision loss.

Detachment of the Retina

Retinal detachment is a partial or complete separation of the retina from the choroid and is characterized clinically by (1) blurred vision or the total loss of sight or (2) the perception of flashes of light and spots before the eyes. The detachment often begins as a small tear in the retina that permits vitreous humor to get behind the retina and separate it from the choroid. Aphakia and myopia are factors that predispose individuals to retinal detachment, although severe trauma can produce retinal detachment even in healthy eyes. In fact, about one-fifth of all detachment cases result from trauma to the patient's head or eye. Retinal detachment may also occur as a result of choroidal hemorrhage, exudate, or tumor.

Treatment of retinal detachment consists of drainage of the vitreous fluid beneath the retina and the intentional creation of a small inflammation of the choroid that produces an exudate at the site of the detachment. After the fluid is drained, the retina falls back against the choroid and adheres to the exudate that has been produced. Surgical procedures such as diathermy, photocoagulation, or cryosurgery can establish a permanent chorioretinal bond. **Surgical diathermy**, which is also called *electrocoagulation,* is a procedure that involves heating body tissues—in this case, the retina—in order to disrupt them and cause the formation of exudate. **Photocoagulation** is the use of an intense beam of light to coagulate tissue. Photocoagulation as a treatment for a detached retina involves focusing a laser made of xenon gas through the patient's pupil to create an inflammatory exudate. This procedure can also use argon gas instead of xenon in order to produce the exudate. **Cryosurgery** is the intentional destruction of tissue by application of extreme cold. In treating a detached retina by means of cryosurgery, the surgeon applies a supercooled probe to the patient's sclera to cause a chorioretinal scar. Each of these surgical methods will correct a retinal detachment. About 80 percent of uncomplicated detachments are corrected after one operation, and an additional 10 percent require a second operation. The remaining 10 percent of these detachments never reattach.

Retinopathy

A *retinopathy* is a general term for any disease of the retina. Some retinopathies result from infections, vascular diseases, or certain drugs. The infection may be viral, bacterial, fungal, or protozoan. *Arteriosclerotic retinopathy* is a vascular disease of the retina that is characterized by the development of thickened, hardened retinal arterioles that can be seen upon ophthalmoscopic examination. Small changes in retinal blood vessels frequently occur in elderly people and cause little reduction in vision, but marked changes, especially those that occur in association with retinal exudates and hemorrhage, do produce a reduction in the patient's visual acuity. *Hypertensive retinopathy* is a disease of the retina that occurs in association with hypertension from any cause and is characterized by retinal hemorrhage and swelling and the development of exudates. The degree of disturbance in the hypertensive retinopathy patient's vision depends on the characteristics of the exudates and hemorrhage. The most common vascular retinopathy is diabetic retinopathy. *Diabetic retinopathy* is a disease of the retina that occurs as a late manifestation of diabetes mellitus and is characterized by the development of tiny hemorrhages, exudates, and capillary aneurysms in the retina. The ophthalmoscopic appearance of the diabetic retinopathy patient's retina is typically divided into five stages: stage I includes slight retinal changes, stages II through IV include advanced changes, and stage V includes hemorrhage and scar tissue, which may lead to total loss of vision. The stage of the retinopathy is related to the duration of time that the patient has had diabetes as well as to the level of control the patient has over the disease. Argon laser treatment has been helpful in partially correcting retinal pathologies and in controlling the progression of these diseases.

Other retinopathies include central serous chorioretinopathy and macular degeneration. *Central serous chorioretinopathy* is a serous detachment of the retina that occurs without obvious cause. This type of detachment occurs more often in men than in women and most often occurs in patients aged 55 and older. Central serous chorioretinopathy may involve both eyes, but usually affects only one at a time, and it may reduce the patient's vision. This retinopathy may resolve without treatment, and initial attacks are usually not treated. However, recurrent attacks require intervention, which typically involves photocoagulation laser therapy. Photocoagulation laser therapy promptly resolves the condition in most cases. *Macular degeneration* is the atrophy or degeneration of the macular disk. Macular degeneration may be secondary to trauma, aging, inherited conditions, or other conditions. Regardless of the cause of the degeneration, damage to a patient's macula may lead to significant, disabling loss of central vision.

Disorders of the Optic Nerve

Disorders of the optic nerve include optic neuritis, papilledema, and optic nerve atrophy.

Optic neuritis is a general term that refers to the inflammation or degeneration of the optic nerve. Two types of optic neuritis are papillitis and retrobulbar optic neuritis. *Papillitis*, which is also called *anterior optic neuritis*, is an inflammation or degeneration of the optic nerve that is confined to the area around the patient's optic disk. *Retrobulbar optic neuritis* is an inflammation of the part of the optic nerve that lies behind the eyeball. Both papillitis and retrobulbar optic neuritis are characterized by the patient's rapid loss of vision, which may be temporary or permanent, in the affected eye. Either type of optic neuritis may arise from the same causes, including multiple sclerosis, lupus erythematosus, viral infection, or other eye inflammations. Furthermore, optic neuritis is the initial manifestation of multiple sclerosis in more than 25 percent of MS patients. The optic neuritis may predate the diagnosis of MS by a number of years. (Multiple sclerosis is discussed in more detail in Chapter 14, *The Nervous System.*)

Papilledema is a noninflammatory swelling of the optic disk. Papilledema typically results from either increased pressure within the cranium or obstruction of the vein that serves the eye. Common causes of papilledema are brain tumors, cerebral hemorrhage, and severe hypertension. Except for creating an enlarged blind spot, papilledema does not affect the patient's visual acuity or visual fields. Treatment of papilledema depends on the underlying cause of the condition.

Optic nerve atrophy is the degeneration and shrinking of the optic nerve and is characterized by the patient's loss of vision. The atrophy may result from glaucoma, trauma, prolonged papilledema, retrobulbular neuritis, obstruction of the central retinal artery and vein, diabetes mellitus, or hemorrhage. The extent of the patient's loss of vision is directly proportional to the degree of atrophy of the optic nerve.

Disorders of the Muscles around the Eyeball

Sometimes the muscles around the eyeballs fail to function properly. The most common disorder of the muscles that attach to the eyeball is strabismus. **Strabismus** is the deviation of an eye caused by the overrelaxation or overcontraction of a muscle that attaches to the eyeball so that the eyes do not move in parallel. People who have vision in both eyes and who develop strabismus typically experience double vision, which is called **diplopia**. People who have had strabismus since infancy experience decreased visual fields and abnormal vision resulting from the suppression of vision in one eye in order to avoid diplopia. Significant strabismus that has an adult onset may be secondary to a neurologic disease.

A strabismus patient's eye may move inward, outward, up, or down. The most common type of strabismus is esotropia. **Esotropia**, which is commonly known as "crossed eyes," is a condition in which one eye deviates inward. The cause of childhood esotropia is often unknown. However, most adult cases of esotropia result from the paralysis of one or more of the muscles that surround the eye. Another type of strabismus is exotropia. **Exotropia**, which is also called *divergent strabismus*, is a condition in which one eye deviates outward. Exotropia may occur intermittently or constantly. Esotropia and exotropia both exhibit strong hereditary tendencies.

Treatment of strabismus generally first involves **occlusive therapy** in which the patient wears an eye patch over his or her good eye. Patching, if undertaken in the patient's infancy, may result in normal vision. If patching does not produce normal vision, surgery to strengthen or weaken the muscles of the affected eye may be necessary.

Tumors of the Eyes and Related Structures

The eyeball and its surrounding structures can be the site of benign and malignant tumors.

Moles and warts are common benign tumors of the eyelids. The most common malignant tumor of the eyelid is the basal cell carcinoma, which is a slowly growing, ulcerative lesion. Basal cell carcinoma is associated with advancing age, and it affects men more often than women. Basal cell carcinoma destroys local areas of eyelid tissue and does not metastasize. The surgical removal of the cancerous lesion in the early stages of its development provides a cure. If the edge of the eyelid is involved in the lesion, however, plastic surgery may be a necessary part of the lesion's removal.

In contrast to basal cell carcinoma, squamous cell carcinoma is less common, grows more rapidly, and is more likely to metastasize. The only treatment for a squamous cell tumor is surgical removal. The prognosis for a patient who has squamous cell carcinoma of the eyelid is good if surgery to remove the lesion includes a wide excision.

Tumors rarely develop within the eyeball, but when they do, they can be fatal if not recognized and treated early. Retinoblastoma is the most common malignant tumor that affects children. Approximately 90 percent of retinoblastoma patients are younger than three, and 70 percent of these patients develop retinoblastoma in only one eye. Malignant melanoma is the most common tumor of the eyeball that affects adults. It frequently develops in the choroid of one eye and most often occurs in Caucasian patients who are older than forty. Skin melanomas tend to metastasize to the eye, and eye melanomas often metastasize to the liver. Most ophthalmologists recommend the removal of the affected eye upon the confirmation of a diagnosis of malignant melanoma. A few ophthalmologists, however, recommend observing the growth of small melanomas before surgical removal of the affected eye, because some melanomas grow slowly and do not interfere with the patient's vision or life for many years. The watchful approach may be preferable for a patient who has only one useful eye or for an elderly patient.

Tumors of the eye socket displace the eyeball, causing it to protrude. These tumors are often characterized by eye pressure, pain, and disturbances of vision. A hemangioma, which was defined in Chapter 5, *The Skin,* as a benign vascular tumor that consists of large blood-filled spaces, is the most common tumor of the eye socket. However, ***rhabdomyosarcoma***, which is a highly malignant tumor of striated muscle tissue, is common in children and has a poor prognosis.

Lymphomas and malignant lacrimal gland tumors may develop in adults, but most eye tumors in adults have metastasized from another location in the body, usually the breast.

ANATOMY AND PHYSIOLOGY OF THE EAR

The ear, which is the organ of hearing, is divided into three parts: the external ear, the middle ear, and the inner ear. The ***external ear*** includes the auricle and the external auditory canal. The ***auricle*** is the fleshy, cartilaginous curved part of the ear that lies on the outside of the head. The auricle collects sound vibrations and channels them into the external auditory canal where they reach the eardrum. The *eardrum*, which is also known as the *tympanic membrane* or *tympanum*, is a thin, semitransparent, oval membrane that lies at the end of the external auditory canal and separates the external ear from the middle ear.

The **middle ear**, which is also called the *tympanic cavity*, is an irregular, air-filled space within the skull and medial to the external ear. Air gains entrance to this space through the eustachian tube. The eustachian tube, which was described in Chapter 8, *The Respiratory System*, extends from the middle ear to the nasopharynx and provides an air passageway for the equalization of air pressure on both sides of the eardrum. If it were not for this tube, the eardrum would bulge outward or inward depending on the relationship between the atmospheric pressure and the pressure in the middle ear. Because the eustachian tube has a tiny channel, air passes through the tube slowly. To reduce the effects of sudden changes in atmospheric pressure, an individual can force air into the middle ear by swallowing or by "blowing" against the resistance of a closed mouth and nose. The middle ear contains a chain of three small, movable bones, which are collectively known as **ossicles** and include the malleus, incus, and stapes. The **malleus** is the bone of the middle ear that lies closest to the external ear. The malleus is attached to the inner surface of the eardrum on one end and to the incus on the other. The **incus** is the middle ear bone that attaches to the malleus on one end and to the stapes on the other end. The **stapes** is the innermost of the auditory bones, and it attaches to the incus on one end and to the oval window of the inner ear on the other. These bones transmit sound impulses that the vibrating eardrum sends to the malleus, which moves them to the incus and then to the stapes. From the stapes, the sound waves travel to the oval opening of the inner ear.

The inner ear extends from an oval opening to the auditory nerve, which carries sound impulses to the brain. The **inner ear**, which is also called the *labyrinth*, is encased in bone and contains three major structures: (1) the vestibule, (2) the cochlea, and (3) three bony semicircular canals. The **vestibule** is a centrally located cavity that has an oval window that lies next to the stapes. The movement of the stapes against the oval window of the vestibule transmits sound impulses. From the vestibule, sound impulses pass to receptor cells in the cochlea. The **cochlea** is a coiled, snail-shell-shaped tube in which branches of the auditory nerve pick up the sound impulses and relay them to the hearing center of the brain. (The auditory nerve is also known as cranial nerve VIII.) Three bony semicircular canals are located at right angles to each other and sit above the vestibule, to which they are attached. The three cavities of the inner ear are filled with a watery fluid called **endolymph**. Movement of endolymph across sensitive nerve endings within the vestibule and the semicircular canals provides the brain with information on the position of the individual's head and provides the person with a sense of balance.

Figure 15–2 provides a cross-sectional view of the parts of the ear.

DISORDERS OF THE EAR

The ear is a common site of infections, some of which can have relatively serious complications, such as loss of hearing. Hearing loss can be quantified by measuring a patient's hearing acuity using an

Figure 15–2.
A Cross-Sectional View of the Parts of the Ear.

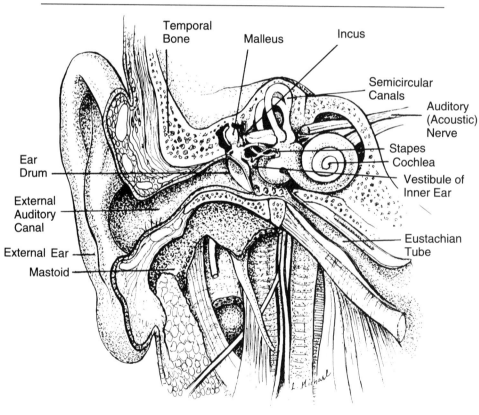

audiometer. An **audiometer** is a medical instrument that generates pure tones that can vary in pitch and intensity, testing seven sound-wave frequencies. The physician measures a patient's hearing loss, in decibels, at each frequency, and tests each ear separately. Normal hearing occurs at 20 or fewer decibels. If an individual's hearing is 40 decibels or fewer, the individual can usually hear well enough for ordinary activities. A noncorrectable hearing loss of more than 40 decibels in both ears may necessitate the use of a hearing aid. Furthermore, a hearing loss of 85 to 90 decibels is generally considered to constitute total deafness.

Hearing loss typically occurs as a result of either of two basic disorders: (1) a defect somewhere in the conduction system in the external ear or middle ear, which causes conductive deafness, or (2) a defect of the cochlea, auditory nerve, or auditory center of the brain, which causes perceptive or sensory-neural deafness. Both basic disorders may arise from a variety of causes.

Conductive hearing loss typically results from thickened, scarred, or perforated ear drums, impacted wax, otitis media (which is discussed later in this chapter), or otosclerosis. Individuals who have a conductive hearing loss can hear well if sounds are amplified, because these individuals have normal inner ear mechanisms. Hearing aids provide this amplification and are best suited for those individuals whose hearing loss is purely conductive in origin, because the loss and the amplification are approximately equal for all tones.

Perceptive hearing loss often results from inner ear, auditory nerve, or auditory center involvement in infection, trauma, diabetes, senile degeneration of these structures, and tumors. Systemic infections, such as meningitis, mumps, measles, or streptococcal infections are very common causes of perceptive hearing loss. Excessive noise that damages the cochlea is a type of trauma and is another common cause of perceptive hearing loss. The loss occurs because loud noises damage the cochlea. Hearing loss may occur following prolonged exposure to excessive amplification of music or persistent industrial noise or following exposure to a single, sudden, extremely loud sound. Some toxic substances, such as alcohol or certain antibiotics, can also cause perceptive hearing loss. Hearing aids help some perceptive hearing loss patients. However, in general, hearing aids are not well-suited for these patients because the aids amplify all tones equally, whereas most of these patients have lost the ability to hear only some tones, usually the high ones. **Presbycusis** is a physiologic loss of hearing associated with aging. It results from arteriosclerosis and other degenerative changes in the receptor cells of the cochlea and in the vessels that supply blood to the branches of the auditory nerve.

Because the structure of the ear also plays an important role in maintaining balance, many disorders of the ear produce disturbances in the individual's sense of equilibrium.

This section will define and discuss four of the most common diseases that affect the ears: otitis media, mastoiditis, otosclerosis, and labyrinthine disorders.

Otitis Media and Mastoiditis

Otitis media is an infection of the middle ear. This infection, which usually originates in the nasopharynx, reaches the middle ear through the eustachian tube. Otitis media may occur as an acute or a chronic disorder. *Acute purulent otitis media*, which is also known as *acute suppurative otitis media*, is a bacterial infection in which pus fills the patient's middle ear and is characterized by throbbing pain in the ear and hearing loss. The acute purulent otitis media patient's eardrum appears fiery red and bulges from the pressure of the pus behind it. Perforation of the eardrum is the most common complication of purulent otitis media, but another complication is that the pus may spread from the inner ear to the adjacent mastoid area.

Administration of antibiotics is the most common method of treating acute purulent otitis media. Before penicillin was available, myringotomy was used extensively. *Myringotomy* is a surgical procedure that involves an incision into the patient's eardrum to release the pus behind it. This procedure is still used occasionally as an adjunct to antibiotic therapy, especially if the patient's eardrum is bulging markedly or if the infection does not respond promptly to antibiotics. After performing a myringotomy, occasionally the surgeon will insert a Teflon button or tube through the patient's eardrum to permit further drainage.

Acute serous otitis media is a condition in which a noninflammatory watery fluid develops in the patient's middle ear in response to allergic phenomena, changes in atmospheric pressure, viral upper respiratory tract infection, or pharyngitis. *Chronic serous otitis media* results from recurrent or neglected acute middle ear infections and is characterized by a chronic discharge and pain. Some loss of hearing usually is present. A *cholesteatoma*, which may result from a persistent middle ear infection, is a collection of old squamous epithelium cells, cellular debris, and other substances. As cholesteatomas enlarge from the accumulation of dead skin and debris, they press upon and cause damage to neighboring structures and may even erode into the brain.

Mastoiditis is an inflammation of the mastoid portion of the temporal bone of the skull that encloses the back side of the middle ear. The mastoid area is filled with air spaces, some of which connect directly with the middle ear. Like otitis media, mastoiditis exists in acute and chronic forms and results from a direct extension of a middle ear infection. Discharge from the ear canal, edema behind the ear, and pain over the mastoid bone are common manifestations of this disease. Treatment of otitis media with antibiotics has greatly reduced the incidence of mastoiditis, although this disorder occasionally occurs in individuals who receive inadequate treatment for middle ear infections.

Chronic ear disease involves an inflammatory process of the middle ear and mastoid—concurrent otitis media and mastoiditis—that persists six or more weeks. Complications of chronic ear disease result from the spread of the infection to neighboring structures. In the past, chronic ear disease frequently led to serious central nervous system complications, such as meningitis and cerebral abscess. To prevent these complications, the surgical removal of the inflamed mastoid air spaces in an operation known as a **mastoidectomy**, often was performed. Furthermore, extensive damage to the middle ear structures from chronic ear infections frequently diminished the patient's hearing. Today, with antibiotics and modern surgical techniques, these complications are much less common and hearing can be restored to many chronic ear disease patients.

If disease destroys a patient's middle ear, the damaged structures must be rebuilt or replaced if the patient's hearing is to be restored. Successful reconstruction of the hearing mechanism may be achieved in a number of ways. A **tympanoplasty** is the surgical restoration of the patient's middle ear and the repair of the patient's eardrum, as well as either the reconstruction of the bony connection between the eardrum and the oval window of the inner ear or the replacement of one or more of the ossicles with an artificial structure. The surgical repair of perforations of the eardrum is called a **myringoplasty**. Tympanoplasties are numbered I to V. A type I tympanoplasty involves only the removal of diseased tissue from the middle ear cavity and the repair of the defect in the eardrum. Tympanoplasties numbered II through V involve progressively more complex reconstructions. For example, a type V tympanoplasty involves the creation of a new opening into the patient's inner ear. The surgeon often will perform a tympanoplasty at the same time as a mastoidectomy.

Otosclerosis

Otosclerosis is a condition of the middle ear that involves the formation of bone around the oval window and is characterized by loss of hearing and tinnitus. **Tinnitus** is a condition characterized by the presence of a constant ringing or buzzing sound in the patient's ear. Otosclerotic tissue formation around the oval window causes ankylosis, or fixation, of the stapes, reducing its vibration in response to soundwave stimuli, thus resulting in conductive hearing loss. In addition, otosclerotic tissue formation in the cochlea can result in perceptive hearing loss. The cause of otosclerosis is unknown, but this disorder shows strong hereditary and familial tendencies. Typically, otosclerosis affects people between the ages of 20 and 40. This condition presents in both ears, although often one ear is more affected than the other, and affects women more often than men.

Several surgical procedures can correct otosclerosis. However, no one of these operations is best for all patients and any one, or a combination of operations in sequence, might be appropriate under a given set of circumstances. A **fenestration** is an operation in which the surgeon creates a new opening. A **fenestra** is a small opening. In treating otosclerosis, the surgeon may create a fenestra through which sound waves may pass into the cochlea. The formation of new bone tissue around the fenestra occurs following a fenestration in approximately 10 percent of these patients.

Another operation to improve hearing in otosclerosis patients is the **stapes mobilization procedure** in which the surgeon frees the stapes from its fixation to the oval window, giving the stapes the opportunity to vibrate more freely. Stapes mobilization requires a shorter period of hospitalization than does fenestration and is usually performed on patients who are under local anesthesia. The patient's hearing improves sooner and more completely following a stapes mobilization than after fenestration. One disadvantage of stapes mobilization is that about half the patients show refixation of the stapes, necessitating a repeat operation.

A third type of corrective operation is a **stapedectomy**, which is the surgical removal of the stapes. The stapes may be replaced either with grafts using veins or fatty tissue or with an artificial stapes made of plastic or wire.

Labyrinthine Disorders

Labyrinthine disorders are diseases of the inner ear and are characterized by hearing loss and vertigo. **Vertigo** is an abnormal sensation of movement. Vertigo patients lose their equilibrium and complain either that objects are spinning, rotating, or twirling around them or that the patients are turning within their surroundings. Disease of the inner ear is present in 85 to 90 percent of patients who have vertigo. **Positional vertigo** is a benign, relatively common condition in which head movements or position produce the typical symptoms of vertigo. The causes of benign positional vertigo usually are disorders of the inner ear or a viral infection of the vestibular nerve. *Dizziness*, on the other hand, refers to subjective symptoms of light-headedness, weakness, giddiness, and faintness. Among the more common causes of dizziness are anemia, anxiety, strenuous exercise, hyperventilation, pregnancy, varicose veins, vitamin deficiency, imbalance of the muscles surrounding the eyes, and cerebral or cardiac disturbances. Although a patient may call the sensations associated with vertigo "dizziness," the physician should obtain a complete medical history of the patient in order to make an accurate diagnosis and to institute proper therapy.

Labyrinthine diseases may arise from

- infection, usually from the spread of otitis media
- trauma, especially trauma that produces a brain concussion or skull fracture
- vascular disturbances, such as arteriosclerosis
- degeneration associated with aging
- drugs
- allergy-producing substances

Endolymphatic hydrops is a condition of generalized dilation of the membranous labyrinth that results from the overproduction of endolymph. *Meniere's disease* is an endolymphatic hydrops of unknown origin in which the patient experiences vertigo, hearing loss, and tinnitus. The vertigo of Meniere's disease may last for minutes to hours, and the patient may enjoy days or weeks of complete relief between attacks. The diagnosis of Meniere's disease should be made only after all other correctable causes of vertigo have been clinically excluded.

An acoustic neuroma is another common labyrinthine disorder. *Acoustic neuroma* is a benign tumor of the acoustic nerve that results in the inability of the patient to hear high-frequency tones and that causes vertigo. The treatment of an acoustic neuroma is surgical removal of the tumor.

16

Psychiatric and Brain Function Disorders

Psychiatry is the branch of medicine that deals with the study, treatment, and prevention of mental impairments. A *psychiatrist* is a medical doctor who specializes in psychiatry and is licensed to prescribe medicine. A *psychiatric disorder* can be any one of several conditions that affect an individual's behavior and/or mental well-being. Each disorder is an independent syndrome and is typically associated with one or more distressful symptoms or signs or with an impairment in one or more activities of the brain. No individual disorder within this group is sharply defined, and no discrete boundaries between one psychiatric disorder and another, or between one disorder and "psychiatric health," exist. Other disorders associated with abnormal brain function include mental retardation and learning disabilities.

PSYCHIATRIC DISORDERS

Psychiatric disorders can be associated with significant morbidity and increased mortality.

- One in three adults in the United States suffers from a psychiatric disorder at some point during the year. Further, more than 50 percent of adults in the United States who required psychiatric care received that care from the general medical care sector.
- Thirty-three percent of the population will suffer from some psychiatric disorder during their lifetimes. This number is 22 percent if alcoholics and other substance abusers are excluded from the calculation.
- Many psychiatric disorders can affect the young and are chronic, recurring illnesses that last a lifetime. Anxiety and depression in association with alcoholism and the abuse of other drugs have a median age of onset of less than 25 years.
- Suicide rates are distinctly higher among persons who are hospitalized for psychiatric disorders, or who were previously hospitalized for psychiatric disorders, than are the rates for the population in general.

Death rates among people who have psychiatric disorders are higher than the death rates for the general population. The excess mortality is greatest in people under age 55. In addition, all causes of death, except neoplasms, occur more often in psychiatric patients than in the general population.

The increase in the number of psychiatric claims has created a need for better understanding and documentation of these disorders. *The Diagnostic and Statistical Manual of Mental Disorders—Revised* (DSM-III-R) of the American Psychiatric Association provides one system for categorizing psychiatric disorders. The DSM-III-R can be used for determining both the diagnosis and the severity of psychiatric disorders. It also tries to differentiate normal human emotions such as "depression" and "anxiety" from psychiatric disorders that share these same names.

The DSM-III-R is written as an outline of diagnostic classes with codes. Five "axes" or categories are used to describe an individual's condition. In Axis I, the psychiatrist codes and defines the patient's clinical syndromes. Axis I includes the identification of the main psychiatric disorder for which the patient is being treated. The DSM-III-R describes the identified condition and provides a list of associated features for the psychiatrist to assess for each patient. These features include the patient's age at the onset of the disorder, the course of the disorder, the frequency of attacks, and any family pattern of the disorder.

Axis II is used to describe developmental and personality disorders that may not limit a patient's ability to function. Often, these conditions will have existed in the patient for several years or for the patient's entire life.

The purpose of Axis III is to indicate any current physical disorder or condition that is potentially relevant to the understanding or management of the patient's psychiatric disorder. For example, a medication for coronary artery disease may be a contraindication for certain medications that treat psychiatric disorders.

In Axis IV, the psychiatrist characterizes the patient's psychosocial stresses. The stresses may be both severe and chronic and may contribute to the development, worsening, or recurrence of the psychiatric disorder. The stresses may include problems in areas such as personal relationships, work, living circumstances, finances, physical illness or injury, or family factors. After characterizing the stresses the patient feels, the psychiatrist rates the severity of the stresses on the patient's life, using a scale in which one is the lowest level of severity and six is the highest level of severity.

Axis V is used to describe the Global Assessment of Function (GAF). In this axis, the psychiatrist indicates the patient's overall level of psychological, social, and occupational function both currently and for the past year. The GAF scale ranges from 1 to 100. Higher numbers indicate less functional impairment, and lower numbers indicate more functional impairment. According to the GAF scale, the ranges of impairment are

- None or Minimal—approximately 71 to 100
- Mild—approximately 61 to 70
- Moderate—approximately 51 to 60
- Serious—approximately 41 to 50
- Severe or Profound—40 or below

The GAF also lists symptoms for each level of the scale. These lists help the psychiatrist determine the patient's level of functional impairment and help standardize diagnoses for all patients.

The World Health Organization (WHO) has also developed a system for classifying medical conditions. The WHO system is called the International Statistical Classification of Diseases, Injuries, and Causes of Death. Because this classification is in its ninth edition, it is called ICD-9. The ICD-9 system can be used for a variety of purposes, including indexing medical records and billing patients. The DSM-III-R and the ICD-9 classification systems are very similar, but the DSM-III-R system is more descriptive and detailed.

A complete psychiatric evaluation includes (1) the patient's psychiatric history, (2) a mental status examination of the patient, (3) the doctor's diagnostic impression of the patient's condition using the DSM-III-R axis system, (4) the doctor's written discussion of the patient's symptoms and signs, (5) the doctor's prognosis of the patient's condition, and (6) the doctor's recommendation for treating the patient.

The doctor must obtain a great deal of information about the patient, including the patient's current psychiatric problem, the history of that problem, the patient's family, work, and school history, any medications the patient is currently taking, and the patient's history of alcohol or other drug abuse. The doctor must also gather information about the patient's personal and social history, including the patient's childhood, recreational activities, employ-ment, religious activities, and living arrangements.

A mental status examination of the patient is necessary in order for the doctor to complete the psychiatric evaluation. The mental status examination is roughly equivalent to a physical examination. During the mental status exam, the doctor pays particular attention to the patient's appearance, behavior, and speech. The doctor will also take note of the patient's perceptions, mood, judgment, and insight.

Usually, the doctor will be able make a diagnosis based on the results of the patient's psychiatric history and mental status exami-nation. However, the doctor may recommend that a patient undergo psychological testing to clarify or validate the diagnosis. In such a case, the doctor will refer the patient to a trained psychologist who then performs the psychological tests and sends the report back to the attending doctor.

A wide variety of therapies are currently available for the treat-ment of the broad range of psychiatric disorders. Three common treatment options are psychotherapy, drug therapy, and electro-convulsive therapy. **Psychotherapy** is a type of treatment that is designed to produce a response by mental, rather than by physical, effects. During psychotherapy, a licensed psychiatrist, psychologist, or social worker may use methods such as suggestion, persuasion, re-education, reassurance, support, analysis, or hypnosis to effect changes in the patient. **Drug therapy**, on the other hand, is a type of treatment in which a substance is administered to alter the physical, mental, or emotional status of a patient. Because drugs can be prescribed only by licensed medical doctors, psychiatrists, not psychologists or social workers, generally use this treatment. More-over, the treatment of mental disorders is often provided by both a psychiatrist and a psychologist or other mental health professional. These people may either work together as a team or may see the patient separately over a period of time. Frequently, the psychiatrist provides drug therapy and the other professional provides psycho-therapy. For many patients, this type of combination therapy is more effective than either drug therapy or psychotherapy alone. ***Electro-convulsive therapy (ECT),*** which is also called *electroshock therapy*, is a form of treatment in which the passage of an electric current through the patient's brain induces brain seizures. Typically, the physician administers a muscle relaxant to the patient prior to the treatment in order to minimize the convulsions to the body. Electro-convulsive therapy is most effective in the treatment of depression.

Psychiatric disorders traditionally have been described as being either organic or functional. ***Organic psychiatric disorders*** are those psychiatric conditions that are associated with the presence of definite brain pathology. The designation ***"organic brain syn-drome"*** is a general term for a group of psychological or behavioral manifestations that arise from a real or presumed physical cause, but without reference to a specific cause. These syndromes are charac-terized by at least one and usually several of the following manifesta-tions: delirium, dementia, impaired consciousness and perception, confusion, depression, disorientation, memory defects, abnormal emotions and behavior, anxiety, hallucinations, and delusions.

Functional psychiatric disorders are those psychiatric condi-tions that are not associated with the clear presence of brain pathology and that pertain to a feeling or a mental state. Psychiatrists are discovering that many psychiatric disorders that previously were thought to be purely "mental" actually result from biological and chemically transmitted abnormalities. The use of the organic/functional classification system, therefore, is becoming less and less common.

This section of the chapter will discuss some of the more common psychiatric disorders.

Anxiety

Anxiety is a feeling of apprehension, uncertainty, fear, unpleasant tension, fatigue, distress, or panic and can be characterized by excessive perspiration, tension headaches, sighing, labored breath-ing, loss of appetite, "butterflies in the stomach," rapid pulse, fainting, impotence, and hyperventilation. ***Hyperventilation*** is rapid or deep breathing in excess of that needed to maintain normal blood levels of oxygen and carbon dioxide. Anxiety can be a normal reaction to certain stimuli, a common manifestation of other psychi-atric disorders, or an independent psychiatric entity. A normal degree of anxiety is proportional to the triggering stimulus and promotes useful action, such as the response to an actual physical threat. Anxiety is excessive if it occurs without appropriate cause or if it is severe, persistent, and produces marked interference with normal daily activities. Under these circumstances, anxiety has a harmful effect. Drug therapy in the form of mild tranquilizers is often useful for relieving the symptoms of anxiety. The treatment of chronic anxiety typically is directed toward removing the stimulus of the attack and can involve psychotherapy, as well as drug therapy.

Depression

Depression consists of a dejected mood, psychomotor retardation, insomnia, weight loss, and, often, excessive feelings of guilt and is characterized by a loss of interest in customary activities, easy fatigability, loss of appetite, lack of interest in sex, obscure aches and pains, and feelings of despondency. Depression, like anxiety, may occur as a normal mood variant, as a symptom of another psychiatric or medical disorder, or as a primary disorder. For example, depression is a normal response to the death of a loved one, the presence of a serious illness, or some other significant misfortune. However, depression can become so excessive as to interfere with the patient's normal functioning. The difference between normal depression and that associated with serious psychiatric disorder is quantitative. **Mood disorders** are those psychiatric disorders that occur when the patient's emotions, typically sadness and happiness, are overly intense and last beyond the normal response to a stressful life event. Two common types of mood disorders are major depressive disorder and bipolar disorder.

Major depressive disorder, which is also called *unipolar mood disorder*, occurs as episodes of depression that are generally recurrent, but may affect the patient only once during the patient's lifetime. **Melancholia** refers to forms of major depressive disorder that are characterized by marked agitation, weight loss, pathologic guilt, morning insomnia, variations in mood and activity throughout the day, and the loss of the ability to experience pleasure.

Bipolar mood disorder commonly begins with a depressive episode and is characterized by at least one manic episode during the course of the illness. A **depressive episode** is a mental state characterized by marked dejection, withdrawal, despondency, slowed thinking and motor activity, and lack of self-confidence. A **manic episode** is a mental state characterized by extreme elation, overtalkativeness, extreme irritability, excitement, an unrestrained flow of ideas, and increased physical activity.

The various mood disorders are second only to anxiety reactions as the most common psychiatric illnesses and the sources of considerable morbidity. Bipolar disorder is less common than major depressive disorder. Major depressive disorders are about twice as common in women as in men, but bipolar disorder is equally common in males and females. The first attack of the manic episode of bipolar disorder usually occurs before age 30, but the first attack of major depressive disorder may occur at any age. Although the etiology of this illness is unknown, it may be seen in individuals who previously have demonstrated cyclic emotional swings from friendly, talkative periods to quiet, reserved periods. Recurrences of attacks of depression are common. The risk of suicide must be considered in all cases of depression.

Treatment of severe cases of depression may include psychotherapy, drug therapy, and/or electroconvulsive therapy. A number of relatively new drugs are now available for the treatment of depression. Each one has a different side-effect profile. Furthermore, one drug may effectively treat some patients, while another drug is more effective for other patients. Antidepressants are the drugs of choice in treating many patients who have severe depression.

Lithium carbonate is an extremely valuable drug that is effective in reducing the incidence of both manic and depressive episodes of bipolar disorder. This drug must be used under highly skilled medical supervision, because it has a wide range of potentially dangerous side effects and drug interactions. These side effects can include neurologic and renal symptoms, which can range from slight to life-threatening. Because the side effects are related to the level of the dosage of lithium carbonate, continued monitoring of the patient's lithium blood levels is necessary. Other medications, such as diuretics and antihypertensives, can affect the patient's lithium blood levels.

Electroconvulsive therapy may be needed for patients who have severe depression and are not responding to psychotherapy or drug therapy. Typically, antidepressant drug therapy is tried before ECT for several reasons. Drugs are easier to prescribe, are less controversial, are more readily accepted by patients, and cause less disruption of patients' lives. Nevertheless, in competent hands, ECT is safe and painless. Complications from ECT, such as dizziness, headache, confusion, and nausea, occur sometimes, but are less serious than the end result of an untreated severe depression. Most ECT patients do experience at least some short-term *amnesia*, which is memory loss, following the procedure. The memory loss is sometimes severe, but the "lost" memory often returns over time. For many patients, the amnesia is generally offset by the procedure's benefits to the patient's emotional and psychological health.

Psychosis

A *psychosis* is a psychiatric disorder that is characterized by gross impairment in the individual's ability to recognize reality. This impairment is evidenced by delusions, hallucinations, incoherent speech, or disorganized and agitated behavior without apparent awareness on the part of the individual of the incomprehensibility of his or her behavior. Genetic, environmental, and biochemical factors may play a role in psychoses.

Hallucination

A *hallucination* is a sensory perception for which there is no logical basis. Auditory hallucinations—hearing voices—are the most common type of hallucinations. Less common are hallucinations of vision, taste, smell, and touch. Hallucinations may occur during the patient's emergence from the effects of a general anesthetic or following periods of prolonged sleep deprivation, starvation, or isolation. Some drugs cause hallucinations. Hallucinations may also occur in association with psychiatric disorders. Treatment of a patient who is hallucinating depends in large part on the cause of the hallucinations. Overcoming the residual effects of the general anesthetic will end the episode of hallucination resulting from that stimulus. Providing sleep, food, and personal communication will effectively treat patients hallucinating from lack of these stimuli. Removal of the hallucinatory drug usually ends hallucinatory episodes that are drug-induced. Ending a hallucinatory episode that occurs as a result of a psychiatric disorder typically involves the treatment of the underlying disorder.

Delirium

Delirium is a dangerous, and sometimes fatal, psychiatric disturbance marked by (1) a reduced clarity of awareness of the environment, (2) the presence of hallucinations and other perceptual disturbances, (3) incoherent speech, and (4) disorientation. The clinical features of delirium usually develop quickly, fluctuate, and last only a short amount of time. Delirium may follow, or be seen in association with, head injury, seizures, high fevers, liver or kidney disease, hypertensive brain disease, other forms of organic brain disease, and alcoholic intoxication and withdrawal, in which case the disorder is called *delirium tremens*. Delirium requires therapy beyond that of any underlying disease. Treatment generally includes administration of large amounts of fluids. Alcohol delirium requires infusions of B-complex vitamins. If the patient has a fever, it should be brought down to at least 102.2 degrees Fahrenheit. Diazepam given intravenously will typically control severe agitation and tremulousness.

Dementia

Dementia is a general designation for mental deterioration characterized by a loss of intellectual abilities, such as memory, judgment, and abstract thinking, of sufficient degree to interfere with social or occupational functioning. Early symptoms of dementia often are poorly defined and may be unrecognizable. As the dementia progresses, the mental disorder becomes more apparent.

Endocrine and nutritional diseases, alcoholism, neoplasms, head trauma, and infection are common causes of dementia. If dementia results from a clearly defined episode of neurological disease, the condition may be acute, short-lived, and followed by recovery. In more than 80 percent of dementia patients, however, the disorder follows a progressive and irreversible downhill course and is untreatable. Dementia occurs predominantly in the elderly, and Alzheimer's disease is the most common cause of senile dementia. However, chronic dementia is not an automatic result of normal aging. Many causes of brain pathology, such as immunologic and hereditary mechanisms, can result in chronic dementia. Vascular disease of the brain, including any disorder that reduces the delivery of oxygen to the brain tissue, accounts for a significant number of cases of chronic dementia.

Dementia is a common problem. Approximately 12 percent of the United States population is over the age of 65, and about 11 percent of these individuals have some form of dementia. People who have chronic dementia occupy hospital and nursing home beds to a disproportionate degree and have decreased longevity. Treatment of acute dementia includes the withdrawal of known toxic drugs and minimal use of drugs that affect brain metabolism. Patients who have any type of dementia respond to treatment that allows them to exist in familiar surroundings with minimal variations in environmental stimuli, but that permits the patients to continue performing as many tasks as possible. Serious problems develop when these patients become aware of their difficulties in concentrating and maintaining a realistic focus. A dementia patient's family will typically receive counseling on encouraging the patient to participate in activities that promote the patient's sense of accomplishment. As the disorder progresses, drug therapy with haloperidol as needed will usually calm the patient without causing excessive drowsiness. Hospitalization or institutionalization may be necessary for patients who have advanced dementia.

Schizophrenic Disorders

Schizophrenic disorders are a group of severe emotional illnesses that are characterized by bizarre and inappropriate behavior and by a regression from a prior level of functioning in such areas as work, social relations, and self-care. Withdrawal, lack of insight, personality disorganization, thought disturbances, and intellectual impairment are common manifestations of schizophrenic disorders. At the height of the active phase of a schizophrenic disorder, the patient suffers from delusions and hallucinations. The affected person may break with reality or be unable to evaluate reality effectively.

Schizophrenic disorders are the most common mental illnesses in which patients show a disturbed sense of reality. Patients who have schizophrenia comprise over one-half of all patients in psychiatric hospitals, and about 25 percent of new admissions to psychiatric hospitals are patients who have a schizophrenic disorder. The causes of schizophrenic disorders are unknown, but hereditary, biochemical, and endocrine factors may contribute. The first symptoms of a schizophrenic disorder usually appear during the patient's adolescence or early adulthood, but can begin in middle or late adult life.

Catatonic schizophrenia is marked by excessive and sometimes violent motor activity and excitement and by generalized motor inhibition. This type of schizophrenic disorder is characterized by alternating mute, passive, stuporous phases and phases of repetitive talking and frenzied, aimless activity. The catatonic patient may experience incoherence, marked loosening of associations, or grossly disorganized or inappropriate behavior.

Patients who have paranoid schizophrenia may have fragmentary delusions or hallucinations and feelings of persecution.

Treatment of all types of schizophrenia with drugs and psychiatric counseling frequently will produce some improvement. Symptoms may begin to subside promptly, or they may subside over the course of a few months. Relapses of schizophrenic attacks are common. The ultimate prognosis depends on the severity of the disease, the duration of the first attack, the adequacy of continued treatment, and the stresses to which the individual is exposed.

Delusional Disorders

A *delusion* is a false belief that cannot be changed by reasonable contradictory evidence. Delusions occur in association with the psychoses, alcohol and other drug intoxication, and cerebral arteriosclerosis. Delusions may take several forms, including (1) feelings of persecution or guilt, (2) thoughts that the individual has an incurable disease, or (3) the belief that the person is an important religious or historic figure or has great power or enormous wealth. *Delusional disorders* are conditions that are characterized by the presence of a persistent false belief that does not result from another mental disorder. Patients who have delusions experience varying amounts of impairment. Some of these patients are able to carry out basic daily activities. A delusional patient's intellectual capability typically is not affected by the disorder, and the patient's behavior is normal in most respects. The various manifestations of delusional disorders overlap without clear distinctions. An *erotomanic delusion* is the false belief that a person is loved by another person. This delusion generally involves romantic love rather than sexual attraction. *Grandiose delusions* involve a person's being convinced that he or she possess some great talent or insight. A *jealous delusion* is present when a person is convinced without due cause that a spouse or lover is unfaithful. A person who has a *persecutory delusion*, which is the most common type of delusion, may feel conspired against, spied upon, poisoned, cheated, followed, obstructed, and/or harassed. *Somatic delusions* may take several forms, but they generally are characterized by the false belief that certain parts of the patient's body are, contrary to all evidence, misshapen, ugly, or nonfunctioning.

Nonpsychotic Psychiatric Disorders

Nonpsychotic psychiatric disorders are conditions that have no known organic origin and have symptoms that are distressing to the affected person and are recognized by that person as being unacceptable. A person who has this type of disorder is in contact with reality, does not show derangement of personality, and does not exhibit delusions and hallucinations. The affected person's behavior usually does not grossly violate social norms, although the disorder may affect the person's relationship to the environment and may impair the person's functioning to some degree.

Adjustment Disorders

Most people respond at times to life's difficult and frustrating situations with symptoms that can be called "neurotic." An *adjustment disorder* is a type of nonpsychotic psychiatric disorder that is characterized by an exaggeration of these neurotic symptoms in response to a real or perceived stressful event. The principal manifestations of adjustment disorder include excessive anxiety and depression.

The degree of departure from normal indicates the severity of the patient's adjustment disorder. A mild adjustment disorder is of short duration, causes little or no interference with the patient's customary activities, and responds to reassurance or simple medications. A severe adjustment disorder interferes significantly with the affected person's normal activities. It may require hospitalization and can lead to, and be associated with, other psychiatric conditions. The symptoms of a severe adjustment disorder are difficult to control. Intensive and usually prolonged psychotherapy is required to treat a patient who has a severe adjustment disorder. Moderate adjustment disorders fall somewhere between the two extremes in duration of symptoms, interference with the patient's activities, and requirements for treatment.

Obsessive-Compulsive Disorder

Obsessions are recurrent unwanted thoughts that intrude upon the individual's consciousness. Compulsions are repetitive acts that the individual feels he or she must perform, no matter how purposeless the acts are. *Obsessive-compulsive disorder*, therefore, is a nonpsychotic disorder characterized by the presence of recurrent ideas and fantasies and repetitive impulses or actions that the patient recognizes as being irrational and toward which the patient feels an inner resistance. Anxiety is created by these thoughts and acts, because the individual is unable to exert any voluntary control over them.

Some individuals have obsessive-compulsive personalities. These individuals typically are disciplined, conscientious, and capable of high achievement. They have a sense of urgency to get things accomplished. As perfectionists, their habits are stereotyped, and they have orderly but inflexible minds. Obsessive-compulsives generally have difficulty relaxing. Obsessive-compulsive disorder is often classified as a personality disorder.

Phobias

A *phobia* is a nonpsychotic disorder characterized by irrational or exaggerated fears of objects, situations, or bodily functions. Typically, the cause of the fear is neither inherently dangerous nor the appropriate target of the associated anxiety, which may be either acute or chronic. Phobias tend to arise in patients who have a family history of anxiety disorders, and the anxiety itself is a reaction that is manifested by excessive activity of the autonomic nervous system. Patients who have phobias generally associate the increasing anxiety they feel with a specific external object or situation, called a phobic symbol, which may or may not have actually caused the original anxiety attack. In fact, sometimes the phobic symbol is determined by the patient's chance exposure to the object or situation at the time of the initial attack. Some common phobias include *agoraphobia*, which is the fear of open, public places or of situations in which crowds are likely to be found; *claustrophobia*, which is the fear of very small or closed spaces; and *acrophobia*, which is the fear of heights. Agoraphobia is the most common phobia, and it often begins with a panic attack in a public place. The fear that a subsequent attack may occur then causes these patients to avoid public places and to confine themselves to their homes or to a limited number of "safe" environments. Many agoraphobic patients can cope with being in public with minimal discomfort only in the presence of another specific person with whom the patient has a close relationship.

Patients who have phobias generally protect themselves from experiencing the associated anxiety by avoiding the stimulus that triggers the attack. This avoidance can lead to a disabling constriction of the patient's daily life and can keep the patient from functioning normally in society. Agoraphobia in particular can be severely disabling and, unlike most other phobias, is not likely to be characterized by periods of significant remission.

Phobias affect females more often than males and typically begin in early adulthood. Most phobias are chronic, but can be treated successfully. The treatment of a phobia commonly involves psychotherapy to force the patient to confront the fear and often also includes drug therapy with a minor tranquilizer or antidepressant to reduce the intensity of the anticipated anxiety.

"Nervous Breakdown"

The term *"nervous breakdown"* is loosely used by the general public but has no precise medical definition. The term is frequently used as a label for an acute episode of schizophrenia or another major disorder or as a substitute for a nonpsychotic disorder of at least moderate severity. The term is also used to designate episodes in which a person's emotional reserves are completely exhausted, especially from continuous stress. Rest, recreation, and removal of the source of the stress usually provide relief from this type of exhaustion.

Personality Disorders

Personality disorders are a wide group of behavior patterns that are acceptable to the affected individuals, but that produce conflict with others. The severity of these conditions ranges from eccentric behavior to borderline psychotic states. Personality disorders are characterized by relatively fixed reactions to some form of distress. Although some behavioral patterns are transient reactions to severe, acute stress, personality disorders have patterns that last for the affected person's lifetime. These personality disorder patterns represent chronic reactions to normal, mild stress encountered daily. Depending on the amount of conflict with others, the symptoms of personality disorders may or may not interfere with the affected person's work. The causes of personality disorders are not known, but these patterns may result from early experiences and conditioning. The personality disorders discussed below are not always easy to distinguish from each other. Many of the characteristics of these disorders overlap. A diagnosis depends on the predominant manifestations the patient is exhibiting.

Individuals who have a **schizoid personality disorder** are timid, aloof, introverted, and self-conscious. Schizoids avoid close relationships and are loners who choose solitary activity. They are not able to express their feelings. Schizoids typically are ambitious, meticulous, and perfectionist. A **hysterical personality disorder** is characterized by shifting emotions, susceptibility to suggestion, impulsiveness, and self-absorption. Overtly, hysterics are theatrical, dramatic, excitable, and their behavior is designed to gain attention. Emotionally, hysterics are unstable and frequently over-react to minor problems or situations. An **antisocial personality disorder**, which is also known as a *psychopathic personality disorder* or a *sociopathic personality disorder*, is characterized by an individual's lack of basic socialization, behavior that results in repeated conflict with society, and the inability to be loyal to individuals, groups, or social codes. Individuals who have an antisocial personality disorder have little foresight, a low tolerance for frustration, a tendency to blame others for inappropriate behavior, and a lack of a sense of guilt. They lack discipline and the ability to learn from experience, and they are callous. Punishment has little or no effect on people who have antisocial personality disorder.

Individuals who have a **passive-dependent personality disorder** avoid responsibility, lack self-reliance, and appear helpless. Passive-dependents find decision-making an almost insurmountably difficult task that they will maneuver to avoid. People who have this personality type are emotionally dependent on others and have a total lack of aggressiveness. On the other hand, a **passive-aggressive personality disorder**, as its name implies, is characterized by aggression that is exhibited passively. For example, a person who is passive-aggressive will show displeasure, get attention, or try to obtain power over a situation by procrastinating, being inefficient, behaving stubbornly, pouting, and being sullen. Passive-aggressives show a resistance to authority.

A *paranoid personality disorder* is characterized by hypersensitivity to, and unwarranted suspicion of, the words and behaviors of others. *Paranoia*, or *paranoid ideation*, is characterized by an individual's believing that someone is intent on causing him or her harm. Mild forms of paranoia occur in many individuals. For example, some people dislike accepting the responsibility for their failures. These people prefer to place the blame for their failures on a parent, business associate, authority figure, employer, or elected official. The distinction between the paranoia seen occasionally in normal individuals and that present in association with a serious psychiatric illness is quantitative. Psychiatrically significant paranoia may be precipitated by stressful situations and is characterized by excessive rigidity, hostility, anxiety, insecurity, mistrust of others, and seclusiveness. Paranoids react poorly to criticism and are excessively envious and jealous of other people. People who have this personality disorder blame others for their misfortunes and show hostility to and belittle the efforts of other people. Patients who have paranoia have an excessive sense of self-importance, which is manifested in the belief that unrelated events and communications are aimed at them.

The course of these personality disorders is often chronic, but, as some patients mature, they outgrow their disorders. Many people who have these problems never obtain psychiatric treatment. Treatment, when it is obtained, is generally painfully slow and prolonged, because individuals often fail to recognize the full effect of a personality trait on their lives. Furthermore, the results of treatment, because they occur over a relatively long period of time, are often difficult to assess.

Eating Disorders

Some types of *eating disorders* are psychiatric disorders that are characterized by a disturbed sense of body image and a morbid fear of obesity. These disorders are manifested by abnormal patterns of food consumption and self-induced, marked weight loss. Eating disorders affect females far more often than males and typically have their onset in adolescence. Many patients come from middle and upper socioeconomic families and, even before the illness, are described as being very meticulous, compulsive, intelligent, and concerned with high achievement and success. Typically, the first indications of an eating disorder are (1) the patient's overly intense concern with obesity, although only about 30 percent of these patients are obese at the onset of the illness, and (2) the beginning of noticeably reduced food intake. Most patients who have an eating disorder deny the existence of the illness and continue to be preoccupied with their weight, even after they have become emaciated. The illness is usually brought to the attention of a physician by the patient's family or by the patient's complaints of constipation, bloating, or abdominal distress. Sometimes, a physician will notice the eating disorder when the patient is examined for some other illness. The two most common types of eating disorders are anorexia nervosa and bulimia.

Anorexia nervosa is a psychologic and physiologic condition that is characterized by a severe and prolonged refusal to eat. "Anorexia" means lack of appetite, but most anorectics retain their appetites, and so "anorexia nervosa" is actually a misnomer. An anorectic is preoccupied with food, as indicated by the patient's (1) intense study of diets and calories, (2) hoarding, concealing, and wasting food, (3) collecting recipes, and (4) preparing elaborate meals for others. Despite the anorectic's preoccupation with food, the patient does not eat and becomes emaciated.

The physical problems associated with anorexia nervosa include amenorrhea in females and impotence in males, bradycardia, low blood pressure, low body temperature, changes in hair patterns and textures, dehydration, and edema. Furthermore, an anorectic's heart usually undergoes a decrease in muscle mass, chamber size, and output. Sudden death as a result of a prolonged case of anorexia nervosa is not uncommon and is associated with ventricular tachyarrhythmias.

Bulimia is a condition that is characterized by episodes of rapidly eating abnormally large amounts of food. Typically, these episodes are followed by self-induced vomiting and/or the use of laxatives and diuretics. The alternating episodes of overeating and forced expulsion of food characterize *binge-purge behavior*. The American Psychiatric Association recognizes bulimia nervosa as a disorder that is separate from, but which may coexist with, anorexia nervosa. *Bulimia nervosa* is a psychologic and physiologic condition that is characterized by recurrent episodes of binge eating, a feeling of the loss of control over eating, self-induced vomiting, the use of laxatives and/or diuretics, or intensive dieting or fasting. Some bulimics follow an eating binge with compulsive strenuous exercise. Bulimics typically express intense concern about weight gain and experience wide fluctuations in weight, but rarely become emaciated. These patients also tend to be more aware of and feel guilty about their behavior than do anorectics.

The binge-purge behavior associated with bulimia can cause several physical problems, including those associated with anorexia nervosa. Binge eating can also lead to acute dilation, and sometimes rupture, of the stomach. Induced vomiting can result in the erosion of the patient's dental enamel, inflammation of the parotid gland, esophagitis, and esophageal rupture. The episodes of forced expulsion of food can also cause *hypokalemia*, which is an abnormally low concentration of potassium in the blood. Hypokalemia is characterized by gastrointestinal disorders, EKG abnormalities, renal disease, and neuromuscular disorders ranging from general weakness to paralysis.

The treatment of an eating disorder usually involves two distinct phases: (1) short-term therapy to deal with the physiologic affects of the disorder and (2) long-term therapy to deal with the psychologic aspects of the disorder. The short-term therapy attempts to restore the patient's body weight and to save the patient's life, and often involves hospitalization, particularly for anorectics. The long-term therapy attempts to solve the patient's underlying psychiatric problems, and it may involve drug therapy for depression, family counseling, and behavioral, as well as other types of individual, psychotherapy.

DISORDERS ASSOCIATED WITH ABNORMAL BRAIN FUNCTION

This last section of the chapter will address disorders, such as mental retardation and learning disabilities, that are associated with abnormal brain function and that do not fall into any of the psychiatric disorder categories.

Mental Retardation

Mental retardation is a condition characterized by significantly subaverage intelligence present from birth or early infancy. Intelligence is a function of the cerebrum and is measured in performance tests by the intelligence quotient (IQ). In the absence of marked cultural differences, which may distort test results, people who have IQs around 100 are considered average in intelligence. An IQ of 70 or below represents mental retardation, which occurs nearly twice as often among males as it does among females. The disorder is associated with impairments in *adaptive behavior*, which is the degree of success with which an individual meets the accepted standards of social responsibility and personal independence.

Mental retardation is commonly classified into four degrees, based on IQ levels:

- Mild retardation: IQ in the 50 to 70 range. Approximately 85 percent of the mentally retarded population is mildly retarded. People who are mildly retarded are educable and may attain fourth grade to sixth grade reading skills. Most adults who are mildly retarded are able to be self-supporting and can live without institutionalization.
- Moderate retardation: IQ in the 35 to 49 range. Approximately ten percent of the mentally retarded population is moderately retarded. People who are moderately retarded are trainable, but have obvious language and motor delays. Many of these people are able to work, but they require sheltered employment and supervised or assisted living arrangements.
- Severe retardation: IQ in the 20 to 34 range. Approximately four percent of the mentally retarded population is severely retarded. People who are severely retarded can be trained to perform some simple tasks, and may be able to communicate using sign language and a few word sounds.
- Profound retardation: IQ below 20. Approximately one percent of the mentally retarded population is profoundly retarded. People who are profoundly retarded usually do not learn to walk and have minimal language skills.

Retarded individuals may have physical defects of a medical, dental, surgical, orthopedic, or cosmetic nature. They may have emotional problems and may require some sheltering from the pressures and stresses of daily living if deep psychiatric problems are to be avoided.

The cause of an individual's mental retardation often is unknown. The major causes of this disorder include hereditary factors, problems during embryonic development, problems during the mother's pregnancy, physical disorders during the individual's childhood, and environmental influences upon the individual, such as deprivation of affection. A large number of cases of mental retardation occur through heredity. Chromosomal abnormalities and metabolic disturbances are the most common hereditary causes of mental retardation.

The level of intellectual impairment of the nonhereditary causes of mental retardation usually is mild. Figure 16–1 provides a brief classification of some of the nonhereditary causes of mental retardation.

Figure 16–1.
Nonhereditary Causes of Mental Retardation.

Cause	Example of Disorder
Maternal illness	Diabetes mellitus or alcoholism during pregnancy
Prenatal disorder	
Medical	Mother has rubella during the first trimester
Obstetrical	Mother has eclampsia
Placental	Abnormality in the functioning of the placenta
Disorder of labor	Prolonged labor, difficult delivery
Illness in the newborn	Erythroblastosis fetalis
Physical disorders in childhood	Trauma, lead poisoning
Environmental influences	Deprivation of food or affection

Learning Disabilities

A *learning disability* is a condition that is characterized by language problems, deficiencies in short-term memory, disordered sequencing of events in time or objects in space, or other subtle distortions in the way in which images and thoughts are processed by the brain. A common manifestation of a learning disability is a subnormal educational performance that cannot be attributed to gross physical handicaps, mental retardation, or an unstable emotional environment. The determination that a person has a learning disability involves the use of IQ testing and measurements of achievement in the areas of reading, spelling, writing, and arithmetic. Reading is the area most commonly affected by learning disabilities. Some people will perform poorly on one achievement test and will perform well on another. For example, it is not unusual for a person who has a language problem to perform well in arithmetic.

Providing help for a person who has a learning disability is difficult and involves a multidisciplinary approach utilizing the combined skills of family, psychiatrists or psychologists, neurologists, and educators. In recent years, progressive school systems have developed resources to identify and test children who have learning disabilities. Two of the most common learning disabilities are attention deficit disorder and dyslexia.

Attention Deficit Disorder

Attention deficit disorder (ADD) is a condition characterized by developmentally inappropriate impulsivity and inattention. *Impulsivity* is characterized by the tendency to act before thinking, difficulty taking turns, problems organizing work, and constant shifting from one activity to another. *Inattention* is characterized by the failure to finish tasks once started, easy distractibility, seeming lack of attention, and difficulty concentrating on tasks that require sustained attention. ADD may or may not include hyperactivity. A *hyperactive*, or *hyperkinetic*, person is typically overactive, restless, and easily distractible. Although most parents describe their children as being "constantly in motion" at various times, a truly hyperactive child's overactivity interferes with the child's normal living and learning and is disruptive to the lives of those living with the child. Some researchers feel that hyperactivity results from *minimal brain damage (MBD),* a condition in which the brain damage is too slight to be measured or identified clinically. When ADD includes hyperactivity, the condition is known as *attention deficit hyperactive disorder (ADHD).*

The cause of ADD is not known. Although the onset of ADD typically occurs between the ages of three and seven, referral to a physician usually occurs when the child is between the ages of eight and ten. The treatment of ADD is difficult. Drugs, such as Ritalin or Dexedrine, help to control some ADD patients' behavior so that the patients can work on improving other functions. However, not all ADD patients show an improvement with these drugs. Furthermore, no method of predicting which patients will benefit from these drugs or how long therapy will be needed currently exists. Role-playing, self-monitoring, and *behavior modification*, which is the rewarding of desirable activity and the discouraging of disruptive activity, and other behavioral and cognitive therapies may be useful alone or in conjunction with drug therapy in treating ADD. Research indicates that many children diagnosed as having ADD do not grow out of their difficulties. Later problems in adolescence and adulthood may be related to academic failure, low self-esteem, and difficulty learning socially appropriate behavior. However, many people who have ADD learn coping skills so that they can function normally in society as adolescents and adults.

Dyslexia

Dyslexia is a group of conditions of unknown origin in which a disparity exists between a person's apparent intellectual potential and that person's ability to read, and often, to spell. The person's inability to read may not affect achievement in other academic areas, such as arithmetic or science. The incidence of dyslexia is higher among males than among females, and the disorder crosses all socioeconomic boundaries. Dyslexics rarely read for pleasure and have difficulty reading aloud. They often experience confusion in the way they perceive letters of the alphabet, and this confusion manifests in several ways. Dyslexics typically

- try to read from right to left, rather than from left to right
- cannot see, and sometimes cannot hear, similarities or differences in letters or words
- lack the ability to "sound out" the pronunciation of unfamiliar words
- reverse letters or words when attempting to read or write
- omit words or lose the place on the page when attempting to read
- have trouble with spatial relationships, such as above, below, in front of, and behind
- are unable to follow a series of oral instructions
- display a better-than-normal ability to mirror-read and mirror-write

Dyslexic children almost always display symptoms of frustration and low self-esteem. A child who has undiagnosed dyslexia is likely to be considered "stupid and lazy." Furthermore, the effects of the dyslexia on the child's learning and school performance can lead to behavioral problems, such as overaggressiveness, self-imposed isolation, and social withdrawal.

Treatment of dyslexia generally involves focused, individualized educational efforts, because no method of correcting perceptual deficits is known. Many programs incorporate exercises that are designed to improve the dyslexic's abilities in problem areas with exercises that are more enjoyable. This type of combination program attempts to balance the dyslexic's educational needs with the individual's emotional needs. Many dyslexic children grow out of their perception deficits or learn methods of coping with the disorder. Other dyslexics, however, never overcome their learning disorder and, thus, do not achieve their intellectual potential.

Substance Abuse

Substance abuse is the use of alcohol and other drugs and chemicals in a manner that may predictably cause harm to the user. Substance abuse is a significant public health problem representing potential morbidity and mortality to the individual and tremendous physical and financial strains on the health care system. Some of the most frequently abused substances include

- alcohol
- cocaine (powder or crystal forms)
- amphetamines
- sedatives
- marijuana
- morphine
- LSD and PCP
- nicotine (tobacco)
- caffeine

Substance abuse problems are not confined to instances of illegal use and may arise in circumstances in which the use is legal or within existing medical practice. For example, most people are dependent to some degree on one or more drugs. Many people use coffee, tea, or tobacco, but do not consider themselves dependent on the drugs, which are usually stimulants, such as the caffeine or nicotine, that are present in these products. Moreover, many proprietary, or so-called "over-the-counter" drugs, such as antihistamines, aspirin, cough syrups, vitamins, cold capsules, antacids, decongestants, mouth washes, throat lozenges, and pain relievers are used to excess. Because so many drugs are consumed, drug-related problems inevitably occur. These problems may be as mild as a minor skin reaction and as severe as death.

This chapter will review some of the problems associated with the abuse of alcohol and the abuse and misuse of other substances. It is beyond the scope of this book to cover all medical and social aspects of substance abuse and misuse, to discuss all drugs that may produce harmful effects, or to deal in any depth with treatment, because treatment often must be multidisciplinary and individualized.

ALCOHOL ABUSE

Alcohol is a drug, and its excessive use can be either acute or chronic. The acute form of alcohol abuse is known as acute alcoholic intoxication, and the chronic form of alcohol abuse is known as alcoholism.

Acute Alcohol Intoxication

Alcohol intoxication, which is also known as *drunkenness*, is a condition of being drunk after ingesting alcohol and results from the rapid absorption into the bloodstream of a large quantity of alcohol. The manifestations of acute intoxication depend on several factors: (1) the level of the alcohol concentration in the individual's blood, (2) the rate at which this level is reached, and (3) the length of time during which this level is maintained. A number of factors influence the body's rate of absorption of alcohol. For example, if the individual has eaten recently before or during the time of ingesting alcohol, the individual will probably take longer to be affected by the alcohol. Furthermore, if the individual is sick, the individual's tolerance of alcohol will probably be lower than normal. In addition, the presence of other drugs in the individual's body can affect the individual's alcohol tolerance levels. Moreover, wide variations among individuals' tolerance levels influence the effects of alcohol on a given person at any blood level.

The diagnosis of acute alcoholic intoxication depends on the individual's history of alcohol consumption, the presence of typical symptoms and signs of intoxication, and the individual's blood alcohol level. However, the odor of alcohol on the breath, coupled with slurred speech, a staggering gait, and other neurological signs do not necessarily indicate alcoholic intoxication. For example, diabetic acidosis, uremia, head injury, and other causes of cerebral impairment can produce a clinical picture that is similar to acute intoxication. Blood tests should be performed in order to identify alcohol intoxication with certainty.

Scientists have not established the minimum blood alcohol level at which an individual will have no apparent effect from alcohol ingestion. However, individuals who have a blood alcohol level of less than 50 milligram (mg) percent, which is also expressed as 0.05 percent, probably will not show any alcohol-related manifestations. Many individuals whose blood alcohol concentration is between 50 and 100 mg percent, or 0.05 to 0.10 percent, will show behavioral changes. Furthermore, all persons show some loss of normal clarity of intellect and muscle control when their blood alcohol concentration levels exceed 150 mg percent, or 0.15 percent.

Figure 17–1 lists some manifestations of acute alcoholic intoxication that are commonly associated with various ranges of blood alcohol levels.

Figure 17–1.
Blood Alcohol Levels and Symptoms.

| Blood Alcohol Levels | | Symptoms | |
Milligrams	Percent	Sporadic Drinkers	Chronic Drinkers
0–50	0–0.05	None	None
50–100	0.05–0.10	Euphoria, gregariousness, incoordination	Minimal or no effect
100–200	0.10–0.20	Slurred speech, exaggerated incoordination, mood swings, drowsiness, nausea	Incoordination, euphoria
200–300	0.20–0.30	Lethargy, combativeness, stupor, incoherent speech, vomiting	Mild emotional and motor changes
300–000	0.30–0.40	Coma	Drowsiness
>400	>0.40	Respiratory problems, depression, death	Lethargy, stupor, coma

Compared to a person who has no alcohol in his or her blood, a person driving a car is 10 times more likely to be involved in an automobile accident when the person's blood alcohol level reaches 100 mg percent and is over 50 times more likely to be involved in an automobile accident when the blood alcohol level reaches 150 mg percent.

Alcoholism

Alcoholism is a chronic illness in which the excessive use of alcohol impairs or interferes with the individual's physical health, social interactions, job performance, and ability to cope with emotions and feelings. People who have this chronic illness are known as *alcoholics*, and they have a pathologic dependence on alcohol. The definition of alcoholism does not include a reference to the quantity of alcohol consumed or the blood level of alcohol. In the latter stages of alcoholism, for example, the alcoholic may require relatively little alcohol to achieve intoxication because of a decreased physiological tolerance to alcohol. An alcoholic's lifespan is shortened on the average by 15 years. Excess mortality among alcoholics is present in all major causes of death, including heart disease, cancer, accidents, and suicide. Doctors and other medical personnel traditionally have been reluctant to cite alcoholism as a cause of death. Therefore, many alcohol-related deaths have not been reported as such.

Physical Effects of Excessive Use of Alcohol

Alcohol affects many body systems and is capable of damaging various organs. This damage is approximately proportional in severity to the amount of alcohol consumed and the amount of time over which it was consumed. The physical effects of alcoholism include malnutrition, liver damage, gastrointestinal disorders, nervous system damage, cardiovascular disease, hematologic abnormalities, and increased risk of cancer.

Malnutrition is common among alcoholics. A typical drink that contains alcohol provides between 70 and 1000 calories from alcohol and carbohydrates. Ten drinks a day will yield many calories, but these calories do not provide any nutrients, such as protein, vitamins, and minerals. In addition, alcohol interferes with the body's ability to absorb vitamins, especially the B vitamins. These nutritional deficiencies lead to neurological and hematological diseases.

Furthermore, alcohol is toxic to liver cells, even if the nutritional status of the individual is good. In the presence of inadequate nutrition, the liver cell damage is more severe. In addition, a steady drinker is more prone to develop liver damage than is a spree drinker.

Liver disease progresses in several stages. The first stage is a fatty liver and is characterized by hepatomegaly, which results from an increased accumulation of fat in the liver cells. Only in rare instances does a fatty liver cause significant abnormalities in liver function tests. In fact, an individual who has a fatty liver may have no symptoms referable to the liver enlargement. This early stage of liver disease is completely reversible. Abstinence from alcohol and the restoration of an appropriately nutritious diet allow the liver to lose its fatty infiltrations and to return to its normal size in about six weeks. The next stage of liver disease is known as alcoholic hepatitis. *Alcoholic hepatitis*, which is considered a precursor of cirrhosis, is characterized by inflammation of liver tissue, the destruction of liver cells, hepatomegaly, and slight jaundice secondary to alcohol ingestion. Alcoholic hepatitis patients typically complain of appetite loss, weakness, and abdominal pain. Liver function test results of alcoholic hepatitis patients generally are elevated. With proper care, this stage of liver disease also is reversible. Cirrhosis, which is a condition in which the liver is shrunken, scarred, and fibrotic as a result of repeated bouts of inflammation, is a late and irreversible stage of liver disease. Cirrhosis develops in about ten percent of heavy drinkers. A liver biopsy will produce a definitive diagnosis and will assist in determining the patient's prognosis.

Esophageal varices sometimes develop in patients who have had cirrhosis for many months when the patient's cirrhotic liver partially obstructs the normal venous blood return to the heart, causing a "back-up" of blood in the venous system. This back-up of blood, in turn, causes the esophageal veins to dilate and causes their walls to become thin as a result of carrying an increased blood volume under greater pressure. Some esophageal varices rupture. A slow leak from a very small rupture of an esophageal varix can produce an anemia, and a massive hemorrhage from a large rupture can result in death.

Alcoholic anemia may also arise from vitamin B-complex deficiency resulting from inadequate nutrition and iron deficiency resulting from gastrointestinal bleeding. Other hematologic disorders associated with alcoholism are a decrease in platelet production and a lowered white blood cell count. The lowered white blood cell count and the toxic effect of the alcohol on the white blood cells decrease the body's resistance to infection. Alcoholics also experience a higher incidence of peptic ulcer, esophagitis, gastritis, and pancreatitis than do nonalcoholics. Although pancreatitis is not a common disorder, it often arises in association with alcohol abuse. Pancreatitis is a very serious condition and may be fatal.

Alcoholism generally causes damage to the alcoholic's brain and peripheral nerves. Among the nervous system effects arising from alcoholism are

- *Korsakoff's syndrome*, which is characterized by rapid mental deterioration
- *Wernicke's encephalopathy*, which is characterized by the failure of muscular coordination, double vision, the paralysis of eye movements, mental deterioration, forgetfulness, and delirium tremens
- degeneration of the part of the brain controlling stance and balance
- loss of sensation, weakness, muscle wasting, and pain and burning in the lower extremities

In addition, excessive use of alcohol increases the risk of several diseases of the heart and vascular system. Hypertension and atrial and ventricular arrhythmias are prominent features of alcohol-related cardiovascular disease, and heavy drinkers are three times more likely to die of stroke than are nondrinkers. Moreover, large amounts of alcohol can cause a disease known as *alcoholic cardiomyopathy*, which is characterized by dilation of the heart chambers. If insufficiency of the valves occurs, congestive heart failure may result.

Furthermore, alcoholism is recognized as a risk factor for certain malignancies. Alcoholics develop cancer ten times more frequently than the general population does. The sites of the greatest increase of cancer risk include the head and neck, esophagus, and cardia of the stomach.

A significant minority of chronic alcoholic men develop irreversible testicular atrophy, shrinkage of the semen-producing and -conveying tubules, and loss of sperm cells. Alcoholic women may experience amenorrhea, decreased ovarian size, infertility, and miscarriage. Moreover, heavy drinking can lead to fetal alcohol syndrome. *Fetal alcohol syndrome (FAS)* is a syndrome in which abnormal prenatal cell growth occurs in infants born to women who were chronically alcoholic during pregnancy. FAS babies often have congenital abnormalities and are mentally retarded. Examples of these congenital abnormalities are abnormally small eyes, stunted growth, incomplete development of facial structures, cardiac defects, inflexible joint muscles, and abnormally small heads. However, no single characteristic is distinctive to FAS and exclusive of other conditions. The number of expressed abnormalities in the infant and the severity of those abnormalities depend upon the degree of the mother's alcohol abuse during the pregnancy.

Addiction to Alcohol

Dependence on a substance can be psychological and/or physical. *Psychological dependence*, which is also called *habituation*, is a compulsion to continue use of the substance despite known adverse consequences. Drugs that induce psychological dependence are said to be habit-forming. *Physical dependence*, which is also called *addiction*, is characterized by (1) the presence of withdrawal symptoms when the substance is withheld and (2) tolerance to the effects of the substance. Withdrawal symptoms usually exist in the form of a group of characteristic symptoms that are specific for each substance and are seen upon abrupt cessation of the use of the substance. Tolerance refers to the fact that repeated administrations of a substance cause the effect of the substance to decline, so that the user must increase the dosage of the drug on repeated administrations in order to achieve the same effect that the drug produced initially. All addictive drugs are habit-forming, but not all habit-forming drugs are addictive.

In alcoholics, the withdrawal syndrome occurs when the individual's alcohol intake is interrupted or decreased without substitution of other sedation. The severity of the withdrawal symptoms varies with both the intensity and the duration of the preceding alcohol exposure. The primary symptoms of mild withdrawal reactions are tremor, sleeplessness, and irritability. These symptoms typically appear within a few hours after alcohol withdrawal and usually disappear within 48 hours. In severe withdrawal reactions, seizures and delirium tremens may also occur. Delirium tremens (DTs), which were discussed in Chapter 16, *Psychiatric and Brain Function Disorders*, commonly begin two to three days after alcohol withdrawal and are characterized by weakness, sweating, confusion, disorientation, irritability, vivid and frightening visual hallucinations, anxiety, and depression. Complications of DTs, including cardiac dysfunction and infections, may lead to death.

Evidence of tolerance to the effects of alcohol is another important diagnostic criterion of alcohol addiction. An individual has developed alcohol tolerance if he or she formerly would show signs of acute intoxication at blood alcohol levels of 100 mg percent, but no longer shows signs of acute intoxication at blood levels of 150 mg percent or higher. However, late in the course of alcoholism, tolerance to the substance decreases, so that signs of intoxication appear at much lower blood alcohol levels.

Certain patterns of drinking are distinctly nonsocial and help to distinguish the alcoholic from the social drinker. An alcoholic (1) uses alcohol as "medicine," (2) is totally preoccupied with the constant use of alcohol, (3) often conceals the supply and consumption of alcohol,

(4) drinks alone, (5) gulps drinks containing alcohol, and (6) frequently drinks in the morning. The National Council on Alcoholism and Drug Dependence, Inc. has established certain criteria for the diagnosis of alcoholism. Figure 17–2 presents these criteria in an abbreviated form. The diagnosis of alcoholism is established when one of the "manifestations clearly associated with alcoholism" in section I of Figure 17–2 is present. The presence of several of the criteria in sections II or III, including at least one item from the physiological and clinical area and one from the behavioral and psychological area, and a history of a steady use of alcohol confirm the diagnosis of alcoholism. A physical examination and laboratory test results must be consistent with the effects of alcoholism in order to ensure a proper diagnosis.

A short four-question screening test called the CAGE test has been used with some success in identifying alcoholism.

C Have you ever felt the need to **Cut** down on drinking?
A Have you ever felt **Annoyed** by criticism of your drinking?
G Have you ever felt **Guilty** about drinking?
E Have you ever taken an **Eye-opener** drink when you woke up?

The predictive value of the CAGE test for alcoholism rises with the number of positive responses to these questions.

Many alcoholics attempt to stop drinking, and many have relapses. The diagnosis of arrested or controlled alcoholism depends on (1) the duration of the patient's abstinence, (2) the patient's regular attendance at and full participation in an active treatment program, such as meetings of Alcoholics Anonymous (AA) or similar program, and (3) the patient's use of professionally guided deterrent medication, such as Antabuse. Antabuse is a drug that, if used properly, causes few adverse effects except when combined with alcohol. Antabuse interferes with the normal metabolism of alcohol, thereby provoking unpleasant physiologic reactions, such as violent retching and vomiting. To be effective, Antabuse must be taken orally each day—an act of commitment generally shown only by those patients who are serious about stopping drinking.

To be considered a recovered alcoholic, an individual must work without absenteeism, accumulate no traffic violations, and refrain from substituting other drugs for alcohol. Most authorities agree that alcohol abstinence is a requirement for recovery, because (1) total abstinence is definitive and easily measured and (2) a little social drinking can easily cause a recovered alcoholic to resume former drinking habits. An alcoholic should never assume that the disease has been completely arrested, but after a ten-year abstinence from alcohol consumption, the alcoholic will probably be able to remain

Figure 17–2.
Criteria for the Diagnosis of Alcoholism.

I. Manifestations clearly associated with alcoholism
   A. Signs of physiological dependence
      1. Withdrawal symptoms
      2. Alcohol tolerance
   B. Presence of alcohol-associated illnesses
      1. Alcoholic hepatitis
      2. Alcoholic cerebellar degeneration
   C. Signs of psychological dependence
      1. Continued drinking despite strong medical or social contraindications known to the patient

II. Manifestations probably associated with and strongly indicating alcoholism
   A. Presence of alcohol-associated illnesses
      1. Fatty degeneration of the liver
      2. Laennec's cirrhosis
   B. Physiological and clinical effects of alcohol
      1. Odor of alcohol on breath at time of visit to doctor's office
      2. Peripheral neuropathy
      3. Laboratory evidence of liver disease
      4. EKG abnormalities, such as arrhythmias
      5. Alcoholic "blackout" periods
   C. Behavioral and psychological effects of alcohol
      1. Frequent absences from work
      2. Surreptitious drinking
      3. Drinking in the morning
      4. Preference for companions who drink

III. Manifestations possibly associated with alcoholism
   A. Presence of alcohol-associated illness
      1. Chronic gastritis
      2. Pancreatitis
   B. Physiological and clinical effects of alcohol
      1. Toxic amblyopia, which is dimness of vision in the absence of a lesion of the eye, resulting from ingesting a substance
      2. Red, flushed face
      3. Iron-deficiency anemia
   C. Behavioral and psychological effects of alcohol
      1. Frequent automobile accidents
      2. Frequent, unexplained changes in residence and in social and business relationships
      3. Depression

Reprinted by permission of The National Council on Alcoholism and Drug Dependence, Inc.

alcohol-free. The longer an alcoholic goes without taking a drink, the greater the chances for a complete and successful recovery.

Alcohol dependency can occur with dependency on other drugs. As many as two-thirds of all alcoholics have another drug addiction.

Interactions of Alcohol and Other Drugs

An *interaction* between two substances is any alteration in the effect of either because of the presence of the other. Interactions between alcohol and other drugs can have important clinical effects and may cause death. Of the 100 most frequently prescribed drugs, more than one-half contain at least one ingredient known to interact adversely with alcohol. Most effects of alcohol-drug interactions depend on the amounts of each substance ingested, especially for those drugs that affect the central nervous system or are metabolized by the liver.

When alcohol reacts in the body with another drug, the effects of the interaction may be either antagonistic or enhanced. Antagonistic effects decrease the action of one of the substances, and enhanced effects, which are also called additive effects, increase the action of one of the substances. For example, alcohol speeds up the metabolism of phenytoin, which is an anticonvulsant and cardiac suppressant that is often used to treat epilepsy. Because alcohol causes an accelerated removal of phenytoin from the body, alcohol has an antagonistic effect on phenytoin. Therefore, if a patient who is taking phenytoin is a chronic alcohol user, the patient will require a larger dose of phenytoin than normal in order to maintain a desired therapeutic effect. In contrast, alcohol enhances the effect of diazepam, which is a tranquilizer that is often sold under the trademark name Valium. Blood plasma levels of diazepam and central nervous system depression are greater after diazepam is taken with alcohol than after it is taken with water.

Figure 17–3 lists some of the adverse effects resulting from the interaction of alcohol and other commonly used drugs.

ABUSE AND MISUSE OF OTHER SUBSTANCES

Abuse of other drugs differs from alcohol abuse in two important respects. First, much smaller quantities of another drug need to be taken over a much shorter period of time, compared with alcohol, to become habit-forming. Second, the relative risk of addiction in an individual is much greater with other drugs than with alcohol. This section will begin with a discussion of psychoactive drugs and then will address other substances that can poison the body.

Psychoactive Drugs

Psychoactive drugs are those substances that affect the mind or senses. The three classes of psychoactive drugs are depressants, stimulants, and psychedelics. Most of the drugs considered in this

Figure 17–3.
Adverse Interactions of Alcohol and Other Drugs.

Interacting Drug	Adverse Effect in Association with Acute Intoxication	Adverse Effect in Association with Chronic Alcohol Abuse
Acetaminophen (Tylenol)		Increased liver damage
Anticoagulants	Increased anticoagulant effect	Decreased anticoagulant effect
Antihistamines	Increased central nervous system depression	
Barbiturates	Increased central nervous system depression	Decreased sedative effect
Antabuse	Abdominal cramps, flushing, vomiting, confusion, psychotic episodes	
Narcotics	Increased central nervous system depression	
Phenytoin	Increased anticonvulsant effect	Decreased anticonvulsant effect
Aspirin	Gastrointestinal bleeding	

section can produce acute poisoning episodes as well as manifestations of chronic abuse. Acute drug poisoning may result from ingestion with suicidal intent, error in dose calculation, variation in drug potency, or unusual sensitivity to the drug. Chronic abuse results in drug dependence. Manifestations of acute and chronic abuse are unique to the class of drugs involved.

Depressants

Depressants are drugs that reduce the activities of the user's central nervous system. Alcohol, narcotics, and sedatives are all depressant drugs. The effects of alcohol were presented in an earlier section of this chapter and, therefore, will not be reconsidered here.

Narcotics are drugs and substances that blunt the senses, relieve pain, induce drowsiness or sleep, and, when taken in large quantities, produce complete insensibility. The narcotic that is most often abused is heroin, but addictions to methadone, morphine, meperidine (Demerol), cocaine, and codeine are also common. Many narcotics contain or are derived from opium, the dried juice of a poppy flower. Narcotics that are derived from opium are called opiates. Morphine and other opiates are usually taken to relieve pain. "Morphine euphoria" refers to morphine's ability to reduce anxiety and to produce a perceived state of well-being. Morphine euphoria induces both psychological and physical dependence. Many morphine users experience tolerance to the effects of the drug and symptoms of withdrawal. The majority of deaths associated with narcotic administration involve an overdose. For people who die suddenly after morphine injection, the cause of death is acute pulmonary edema, although overdosage also causes central nervous system and respiratory depression.

Sedatives are drugs that exert a calming effect, relieve irritability or excitement, ease mild pain, and, in larger doses, produce sleep. Barbiturates and tranquilizers are examples of sedatives. Barbiturates induce sedation and hypnosis or sleep in patients before surgery. Barbiturates are also used in anticonvulsant therapy, but they have been replaced by other drugs in the treatment of anxiety. The several types of barbiturate drugs differ in the duration of their action. Overdosages of barbiturates cause inappropriate behavior, poor mental function, and impaired muscular coordination. Tolerance develops, and withdrawal symptoms, such as increasing anxiety and nervousness, tremors, delusions, and hallucinations, occur upon discontinuance of the drug.

Many nonbarbiturate, sedative-hypnotic drugs, generally referred to as tranquilizers, are used extensively to control anxiety and are more effective and safer than barbiturates if properly used for this purpose. Some of the most widely used tranquilizers are chlordiazepoxide (Librium), diazepam (Valium), and methaqualone (Quaalude). The toxic effects of these drugs include slurred speech, a stumbling gait, drowsiness, confusion, and coma. The advantages of tranquilizers are their relatively low toxicity and low potential for addiction. Nevertheless, all sedatives, to varying degrees, cause problems in dependence, tolerance, and abuse.

Stimulants

A second category of psychoactive drugs consists of the stimulants, which act primarily upon the central nervous system and have a limited therapeutic use. One group of stimulants is the ampheta-mines, including Dexedrine and methamphetamine, which is com-monly called "speed." Amphetamines elevate the users' moods, reverse fatigue, and depress appetites. These drugs are useful in the management of narcolepsy, because they postpone the need for sleep. Amphetamines have also been used indiscriminately for weight control and avoidance of fatigue. Overdosage or continued use of amphetamines leads to irritability, tension, anxiety, tremors, muscular incoordination, and, in some cases, psychosis. The devel-opment of psychologic dependence on and tolerance of ampheta-mines often occur, but the abrupt withdrawal of these drugs does not produce marked symptoms.

Psychedelics

The third group of psychoactive drugs is called psychedelics. *Psychedelics*, which are also called *hallucinogens*, are drugs that produce visual hallucinations, intensified perceptions, delusions, euphoria, dream-like states, distortion of time, and other psychotic manifestations. Although psychologic dependence on these drugs is common, tolerance and physical dependence are not. Two examples of psychedelics are lysergic acid diethylamide (LSD) and marijuana.

Following ingestion of LSD, an individual will (1) experience distorted color, time, and space perception, (2) have unusual dreams, (3) experience an increase in auditory acuity, and (4) develop mood changes and psychiatric disorders characterized by panic and rage. The development of psychoses and attempts at suicide have resulted from some LSD "trips." Tolerance to LSD may develop, but it disappears rapidly, permitting repeated trips without progressive increases in dosage. Withdrawal symptoms are not associated with LSD. The use of this drug had declined through the 1980s, but is undergoing a resurgence in popularity. Often, a liquid form of LSD is spread on blotter paper and allowed to dry. Users then place a piece of this paper, which is typically perforated by a hole-puncher, on their tongues. The user's saliva activates the drug.

Marijuana is derived from the plant Cannabis sativa, the parts of which vary in psychoactive potency. The most active ingredient of this plant is tetrahydrocannabinol (THC). The effects of marijuana may be produced by several routes of administration, but the drug produces its greatest effect when inhaled. Smoking one or two marijuana cigarettes, which are commonly called "joints," will pro-duce the desired euphoria. After a person smokes marijuana, eupho-ria appears within twenty minutes and disappears within three hours. The marijuana experience is variable and includes dreamlike states, distortions of time and space perception, and impairments of judgment and memory. The effect of a single use of marijuana is transient and wears off leaving no significant after-effect. However, repeated usage of marijuana may cause confusion, anxiety, apathy, sleep disturbances, and sluggish physical and mental responses. High doses may cause confusion, disorientation, and paranoia. The intensity of the symptoms is related to the frequency and length of time of use.

Although marijuana is not physically addictive, its use can cause many medical problems. Bronchial and pulmonary irritation and other respiratory reactions are common results of marijuana use. Marijuana also produces an increase in heart rate and conjunctivitis. The physical complications of long-term, regular use of marijuana include cerebral atrophy and obliterative arteritis, which may be fatal. In males, the excessive use of marijuana may lead to impotence. Because marijuana impairs reaction time and motor coordination and distorts visual perception, people who drive a vehicle or operate machinery after smoking marijuana present a higher risk of accident than do people who do not smoke marijuana. Regular users of marijuana, like regular users of other psychoactive drugs, appear tired and older than their actual ages.

The hazards of marijuana generally outweigh its therapeutic potentials. However, in carefully selected and controlled instances, marijuana has been successful in lessening the extreme nausea resulting from cancer chemotherapy that other antinauseants have not effectively treated.

Figure 17–4 provides examples of each class of psychoactive drugs.

Poisons

Almost all drugs or chemicals are capable of poisoning the human body. Whether the drug or chemical acts as a poison depends on (1) the pharmacological properties of the substance, (2) the individual's sensitivity to the particular substance, and (3) the amount of the substance absorbed by the body. In the United States, each year more than two million poisonings occur and approximately 5,000 people die as a result. Many people who survive poisonings are left with a permanent disability from the act of swallowing a caustic substance or from the effect of the substance on the hepatic, renal, or central nervous system. Over 50 percent of poisonings involve children under the age of five. Medicines are involved in 50 percent of all poisonings; cosmetics, pesticides, petroleum products, and turpentine paints are involved in 20 percent of all poisonings; and

Figure 17–4.
Psychoactive Drugs.

Class of Drug	Examples
Depressants	
Alcohol	Ethyl alcohol
Narcotics or opiates	Morphine, heroin, Demerol
Sedatives	
Barbiturates	Nembutal, Seconal
Tranquilizers	Valium, Librium
Stimulants	
Amphetamines	Dexedrine, Methamphetamine
Synthetics	Preludin
Cocaine	"Crack," "snow"
Psychedelics	LSD, marijuana

Figure 17–5.
Manifestations of Common Poisons.

Organs Affected	Symptoms and Signs
Skin, mucous membranes	Itching, rash, cyanosis, jaundice, redness
Central nervous system	Lack of coordination, coma, delirium, hallucinations, headache, convulsions, drowsiness, depression
Gastrointestinal system	Enteritis, constipation, increased salivation
Respiratory system	Breathing disorders, pulmonary edema
Cardiovascular system	Hypertension, shock, hemolysis, abnormal heartbeats and heart rates
Eyes, ears	Blurred or double vision, dilated or contracted pupil, disturbed equilibrium, deafness, tinnitus
General	Fever, weight loss, weakness, muscular pain

cleaning and polishing agents are involved in 15 percent of all poisoning cases.

Drugs and chemicals are capable of producing a wide spectrum of systemic manifestations. No system of the body is immune to drug reactions. Generally, the manifestations of poisoning are nonspecific. In fact, no commonly used substances produce distinctive symptoms and signs. In some cases, a physician will have difficulty determining if the patient's manifestations arise from an underlying disease or the drugs used to treat the disease.

Figure 17–5 lists some common symptoms and signs of poisoning.

In many cases of poisoning, the substance responsible for the ill effects is known. In these cases, the physician must determine the degree of the patient's exposure to the substance so that appropriate therapy can begin. In disease states of questionable cause, the physician can establish a diagnosis after carefully obtaining the patient's medical history, giving the patient a complete physical examination, and ordering routine and specialized toxicologic laboratory tests on the patient.

CHAPTER

18

Duration of Disability

One of the most important tasks disability claims examiners must perform is estimating the amount of time that an insured will be away from work because of a disabling injury or illness. Estimating the length of a person's disability is difficult, because the duration of a disability depends on many factors. This chapter will discuss the important factors that affect the duration of an insured's disability and then will address the investigation of disability claims.

ESTIMATING THE DURATION OF DISABILITY

Both medical and nonmedical factors play a role in determining the duration of an insured's disability. Separating the two types of factors as causes of continuing disability is often a difficult task.

Medical Factors

The starting point in any determination of the expected duration of a person's disability is the evaluation of the objective evidence of disease, including the diagnosis of the condition, the findings in a physical examination of the person, the person's relevant medical history, and laboratory test results. Other medical factors that are also relevant in making a diagnosis are

459

- The patient's age and general physical condition
- The degree of severity of the primary cause of the patient's disability
- The presence of complications
- The presence of pre-existing or co-existing medical conditions
- The status of the patient's general health
- The type of treatment, such as surgery or specialized care, required for the patient's condition

Many of these factors have been discussed in the preceding chapters, and so this chapter will concentrate on the effect certain nonmedical factors have on the length of disability.

Nonmedical Factors

Sometimes nonmedical factors are even more important in assessing the duration of a patient's disability than the underlying medical problem is. Nonmedical factors that affect the duration of a person's disability include

- The patient's internal motivation to return to work
- The patient's economic need to return to work
- Pending litigation that affects the patient
- General availability of work
- The patient's occupation
- The definition of disability in the patient's insurance contract

Physicians generally recognize the role of a person's internal motivation in predicting when a disabled person will return to work. However, an individual's motivation is subjective, and so, is difficult to assess. Some individuals possess an inner discipline that, despite most other factors, reduces the duration of a medical disability. Other patients, however, lack this internal motivation, and so take longer to recover from the same type of disability.

Economic need often influences a person's motivation to return to the workplace, and may be the most important nonmedical factor in determining the length of a patient's disability. Individuals who have mounting financial obligations and who lack other sources of financial support must return to work at the earliest possible moment after the acute phase of an illness passes. These individuals may have a shorter duration of disability than those who have other sources of income. If a patient's financial needs are satisfied without working, economic motivation to return to work will be minimized.

A patient who is involved in a lawsuit because of an injury that resulted in disability may not be motivated to return to work because he or she may fear that resuming employment activities will negatively influence the outcome of the lawsuit. The individual's "symptoms," and hence the disability, are often prolonged in such cases and may not "subside" until the litigation is settled.

The availability of work is another important factor that can influence the duration of a person's disability. Research has shown that during a recession and other situations in which the unemployment rate is relatively high, the number and duration of claimed disabilities increase. Thus, the lack of employment opportunities in the general economy has some relation to health insurers' disability claims experience.

A disabled worker's occupation is another major factor in determining the length of a person's disability. A laborer whose job requires strenuous physical activity may necessarily have a longer period of disability than a sedentary worker who has a similar medical problem. For example, a patient who has had arthroscopic surgery on a knee will probably be able to return to work sooner if the patient is a claim processor than if the patient does heavy industrial construction work. A physician cannot predict the duration of a patient's disability without an understanding of the tasks the patient customarily completes on the job and the physical and emotional demands these tasks place on the patient. If the patient's occupation is a common one that has easily understood responsibilities, or if the tasks involved can be described clearly, the decision as to when disability has ceased is easier to evaluate than if the occupation is less common or more complex.

A decision regarding the duration of a patient's disability should only be made with knowledge of the definition of disability contained in the patient's insurance policy. Some disability insurance contracts define disability in two stages. Initially, disability, as defined in these contracts, is the inability of the insured to perform the tasks of the insured's own occupation. After an initial period of disability, usually two years, the insured is considered to be totally disabled if the disability prevents the insured from performing the duties of any occupation for which he or she is reasonably fitted by education, training, or experience. For individuals who work at jobs that require a low level of physical activity, the distinction between "own occupation" and "any occupation" is difficult to make. Thus, if these patients are physically disabled for their own occupations, often they are also disabled for any occupation as well. However, under this type of contract, an insured individual who works at a job that requires a high level of physical activity will no longer be considered disabled if he or she is recovered enough to perform a less strenuous task. If, for example, a disabled police officer cannot return to patrol duty but is physically able to work a "desk job," his or her condition would no longer fit the definition of disability as stated in the policy.

Sometimes, a disability insurance contract will specify a definition of disability that refers only to the inability of the insured to perform the tasks of his or her own occupation. If the person insured under such a policy works at a job that requires special knowledge, education, or skill, insurance benefits may continue for a longer period of time than they would under a policy that had the two-stage definition of disability described above. For example, a surgeon who loses the use of a hand may not be able to perform surgery, but may be able to secure a position teaching at a medical college. If the definition of disability in the surgeon's contract specifies only the insured's "own previous occupation," the surgeon would continue to receive policy benefits even though he or she was physically able to perform the duties of the other job.

The definition of disability in many policies specifies that the disabled worker must be unable to perform any occupation that will produce approximately the same livelihood the insured had enjoyed before the impairment and for which the insured's education, training, and experience are appropriate. Thus, an individual need not be bedridden to be considered totally disabled.

In some instances, disability claim examiners should also have knowledge of the court decisions regarding disability definitions in the insured's state of residence. On occasion, court rulings have modified policy language, generally with liberalizations that benefit the insured.

One reason that estimating the potential duration of a disabled person's disability is difficult is that physicians may not agree on what constitutes significant impairment, and so any assessment of a given patient is somewhat subjective. Two or more competent physicians may examine the same individual and disagree on the existence of impairment and on the impairment's probable duration. Furthermore, some individuals who have hypertension, angina, diabetes, heart disease, arthritis, low back pain, or other acute or chronic conditions continue to work or resume work after the acute phase of their illness passes. Other patients who have one or more of these conditions will seek disability status.

Recognizing that many exceptions exist, the following general statements are useful:

- The shorter the average duration of disability for a given diagnosis, the more accurate the prediction of the length of disability for a given disability caused by that condition will be. Average expected durations of disability for many conditions are published. (The Appendix to this text contains a chart that provides average expected disability durations for several illnesses, operations, and conditions. *The State of California's Medical Yardsticks—Disability Insurance* is an even more extensive source that many claim personnel find helpful.)

- Predicting when the patient can return to work following operations or fractures is generally more accurate than predicting when the patient can return to work after most illnesses. Illnesses often have subacute or chronic stages that, for varying periods, affect an individual's ability to perform selected tasks.

- Predicting when the patient can return to work following a condition that presents substantial objective clinical evidence is more accurate than predicting when a patient can return to work following a condition that presents few objective signs. If a patient makes many subjective complaints, the cause for which cannot be supported by firm objective evidence, the patient's disability associated with these symptoms is generally of unpredictable duration. For example, the duration of disability resulting from many psychiatric illnesses is unpredictable, and the range of possible durations of disability associated with a given psychiatric diagnosis is broad. Any estimate of a return-to-work date by an attending physician at the onset of a psychiatric illness is often inaccurate.

THE ROLE OF MEDICAL PERSONNEL IN THE INVESTIGATION OF DISABILITY CLAIMS

The period over which the disability income benefits are payable is of great importance to both the insured, who may depend on the benefits for living expenses, and the insurance company, which in fairness to other policyowners should pay only valid claims. Thus, the listing of a potentially serious diagnosis on the claim form should not lead the claim reviewer to conclude automatically that the basis for the disability claim is valid. The claim reviewer should conduct a full investigation of every claim, including a careful evaluation of the attending physician's statement. In some cases, the reviewer should obtain corroborative data in the form of an examination by a consultant, who is usually an independent medical examiner and is a specialist in a particular field of medicine. The claim examiner also depends on the advice and expertise of the insurer's medical director.

Evaluating the Attending Physician's Report

In estimating the time at which a patient may return to work, attending physicians, under the stresses of maintaining strong doctor-patient relationships, sometimes have difficulty in being totally unbiased. Moreover, these attending physicians may not recognize their lack of objectivity. A growing philosophical concern among physicians is the ethical question of whether a physician should be placed in the position of predicting the extent of his or her patient's disability. Physicians should be able to evaluate and describe the extent of the impairment resulting from the patient's medical condition, while still leaving the decision regarding the patient's disability to the claim reviewer. Because some doctors leave the return-to-work date to the discretion of their patients, the claim reviewer may require a statement from the attending physician explaining specifically why a particular patient's condition interferes with that person's completion of assigned daily job responsibilities. In fairness to physicians, however, claim reviewers must recognize that not all illnesses can be objectively measured. Subjective complaints and patients' statements that they are not ready to return to work often are difficult for physicians to challenge.

The claim reviewer should make no assumptions about the attending physician's comments in a medical report. If the attending physician's report is too abbreviated or vague for an accurate assessment of a disabled worker's status, the claim reviewer must ask for more medical data. A review of copies of office records, hospital discharge summaries, and/or certain laboratory test results may help clarify the patient's medical condition. Some claims, upon investigation, prove to be based on erroneous or fraudulent information.

Consulting an Independent Physician

A claims reviewer will sometimes need to consult with an independent physician, usually a specialist who is familiar with the diagnosis and treatment of the type of medical problem under review. The consulting physician should provide a knowledgeable, impartial, and objective opinion and should clarify the extent of the patient's impairment. The consultant will be able to provide this information only if the claim reviewer gives the consultant all the information the insurance company has on file regarding the insured's job and copies of all medical reports the insurance company has received from the attending physician.

Knowledge of the insured's job responsibilities is necessary if the consultant is to give an informed decision concerning the extent to which the insured's impairment may preclude the insured from returning to work. A consultant's opinion is not authoritative unless the consultant is aware of the specific requirements of the insured's job. The claim reviewer should encourage the consultant to question the insured about the scope of his or her assigned duties, especially if these duties require lifting, bending, prolonged standing, and other acts demanding physical stamina.

Within limits, the reviewer should authorize the specialist to complete selected tests on the insured if these tests are necessary for clarification of the insured's problem. The insured's medical history and the results of previous tests, examinations, and laboratory studies are essential to the consulting physician in evaluating the findings of examinations the consultant has administered to the insured. These additional tests may be important, particularly if the consultant has reached a conclusion regarding the insured's impairment and that conclusion differs from the one the attending physician reached.

In selecting a consultant specialist for an independent examination, the insurance company should be certain that the medical problem lies within the specialist's field of expertise. In complex cases, the insurer may be wise to obtain opinions from more than one consultant, each knowledgeable in a particular specialty. Sometimes the attending physician will have asked for the opinions of several consultants. The insurance company should obtain these consultants' reports before making a decision or ordering further consultations.

Consulting the Insurer's Medical Director

The responsibility for the decision to pay a disability claim rests with the claim reviewer. However, the insurer's medical director provides insight and helps the claim reviewer interpret reports and make referrals.

The role of the insurance company's medical director in assessing disability claims consists of two main tasks: assisting in the investigation of the disability and assisting in the evaluation of medical data. In assisting in the investigation of the disability, the medical director should indicate what an investigation of the claimant's disability should focus upon. The medical director can advise the claim reviewer in developing medical data, suggesting probing questions to ask the attending physician, determining the tests and studies to undertake, and preparing the framework for the consultant's examination. Sometimes the claimant's medical problems extend into more than one medical discipline. In such instances, the medical director will advise the claim reviewer as to the order of examinations the reviewer should seek from the appropriate specialists. In assisting in the evaluation of medical data, the medical director should advise the claim reviewer if the insured's medical history, physical examination and laboratory test results, and reports from the attending physician and the consultant support the attending physician's diagnosis. Furthermore, the medical director should assist the reviewer in the interpretation of symptoms, physical findings, and laboratory data, especially concerning the extent to which this medical evidence actually contributes to the insured's inability to perform all assigned job duties. In short, the medical director must assist the claim reviewer in deciding if the given diagnosis is reasonable based upon available evidence, if the insured's medical condition might be expected to produce an impairment that precludes the insured's return to work, and if the duration of the insured's disability corresponds with the duration anticipated from a review of all medical data.

In arriving at an opinion, the medical director should give serious consideration to the opinion of the attending physician, because the attending physician has observed the insured on several occasions over a period of time, whereas the company's consultant has had only a single, brief contact with the claimant. If a significant difference of opinion exists between the attending physician and the consultant, the medical director may consider getting the opinion of a second independent examiner.

The medical director's role is to advise on medical issues and does not include ruling directly on the question of disability. Physicians, in general, assess disease and its consequent impairment. The claim examiner, on the other hand, determines if an insured's condition falls within the insurance policy's definition of disability. The medical director's role is distinct from the role of the attending physician and the consulting examiner. And none of the medical professionals can effectively function as experts regarding the insured's job requirements. All medical personnel, therefore, including the medical director, advise the claim examiner so that the claim examiner can properly assess all relevant evidence in making a claim decision about an insured's duration of disability.

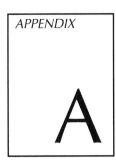
Medical Word Parts

PREFIXES AND ROOTS

a-	lack of, without, deficient; may be used as an- (amenorrhea: absence of menstral flow)
ab-	away from, from, out of, separate; may be used as ap- or apo- (abduct: move away from the middle point)
acou-	hearing (acoustic: pertaining to the sense of hearing)
acro-	extremes, extremity (acrophobia: fear of heights)
ad-	to, toward, near (adduct: move toward the middle point)
aden-	gland (adenitis: inflammation of a gland)
aer-	air (aerated: filled with air)
alg-	pain (analgesia: pain relief)
ambi-	both, on both sides (ambidextrous: able to use either hand effectively)
andro-	male (androgen: male hormone)
angi-	related to blood vessel or lymphatic vessel (angiogram: x-ray study of a vessel)
ankyl-	stiff (ankylosis: frozen, immovable joint)
ante-	before (anterior: in front of)

antero-	before, in front of (anteroposterior: from the front to the back)
anti-	against (antiseptic: substance that combats infection)
arterio-	related to arteries (arteriography: x-ray study of an artery)
arthro-	related to joint (arthrotomy: incision into a joint)
asthen-	weakness, exhaustion (neurasthenia: nervous exhaustion)
audio-	related to hearing; may be used as audito- (audiometer: instrument for measuring hearing acuity)
auri-	related to the ear (auricle: ear-shaped structure or appendage)
auto-	self (autograft: tissue removed from one area and grafted onto another part of the same body)
bi-	two, twice, double; may be used as bis- or bin- (bilateral: having two sides)
bil-	bile (biliary: related to bile ducts)
bio-	related to living, life (biopsy: excision of tissue during life to establish a diagnosis)
blepharo-	related to eyelids (blepharoplasty: corrective surgery on the eyelids)
brachi-	related to the arm (brachial plexus: network of nerves that distribute branches to the arm)
brachy-	short (brachycephalic: shortness of the head)
brady-	slow (bradycardia: slow heart rate)
broncho-	related to a bronchus (bronchodilator: a drug or instrument that dilates the bronchus)
bucco-	related to the cheek; may be used as bucca- (buccolingual: related to the cheek and the tongue)
carcino-	related to cancer (carcinogen: substance with cancer producing potential)
cardio-	related to the heart (electrocardiogram: record of the heart's electrical activity)
cata-	down, lower, against (catabolite: a break-down product of the metabolic process)
cente-	related to a puncture (paracentesis: a tapping of a cavity to withdraw fluid)
centi-	related to 100, usually $1/100$ (centimeter: one hundredth of a meter)
cephal-	related to head (cephalalgia: headache)

cerebro-	related to the brain (cerebrovascular: related to the blood vessels of the brain)
cervic-	related to the neck of an organ (cervicitis: inflammation of the cervix; cervicodynia: pain in the neck)
chole-	related to bile (cholecystectomy: surgical removal of the gallbladder)
chondro-	related to cartilage (chondrosarcoma: malignancy of cartilage)
cine-	motion picture (cineroentgenography: motion picture record of the successive images appearing on a fluoroscope screen)
co-	with, together; may be used as col-, com-, or con- (coagulate: to clot)
colo-	related to the colon (colostomy: surgically created opening of the colon on the surface of the body)
colpo-	related to the vagina (colporrhaphy: reconstructive surgery on the vagina)
contra-	against, opposed (contralateral: situated on the opposite side)
costa-	related to a rib; may be used as costo- (intercostal: between the ribs)
cranio-	related to the skull (cranioplasty: plastic operation on the skull)
cryo-	related to cold (cryosurgery: destruction of tissue by application of extreme cold)
crypto-	related to a crypt; hidden, concealed (cryptorchidism: undescended testicles)
cuta-	related to skin; may be used as cuti- (subcutaneous: under the skin)
cyano-	bluish color (cyanosis: blue discoloration of skin)
cyst-	related to any fluid-filled sac (cystitis: inflammation of the urinary bladder)
cyto-	related to cells (cytogenesis: the origin and development of cells)
dacr-	related to tear glands (dacryocystitis: inflammation of the tear glands)
de-	down, from (dehydrate: to remove water from)
deca-	ten times (decaliter: ten liters)
deci-	one tenth (decimeter: one-tenth of a meter)
dent-	teeth; may be used as dento-, denta-, denti-, dentia- (dentition: an entire set of teeth)

derma-	skin; may be used as dermato- (dermatome: an instrument used in obtaining thin skin grafts)
dextro-	right (dextromanual: right-handed)
di-	two, twice (dioxide: a molecule containing two atoms of oxygen)
dia-	through, apart, across, between (diaphragm: muscle separating thorax and abdomen)
diplo-	two, twice, double, twin (diplopia: double vision)
dis-	apart, away from, separation (dislocation: displacement of any part)
dorsi-	related to the back; may be used as dorso- (dorsiflexion: backward flexion or bending)
dys-	difficult, painful (dysmenorrhea: painful menstruation)
e-	out, from, without; may be used as ec- or ex- (edentulous: without teeth)
ec-	out of (eccentric: away from the center; odd)
ecto-	outside of, without (ectoderm: outer layer of the embryo)
ectop-	misplaced (ectopic pregnancy: pregnancy in which the fetus grows outside the uterus)
en-	in, on (encapsulate: enclose in a capsule)
encephal-	brain (anencephalic: having no brain)
endo-	inside (endometrium: lining of uterine cavity)
enteri-	small intestine; may be used as entero- (gastroenteritis: inflammation of stomach and small intestine)
epi-	on top of, upon, on (epidermis: outer layer of skin)
erythro-	red (erythrocyte: red blood cell)
eso-	inside, inward, within (esotropia: one eye fixes on an object while the other deviates inward)
eu-	normal, well (euthyroid: normal thyroid function)
ex-	out of, from (excise: to surgically cut out)
exo-	outside, outward, away from (exocervix: portion of uterus protruding into the vagina)
extra-	outside, beyond, in addition (extrasystole: an additional contraction of the heart)
fibro-	fiber, fibrous tissue (adenofibroma: a tumor composed of glandular and fibrous connective tissues)
gastr-	denoting a relationship to the stomach (gastrectomy: surgical removal of the stomach)
gingiv-	related to the gums (gingivitis: inflammation of the gums)

glosso-	tongue (glossoplegia: paralysis of the tongue)
glyc-	sugar (hyperglycemia: elevated blood sugar)
gyneco-	female; may be used as gyn-, gyne-, or gyno- (gynecoid: resembling a female)
hemo-	blood; may be used as hemato-, hem-, haem-, or hema- (hemoglobin: oxygen-carrying pigment in red blood cells)
hemi-	one-half (hemianopia: defective vision in one-half of the visual field)
hepato-	liver; may be used as hepa- (hepatomegaly: enlargement of the liver)
hetero-	other, opposite, different (heterosexual: directed toward the opposite sex)
histo-	tissue (histotoxic: poisonous to tissues)
homeo-	constant, unchanging, the same (homeostasis: stability in the body's internal environment)
homo-	same (homograft: a graft obtained from the body of another animal of the same species)
hydro-	water (hydrocele: an accumulation of fluid in a sac around the testis)
hyper-	above, greater, excessive (hypertension: blood pressure above the normal range)
hypo-	below, under, insufficient (hypoglycemia: blood sugar level below normal)
hyster-	uterus (hysterectomy: surgical removal of the uterus)
im-	in, within, not; may also be used as in- (impalpable: not able to be detected by touch; incision: cut into)
infra-	beneath, below, downward (infraorbital: located below the orbit or eye)
irid-	iris (iridectomy: removal of the iris)
kerat-	horny tissue; cornea (keratoma: a growth of horny tissue; keratoconus: a conical protrusion of the cornea)
kilo-	one thousand (kilogram: one thousand grams)
lacrim-	tears (lacrimal gland: tear-producing gland)
laparo-	flank, loin; more loosely, the abdomen (laparoscope: an instrument introduced into the abdominal cavity for viewing the contents of that cavity)
latera-	to one side (lateral: located on one side of the midline)
leio-	smooth (leiomyoma: a benign tumor consisting primarily of smooth muscle cells)

lepto-	thin, small, weak, fine (leptomeninges: the arachnoid and pia, thin membranes around the brain)
leuco-	white; may be used as leuko- (leucocyte: a white blood cell)
levo-	left (levorotation: rotation to the left)
lipo-	fat (lipoprotein: a group of proteins consisting of a protein combined with a fat)
litho-	stone (pyelolithotomy: a surgical incision into the kidney pelvis to remove a stone)
macro-	large, elongated (macrocyte: a giant cell found in the blood in certain anemias)
mal-	ill, bad (malaise: a general feeling of illness)
mammo-	breast (mammography: x-ray of the breast)
mast-	breast (mastitis: inflammation of the breast)
medi-	middle, midline (medial: closer to the midline)
mega-	great size; one million; may be used as megalo- (megacolon: an abnormally large colon; megavolt: one million volts)
melano-	black, dark color; related to melanin (melanodermic: having a dark skin)
meno-	month (menopause: cessation of monthly menstrual periods)
meso-	middle (meso-aortitis: inflammation of the middle muscular coat of the aorta)
meta-	change, after (metastasis: transfer of disease from one organ to another)
metro-	uterus (metrorrhagia: abnormal uterine bleeding)
micro-	small, tiny (microtome: an instrument for cutting thin slices of tissue for microscopic examination)
milli-	one-thousandth (milligram: one-thousandth of a gram)
mono-	one, single (mononuclear: having one nucleus)
morpho-	shape, form (morphology: the science that deals with structure and form)
muc-	mucus (mucosa: the lining tissue of the mouth and other organs of the intestinal tract)
multi-	many, much (multilobular: having many lobes)
myel-	bone marrow; spinal cord (osteomyelitis: inflammation of bone; myelogram: x-ray of the spinal cord and surrounding structures)
myo-	muscle (myocardium: the heart muscle)
necro-	corpse; death (necrosis: death of tissue)
neo-	new (neoplasm: a new growth of tissue, a tumor)

nephro-	kidney (nephrosclerosis: hardening of the kidney seen in hypertensive vascular disease)
neuro-	nerve (neurotoxic: poisonous or destructive to nerve tissue)
ocul-	eye (oculus dexter: the right eye)
odonto-	tooth (odontonecrosis: decay of the teeth)
oligo-	few, scant, deficiency (oligomenorrhea: abnormally infrequent menstruation)
onco-	tumor; may be used as oncho- (oncology: the study and treatment of tumors)
onych-	nail (paronychia: infection around the base of the nail)
oo-	egg (oogenesis: the process of origination and maturation of the ovum)
oophor-	ovary (oophorectomy: the surgical removal of an ovary)
ophthalmo-	eye (ophthalmoscope: an instrument for examining the interior of the eye)
orchi-	testis (orchitis: inflammation of the testis)
ortho-	straight, normal, true (orthodontics: the branch of dentistry concerned with malocclusion)
osteo-	bone; may be used as oss- (osteomalacia: softening of bone)
oto-	ear (otosclerosis: formation of spongy bone around the oval window of the inner ear)
ovari-	ovary (ovariectomy: excision of an ovary; oophorectomy)
ovi-	ovum, egg (oviduct: the tube serving to transport the ovum from the ovary to the uterus)
pan-	all (panhysterectomy: removal of the entire uterus)
para-	beside, near, closely resembling (paramedical: having an adjunctive relationship to the practice of medicine)
patho-	disease (pathogen: a disease-producing agent)
ped-	child; foot (pediatrics: the branch of medicine dealing with illnesses of childhood; pedicle: a foot-like or stem-like part)
per-	by way of, through (per os: by mouth)
peri-	around (pericardium: membranous sac surrounding the heart)
pex-	fixation (oophoropexy: surgical fixation of an ovary in a new position)
phago-	eat (phagocyte: any cell that ingests microorganisms or other cells)

phleb- vein (phlebitis: inflammation of a vein)

phren- diaphragm (phrenic nerve: nerve passing through the diaphragm)

pleuro- rib; pleura (pleurodynia: pain in the intercostal muscles)

pneumo- lung; air, breath (pneumonectomy: surgical removal of a lung; pneumoencephalogram: x-ray of the brain after replacement of some cerebrospinal fluid with air)

pod- foot (podagra: gouty pain in the big toe)

polio- gray matter of the nervous system (poliomyelitis: inflammation of the gray matter of the spinal cord)

poly- many (polycythemia: a condition characterized by an excessive number of circulating blood cells)

post- after, behind (postpartum: after delivery)

pre- before, in front of (premature: occurring sooner than anticipated)

presby- old (presbyopia: a condition of the elderly in which the near point of distant vision is removed farther from the eye)

pro- before, in front of (progenitor: a parent or ancestor)

procto- anus, rectum (proctoscope: an instrument for examination of the anus and rectum)

pseudo- false (pseudotumor: a nontumorous condition that produces the symptoms of a tumor)

psycho- mind, mental processes (psychosis: severe mental disorder)

pyelo- kidney pelvis (pyelocaliectasis: dilation of the kidney pelvis and calyces)

pyo- pus (pyoderma: any skin disease associated with the formation of pus)

ren- kidney (renal artery: artery going to the kidney)

retro- behind, backward (retrocecal: behind the cecum)

rhino- nose (rhinoplasty: plastic surgery on the nose)

salping- auditory tube or fallopian tube (salpingectomy: surgical removal of a fallopian tube)

schizo- divided, split (schizophrenia: a psychosis characterized by inappropriate responses to emotional stimuli, inappropriate mood, and unpredictable behavior)

sclero- hard; white of eye (scleroderma: a systemic disease that produces a hardening of the connective tissue in several organs; sclerokeratitis: inflammation of the sclera and cornea)

semi-	one-half (semipermeable: permits passage of certain substances and hinders others)
sinistro-	left (sinistrocular: having the left eye as the dominant eye)
spermato-	sperm (spermatogenesis: sperm formation)
spleno-	spleen (splenomegaly: enlargement of the spleen)
spondylo-	vertebrae (spondylolisthesis: forward displacement of one vertebrae over another)
steato-	fat; may be used as stearo- (steatorrhea: the excessive loss of fat in the stool)
steno-	contracted, narrow (stenosis: constriction of a channel or aperture)
stomat-	mouth, opening (stomatitis: inflammation of the oral mucosa)
sub-	under, beneath, almost (subtotal: less than complete)
super-	above, excessive (superficial: being at or near the surface)
supra-	above, over (supraorbital: above the orbit)
syn-	with, union, together (syndrome: a set of symptoms that occur together)
tachy-	rapid (tachycardia: a rapid heart beat)
thoraco-	chest (thoracotomy: surgical incision into the chest wall)
thyro-	thyroid gland (thyroidectomy: surgical removal of the thyroid gland)
toxi-	poison (toxicology: the study of poisons)
tracheo-	trachea (tracheobronchitis: an inflammation of the trachea and bronchi)
trans-	across, through (transurethral: performed through the urethra)
tricho-	hair (trichobezoar: a concretion formed of hairs located within the intestinal tract)
un-	not (unconscious: not conscious)
uni-	one, single (unicellular: composed of one cell)
uretero-	ureter (ureterocele: a dilation of the ureter)
ur-	urine, urinary tract (uremia: the presence of urinary constituents in the blood)
utero-	uterus (utero-ovarian: pertaining to the uterus and ovary)
vaso-	vessel, duct (vasodilator: an agent causing dilation of blood vessels)

vesico-   bladder (vesicoureteral: pertaining to the bladder and ureter)

xanthe-   yellow (xanthelasma: yellowish spots or plaques on the eyelids)

SUFFIXES

-agra   painful seizure (podagra: pain in the great toe caused by gout)

-algia   painful condition (arthralgia: pain in a joint)

-ase   enzyme (diastase: an enzyme that assists in the breakdown of complex starches)

-asis   state, condition (bronchiectasis: dilation of bronchi from an inflammatory or degenerative process)

-cele   tumor, swelling, cavity (spermatocele: a cystic distention of the epididymis)

-centesis   tapping, puncture (thoracocentesis: tapping the pleural cavity to withdraw fluid)

-cide   cut, kill (bactericide: an agent that kills bacteria)

-clysis   injection, washing out (hypodermoclysis: injection of fluid into the subcutaneous tissue)

-cyte   cell (erythrocyte: red blood cell)

-dynia   pain (pleurodynia: pain originating in the pleura)

-ectasis   dilation, stretching (caliectasis: dilation of a calix of the kidney)

-ectomy   excision, cutting out (colectomy: surgical removal of the colon)

-em   blood (septicemia: a blood infection)

-esis   state, condition (pathogenesis: development of disease)

-esthesia   a feeling (anesthesia: absence of feeling or sensation)

-gen   productive of (allergen: substance causing an allergic reaction)

-gram   record (electrocardiogram: record of the electrical activity of the heart)

-graph   recording instrument (polygraph: an instrument for recording respiratory movements, pulse rate, blood pressure, etc.)

-ia	state, condition (pneumonia: infection of the lungs)
-iasis	process, condition (amebiasis: infected with amebae)
-ic	of, pertaining to (hepatic: pertaining to the liver)
-itis	inflammation (pneumonitis: inflammation of the lung)

-logy	study of (neurology: study of the nervous system and the diseases affecting this system)
-lysis	dissolving (hemolysis: destruction of red blood cells with the release of hemoglobin)

-malacia	softening (osteomalacia: softening of bones)
-megaly	enlargement, big, great (cardiomegaly: an enlargement of the heart)

-oid	like, resembling (schizoid: resembling schizophrenia)
-oma	tumor (neuroma: a tumor composed of nerve tissue)
-opia	defect of the eye (hemianopia: defective vision or blindness in half of the visual field)
-orrhagia	hemorrhage (menorrhagia: heavy menstrual flow)
-orrhea	flow (amenorrhea: absence of menstrual flow)
-osis	condition, disease; abnormal increase (pneumoconiosis: a chronic disease of the lungs)

-pathy	disease (myopathy: disease of muscle)
-penia	want, decrease (leukopenia: a decrease in the normal count of white blood cells in the blood)
-pepsia	digestion (dyspepsia: indigestion)
-pexy	fix in place (vaginopexy: corrective fixation of the vagina)
-phasia	speech (aphasia: loss of speech)
-philia	tendency, toward, attraction (hydrophilia: property of absorbing water)
-phobia	fear (claustrophobia: fear of being shut up in a confined space)
-plasia	growth, development (hyperplasia: marked increase in tissue formation)
-plasty	forming, repair, reconstruction (arthroplasty: surgical repair of a joint)
-plegia	paralysis, stroke (paraplegia: paralysis of the lower trunk and legs)
-pnea	breathing (dyspnea: difficult, labored breathing)
-poiesis	making, forming (hematopoiesis: formation of blood cells)
-ptosis	downward displacement (nephroptosis: prolapse of the kidney)

-rrhage	flowing, bursting forth (hemorrhage: any abnormally heavy bleeding from any site)
-rrhaphy	suturing together (herniorrhaphy: surgical repair of a hernia)
-rrhea	discharge, excessive flow (rhinorrhea: discharge of watery nasal mucus)
-rrhexis	rupture (karyorrhexis: rupture of the cell nucleus)
-scope	optical instrument (otoscope: instrument for examining the ear)
-scopy	inspection, examination by viewing through a specialized optical instrument (sigmoidoscopy: examination of the sigmoid colon through a sigmoidoscope)
-sis	condition, state (hemoptysis: coughing up blood)
-spasm	sudden, involuntary contraction (laryngospasm: spasm of the glottis and vocal cords in the larynx)
-stasis	standing still, stopping (hemostasis: stopping the flow of blood)
-stomy	make an opening or mouth into (ileostomy: a surgical opening of the ileum on the abdominal wall)
-tome	instrument for cutting (dermatome: instrument for removing a thin layer of skin for use in grafting)
-tomy	incision into (tracheotomy: cutting into the trachea)
-trophy	growth, nourishment (hypertrophy: excessive growth or enlargement of an organ)
-uria	urine (hematuria: red blood cells in the urine)

B

Medical Abbreviations

A	albumin; artery
A_2	aortic valve second sound
AA	Alcoholics Anonymous; aortic arch; autoanalyzer; automobile accident; acute abdomen
AAA	abdominal aortic aneurysm
AAL	anterior axillary line
Ab	antibody
ABD	abdomen
ABE	acute bacterial endocarditis
ABG	arterial blood gases
AC	*ante cibum* (before meals)
ACB	aortocoronary bypass
ACBG	aortocoronary bypass graft
ACC	accident
ACE	angiotensin converting enzyme
ACG	angiocardiography
ACLS	advanced cardiac life support
ACTH	adrenocorticotropic hormone
AD	right ear
ADA	American Dental Association; American Diabetic Association; Americans with Disabilities Act
ADD	attention deficit disorder
ADH	antidiuretic hormone

ADHD	attention deficit hyperactivity disorder
AF	atrial fibrillation; atrial flutter
AFB	acid-fast bacillus
AFIB	atrial fibrillation
AFL	atrial flutter
AFP	α -Fetoprotein
Ag	silver; antigen
A/G	albumin/globulin ratio
AGS	adrenogenital syndrome
AHF	antihemophilic factor
AHG	antihemophilic globulin
AI	aortic insufficiency
AIDS	acquired immunodeficiency syndrome
ALB	albumin
ALL	acute lymphoblastic leukemia
ALS	amyotrophic lateral sclerosis; advanced life support
ALT	alanine aminotransferase (formerly SGPT)
AMA	against medical advice; American Medical Association
AMI	acute myocardial infarction; anterior myocardial infarction
AML	acute myelocytic leukemia
ANA	antinuclear antibody
ANS	autonomic nervous system
ANT	anterior
anti-HAV	antibody to the hepatitis A virus
anti-HB$_c$	antibody to the hepatitis B core antigen
anti-HB$_e$	antibody to the hepatitis B$_e$ antigen
anti-HB$_s$	antibody to the hepatitis B surface antigen
anti-HCV	antibody to the hepatitis C virus
AOD	arterial occlusive disease
AODM	adult onset diabetes mellitus
AOM	acute otitis media
A&P	auscultation and percussion
AP	alkaline phosphatase; anterior-posterior; attending physician
APC	aspirin, phenacetin, caffeine; atrial premature contraction
APKD	adult polycystic kidney disease
APS	attending physician's statement
APTT	activated partial thromboplastin time
ARDS	adult respiratory distress syndrome
ARF	acute renal failure; acute respiratory failure; acute rheumatic fever
AS	aortic stenosis; left ear

ASA	aspirin
ASCVD	arteriosclerotic cardiovascular disease
AST	aspartate aminotransferase (SGOT)
ASD	atrial septal defect
ASH	asymmetric septal hypertrophy
ASHD	arteriosclerotic heart disease
ASO	antistreptolysin O; atherosclerosis obliterans
ASPVD	arteriosclerotic peripheral vascular disease
AST	aspartate aminotransferase (formerly SGOT)
AS_X	asymptomatic
ATN	acute tubular necrosis
ATS	anxiety-tension state
AU	both ears
Au	gold
AV	arteriovenous; atrioventricular
AVM	arteriovenous malformation
AVN	arteriovenous nicking
AWMI	anterior wall myocardial infarction
B	bacillus
Ba	barium
BBB	bundle branch block
BCC	basal cell carcinoma
BCG	vaccination to prevent tuberculosis
BCP	birth control pill
BE	barium enema
BID	twice a day
BLS	basic life support
BM	bone marrow; bowel movement
BMR	basal metabolic rate
BOM	bilateral otitis media
BP	blood pressure
BPH	benign prostatic hypertrophy
BPM	beats per minute
BS	blood sugar; bowel sounds; breath sounds
BSER	brain stem evoked response
BSO	bilateral salpingo-oophorectomy
BSP	Bromsulphalein test
BSS	black silk sutures
BSTT	blood sugar tolerance test
BT	bleeding time
BTB	breakthrough bleeding
BTL	bilateral tubal ligation
BTS	brady-tachyarrhythmia syndrome

BU	Bodansky units
BUN	blood urea nitrogen
B_X	biopsy
C	centigrade; cervical; chronic; colored; complete
$\bar{c}$	with
Ca	calcium; cancer; carcinoma
CABG	coronary artery bypass graft
CAD	coronary artery disease
C&E	cautery and excision
C&S	culture and smear; culture and sensitivity
CAPD	continuous ambulatory peritoneal dialysis
CAT	catamenia; computerized axial tomography
CB	cell block
CBC	complete blood count
CBS	chronic brain syndrome
CBT	computerized body tomography
CC	chief complaint
cc	cubic centimeter
$\overline{cc}$	with correction
CCHB	congenital complete heart block
CCT	computerized cranial tomography
CCU	coronary care unit; critical care unit
CD	childhood diseases
CDC	chenodeoxycholic acid; Centers for Disease Control
CEA	carcinoembryonic antigen
CF	cephalin flocculation; complement fixation; count fingers; cystic fibrosis
CG	chorionic gonadotropin
CGD	chronic granulomatous disease
CHB	complete heart block
CHD	congenital heart disease; coronary heart disease
CHF	congestive heart failure
CHO	carbohydrate
CHOL	cholesterol
CHR	chronic
CIBD	chronic inflammatory bowel disease
CIN	cervical intraepithelial neoplasia
CIS	carcinoma-in-situ
CK	creatinine kinase
CLL	chronic lymphatic leukemia
cm	centimeter
CMI	cell-mediated immunity
CMK	congenital multicystic kidney

CML	chronic myelogenous leukemia
CMV	cytomegalovirus
CNS	central nervous system
CO	carbon monoxide; cardiac output
COC	coccygeal; coccyx
COLD	chronic obstructive lung disease
CONG	congenital
COPD	chronic obstructive pulmonary disease
CP	carotid pressure; chest pain; cerebral palsy; cor pulmonale
CPAP	continuous positive airway pressure
CPE	complete physical examination
CPK	creatine phosphokinase
CPKD	childhood polycystic kidney disease
CPR	cardiopulmonary resuscitation
CR	cardiorespiratory
CREST	calcinosis, Raynaud's phenomenon, esophageal dysfunction, sclerodactyly, telangiectasia (syndrome)
CRF	chronic renal failure
CRP	C-reactive protein
CSF	cerebrospinal fluid
CST	convulsive shock treatment
CT	cardiothoracic; clotting time; computerized tomography
CTGs	curettings
CTM	chlortrimeton®
CTR	cardiac-thoracic ratio
CTS	carpal tunnel syndrome
CUC	chronic ulcerative colitis
CV	cardiovascular
CVA	cerebrovascular accident; costovertebral angle
CVD	cardiovascular disease
CVI	cerebrovascular insufficiency
CVP	central venous pressure
CVRD	cardiovascular-renal disease
CVS	chorionic villi sampling
CWP	coalworkers' pneumoconiosis
D	disease; dorsal
D&C	dilation and curettage
D&E	dilation and evacuation
dB	decibel
DC	discontinue
DEF	definition

DES	diethylstilbestrol
DGI	disseminated gonococcal infection
DH	dehydrogenase
DI	diabetes insipidus
DIC	disseminated intravascular coagulation
DIFF	differential blood count
DILD	diffuse infiltrative lung diseases
DIP	distal intraphalangeal (joint)
DIS	disease
DJD	degenerative joint disease
DKA	diabetic ketoacidosis
DLE	discoid lupus erythematosus; disseminated lupus erythematosus
DM	diabetes mellitus; diastolic murmur
DMI	diaphragmatic myocardial infarction
DNA	deoxyribonucleic acid
DNKA	did not keep appointment
DNR	do not resuscitate
DOA	dead on arrival
DOE	dyspnea on exertion
DPT	diphtheria-pertussis-tetanus (vaccine)
DRG	diagnosis-related group
DSM	Diagnostic and Statistical Manual
DTR	deep tendon reflex
DT	delirium tremens; diphtheria tetanus (vaccine)
DU	duodenal ulcer
DVI	digital vascular imaging
DVT	deep venous thrombosis
DX	diagnosis
EBV	Epstein-Barr virus
ECC	emergency cardiac care
ECG	electrocardiogram
ECF	extracellular fluid
ECHO	echocardiogram; virus affecting humans
ECT	electroconvulsive therapy
EDC	expected date of confinement
EDD	expected date of delivery
EDV	end diastolic volume
EEE	eastern equine encephalitis
EECG	exercise electrocardiogram
EEG	electroencephalogram
EEKG	exercise electrocardiogram
EENT	eye, ear, nose, throat

EF	ejection fraction
EGD	esophagogastroduodenoscopy
EHH	esophageal hiatus hernia
EKG	electrocardiogram
ELISA	enzyme-linked immunosorbent assay (test)
EM	electron microscopy; erythema multiforme
EMD	electromechanical dissociation
EMG	electromyogram
ENG	electronystagmograph
ENL	enlarged
ENT	ear, nose, throat
EOM	extraocular movement; extraocular muscles
EP	examining physician
EPM	electronic pacemaker
EPS	electrophysiological studies
ER	emergency room; estrogen receptor
ERA	estrogen receptor assay (test)
ERCP	endoscopic retrograde cholangiopancreatography
ESP	extrasensory perception
ESR	erythrocyte sedimentation rate
ESRD	end stage renal disease
EST	electroshock therapy
ET	and
ETOH	alcohol
ETT	exercise tolerance test
EU	etiology unknown
EUA	examination under anesthesia

F	Fahrenheit
FA	fluorescent antibody (test); fatty acid
FANA	fluorescent antinuclear antibody
FAS	fetal alcohol syndrome
FB	foreign body
FBD	functional bowel disorder
FBS	fasting blood sugar
Fe	iron
FEF	forced expiratory flow
FEV_1	forced expiratory volume in one second
FFB	flexible fiberoptic bronchoscopy
FH	family history
FH_X	family history
FMF	Familial Mediterranean fever
FNA	fine needle aspiration
Fr	french ($1/3$ mm)

FS	frozen section
FSH	follicle stimulating hormone
FT	full term
FTA	fluorescent treponemal antibody
FTA-ABS	fluorescent treponemal antibody absorption
FTI	free thyroxin index
FTND	full term normal delivery
FU	follow-up
FUO	fever of unknown origin
FVC	forced vital capacity
F_X	fracture
G	gravida
GB	gallbladder
GBS	Guillain-Barré syndrome
GC	gonococcus; gonorrhea
GDM	gestational diabetes mellitus
GERD	gastroesophageal reflux disease
GFR	glomerular filtration rate
GG	gamma globulin
GH	growth hormone
GI	gastrointestinal
GLU	glucose
GM	grand mal
gm	gram
GNID	gram negative intracellular diplococci
GOT	glutamic oxalacetic transaminase (AST)
G6PD	glucose-6-phosphate dehydrogenase
GPT	glutamic pyruvic transaminase
gr	grain
GSW	gun shot wound
gt (gtt)	drop (drops)
GTT	glucose tolerance test
GU	gastric ulcer; genitourinary
GXT	graded exercise test
GYN	gynecological; gynecology
H	hydrogen
H&E	hematoxylin and eosin (stain)
HAV	hepatitis A virus
HB	hemoglobin
HB_sAg	hepatitis B surface antigen
HBO	hyperbaric oxygenation
HBP	high blood pressure

HBV	hepatitis B virus
HCG	human chorionic gonadotropin
HCT	hematocrit
HCVD	hypertensive cardiovascular disease
HD	heart disease; Hodgkin's disease
HDL	high density lipoprotein
HDN	hemolytic disease of the newborn
HEENT	head, ears, eyes, nose, throat
HGB	hemoglobin
HGH	human growth hormone
HH	hiatus hernia
HHD	hypertensive heart disease
HIV	human immunodeficiency virus
HM	hand movement
HNP	herniated nucleus pulposus
HO	history of
HPF	high power field
HPV	human papilloma virus
HS	heart sounds; heat stroke; hereditary spherocytosis; hernial sac; hour of sleep
HSE	herpes simplex encephalitis
HSV	herpes simplex virus
HT	heart; hematocrit
HTN	hypertension
HVD	hypertensive vascular disease
HVS	hyperventilation syndrome
H_X	history
I	iodine
I&D	incision and drainage
IASD	intra-atrial septal defect
IBD	inflammatory bowel disease
IBS	irritable bowel syndrome
IC	intensive care
ICCE	intracapsular cataract extraction
ICH	immunocompromised host
ICP	intracranial pressure
ICS	intercostal space; irritable colon syndrome
ICU	intensive care unit
IDDM	insulin-dependent diabetes mellitus
IGT	impaired glucose tolerance
IH	infectious hepatitis (hepatitis A); in hospital
IHD	ischemic heart disease
IHSS	idiopathic hypertrophic subaortic stenosis

IM	infectious mononucleosis; intramuscular
IMA	internal mammary artery
INF	inferior
INH	isoniazid
IOL	intraocular lens
IOP	intraocular pressure
IPF	idiopathic pulmonary fibrosis
IPPD	intermittent positive pressure breathing
IPV	inactivated poliovirus vaccine
ISG	immune serum globulin
IST	insulin shock therapy
ITP	idiopathic thrombocytopenic purpura
IUCD	intrauterine contraceptive device
IUD	intrauterine device; IUCD
IUP	intrauterine pregnancy
IV	intravenous
IVC	inferior vena cava
IVP	intravenous pyelogram
IVSD	interventricular septal defect
IVU	intravenous urogram
JRA	juvenile rheumatoid arthritis
JVD	jugular venous distention
K	potassium
KA	King-Armstrong (units)
kg	kilogram
KS	Kaposi's sarcoma
KUB	kidney, ureter, bladder
KW	Keith-Wagener; Kimmelstiel-Wilson
L	left; lumbar
L&A	light and accommodation
L&W	living and well
LA	left atrium
LAD	lactic acid dehydrogenase; left axis deviation; left anterior descending
LAH	left anterior hemiblock
LBBB	left bundle branch block
LBCD	left border of cardiac dullness
LBP	low back pain
LCB	left cardiac border
LDH	lactic acid dehydrogenase
LDL	low density lipoprotein

LE	lupus erythematosus
LF	low forceps
LFT	liver function test
LGL	Lown-Ganong-Levine (syndrome)
LGV	lymphogranuloma venereum
LH	luteinizing hormone
LKS	liver, kidney, spleen
LLE	left lower extremity
LLL	left lower lobe
LLQ	left lower quadrant
LMD	local medical doctor
LMP	last menstrual period
LNMP	last normal menstrual period
LOC	loss of consciousness
LOM	left otitis media
LP	light perception; lumbar puncture
LPF	low power field
LPH	left posterior hemiblock
LS	lumbosacral
LSB	left sternal border
LSD	lysergic acid diethylamide
LSK	liver, spleen, kidney
LSS	lumbosacral strain
LT	left
LUE	left upper extremity
LUL	left upper lobe
LUQ	left upper quadrant
LV	left ventricle
LVD	left ventricular dysfunction
LVEDV	left ventricular end diastolic volume
LVET	left ventricular injection time
LVH	left ventricular hypertrophy
LVS	left ventricular strain
M	male; minute; murmur; muscle; one thousand
M_1	mitral valve first sound
MA	mental age
MAL	midaxillary line
MAO	monoamine oxidase
MAX	maximum
MBD	minimal brain damage/dysfunction
mcg	microgram (0.001 mg)
MCH	mean corpuscular hemoglobin
MCHC	mean corpuscular hemoglobin concentration

mcl	microliter (0.001 ml)
MCL	midclavicular line
MCT	medullary carcinoma of thyroid gland; medium chain triglycerides
MCTD	mixed connective tissue disease
MCV	mean corpuscular volume
MED	medial; median
MEN	multiple endocrine neoplasia
mEq	milliequivalent
mg	milligram (0.001 grams)
MHB	maximum hospital benefit
MI	maturation index; mitral insufficiency; myocardial infarction; myocardial ischemia
MIN	minimum; minute
ml	milliliter
mm	millimeter
MODM	maturity onset diabetes mellitus
MP	metacarpal phalangeal
MRI	magnetic resonance imaging
MS	multiple sclerosis; mitral stenosis; morphine sulfate
MSL	midsternal line
MTC	medullary thyroid gland carcinoma
MUGA	multiple gated acquisition
MVA	motor vehicle accident
MVP	mitral valve prolapse
MVV	maximal voluntary ventilation
N	nerve; nitrogen
Na	sodium
NAD	no apparent disease; no abnormality discovered
NC	no complaints; no complications
NCNS	no complications, no sequelae
NDAR	no diagnostic abnormality recognized
NEAD	no evident active disease
NEC	necrotizing enterocolitis
NED	no evident disease
NEG	negative
NF	neurofibromatosis
NG	nasogastric; no good
NGU	nongonococcal urethritis
NHL	non-Hodgkin's lymphoma
NIDDM	non-insulin dependent diabetes mellitus
NKA	no known allergies

NL	normal
NMI	nuclear magnetic imaging
NMR	nuclear magnetic resonance
NOS	not otherwise specified
NP	neuropsychiatric; not palpable; nurse practitioner
NPC	nodal premature contraction
NPH	intermediate-acting insulin
NPN	non-protein nitrogen
NPO	nothing by mouth
NREM	non-rapid eye movements
NSA	no significant abnormality
NSAID	nonsteroidal anti-inflammatory drug
NSD	no significant disease
NSR	normal sinus rhythm
NSSTT	nonspecific ST-T wave (abnormalities)
NSU	nonspecific urethritis
NSV	nonspecific vaginitis
NT	nodal tachycardia
NTG	nitroglycerine
N&V	nausea and vomiting
O	oxygen
O_2	oxygen
OA	osteoarthritis
OB	obstetrics
OBG	obstetrics/gynecology
OBS	obstetrics; organic brain syndrome
OC	oral contraceptives
OD	overdose; right eye
OGTT	oral glucose tolerance test
OM	otitis media
OMPA	otitis media, purulent, acute
OMT	osteomanipulative treatment
OP	operation; operative
OPD	outpatient department
OPV	oral polio vaccine
OR	open reduction; operating room
OS	left eye
OT	occupational therapy; otology; oxaloacetic transaminase
OTC	over the counter (drug)
OU	both eyes
OV	office visit
oz	ounce

P	parity; phosphorus; pulse; pressure
$\bar{p}$	after
P_2	pulmonic valve second sound
PA	pernicious anemia; postero-anterior; physician's assistant; pulmonary artery
PAC	premature atrial contraction
PAF	paroxysmal atrial fibrillation
PAOD	peripheral arterial occlusive disease
PAP	Pap smear
PAS	para-aminosalicylic acid
PAT	paroxysmal atrial tachycardia
PATH	pathology
Pb	lead
PB	Phenobarbital
PBI	protein bound iodine
pc	*post cibum* (after meals)
PCN	penicillin
PCP	pneumocystis carinii pneumonia; phencyclidine hydrochloride
PCV	packed cell volume
PCWP	pulmonary capillary wedge pressure
PE	physical examination; polyethylene; pulmonary embolism
PED	pediatrics
PEEP	positive end-expiratory pressure
PEF	peak expiratory flow
PEG	pneumoencephalogram
PERLA	pupils equal, react to light and accommodation
PES	pre-excitation syndrome
PET	positron emission tomography
PETT	positron emission transaxial tomography
PFT	pulmonary function test
PG	pregnancy; pregnant
PH_X	previous history
pH	hydrogen ion concentration
PR_X	previous history
PI	present illness; proposed insured
PID	pelvic inflammatory disease
PIE	pulmonary infiltrate with eosinophilia
PIP	proximal interphalangeal joint
PKU	phenylketonuria
PM	petit mal; polymyositis
PMA	progressive muscular atrophy
PMD	private medical doctor; papillary muscle dysfunction

PMI	point of maximum impulse; posterior myocardial infarction
PMN	polymorphonuclear neutrophil
PMR	polymyalgia rheumatica
PMS	premenstrual syndrome
PMV	prolapse of the mitral valve
PNA	perennial nasal allergy
PND	paroxysmal nocturnal dyspnea; post-nasal drip
PNH	paroxysmal nocturnal hemoglobinuria
PNS	partial nonprogressing stroke; peripheral nervous system
PO	*per os* (by mouth); post-operative
POC	products of conception
PP	postpartum; postpone; postprandial; pulse pressure
PP&A	palpation, percussion, and auscultation
PPD	purified protein derivative
PPLO	pleuropneumonia-like organisms (mycoplasma species)
PRN	*pro re nata* (whenever required, as needed)
PS	prostate smear
PSA	prostate-specific antigen
PSS	progressive systemic sclerosis
PSVT	paroxysmal supraventricular tachycardia
PT	patient; physical therapy; prothrombin time; pyruvic transaminase
PTA	percutaneous transluminal angioplasty; plasma thromboplastin antecedent; prior to admission
PTC	percutaneous transhepatic cholangiography; plasma thromboplastin component
PTCA	percutaneous transluminal coronary angioplasty
PTE	pretibial edema; pulmonary thromboembolism
PTH	parathyroid hormone
PTS	premenstrual tension syndrome
PTT	partial thromboplastin time (test)
PTU	propylthiouracil
PU	peptic ulcer
PUD	peptic ulcer disease
PUVA	psoriasis treatment with a psoralen compound and ultraviolet A irradiation
PV	polycythemia vera
PVB	premature ventricular beat
PVC	premature ventricular contraction
PVD	peripheral vascular disease
P_X	physical examination
PZI	prolamine zinc insulin

Q	each, every
QD	once daily
QH	every hour
QID	four times daily
QNS	quantity not sufficient
QOD	every other day
QRS	QRS segment of an EKG
QV	*quod vide* (which see)

R	respiration; right
Ra	radium
RA	rheumatoid arthritis; right atrium
RAD	right axis deviation
RAI	radioactive iodine
RBBB	right bundle branch block
RBC	red blood cell; red blood (cell) count
RCA	right coronary artery
REM	rapid eye movement
RESP	respiration; respiratory
RF	rheumatic fever; rheumatoid factor
Rh	Rhesus factor (blood group)
RHD	rheumatic heart disease
RLE	right lower extremity
RLF	retrolental fibroplasia
RLL	right lower lobe
RLQ	right lower quadrant
RML	right middle lobe
RNA	ribonucleic acid
RND	regional node dissection
RNS	radionuclide scan
RO	rule out
ROM	range of motion; right otitis media
ROS	review of systems
RPF	renal plasma flow
RPR	rapid plasma reagin
RRR	regular rate and rhythm
RS	Reed Sternberg (cells); Reye's syndrome
RSR	regular sinus rhythm
RSV	respiratory syncytial virus
RT	radiotherapy; right; rubella titer
RTA	renal tubular acidosis
RTC	return to clinic
RTW	return to work
RUE	right upper extremity

RUL	right upper lobe
RUQ	right upper quadrant
RV	right ventricle
RVH	right ventricular hypertrophy
RVS	relative value system; right ventricular strain
R_X	prescription; treatment
S	sacral; serum; sugar; systolic
$\bar{s}$	without
SA	sino-atrial; sinus arrest
SAH	subarachnoid hemorrhage; systolic arterial hypertension
S&C	smear and culture
SB	sinus bradycardia
SBE	scleral buckling procedure; self breast examination; subacute bacterial endocarditis
SBP	systolic blood pressure
$\overline{sc}$	without correction
SC	sickle cell; subcutaneous
SCA	sickle cell anemia
SCD	sudden cardiac death
SCID	severe combined immunodeficiency disorder
SCL	scleroderma
SED	sedimentation
SEM	systolic ejection murmur
SF	spinal fluid
SG	specific gravity
SGOT	serum glutamic oxalacetic transaminase
SGPT	serum glutamic pyruvic transaminase
SH	serum hepatitis
SI	sacroiliac; saline instillation
SIDH	syndrome of inappropriate antidiuretic hormone
SIDS	sudden infant death syndrome
SLD	specific learning disorder/disability
SLE	St. Louis encephalitis; slit lamp examination; systemic lupus erythematosus
SLR	straight leg raising
SM	streptomycin; systolic murmur
SMA	Sequential Multiple Analyzer
SMR	submucous resection
SOB	shortness of breath
SOM	secretory otitis media
SQ	subcutaneous
SP	sinus pause; systolic pressure

SpGr	specific gravity
SR	sedimentation rate; sinus rhythm; Sternberg-Reed (cells); system review
SS	systemic sclerosis
SSE	soap suds enema
SSS	sick sinus syndrome; scalded skin syndrome
ST	ST segment of EKG; sinus tachycardia; spinal tap
STD	sexually transmitted disease
STS	serologic test for syphilis
STSG	split thickness skin graft
SUP	superior
SVBG	saphenous vein bypass graft
SVCS	superior vena cava syndrome
SVT	supraventricular tachycardia
S_X	symptom
T	temperature; total
T_3	triiodothyronine
T_4	tetraiodothyronine (thyroxine)
T&A	tonsillectomy and adenoidectomy
TAH	total abdominal hysterectomy
TAL	tendo-achilles lengthening
TAO	thromboangiitis obliterans
TAPVC	total anomalous pulmonary venous connection
TAT	tetanus antitoxin
TB	total bilirubin; tubercle bacillus; tuberculosis
TBB	transbronchial biopsy
TBC	tuberculosis
TBE	tick-borne encephalitis
TBG	thyroxin-binding globulin
TCD	transverse chest diameter
TCI	transient cerebral ischemia
TCN	tetracycline
TD	transverse diameter (of the heart); tetanus diphtheria (vaccine)
TENS	transcutaneous electronic nerve stimulation (pain management)
TFT	thyroid function test
TH	thoracic
THC	tetrahydrocannabinol (marijuana)
THR	total hip replacement
TIA	transient ischemic attack
TIBC	total iron binding capacity
TID	three times a day

TIFD	tissue insufficient for diagnosis
TLC	tender loving care; thin layer chromatography
TM	tympanic membrane
TMJ	temporomandibular joint
TNG	nitroglycerine
TNTC	too numerous to count
TP	total protein
tPA	tissue plasminogen activator
TPCF	treponema pallidum complement fixation
TPI	treponema pallidum immobilization
TPN	total parenteral nutrition
TPR	temperature, pulse, respiration
TSH	thyroid stimulating hormone
TSS	toxic shock syndrome
TTP	thrombotic thrombocytopenic purpura
TUR	transurethral resection
TURP	transurethral resection of the prostate
TV	tidal volume; total volume; Trichomonas vaginalis
TVC	timed vital capacity
TVD	three vessel disease
TVH	total vaginal hysterectomy
T_x	treatment
UA	uric acid; urinalysis
UCD	usual childhood diseases
UCG	urine chorionic gonadotropin
UGI	upper gastrointestinal
UPT	urine pregnancy test
URI	upper respiratory infection
US	ultrasonography
UTI	urinary tract infection
UV	ultraviolet
UVA	ultraviolet light (of long wave length)
UVB	ultraviolet light (of intermediate wave length, the spectrum involved in sunburn)
UVC	ultraviolet light (of short wave length)
V	vein
VA	ventricular arrest; visual acuity
V&D	vomiting and diarrhea
VB	ventricular bradycardia
VC	vena cava; vital capacity
VCG	vector cardiogram
VCU	voiding cystourethrogram

VD	venereal disease; vessel disease
VDH	valvular disease of the heart
VDRL	venereal disease research laboratory
VDRR	vitamin D resistant rickets
VEA	ventricular ectopic activity
VEE	Venezuelan equine encephalitis
VF	ventricular fibrillation; ventricular flutter
VFib	ventricular fibrillation
VFl	ventricular flutter
VHD	valvular heart disease
VLDL	very low density lipoprotein
VMA	vanillylmandelic acid
VP	ventricular pause
VPC	ventricular premature contraction
VPS	ventricular-peritoneal shunt
VSD	ventricular septal defect
VT	ventricular tachycardia
VV	varicose veins; vulvo-vaginal

w/	with
WBC	white blood cell; white blood (cell) count
WDWN	well developed, well nourished
WEE	western equine encephalitis
WLE	wide local excision
WNL	within normal limits
w/o	without
WPW	Wolff-Parkinson-White (syndrome)
WV	whispered voice

X	sex chromosome (for female characteristics)
XRT	radiation therapy
XS	excess
XU	extrauterine pregnancy

| Y | sex chromosome (for male characteristics) |

Medical References

This appendix provides a list of medical text references that will be helpful for insurance personnel.

American Cancer Society Textbook of Clinical Oncology, 1st Ed., 1991
Current Obstetric and Gynecologic Diagnosis and Treatment, 7th Ed., Appleton and Lange, 1991
Diagnostic and Statistical Manual of Mental Disorders, 3rd Ed., revised ("DSM-III-R"), American Psychiatric Association, 1987
Disability Evaluation Under Social Security, U.S. Department of Health and Human Services, SSA Publication No. 05–10089, Feb. 1986
Medical Yardsticks for Disability Insurance, Volume XXI, State of California, Employment Development Department, 1980
Merck Manual, 16th Ed., 1992
Outline of Orthopedics, by Adams and Hamblen, 11th Ed., Churchill Livingstone, 1990
Physician's Desk Reference (PDR), 48th Ed., Medical Economics Data Production Co., Montvale, NJ 07645–1742, 1994
Pocket Handbook of Clinical Psychiatry, by Kaplan and Sadock, Williams and Wilkins, 1990

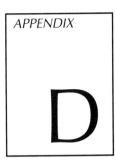

Cranial Nerves

Number and Name of Nerve	Major Type of Stimuli Transmission	Major Functions
I. Olfactory	sensory	transmission of sense of smell
II. Optic	sensory	transmission of sense of sight
III. Oculomotor	motor	movement of eyeball and upper eyelid; change in shape of lens and pupil
IV. Trochlear	motor	movement of eyeball
V. Trigeminal	motor	movement of muscles for chewing
	sensory	transmission of sensations from face
VI. Abducens	motor	movement of eyeball

Number and Name of Nerve	Major Type of Stimuli Transmission	Major Functions
VII. Facial	motor	movement of facial muscles; control of glands of nose; mouth and jaw muscles
	sensory	transmission of sense of taste and other sensations from nose and palate
VIII. Acoustic	sensory	transmission of sense of sound and equilibrium
IX. Glossopharyngeal	motor	movement of muscles of pharynx; control of parotid gland
	sensory	transmission of sense of taste and other sensations from palate, tongue, pharynx and ear
X. Vagus	motor	movement of muscles of pharynx, larynx; control over certain functions of the heart, liver, intestinal tract and pancreas
	sensory	transmission of sensations from organs in thorax and abdomen
XI. Accessory	motor	movement of neck and shoulder muscles
XII. Hypoglossal	motor	movement of tongue

E

Duration of Disability

The purpose of the following lists is to give the claim reviewer a broad sampling of durations of disability for many common conditions. It is not the authors' intent to make the lists all-inclusive. Furthermore, if a claimant's duration of disability exceeds the stated limit, the reviewer should not assume that the claimant is malingering. The claim reviewer should, however, make a prompt and thorough review of all facts bearing on the claimant's illness.

For the purpose of these lists, a disability is considered to have terminated when an average middle-aged adult, under normal circumstances, would be capable of returning to a full-time job that may involve some light physical activity. The listed disability durations are averages and should be used only as guides. Some adults may return to work sooner and others later than the stated durations. A longer convalescence may be necessary for those claimants whose jobs require manual labor.

The given duration of disability for a fracture is based on the assumption that the fracture is a simple (non-compound) one. For an illness that does not require surgical treatment, the duration of disability is based on an acute attack of average severity. However, many illnesses have subacute or chronic stages that may affect an individual's ability to perform selected tasks for varying periods. The given duration of disability for a surgical procedure is based on the assumption that the claimant experiences no postoperative complication.

FRACTURES

Bone fractured	Duration of Disability
Carpal bones	
except navicular	6–8 weeks
navicular	14–20 weeks
Clavicle	4–8 weeks
Femur	
near hip	8–12 months
near knee	6–10 months
Fibula	
shaft	6 weeks
lateral malleolus	9–12 weeks
Finger	3–4 weeks
Humerus	
neck	8–10 weeks
shaft	10–14 weeks
Metacarpal	4–6 weeks
Metatarsal	4–8 weeks
Os calcis	5–6 months
Patella	10–16 weeks
Pelvis	10–12 weeks
Radius	
head	6–8 weeks
shaft	10–16 weeks
and ulna, shafts	4–6 months
Ribs	0–2 weeks
Scapula	6–10 weeks
Tarsal bones	
except os calcis	8–12 weeks
os calcis	5–6 months
Toe	2–4 weeks
Tibia	
upper end	4–8 months
lower end	8–12 months
medial malleolus	10–16 weeks
Ulna	
near wrist	8–10 weeks
shaft	12–18 weeks
Vertebra	
body	2–8 months
spinous process	3–4 weeks

OPERATIONS

Operation/condition	Duration of disability
Abdomino-perineal resection	3–4 months
Anterior-posterior colporrhaphy	6 weeks
Aortic aneurysm, abdominal aorta	6–8 weeks
Appendectomy	4 weeks

OPERATIONS

Operation/condition	Duration of disability
Arthroscopy, knee	
diagnostic	7–10 weeks
resection of plica	2 weeks
removal of loose bodies	3 weeks
partial medial/lateral meniscectomy	6 weeks
repair medial/lateral meniscus	12–16 weeks
repair anterior cruciate ligament	up to 1 year
repair posterior cruciate ligament	up to 1 year
chondroplasty	4–6 weeks
debridement	4–8 weeks
Arthroscopy, shoulder	
diagnostic	2 weeks
impingement syndrome	12–16 weeks
excision of a detached glenoid labrum	6–8 weeks
repair rotator cuff	12–16 weeks
debridement	4 weeks
Bowel resection with colostomy	3–4 months
Breast cyst	
aspiration	none
excision	2 weeks
Breast adenoma, excision	2 weeks
Caesarean section	6–8 weeks
Caldwall-Luc operation	3–4 weeks
Carotid endarterectomy	6 weeks
Carpal tunnel surgery	4–6 weeks
Cataract extraction	3–6 weeks
Cholecystectomy	8–10 weeks
Colostomy	8–10 weeks
Colporrhaphy, anterior and posterior	6 weeks
Commissurotomy, mitral valve	3 months
Cone biopsy of cervix	2 weeks
Coronary artery bypass	3 months
Cystocele repair	6 weeks
Cystoscopy	0–2 weeks
Cystotomy	6 weeks
Dilation and curettage	1–2 weeks
Gastroenterostomy	8 weeks
Gastrectomy	8–10 weeks
Hallux valgus surgery	6 weeks
Heart valve replacement	3 months
Hemorrhoidectomy	
external	2–3 weeks
internal and external	3–4 weeks
Herniorrhaphy	4–8 weeks
Hip replacement, total	
protective weight-bearing	4–6 weeks
with partially increasing activity as tolerated and expected end result	3–6 months

OPERATIONS

Operation/condition	Duration of disability
Hysterectomy	
abdominal	8–10 weeks
radical abdominal	3–4 months
vaginal	6–8 weeks
Ileostomy	8–10 weeks
Iridectomy	3–5 weeks
Knee cartilage, excision of	6 weeks
Knee replacement, total	
protective weight-bearing	4–6 weeks
with partially increasing activity as tolerated and expected end result	3–6 months
Laminectomy	6–12 weeks
Laparoscopy	0–3 days
Laryngectomy	
partial	6–8 weeks
total	3–4 months
Laser therapy for retinal detachment	0–2 weeks
Lobectomy, pulmonary	8–10 weeks
Lumbar disc surgery	2–3 months
Mastectomy	
simple	6–8 weeks
radical	2–3 months
Nephrectomy	8–10 weeks
Nephrolithotomy	8–10 weeks
Oophorectomy	4–6 weeks
Pacemaker insertion	3 weeks
Pilonidal cyst, excision	3–5 weeks
Pneumonectomy	2–4 months
Prostatectomy	6–8 weeks
Pyelolithotomy	8–10 weeks
Salpingectomy	4–6 weeks
Scleral buckling for retinal detachment	6 weeks
Spinal fusion	4–6 months
Splenectomy	6–8 weeks
Stapedectomy	2 weeks
Sympathectomy, lumbar	4 weeks
Thyroidectomy	4–6 weeks
Tonsillectomy	1–2 weeks
Tubal ligation	
laparoscopic	0–3 days
laparotomic	4 weeks
Ureterolithotomy	8–10 weeks
Vagotomy	8 weeks
Vein stripping	3–5 weeks
Vulvectomy	
simple	6–8 weeks
radical	3–4 months

ILLNESSES

Illness	Duration of disability
Asthma	0–2 weeks
Bronchiectasis	1–6 weeks
Bronchitis	0–1 week
Bursitis	0–2 weeks
Cholecystitis	2–4 weeks
Colitis, spastic (mucous)	0–2 weeks
Cystitis	0–2 weeks
Diverticulitis	2–4 weeks
Empyema	4–12 weeks
Endocarditis	2–6 months
Glomerulonephritis	2–8 weeks
Gout	0–2 weeks
Hay fever	usually none
Hepatitis	3–8 weeks
Infectious mononucleosis	1–4 weeks
Influenza	1–3 weeks
Kidney stone	2–4 weeks
Meningitis	3–10 weeks
Osteomyelitis	none–months
Pancreatitis	3–8 weeks
Pericarditis	4–12 weeks
Pharyngitis	0–1 week
Phlebitis	2–6 weeks
Pleurisy	
without effusion	1–3 weeks
with effusion	2–6 weeks
Pneumonia	2–6 weeks
Pulmonary abscess	4–12 weeks
Pyelonephritis	1–3 weeks
Regional enteritis	4–12 weeks
Salpingitis (PID)	1–3 weeks
Ulcer, peptic	2–6 weeks
Ulcerative colitis	4–12 weeks

The following illnesses may cause minimal disability in their mild forms, but may, in their severe and chronic forms, be associated with permanent partial or total disability.

Angina pectoris
Arteriosclerosis obliterans
Arteriosclerotic heart disease
Buerger's disease
Cerebral vascular accident
Cirrhosis
Congestive heart disease
Coronary artery disease

Emphysema, obstructive
Glomerulonephritis
Hypertensive heart disease
Multiple sclerosis
Paraplegia
Pyelonephritis
Retinitis

Glossary

This glossary is intended to give concise definitions of medical terms as a study tool and as a quick reference source for insurance personnel and others who are not medical professionals. For more complete and technical medical definitions, please consult a medical dictionary or other medical reference.

abdomen The largest cavity in the body, it contains the greater part of the digestive tract, some of the accessory organs of digestion, the spleen, the kidneys, and the adrenal glands.

abdominal laparoscopy The inspection of a patient's abdominal and pelvic organs using a fiberoptic scope, known as a laparoscope, that a surgeon inserts through a small incision in the front wall of the patient's abdomen.

abduction Movement away from the midline.

abortion The termination of pregnancy before the conceptus, embryo, or fetus is capable of living outside the uterus.

abruptio placenta A condition in which the placenta begins to separate from its implanted position in the mother's uterus before the birth of the baby.

absence seizure A generalized epileptic episode characterized by a brief lapse of consciousness that is often so fleeting that the affected person may be unaware of the seizure, even if several of these seizures occur per day.

509

accelerated hypertension   A condition characterized by markedly and increasingly elevated blood pressure accompanied by vascular changes in the retina.

accidental proteinuria   A condition in which protein is present in the urine as a result of contamination.

accommodation   The process by which ciliary muscles change the shape of the lens in the eye to accomplish precise focusing of near and distant objects.

acetabulum   A cup-shaped socket in and around which the ilium, the ischium, and the pubis join together.

achalasia   A disorder in which the esophageal contracture is markedly ineffective and the lower esophageal sphincter over-contracts and does not permit food to enter the stomach.

achlorhydria   A condition in which the patient's gastric mucosa fails to produce any hydrochloric acid.

acne   A common skin condition characterized by the presence of blackhead pimples, papules, pustules, and cysts. Also known as acne vulgaris.

acne vulgaris   *See* acne.

acoustic nerve   The nerve responsible for the sense of balance and hearing. Also known as cranial nerve VIII.

acoustic neuroma   A benign tumor of the acoustic nerve that results in the inability of a patient to hear high-frequency tones and causes vertigo.

acquired immune deficiency syndrome   A condition that is caused by the human immunodeficiency virus and which results in the suppression of the patient's immune system and in an irreversible defect in the patient's cell-mediated immunity. Also known as AIDS.

acro lentiginous melanoma   A type of melanocarcinoma that involves moles arising on palms or soles or under nails.

acromegaly   A chronic, often disabling disorder caused by an adenoma of the anterior pituitary lobe that produces an excessive amount of growth hormone.

acrophobia   The fear of heights.

ACTH   *See* adrenocorticotropic hormone.

actinic keratosis   A common precancerous lesion of the skin. It is characterized by irregular red patches of epidermis that are covered by rough scales.

active immunity   Immunity that results from the presence of either antibodies or immune lymphoid cells that were formed in response to an antigen.

acute bronchitis   An acute inflammation of the tracheobronchial tree.

acute diffuse glomerulonephritis   An acute form of glomerulonephritis that typically is characterized by fever, massive proteinuria, hematuria, anemia, hypertension, decreased urinary output, and generalized retention of tissue fluids.

acute disease   A disease of any type that is generally characterized by a sudden onset and a relatively short course of illness.

acute enteritis   An inflammation of the lining of the small intestine that usually has a sudden onset and is of short duration.

acute gastritis   An acute inflammation of the lining of the stomach.

acute idiopathic polyneuritis   *See* Guillain-Barré syndrome.

acute laryngotracheobronchitis   An acute respiratory infection in which the mucous membranes of the larynx, trachea, and bronchi are acutely inflamed and swollen.

acute myocardial infarction   The death of heart muscle that is characterized by the sudden onset of severe, persistent chest pain, often associated with excess perspiration, pallor, restlessness, and a sense of impending doom. It is usually secondary to coronary artery atherosclerosis.

acute prostatitis   A bacterial infection of the prostate, characterized by (1) an abrupt onset of fever, (2) pain at the base of the penis, (3) rectal aching, (4) frequent, urgent, and painful urination, and (5) an uncontrolled discharge of cloudy fluid from the urethra.

acute purulent otitis media   A bacterial infection in which pus fills a patient's middle ear. This condition is characterized by throbbing pain in the ear and hearing loss. Also known as acute suppurative otitis media.

acute pyelonephritis   A bacterial infection of the kidney that appears suddenly and is characterized by high fever, chills, rapid pulse, flank pain, frequency of urination, and dysuria.

acute rheumatic fever   A delayed, non-pus producing, inflammatory reaction that occurs principally in the joints, heart, and subcutaneous tissues, and is secondary to a streptococcal oropharynx infection.

acute rhinitis   A condition caused by one of many viruses that produce manifestations including inflammation of the mucous membrane of the nose with large amounts of nasal discharge, mild fever, sore throat, headache, and a general feeling of discomfort.

acute serous otitis media   A condition in which a noninflammatory watery fluid develops in a patient's middle ear in response to allergic phenomena, changes in atmospheric pressure, or pharyngitis.

acute suppurative otitis media   *See* acute purulent otitis media.

acute tubular necrosis   The sudden death of the cells of the renal tubules.

adaptive behavior   The degree of success with which an individual meets the accepted standards of social responsibility and personal independence.

ADD *See* attention deficit disorder.

addiction *See* physical dependence.

Addison's disease A condition in which the adrenal glands under-produce corticosteroids and mineralocorticoids and which is characterized by progressive weakness, brownish pigmentation of the skin, low blood pressure, dizziness, fainting spells, diarrhea, and weight loss.

adenocarcinoma A general name given to a group of malignancies derived from the epithelium of glands or ducts.

adenoma A benign tumor composed of glandular cells that may manufacture and secrete hormones and other substances.

adenomyosis A condition in which the endometrial implants are located in the myometrium.

ADH *See* antidiuretic hormone.

ADHD *See* attention deficit hyperactive disorder.

adhesion A thin, narrow, thread-like band or broad fold of tissue.

adhesive capsulitis A condition that involves an adhesive inflammation between a joint capsule and the peripheral cartilage of the joint.

adipose tissue Connective tissue that contains many fat cells.

adjustment disorder A type of non-psychotic psychiatric disorder that is characterized by an exaggeration of neurotic symptoms in response to a real or perceived stressful event.

adrenal gland A small, flattened, cup-shaped structure that lies immediately above and in front of the upper end of a kidney.

adrenal virilism An overproduction of adrenal cortical androgen caused by Cushing's disease or an adenoma.

adrenalin *See* epinephrine.

adrenocorticotropic hormone (ACTH) A pituitary hormone that stimulates the production of hormones from the adrenal cortex.

adynamic ileus The loss of normal activity of the ileum.

afferent nerves Nerves that convey sensations from peripheral nerve endings over sensory pathways to the spinal cord and the brain.

agoraphobia The fear of open, public places or of situations in which crowds are likely to be found.

AIDS *See* acquired immune deficiency syndrome.

air embolism An air bubble that occludes a blood vessel.

air space *See* alveolus.

akinesia The absence of muscular contraction.

alcoholic An individual who has the chronic illness of alcoholism and has a pathologic dependence on alcohol.

alcoholic cardiomyopathy   A disease that is characterized by dilation of the heart chambers. It is caused by the consumption of large amounts of alcohol.

alcoholic cirrhosis   A type of degenerative liver disease that involves the progressive destruction of liver cells resulting from long-term abuse of alcohol.

alcoholic hepatitis   A condition characterized by inflammation of liver tissue, the destruction of liver cells, hepatomegaly, and slight jaundice secondary to alcohol ingestion.

alcohol intoxication   A pathologic condition caused by ingesting alcohol. Also known as drunkenness.

alcoholism   A chronic illness in which the excessive use of alcohol impairs or interferes with an individual's physical health, social interaction, job performance, and ability to cope with emotions and feelings.

aldosterone   A hormone that is secreted by the adrenal cortex and regulates the body's water and salt balance.

aldosteronism   The secretion of aldosterone in excessive amounts.

allergy   A hypersensitive reaction to a particular antigen.

alopecia   The loss of hair.

ALS   *See* amyotrophic lateral sclerosis.

alveolar duct   A fine air passage that connects a bronchiole and an alveolus.

alveolar edema   A condition in which serous fluid from the capillaries surrounding the alveoli escapes and enters the alveolar space.

alveolus   A rounded projection that lies at the end of an alveolar duct. Also known as an air space.

Alzheimer's disease   A slowly progressive disorder that is characterized by loss of intellectual, speech, and motor function that may progress to total helplessness.

amebiasis   A protozoan disease which is typically characterized by abscesses of the liver and ulcers of the colon.

amebic dysentery   An infectious colitis that is caused by the protozoan Entamoeba histolytica, which is primarily found in tropical or subtropical climates.

amenorrhea   The absence of menstruation.

AMI   *See* acute myocardial infarction.

aminotransferase   An enzyme that is normally present in the blood serum and various body tissues, especially the heart and liver. Also known as a transaminase.

amniocentesis   A procedure by which amniotic fluid is withdrawn from a pregnant woman and tested to determine if a genetic disease is present in the growing fetus.

amyloid   A type of abnormal complex protein.

amyloidosis A condition in which amyloids infiltrate multiple organs such as the liver, heart, stomach, and kidney.

amyotrophic lateral sclerosis (ALS) A slowly progressive disease that is characterized by impairment of the patient's motor function, spasticity of all extremities, muscle weakness, and wasting of tissues. Also known as Lou Gehrig's disease.

anal fissure An open, ulcerated crevice in the mucosa of the anus. Also known as fissure-in-ano.

analgesic An agent that relieves pain without causing a loss of consciousness.

anaphylaxis An unusual or exaggerated allergic reaction to a foreign protein or other substance.

anatomic pathology The gross and microscopic study of changes in the structures of diseased organs.

androgen Any substance that possesses masculinizing activities.

anemia A condition in which the amount of hemoglobin or the number of erythrocytes in the blood is below the normal level.

anesthesia An artificially induced insensibility to the pain caused by surgery, other painful procedures, injury, or disease.

anesthesia by local infiltration The induced loss of sensation of a part of the body resulting from the injection of an anesthetic agent into the patient's skin and subcutaneous tissues.

anesthesiology The study of ways of producing an absence of sensation.

aneurysm A sac that forms from a weakened section in the wall of an artery, a vein, or the heart.

angina pectoris Chest pain of cardiac origin, which results from an inadequate supply of oxygen to the myocardium.

angiography A diagnostic technique involving the introduction of a contrast material into a patient's blood vessel, followed by a series of x-rays, usually taken in rapid sequence.

angioneurotic edema A skin condition that involves swelling of deeper skin and fat. Also known as giant hives.

angulation A bone deformity in which the bone no longer lies in a straight line.

anions Negatively-charged ions.

ankylosing spondylitis A chronic, slowly progressive form of arthritis, which primarily involves the spine and sacroiliac joints. Also known as Marie Strumpell disease.

annulus fibrosus The fibrocartilage that surrounds the intervertebral disc.

anorectal abscess A condition which begins as an infection in the rectal glands that later invades the surrounding tissue. Also known as perirectal abscess or perianal abscess.

anorexia nervosa   A psychologic and physiologic condition that is characterized by a severe and prolonged refusal to eat.

anovulation   The absence of ovulation.

anoxia   A condition that is characterized by an absence of oxygen to the tissues.

anterior cruciate   A ligament that lies on the front of the knee joint and helps to control that joint.

anterior optic neuritis   *See* papillitis.

anthracosis   A type of pneumoconiosis caused by inhaling coal dust.

antibody   A complex protein that a body generates in response to the presence of an antigen that does not normally inhabit the body.

antidiuretic hormone (ADH)   A hypothalamus hormone that causes the kidney tubules to increase their reabsorption of water, leading to decreased urine output, and causes the constriction of the smooth muscle found in the walls of blood vessels.

antigen   A molecule or a part of a molecule found on the surface of a foreign substance in a body, and used by the immune system to identify the substance as being foreign.

antihemophilic factor   A type of coagulation factor found in plasma. Also known as Factor VIII.

antihypertensive   A drug that reduces elevated blood pressure.

antisocial personality disorder   A condition characterized by an individual's lack of basic socialization, behavior that results in repeated conflict with society, and the inability to be loyal to individuals, groups, or social codes. Also known as psychopathic personality disorder or sociopathic personality disorder.

antrectomy   The surgical removal of part of the pylorus.

anus   The distal opening of the digestive system to the outside of the body.

anxiety   A feeling of apprehension, uncertainty, fear, unpleasant tension, fatigue, distress, or panic, that is characterized by excessive perspiration, tension headaches, sighing, labored breathing, loss of appetite, "butterflies in the stomach," rapid pulse, fainting, impotence, and hyperventilation.

aortic regurgitation   A failure of the aortic valve to close properly in diastole, thus allowing blood from the aorta to flow back into the left ventricle leading to excessive blood volume in that chamber.

aortic stenosis   An obstructive lesion of the aorta that is usually secondary to an abnormal valve, and presents in childhood or in later life as the valve undergoes progressive degeneration, fibrosis, and calcification.

aphakia   A condition in which an individual does not have a lens in his or her eye, for any reason, and is a common result of cataract surgery.

aplastic anemia   A disorder characterized by a condition called pancytopenia, which is a reduction in the number of red blood cells, white blood cells, and platelets.

appendectomy   The surgical removal of the appendix.

appendicitis   An inflammation of the appendix.

appendix   A long, narrow, worm-like tube that arises from the cecum.

aqueous humor   A fluid that fills the chamber that lies between the cornea and the iris of the eye.

arachnoid   The delicate middle meninge.

arrhythmia   Any alteration in the pattern or rate of normal cardiac sinus rhythm.

arteriography   The x-ray visualization of an artery after the injection of radiopaque dye.

arteriosclerosis   The thickening, with loss of elasticity, of small, medium, and large arteries.

arteriosclerosis obliterans   Obstruction of the peripheral vessels in the lower extremities leading to bloodflow deficiency.

arteriosclerotic retinopathy   A disease of the retina that is characterized by the development of thickened, hardened retinal arterioles that can be seen upon ophthalmoscopic examination.

arteritis   A condition characterized by an inflammation of the arterial wall.

arthralgia   A condition in which pain occurs in a joint without anatomic change.

arthritis   A general term for several disorders in which anatomic change produces pain and stiffness in joints.

arthrocentesis   The needle puncture of a joint for the removal of joint fluid.

arthrodesis   The surgical fixation of a joint through a procedure that causes the joint surfaces to fuse by promoting the proliferation of bone cells. Also known as artificial ankylosis.

arthrogram   An x-ray of a joint taken after a dye has been injected into the joint.

arthroscopy   A diagnostic procedure that permits direct visualization of a joint through fiberoptic imaging that is visualized on a monitoring cathode-ray tube screen.

arthrotomy   A procedure in which a surgeon makes an incision through the patient's skin and into the joint for direct visualization and manipulation of the structure.

articular capsule   A sac-like envelope that encloses the cavity of a joint.

articulation   See joint.

artificial ankylosis   See arthrodesis.

asbestosis   A type of pneumoconiosis caused by inhaling asbestos.

ascending colon   The part of the large intestine that ascends from the cecum.

ascites   A condition in which the patient accumulates fluid in the abdomen.

ASD   *See* atrial septal defect.

asthmatic bronchitis   A condition characterized by asthma-like attacks that occur during the course of a bronchitis or other respiratory tract infection.

asthmatic crisis   *See* status asthmaticus.

asthmatic shock   *See* status asthmaticus.

astigmatism   A refractive error of the eye in which rays of light are brought to a focus at different points along the retina.

asymptomatic   A patient or a disease that does not manifest any symptoms.

atelectasis   A condition of airlessness resulting from a collapse of lung tissue.

atherosclerosis   A disease of lipid, or fat, in the medium and large muscular and elastic arteries.

athetoid movement   A ceaseless, slow, involuntary writhing motion, especially of the hands, common in cerebral palsy patients.

athlete's foot   A common fungal infection of the skin, hair, and nails.

atonic seizure   A seizure characterized by a transient loss of postural tone, causing the affected person to fall suddenly.

atopic dermatitis   A noncontagious inflammation of the skin that is characterized by lesions which redden, ooze, scale, and crust. Also known as atopic eczema.

atopic eczema   *See* atopic dermatitis.

atria   The two upper chambers of the heart.

atrial fibrillation   An irregular, chaotic rhythm in the atria with a rapid irregular ventricular response.

atrial flutter   A regular supraventricular tachycardia that rarely occurs in normal hearts.

atrial septal defect   An opening in the atrial septum allowing an abnormal shunt between the two atria.

atrophic vaginitis   A form of vaginitis that occurs in postmenopausal women. It is associated with an estrogen deficiency. Also known as senile vaginitis.

attention deficit disorder (ADD)   A condition characterized by developmentally inappropriate impulsivity and inattention.

attention deficit hyperactive disorder (ADHD)   A condition that includes attention deficit disorder and hyperactivity.

audiometer   A medical instrument that tests hearing acuity by generating pure tones that can vary in pitch and intensity.

auditory tube   *See* eustachian tube.

aura   The warning symptoms that precede a migraine.

auricle   The fleshy, cartilaginous curved part of the ear that lies on the outside of the head.

autoimmune disease   Any one of several disorders in which the body attacks its own tissue.

autonomic nervous system   The part of the peripheral nervous system that regulates the activities of cardiac muscle, smooth muscle, and glands.

autosome   Any ordinary paired chromosome, as distinguished from a sex chromosome. Humans have 22 pairs of autosomes.

avulsion fracture   A fracture that occurs as the result of a sudden, severe muscle pull that tears the ligaments and muscles from the bone.

B lymphocyte   A type of lymphocyte that is primarily involved with antigen identification and antibody production.

bacillary bacterium   *See* rod bacterium.

bacillary dysentery   An acute bacterial infection that is characterized by fever and bloody diarrhea.

backbone   *See* spine.

bacteremia   A transient bacterial invasion of the blood stream.

bacterial endocarditis   An infection that primarily affects the endocardium overlying the heart valves.

bacteriology   The study of bacteria.

bacterium   A microscopic unicellular organism that occurs in several shapes.

ball and socket joint   A joint that permits motion in an indefinite number of axes.

Bartholin's gland   One of two small glands that are situated on either side of the vaginal opening.

Bartholin's gland abscess   A condition in which an infection involves an entire Bartholin's gland, and a collection of pus distends the gland.

basal cell carcinoma   The most common skin malignancy in whites, it is characterized by a smooth, slightly elevated papule, and most often occurs on the patient's face as a single lesion or multiple lesions. Also known as basal cell epithelioma.

basal cell epithelioma   *See* basal cell carcinoma.

behavior modification   The rewarding of desirable activity and the discouraging of disruptive activity.

Bell's palsy   A unilateral facial paralysis of sudden onset, caused by a lesion of the facial nerve and resulting in characteristic distortion of the face.

benign prostatic hypertrophy   A condition that involves the noncancerous enlargement of the prostate gland.

benign tumor   A slow growing tumor which does not invade neighboring tissues or spread to distant parts of the body, and that does
not recur after complete removal.

bifocal lenses   Lenses for eyeglasses that consist of two sections—
one section corrects hyperopia and the other corrects myopia.

bilateral adrenocortical hyperplasia   A condition in which the
cortexes of both adrenal glands are the sites of abnormal multiplication of cells in a normal arrangement.

bilateral oophorectomy   The surgical removal of both ovaries.

bile   An orange-brown or greenish-yellow solution that contains bile
pigments, bile salts, cholesterol, minerals, and other organic substances.

bilirubin   An end-product of the destruction of aged red blood
cells.

binge-purge behavior   Alternating episodes of over-eating and
forced expulsion of food.

biopsy   A diagnostic procedure in which a small piece of tissue is
obtained for pathologic study.

bipolar mood disorder   A condition that commonly begins with a
depressive episode and which is characterized by at least one
manic episode during the course of the illness.

birth control pills   Hormonal compounds that women take orally
in order to block ovulation and thus prevent pregnancy. Also
known as oral contraceptives.

blepharitis   An inflammation of the eyelid edges, in which a patient's
eyes are red-rimmed and the lid edges are covered with crusts.

blindness   A condition in which an individual whose vision has
been corrected with glasses or contact lenses has distance vision
of 20/200 or worse in the better eye or a visual field restricted to 20
degrees or less in the better eye.

blood   The liquid that transports vital substances to body tissues
and removes the waste products of the tissues' metabolism.

blood corpuscle   One of the three types of cellular elements of
blood which are suspended in the plasma.

blood pressure   The pressure that the blood exerts on the walls of
the arteries.

blood pressure cuff   *See* sphygmomanometer.

blood typing   A procedure for testing blood to determine to which
blood group an individual's blood belongs.

blood urea nitrogen (BUN)   The concentration of urea nitrogen in
the blood.

body (of stomach)   The largest part of the stomach. It lies between
the fundus and the pylorus.

Boeck's sarcoid   *See* sarcoidosis.

boil   *See* furuncle.

bone   A dense form of connective tissue that is made rigid by deposits of large amounts of calcium.

bone grafting   The implanting or transplanting of bone tissue from one site to another.

Bowen's disease   An intraepidermal in-situ squamous cell carcinoma usually occurring as a single lesion that spreads slowly by peripheral extension.

brain   The organ of the CNS that is contained within the cranium and consists of the cerebrum, cerebellum, midbrain, pons, and medulla.

breast augmentation   The surgical enlargement of a breast.

breast reconstruction   The surgical reformation of a breast, typically following any type of mastectomy.

breathing   The process by which air, with its supply of oxygen, is taken into the lungs during inspiration and is expelled with carbon dioxide during expiration.

bronchial asthma   A symptom-complex that is characterized by shortness of breath and wheezing and is caused by constriction of the smaller bronchi and bronchioles.

bronchiectasis   A chronic inflammatory pulmonary disease characterized clinically by a cough productive of large amounts of foul-smelling or bloody sputum, chest pain, and shortness of breath.

bronchiole   A tiny air tube which branches off a bronchus.

bronchography   A diagnostic procedure in which a radiopaque dye is introduced into the bronchial tree, followed by a chest x-ray.

bronchoscopy   A diagnostic procedure involving a fiberoptic scope that is used to look at the trachea and bronchi.

bronchus   A large air passage in the lungs.

Buerger's disease   Inflammation of segments in the small and medium arteries and veins in the upper and lower extremities leading to obstruction of these vessels. Also known as thromboangiitis obliterans.

bulimia   A condition that is characterized by episodes of rapidly eating abnormally large amounts of food. Typically, these episodes are followed by self-induced vomiting and/or the use of laxatives and diuretics.

bulimia nervosa   A psychologic and physiologic condition that is characterized by recurrent episodes of binge eating, a feeling of the loss of control over eating, and self-induced vomiting, the use of laxatives and/or diuretics, or intensive dieting or fasting.

bulla   *See* bullous lesion.

bullous emphysema   A condition in which localized, large solitary air cysts occur in the lung.

bullous lesion   A large skin blister. Also known as a bulla.

BUN   *See* blood urea nitrogen.

bursa   A two-layered sac that is filled with fluid. Bursae surround many freely movable joints.

bursitis   An inflammation of a bursa.

byssinosis   A type of pneumoconiosis caused by inhaling cotton dust.

cachexia   A condition of general ill health and malnutrition.

calcific tendinitis   An inflammation and calcification of the bursa in a joint, resulting in pain, tenderness, and limitation of motion in that joint.

calcitonin   A hormone secreted by cells within the thyroid gland.

Caldwell-Luc procedure   A procedure used to relieve chronic sinusitis by creating a window in the affected sinus for drainage and removal of the diseased contents.

callus bone   New bone tissue that is formed in the healing process following a fracture.

cancellous bone   A spongy latticework-like tissue that composes the central core of a bone.

cancer   *See* malignant tumor.

cancer-in-situ   *See* carcinoma-in-situ.

CAPD   *See* continuous ambulatory peritoneal dialysis.

capillaries   Microscopic blood vessels.

carbuncle   A collection of furuncles organized into one lesion.

carcinoma   A malignant tumor that arises from epithelial tissue.

carcinoma-in-situ   A lesion that has all the characteristics of malignancy under microscopic analysis except that of invasion. Also known as cancer-in-situ or intraepithelial cancer.

cardia   The part of the stomach that surrounds the esophagogastric junction.

cardiac catheterization   The insertion of a catheter in order to obtain precise functional and anatomic information about a patient's heart prior to cardiac surgery.

cardiac ischemia   A reduction in the bloodflow to the heart.

cardiac muscle   A type of muscle that appears only in the heart and is not under the individual's voluntary control.

cardiomyopathies   Primary diseases of the heart muscles that are not associated with any other disease of the heart.

cardiovascular system   *See* circulatory system.

carotid arteries   The arteries that furnish the principal arterial blood supply to the head and neck.

carpal bones   The wrist bones.

carpal tunnel syndrome   A condition that arises when the median nerve that crosses the carpal tunnel is entrapped as a result of repetitive motion, injury, pregnancy, or endocrine diseases such as diabetes mellitus or thyroid disease.

carrier An individual who has a recessive gene on one chromosome and not on the other chromosome of a pair. A carrier does not exhibit the characteristic of the recessive gene.

cartilage A specialized type of connective tissue that forms most of an embryo's temporary skeleton, providing a model in which most of the bones develop. In adults, cartilage is found in the nasal septum, larynx, trachea, bronchi, external ear, intervertebral disks, and at the ends of long bones.

casts Cylindrical structures found in the urine that are composed of protein, red blood cells, white blood cells, and fat, in varying proportions.

CAT scan *See* computerized axial tomography.

cataplexy A condition characterized by muscle weakness and a transient loss of muscle tone.

cataract Any opacity or cloudiness in the lens of the eye. It is characterized by blurred distance and near vision that cannot be corrected by optical devices.

catatonic schizophrenia A condition characterized by excessive and sometimes violent motor activity and excitement, and by generalized motor inhibition.

catheter A hollow, flexible tube used for withdrawing fluids from or introducing fluids into a body cavity or blood vessel.

cation A positively-charged ion.

cecum A dilated pouch found at the beginning of the large intestine.

cellular immunity An immune response that results from the interaction of an antigen with sensitized lymphocytes or other sensitized cells.

central nervous system (CNS) The part of the human nervous system that is highly developed and specialized and that includes the brain and the spinal cord.

cephalopelvic disproportion A condition in which the mother's pelvis is too small for the size of the baby's head.

cerebellum The second largest division of the brain, it lies beneath the cerebral hemispheres in the back of the cranial cavity. It coordinates muscle movements, especially to maintain posture, and provides muscle contractions to control equilibrium.

cerebral contusion A bruise of the brain.

cerebral cortex The surface of the cerebrum.

cerebral embolism The occlusion of a cerebral vessel by a traveling blood clot, air bubble, tumor, or other material.

cerebral palsy (CP) A general term for nonprogressive disorders of the central nervous system resulting from damage sustained by the infant during the mother's pregnancy, at delivery, or shortly after the infant's birth.

cerebral thrombosis A condition in which a blood clot develops in a cerebral artery and blocks the flow of blood to the area of the brain served by that artery.

cerebral vascular accident (CVA) Any disease of the cerebral vascular system that results in cerebral, cerebellar, or brain stem anoxic damage. Also known as a stroke.

cerebrospinal fluid A clear, watery liquid that is contained in the ventricles of the brain and in the meninges of the brain and spinal cord. It cushions the brain and spinal cord against mechanical jolts and sudden changes in pressure.

cerebrum The upper part of the brain. It is the largest part of the human central nervous system.

cervical radiculitis An irritation of a nerve root at the point at which the root emerges from the cervical spine.

cervical rib An extra rib resulting from a congenital overdevelopment of the seventh cervical vertebra.

cervical vertebrae Vertebrae that lie at the top end of the spine, supporting the head and neck.

cervix The lower constricted neck of the uterus.

cesarean section A surgical procedure in which an incision is made through the mother's abdominal and uterine walls in order to deliver a fetus.

chalazion A localized enlargement of a lacrimal gland that results from blockage of its duct.

chemotherapy The treatment of disease using chemical agents.

chicken pox See varicella.

cholangitis The inflammation of the bile ducts.

cholecystectomy The removal of a patient's gallbladder.

cholecystitis An inflammation of the gallbladder.

cholecystogram An x-ray of the gallbladder.

cholelithiasis A condition characterized by the formation or presence of gallstones.

cholesteatoma A condition which may result from a persistent middle ear infection and that is characterized by a collection of old squamous epithelium cells, cellular debris, and other substances.

chondrosarcoma A malignant tumor arising from cartilage.

chorea A condition which is characterized by involuntary, purposeless muscle movements, and/or personality changes.

chorionic gonadotrophin A hormone secreted by a woman's placenta very early in pregnancy to stimulate the ovaries and prevent the degeneration of the corpus luteum.

chorionic villi Thread-like projections that grow in tufts on the external surface of the membrane that surrounds a fetus.

chorionic villi sampling A prenatal diagnostic test which involves the removal of some chorionic villi with a needle aspiration. Also known as CVS.

choroid The middle section of the eyeball that contains a dense network of blood vessels that serve the structures of the eye.

Christmas disease *See* hemophilia B.

chromosome A complex structure which is composed of genes and is found in the nucleus of each cell in the body. Humans have 46 chromosomes.

chronic bronchitis A chronic inflammation of the tracheobronchial tree.

chronic diffuse glomerulonephritis A progressive disease that is characterized by irreversible damage to the renal glomeruli and tubules.

chronic disease A disease of any type that is generally characterized by a slow onset and a relatively long and progressive course of illness.

chronic obstructive pulmonary disease A varied group of chronic respiratory disorders that are associated with varying degrees of obstruction to the flow of air during expiration.

chronic prostatitis A recurrent, low grade infection or inflammation of the prostate that is difficult to treat because often no bacterium can be identified as the certain cause of the disorder.

chronic pyelonephritis A slowly progressive infection that usually affects both kidneys.

chronic renal failure A progressive condition that is characterized by disorders in all aspects of renal function.

chronic serous otitis media A condition which occurs from recurrent or neglected acute middle ear infections and that is characterized by a chronic discharge and pain.

cilia Microscopic hair-like structures.

ciliary muscle The muscle that joins the sclera and the outer ring of the iris, is continuous with the choroid, and suspends the iris.

cineangiography A diagnostic procedure for complex cardiac problems that involves the selective injection of contrast media into the heart and coronary vessels combined with exposure of high-speed x-ray motion pictures.

circulatory system An organ group that consists of the heart and blood vessels and is responsible for the flow of blood throughout the body. Also known as the cardiovascular system.

circumduction Movement in a circle.

cirrhosis A chronic degenerative liver disease that involves the progressive destruction of liver cells.

claustrophobia The fear of very small or closed spaces.

clavicle The bone that forms the front of the shoulder girdle. Also known as the collar bone.

clinical pathology The chemical, hematologic, bacteriologic, microscopic, and other laboratory analyses of blood, urine, and specimens from other tissues and fluids.

clitoris A small, cylindrical erectile structure that is located above the urethral opening at the most forward position of the vulva and is partly concealed by the labia.

clonic convulsion A seizure characterized by rhythmic, generalized, involuntary contractions and relaxations of muscles.

closed fracture A fracture in which the overlying skin and soft tissues remain intact after the bone surface has been broken.

closed head injury An injury in which a patient's skull has not received injury or at most has incurred a simple, nondisplaced, linear fracture without scalp laceration.

cluster headache A vascular headache that is characterized by severe pain of a short duration, located behind or near one eye.

CNS *See* central nervous system.

coagulation factors Substances found in plasma that are essential to the clotting process.

coarctation of the aorta A congenital narrowing of the aorta just beyond the point at which the arteries that supply the upper extremities leave the aorta.

coccus bacterium A form of bacterium that is round or oval.

coccygeal vertebrae Vertebrae that form the lowest segments of the spine.

coccyx The bone at the very base of the adult spine. It is formed by the fusing of the four coccygeal vertebrae.

cochlea A coiled, snail shell-shaped tube in which branches of the auditory nerve pick up sound impulses and relay them to the hearing center of the brain.

coitus interruptus A contraceptive method that involves the male's removal of his penis from the woman's vagina just prior to ejaculation. Also known as the withdrawal method.

colectomy The surgical removal of the colon.

colitis An inflammation of the large intestine.

collagen-vascular disorders A diverse group of diseases that have in common widespread alterations of connective tissues. Also known connective tissue disorders.

collar bone *See* clavicle.

Colles' fracture A fracture of the distal end of the radius.

colon   *See* large intestine.

colonoscopy   The inspection of the interior of the large intestine by means of a flexible, fiberoptic colonoscope.

colostomy   A surgically created opening between the colon and the surface of the patient's body.

colposcopy   An office procedure that involves the insertion of an instrument called a colposcope into a patient's vagina for the examination of the patient's cervical and vaginal tissues.

columnar epithelium   A type of epithelial tissue that is composed of long, cylindrical cells, and is the chief secretory tissue of the body.

comminuted fracture   A fracture that involves more than two bone fragments.

commissure   The juncture between one valve leaflet and another.

compact bone   The very dense tissue that composes the outside layer of a bone.

complex partial seizure   A behavioral seizure in which a patient loses consciousness, but experiences involuntary movements during the loss of consciousness. Also known as a psychomotor seizure or a temporal lobe seizure.

complicated hypertension   The presence of hypertension and one of its common complications, such as stroke, congestive heart failure, myocardial infarction, and renal failure.

compulsion   A repetitive act that an individual feels he or she must perform, no matter how purposeless the act is.

computerized axial tomography   A noninvasive technique in which a special machine that is linked to a computer examines a section of a patient's body, records multiple x-ray images and then analyzes, reconstructs, and displays those images to give an accurate visualization of structures deep within the body that are inaccessible to conventional x-ray techniques. Also known as CT scanning or CAT scanning.

conceptus   The product of conception during the first two weeks of pregnancy. Also known as a zygote.

concussion   A brief loss of consciousness without permanent neurologic changes.

cone   One of two types of highly specialized light-sensitive cells in the eye. A cone contains compounds that are responsible for color vision.

congenital disorder   A disorder that is present at a child's birth and that may result from heredity or from disease or injury to the fetus before delivery.

congenital glaucoma   *See* developmental glaucoma.

congenital hydrocephalus   An enlargement of the ventricles of the brain arising from the excess accumulation of cerebrospinal fluid that first appears before birth or shortly thereafter.

congestive heart failure   The inability of the heart to pump an adequate supply of blood to the peripheral tissues for their metabolic needs, leading to vascular congestion.

congestive splenomegaly   An enlargement of the spleen resulting from an engorgement or "back-up" of blood within the portal veins that connect the spleen with the liver.

conization   A procedure in which a physician removes a cone of tissue from a patient's cervical canal for microscopic evaluation by a pathologist.

conjunctiva   A thin mucous membrane that lines the front of the sclera and cornea, as well as the back of the eyelids.

conjunctivitis   An inflammation of the conjunctiva that is characterized by a watery or mucous discharge. Also known as pinkeye.

connective tissue   Tissue that helps to support the body by binding tissues and organs to each other, forming the framework of most organs, and surrounding blood vessels.

connective tissue disorders   *See* collagen-vascular disorders.

contact dermatitis   A common skin disorder in which a rash is produced by contact with either a primary skin irritant or a sensitizing agent.

contact lenses   Corrective lenses that, unlike traditional eyeglasses, sit directly on a patient's cornea.

continuous ambulatory peritoneal dialysis (CAPD)   A procedure that involves an indwelling peritoneal catheter that permits the addition of dialysis fluid to the peritoneal cavity followed by drainage of fluid containing nitrogenous wastes three to five times daily.

contraception   The intentional prevention of pregnancy.

contraindication   A piece of evidence present in the patient, or in the patient's medical history, that warns against a particular procedure or treatment.

control of breathing   The process by which the rate and depth of ventilation is maintained during periods of exercise, rest, and stress; in environments having reduced atmospheric pressure; and in the presence of changing metabolic needs.

convolutions   Folds on the surface of the cerebrum. Also known as gyri.

convulsion   An episode of neurologic dysfunction that involves the patient's motor activity.

COPD   *See* chronic obstructive pulmonary disease.

cor pulmonale   A form of heart disease caused by high pressure in the pulmonary blood vessels, secondary to increased pulmonary vascular resistence.

corium *See* dermis.

cornea A transparent convex structure that forms the very front section of the eyeball.

coronary arteriography The injection of a contrast medium through a catheter directly into each of a patient's coronary arteries.

coronary artery bypass grafting A procedure which involves an incision into the patient's chest to allow for the insertion of a graft, usually consisting of a segment of a leg vein, from the ascending aorta to a coronary artery.

corpus luteum An empty ovarian follicle. It manufactures progesterone.

corticotropin-releasing hormone (CRH) A releasing factor from the hypothalamus that causes the release of ACTH from the pituitary.

CP *See* cerebral palsy.

cranial nerve I *See* olfactory nerve.

cranial nerve II *See* optic nerve.

cranial nerve V *See* trigeminal nerve.

cranial nerve VIII *See* acoustic nerve.

cranial nerve IX *See* glossopharyngeal nerve.

cranial nerve X *See* vagus nerve.

cranial nerves The twelve pairs of nerves that originate in nuclei found in the brain. Each of these nerves is designated by a roman numeral in addition to a specific name, and each has a specific function.

cranium The skull.

creatinine A metabolic end-product that is derived primarily from muscle metabolism, and, to a lesser degree, dietary intake.

cretinism Fully developed and advanced hypothyroidism in infants and small children.

CRH *See* corticotropin-releasing hormone.

Crohn's colitis *See* granulomatous colitis.

Crohn's disease *See* regional enteritis.

Crohn's disease of the colon *See* ileocolitis.

crossed eyes *See* esotropia.

cryosurgery The intentional destruction of tissue by application of extreme cold.

cryptorchidism A condition in which a male has an undescended testis. It is the most common congenital anomaly of the male reproductive system. Also known as cryptorchism.

cryptorchism *See* cryptorchidism.

CT scan *See* computerized axial tomography.

cuboidal epithelium A type of epithelial tissue that is composed of cube-shaped cells, and which forms the lining of gland ducts, kidney tubules, and bronchi.

culture The intentional growth of microorganisms or cells in special substances that provide good environments for the microorganisms' or cells' growth.

cumulative drug effect A condition that produces heightened pharmacologic action, and occurs when the rates of detoxification and excretion are lower than the rate of administration.

curettage Scraping.

Cushing's syndrome A condition in which hormones that affect metabolism exist in excessive amounts, as a result of either overproduction or oral administration, for a sustained period of time.

cutaneous T cell lymphoma *See* mycosis fungoides.

CVA *See* cerebral vascular accident.

CVS *See* chorionic villi sampling.

cylindruria A condition in which casts are present in the urine.

cyst Any closed cavity or sac, normal or abnormal, lined by epithelium.

cystadenoma A type of benign tumor that is formed when secretions from the glandular cells of the tumor are retained, leading to its dilation and cyst formation.

cystectomy The surgical removal of the bladder.

cystic fibrosis An inherited disease in which a patient's pancreas develops an obstruction of its ducts, resulting from fibrosis and degeneration of the exocrine cells. Also known as mucoviscidosis or fibrocystic disease of the pancreas.

cystitis A common acute inflammation of the bladder epithelium that is characterized by frequency of urination, fever, and dysuria.

cystocele A sagging of the bladder into the vagina.

cystogram A diagnostic procedure in which a small amount of a radiopaque dye is passed through a catheter into the patient's bladder, followed by a series of x-rays.

cystoscope A fiberoptic instrument that permits a surgeon to view the interior of a patient's bladder.

cystoscopy A procedure that permits a surgeon to view the interior of a patient's bladder through a fiberoptic instrument known as a cystoscope.

cystourethrocele A sagging of the urethra and the bladder into the vagina.

cytology The microscopic study of cells, including the study of their origin, structure, function, and pathology.

cytoplasm A colorless semiliquid substance in which many of a cell's vital activities take place.

D&C   *See* dilation and curettage.

degenerative arthritis   *See* osteoarthritis.

degenerative joint disease   *See* osteoarthritis.

deglutition   The act of swallowing.

delayed hypersensitivity reaction   An antigen-lymphocyte reaction that requires 12 to 28 hours for the immune reaction to develop.

delirium   A dangerous, and sometimes fatal, psychiatric disturbance marked by (1) a reduced clarity of awareness of the environment, (2) the presence of hallucinations and other perceptual disturbances, (3) incoherent speech, and (4) disorientation.

delirium tremens   Delirium associated with alcoholic intoxication and withdrawal.

deltoid muscle   The triangular muscle at the shoulder joint.

delusion   A false belief that cannot be changed by reasonable contradictory evidence.

delusional disorders   A group of conditions that are characterized by the presence of a persistent false belief that does not result from another mental disorder.

dementia   A general designation for mental deterioration characterized by a loss of intellectual abilities, such as memory, judgment, and abstract thinking, of sufficient degree to interfere with social or occupational functioning.

depressants   Drugs that reduce the activities of a user's central nervous system.

depression   A condition that consists of a dejected mood, psychomotor retardation, insomnia, weight loss, and, often, excessive feelings of guilt. This condition is characterized by a loss of interest in customary activities, easy fatigability, loss of appetite, lack of interest in sex, obscure aches and pains, and feelings of despondency.

depressive episode   A mental state characterized by marked dejection, withdrawal, despondency, slowed thinking and motor activity, and lack of self-confidence.

DeQuervain's disease   A wrist disorder characterized by a painful inflammation of the abductor and extensor muscles of the thumb.

dermatitis   A general term for skin inflammation.

dermatochalasis   A condition characterized by bagginess and loss of elasticity in the skin of the patient's eyelids.

dermatomyositis   A connective tissue disorder that affects the skin, subcutaneous tissues, and skeletal muscles.

dermis   The portion of the skin that lies beneath the epidermis. Also known as corium.

dermoid cyst   A tumor that is composed of several different types of tissue, none of which is native to the location of the growth.

descending colon The part of the large intestine that extends downward from the transverse colon.

developmental glaucoma A type of primary glaucoma that results from an abnormality in the growth of embryonic tissue that produces an anterior chamber angle defect in the child when it is born. Also known as congenital glaucoma.

diabetes insipidus A condition that is characterized by a excessive excretion of very dilute urine, and which results from a deficiency of ADH.

diabetes mellitus (DM) A heterogeneous group of disorders that, because of the body's inability to metabolize glucose properly, are characterized by hyperglycemia.

diabetic retinopathy A disease of the retina that occurs as a late manifestation of diabetes mellitus and is characterized by the development of tiny hemorrhages, exudates, and capillary aneurysms in the retina.

dialysis The process of separating substances that are suspended in a solution by diffusing the substances through a semipermeable membrane.

diaphragm (1) A thin, dome-shaped muscle that is attached to the spinal column and to the lower ribs and rib cartilages and forms the lower boundary of the thoracic cavity. It is the major muscle of the respiratory system. (2) A contraceptive device that is made of molded rubber or soft plastic and has a metal spring rim.

diaphragmatic hernia *See* hiatus hernia.

diaphysis The shaft of a bone.

diastole The period of the heart cycle during which the ventricles relax and fill with blood.

diastolic pressure The point at which the sound produced by the systolic pulse disappears as the pressure in the blood pressure cuff falls.

DIC *See* disseminated intravascular coagulation.

diffuse scleroderma A generalized disorder of connective tissue characterized by inflammatory, fibrotic, and degenerative changes in the patient's skin, esophagus, intestinal tract, heart, lungs, and kidneys. Also known as progressive systemic sclerosis or PSS.

diffuse spasm of the esophagus A condition that is characterized by repetitive, nonperistaltic, and often powerful contractions of the esophagus.

diffuse toxic goiter A smooth, generalized enlargement of the thyroid gland, associated with the overproduction of thyroid hormone.

diffusion of gases in the lungs The process by which oxygen from the inspired air crosses the alveoli to enter the blood in the lung's capillaries, and carbon dioxide, a product of cellular metabolism, is released from the blood to become part of the expired air.

diffusion of gases in the tissues   The process by which oxygen is released to the cells and carbon dioxide enters the small peripheral capillaries.

digestive system   The group of organs that converts food into chemical substances that the body can absorb and assimilate. Also known as the digestive tract.

digestive tract   *See* the digestive system.

dilated cardiomyopathy   A class of primary heart diseases that is characterized by an increase in the internal diameter of the ventricles, principally the left ventricle, without a corresponding increase in the size of the chamber wall.

dilation and curettage   An operative procedure in which a physician dilates the canal of a patient's cervix with a series of graduated dilators, followed by a scraping of the patient's uterine cavity. Commonly called a D&C.

dip-stick test   A diagnostic procedure in which a narrow plastic strip, onto which one or more small test pads are affixed, is dipped into a patient's urine specimen and then removed from the specimen. Alternatively, drops of the urine specimen may be placed on the pads.

diplopia   Double vision.

discoid LE   *See* discoid lupus erythematosus.

discoid lupus erythematosus   A collagen-vascular disorder that is limited to the skin and which is characterized by a scarring eruption with hair loss. Also known as discoid LE.

disease   A condition in which the body, or part of it, deviates from health.

dislocation   A total displacement of one or more bones that comprise a joint, causing a complete change in the normal relationship between these bony surfaces. Also known as luxation.

displacement   A change from a normal position or relationship.

disseminated intravascular coagulation (DIC)   An acquired disorder in which fibrin is abnormally generated in circulating blood.

diuretic   A drug that promotes the excretion of urine.

divergent strabismus   *See* exotropia.

diverticulitis   Inflammation of a diverticulum.

diverticulosis   A condition characterized by the presence of several diverticula, particularly in the intestines.

diverticulum   A mucous membrane-lined pouch or sac that protrudes outward through the wall of a tubular organ.

dizziness   A condition characterized by subjective symptoms of light-headedness, weakness, giddiness, and faintness.

DM   *See* diabetes mellitus.

dominant trait   A trait that requires the presence of a specific gene on only one of a pair of chromosomes in order to produce the trait.

Down's syndrome   A condition which results from an abnormal number of a specific chromosome—chromosome 21—or from abnormalities of that chromosome's structure. It is characterized by mental retardation and a variety of physical malformations. Also known as mongolism.

drug therapy   A type of treatment in which a substance is administered to alter the physical, mental, or emotional status of a patient.

drug tolerance   A condition wherein repeated administration of the same quantity of a drug will produce a lessened pharmacologic effect.

drunkenness   *See* intoxication.

dual pathogenicity   The ability to cause disease in two ways.

Duchenne's muscular dystrophy   A type of muscular dystrophy that is characterized by weakness and the eventual atrophy of affected muscles. A Duchenne's patient's gait and posture are noticeably abnormal.

dumping syndrome   A condition that is characterized by symptoms including palpitations, light-headedness, and extreme perspiration after eating.

duodenitis   A general, nonspecific term that describes any inflammation of the duodenum.

duodenum   The shortest, widest, most fixed part of the small intestine. It is connected to the stomach.

dura   The outermost meninge. It is thick and tough.

dynamic ileus   An overly active ileum.

dysentery   A type of colitis that is characterized by abdominal cramps and pain, and frequent, watery stools containing pus, mucus, or blood.

dyskinesia   An abnormal muscular contraction.

dyslexia   A group of conditions of unknown origin in which a disparity exists between a person's apparent intellectual potential and that person's ability to read, and often, to spell.

dysmenorrhea   Painful menstruation that is commonly associated with lower abdominal cramps.

dyspepsia   A common nonspecific designation for discomfort resulting from a wide variety of diseases that originate in the gastrointestinal tract, other abdominal organs, or elsewhere in the patient's body. Also called indigestion.

dysphagia   Difficulty in swallowing from any cause, often associated with discomfort or mild pain beneath the breastbone.

dysplasia   A condition in which the size, shape, and organization of adult cells are altered.

dysplastic cells   Adult cells that display an alteration in their size, shape, or organization.

dysplastic nevus   A premalignant skin tumor that is larger and more variegated in pigmentation than other moles. It is the precursor of malignant melanoma.

dystocia   Abnormal labor or childbirth.

dysuria   Pain upon urinating.

ear drum   A thin, semitransparent, oval membrane that lies at the end of the external auditory canal and separates the external ear from the middle ear. Also known as the tympanic membrane or the tympanum.

eating disorders   Psychiatric disorders that are characterized by a disturbed sense of body image and a morbid fear of obesity, and are manifested by abnormal patterns of food consumption, and self-induced marked weight loss.

ecchymosis   A large hemorrhage into the skin, recognizable by "black and blue" marks.

echocardiogram   The recorded image produced by an echocardiograph.

echocardiograph   A machine that directs high-frequency sound waves into the patient's body and has a mechanism that records the sound waves as they reflect off the patient's heart walls, chambers, valves, and red blood cells.

echocardiography   A ultrasound procedure that is used to study the heart and to aid in the diagnosis and management of heart disease.

eclampsia   A disorder of pregnancy that results from preeclampsia that is not properly treated. Eclampsia is associated with convulsions and coma.

ECT   *See* electroconvulsive therapy.

ectopic pregnancy   A condition in which a fertilized ovum implants and develops outside the mother's uterine cavity. Also known as tubal pregnancy.

ectropion   A condition characterized by the outward relaxation of part or all of the patient's eyelid edges.

efferent nerves   Nerves that convey impulses from the central nervous system to the peripheral nervous system.

ejection fraction   The ratio of stroke volume to the volume of the left ventricle at the end of diastole.

electrocardiogram   The recording produced by an electrocardiograph.

electrocardiograph   An instrument that records the electrical current generated by the heart muscle.

electrocoagulation   *See* surgical diathermy.

electroconvulsive therapy (ECT)   A form of treatment in which the passage of an electric current through a patient's brain induces unconsciousness and/or convulsions. Also known as electroshock therapy.

electroencephalography   The study of the electrical activity of the brain.

electromyography (EMG)   A diagnostic procedure which utilizes the natural electrical properties of skeletal muscle by recording the electrical activity evoked in a muscle by the electrical stimulation of its nerve.

electroshock therapy   *See* electroconvulsive therapy.

ELISA test   A test for a disease in which a pathologist places a blood serum or plasma sample from a person being tested in contact with antigen-coated cells. If antibodies are present in the sample, they link to the corresponding antigens in the prepared cell. This test is often used to test for HIV antibodies.

embolism   A circulatory system obstruction resulting from an embolus becoming lodged in a blood vessel.

embolus   A clot, bubble, or tumor that consists of blood, fat, air, infected tissue, or other material that travels in the blood stream to a distant location where it obstructs circulation.

embryo   The product of conception from the third to the fifth week of pregnancy.

embryonal nephroma   A malignant tumor of the kidney. It is the most common kidney cancer occurring in patients younger than age five. Also known as Wilms tumor.

EMG   *See* electromyography.

emphysema   An irreversible condition of the lung characterized by an increase in the size of the alveoli with destructive changes in their walls.

empyema   A condition that is characterized by the presence of pus in the pleural cavity.

encephalitis   An acute inflammation of the brain that may be caused by many different strains of viruses or other infectious organisms and that is generally characterized by high fever, headache, lethargy, tremors, and delirium.

end-stage heart disease   A condition of chronic intractable congestive heart failure no longer amenable to drug therapy.

endocardium   A thin, strong membrane that lines the chambers of the heart.

endocrine gland   A type of gland that does not have ducts.

endocrine system   The group of glands and other structures in the body that create hormones and release the hormones directly into the circulatory system.

endolymph   A watery fluid that fills the three cavities of the inner ear.

endolymphatic hydrops   A condition of generalized dilation of the membranous labyrinth that results from the overproduction of endolymph.

endometrial cavity   A small triangular space within the uterine corpus.

endometriomas   Pieces of endometrial tissue that become implanted and grow in areas outside their normal location in the lining of the uterine cavity.

endometriosis   A condition in which very small pieces of endometrial tissue become implanted and grow in areas outside their normal location in the lining of the uterine cavity.

endometrium   The inner, thin layer of tissue that lines the cavity of the uterine corpus.

endoscopic retrograde cholangiopancreatography   A procedure which allows medical personnel to directly visualize a patient's common bile duct and pancreatic duct through a flexible fiberoptic endoscope following the injection of a radiopaque substance into the area in a direction opposite to the normal flow of bile. The endoscope is passed down the patient's esophagus, through the stomach, and into the duodenum. Also known as endoscopic retrograde cholangiography or ERCP.

endoscopic retrograde cholangiography   *See* endoscopic retrograde cholangiopancreatography.

endoscopy   An invasive technique that permits the visual inspection of a cavity or hollow organ with a specially designed tubular instrument that incorporates fiberoptics.

enthesis   The site of ligamentous attachment to bone.

entropion   A condition characterized by the inward relaxation of the patient's eyelid edges.

enzyme   An organic substance capable of accelerating or producing by catalytic action some chemical change in another substance.

enzyme-linked immunosorbent assay test   *See* ELISA test.

epidermis   The outermost, nonvascular portion of the skin.

epididymis   A long, narrow, highly coiled duct through which sperm cells and fluids produced in the testis pass.

epididymitis   An inflammation of the epididymis.

epididymo-orchitis   An inflammation of the epididymis and the testes.

epidural anesthesia   The inhibition of nerve impulses in the area outside the patient's dura.

epidural hematoma   A localized collection of clotted blood around and above the dura. It can be fatal if not treated promptly.

epiglottis   One of the cartilages of the larynx. During the ingestion of food, the epiglottis forms a lid over the opening to the larynx to prevent the entrance of food into the larynx and trachea.

epiglottitis   An inflammation of the epiglottis.

epilepsy   Any one of a group of neurologic disorders resulting from the abnormal electrical activity of the patient's brain.

epinephrine   An adrenal hormone that causes acceleration of the individual's heart rate, relaxation of the smooth muscle of the bronchial tubes, and constriction of the peripheral blood vessels. Also known as adrenalin.

epispadias   A condition affecting some males in which the urethra opens on the upper, or dorsal, surface of the penis.

epithelial tissue   A type of tissue that covers or lines most organs of the body.

ERCP   *See* endoscopic retrograde cholangiopancreatography.

erotomanic delusion   The false belief that a person is loved by another person.

erysipelas   A serious bacterial infection that primarily affects the patient's face and head with a red, hot, fluid-filled spreading lesion that may involve large areas of the patient's skin.

erythema   A skin condition characterized by redness.

erythema infectiosum   A mildly contagious disease that is marked by a rose-colored macular rash. Also known as fifth disease.

erythema multiforme   A skin eruption that involves different types of reddish lesions.

erythema nodosum   A skin eruption characterized by painful, deep-seated, reddened nodules.

erythrocyte   One of the three types of corpuscles. Also known as a red blood cell.

erythrocytosis   *See* secondary polycythemia.

esophageal manometry   A diagnostic procedure that measures muscular pressures and dysfunctions of peristalsis in the patient's esophagus.

esophageal ring   A thin ridge of mucosa that projects into the channel of the lower esophagus, usually at or near the gastroesophageal junction.

esophageal varix   A dilated, or varicose, vein that surrounds the lower part of the esophagus and that is prone to rupture.

esophagitis   An inflammation of the lining of the esophagus.

esophagus   A muscular canal about ten inches long that extends from the pharynx and connects the oral cavity with the stomach.

esotropia   A condition in which one eye deviates inward. Commonly known as "crossed eyes."

essential hypertension   Hypertension of unknown cause. Also known as primary hypertension.

estrogen   A female hormone that stimulates growth of the endometrium and myometrium, cervix, vaginal mucosa, and the ducts and glands of the breasts.

etiology   The study of the causes of disease.

eustachian tube   A canal leading from the middle ear to the nasopharynx. Also known as an auditory tube.

euthyroidism   The clinical condition of normal thyroid function.

Ewing's tumor   A malignant tumor of the bone that always arises in bone marrow.

excisional biopsy   An open biopsy method in which a surgeon removes an entire lesion for pathologic examination.

excoriation   A scratch mark on the skin.

exfoliative cytology   The study of cells normally shed from the skin and other body surfaces in order to detect malignant changes.

exocrine gland   Any gland that has ducts.

exophthalmos   A condition in which the patient has abnormally protruding eyeballs.

exotropia   A condition in which one eye deviates outward. Also known as divergent strabismus.

expiratory reserve volume   The volume of air that, after a maximum inspiration, can be exhaled with maximum effort in excess of both tidal air and the inspiratory reserve volume air.

exstrophy   A rare, but treatable urinary tract malformation in which the front wall of the bladder is absent.

extension   The movement by which the two ends of a joint are drawn away from each other.

external bridging   A process in which new bone tissue grows over the area of a break on the outer layer of bone.

external ear   The part of the ear that includes the auricle and the external auditory canal.

external hemorrhoid   A varicose vein in the skin and subcutaneous area surrounding the anus.

extracapsular lens extraction   The surgical removal of only the front of the lens.

exudate   Any material, such as fluid, cells, or cellular debris, which has escaped from blood vessels and has been deposited in tissues or on tissue surfaces, usually as a result of inflammation.

eye socket   *See* orbit.

eyeball   A spherical organ of sight.

Factor I   *See* fibrinogen.

Factor VIII   *See* antihemophilic factor.

Factor IX   *See* plasma thromboplastin component.

fallopian tube   An open passageway that functions to move ova from the surface of the ovary into the uterus. Also known as an oviduct.

FAS   *See* fetal alcohol syndrome.

fasting hypoglycemia   Hypoglycemia that occurs after abstinence from eating so that all glucose contents of the intestines have been absorbed.

fat embolism   A particle that consists of fat and that occludes a blood vessel.

febrile seizure   A type of seizure that occurs in association with a high fever.

feces   Excretions from the bowel consisting in part of indigestible matter and bacteria.

femur   The long bone in the upper leg. It is the strongest and longest bone in the body.

fenestra   Any small opening.

fenestration   An operation in which a surgeon creates a new opening.

fertilization   The union of an ovum and a spermatozoa, including the fusion of male and female chromosomes.

fetal alcohol syndrome (FAS)   A syndrome in which abnormal prenatal cell growth occurs in infants born to women who were chronically alcoholic during pregnancy.

fetus   The product of conception after the fifth week of pregnancy.

fiberoptic bronchoscope   A flexible instrument used to examine a patient's endobronchial tree, to establish a tissue diagnosis by biopsy, and to collect washings and other secretions for bacterial culture and cytology.

fiberoptic endoscopy   An investigative diagnostic procedure in which the physician directly views the patient's esophagus through a fiberoptic endoscope that has been inserted through the patient's mouth.

fiberoptic strand   A tiny, flexible glass filament that can transmit light without distortion and without a reduction in the light's intensity.

fibrin   A protein blood component that is essential for blood coagulation.

fibrinogen   A plasma protein that is converted to fibrin in a complex sequence of steps in the clotting process. Also known as Factor I.

fibrocartilage A type of connective tissue that consists of typical cartilage cells and parallel thick, compact collagenous bundles.

fibrocystic disease of the breast A condition that usually affects both breasts and is characterized by the formation of multiple, benign, painful lumps that become increasingly tender just prior to and during menstruation.

fibrocystic disease of the pancreas *See* cystic fibrosis.

fibroid A benign tumor that is composed primarily of uterine muscle that has undergone excessive growth. Also known as a myoma or leiomyoma.

fibroma A benign tumor of the dermis which is composed of fibrous or fully developed connective tissue.

fibrosarcoma A malignant tumor arising from fibrous connective tissue.

fibrous tissue The ordinary connective tissue of the body.

fibula The calf bone.

fifth disease *See* erythema infectiosum.

filtrate A liquid that has passed through a filter.

fimbriae Finger-like, or fringed, ends of each fallopian tube that drape down over the ovary.

first degree relatives An affected individual's parents, siblings, or children with regard to a family medical history.

fissure-in-ano *See* anal fissure.

fissuring The development of an ulcerated, narrow, deep crevice.

fistula An abnormal passage between an internal organ and the exterior of the body, or between two internal organs.

flexion The act of bending a joint.

focal glomerulonephritis A kidney condition in which only some glomeruli show inflammatory changes, and other glomeruli appear to be normal.

focal seizure *See* partial seizure.

follicle-stimulating hormone (FSH) A pituitary hormone that causes maturation of the ovum and induces estrogen production in the female and induces the production of sperm in the male.

forced vital capacity The volume of air expired as forcefully and completely as possible after maximum inspiration.

fovea A small depression at the center of the macula which is the location of sharpest vision.

fracture A break in the surface of a bone.

frontal lobe One of the four main lobes of the cerebrum. It lies at the forward part of the cerebrum.

frozen section biopsy method A method of preparing excised tissue for microscopic examination in which a biopsy specimen is removed, frozen by a special quick freezing method, stained, and promptly interpreted.

FSH   *See* follicle-stimulating hormone.

functional psychiatric disorder   Any psychiatric condition that is not associated with the presence of brain pathology and which pertains to a feeling or a mental state.

fundus   (1) The upper, expanded portion of the stomach. It lies above and to the left of the esophageal opening. (2) The part of the uterus that lies above the fallopian tubes' points of entrance.

furuncle   An acute, tender, localized collection of pus, generally caused by a staphylococcus bacterium. Also known as a boil.

FVC   *See* forced vital capacity.

galactorrhea   Abnormal discharge of milk from the breast.

gallbladder   A four-inch long pear-shaped sac that stores bile and is located under the right lobe of the liver.

ganglion   (1) A benign cyst on the back of the wrist. (2) A group of nerve cell bodies.

gangrene   Tissue death and decomposition.

gas-permeable contact lenses   Contact lenses that allow oxygen and carbon dioxide to pass across the cornea freely, but also offer high visual quality. Also known as semi-rigid contact lenses.

gastric antrum   The distal portion of the body of the stomach. It ends at the pylorus.

gastric juice   A liquid secreted by the stomach lining that contains hydrochloric acid and digestive enzymes and assists the digestive process.

gastroenteritis   An inflammation of the lining of the small intestine and the stomach.

gastroenterocolitis   An inflammation of the lining of the entire gastrointestinal tract.

gastroesophageal junction   The lower portion of the esophagus. It lies at the junction of the esophagus with the stomach.

gastroesophageal reflux   *See* reflux esophagitis.

GDM   *See* gestational diabetes mellitus.

gene   The basic unit of heredity. Each gene holds the information for the transmission of a trait from one generation of living organisms to another.

general anesthesia   A reversible, drug-induced depression of the central nervous system that renders the patient unconscious.

generalized seizure   An epileptic seizure that affects several areas of the brain from the beginning of the attack.

German measles   *See* rubella.

gestational diabetes mellitus (GDM)   Diabetes mellitus that develops only during a woman's pregnancy.

giant hives   *See* angioneurotic edema.

glandular fever   *See* infectious mononucleosis.

glaucoma   A condition in which an increase in the pressure within a patient's eyeball is sufficient to damage the optic nerve and interfere with that patient's vision.

gliding joint   A joint that permits only gliding movements.

glioma   A tumor of the supporting tissues that typically is not well encapsulated and is difficult to remove completely.

glomerulonephritis   A widely distributed inflammatory disease of the kidney that is characterized by pathologic changes in the glomeruli and smaller arterioles of the kidney.

glomerulus   A tuft or looped coil of capillaries in a kidney formed from successively smaller branches of the renal artery.

glossopharyngeal nerve   The cranial nerve that serves the area of the tonsils, the back of the pharynx, the back of the tongue, and the middle ear. Also known as cranial nerve IX.

glossopharyngeal neuralgia   A condition of unknown cause that is characterized by sudden intense pain in the area of the tonsils, the back of the pharynx, the back of the tongue, and the middle ear.

glucocorticoid   *See* glucosteroid.

glucose   The form in which complex sugars appear in the blood. It is the end product of carbohydrate metabolism and is a major source of energy in living organisms.

glucosteroid   A steroid secreted by the adrenal gland that assists in regulating the body's sugar metabolism and numerous other functions. Also known as glucocorticoids.

glycosuria   A condition in which an excessive amount of glucose is excreted in the patient's urine.

goiter   An enlargement of the thyroid gland.

gonioscopy   An examination of (1) the angle of the anterior chamber of the eye and (2) the ability of the eye to move normally.

gonorrhea   An infection that is caused by the Neisseria gonorrhoeae, which is commonly called the gonococcus bacteria.

gout   A hereditary form of arthritis that is characterized by an excess of uric acid in the blood and recurrent acute attacks of arthritis in the peripheral joints.

grade I tumor   A tumor which has cells that closely resemble the normal parent cells. Also known as a low grade tumor.

grade IV tumor   A tumor which has bizarre cells that do not resemble the parent cell. Also known as a high grade tumor.

grading A method of evaluating a tumor by describing its microscopic appearance.

grandiose delusions A type of delusion which involves a person's being convinced that he or she possesses some great talent or insight.

granulomatous colitis A regional enteritis that affects the colon. Also called Crohn's colitis.

granulosa cell tumor A malignant neoplasm that arises out of the cells that surround the ovarian follicles.

Graves' disease An autoimmune disease of unknown cause that is characterized by hyperthyroidism, exophthalmos, and characteristic skin changes.

GRH See growth hormone-releasing hormone.

gross hematuria A condition in which large amounts of red blood cells are constantly and readily apparent in a patient's urine.

growth hormone-releasing hormone (GRH) A releasing factor that causes the release of HGH from the pituitary.

Guillain-Barré syndrome A disorder involving both cranial and peripheral nerves that is characterized initially by acute weakness and paralysis of the patient's legs. Also known as acute idiopathic polyneuritis.

gynecology The branch of medicine that treats diseases of the genital tract in females.

gyri See convolutions.

habituation See psychological dependence.

hallucination A sensory perception for which there is no logical basis.

hallucinogens See psychedelics.

hard contact lenses The oldest type of contacts. They are made of a rigid plastic.

Hashimoto's thyroiditis An autoimmune disease of the thyroid that may be associated with other autoimmune diseases such as pernicious anemia and systemic lupus erythematosus.

health The normal functioning of the human body.

heart A hollow, muscular organ that pumps blood to all parts of the body.

heartburn A burning or fiery sensation located beneath the sternum or in the upper middle area of the abdomen and is usually caused by disease of the esophagus. Also known as pyrosis.

hemangioma A benign vascular tumor that consists of large blood-filled spaces.

hemarthrosis An episode of spontaneous bleeding into joints characteristic of hemophilia A.

hematemesis Bloody vomiting.

hematochezia The passage of bloody stools.

hematologic disorder Any abnormal or pathological condition of the fluid, chemical, or cellular components of blood or of the blood-forming organs.

hematology The medical science that deals with the study of the origin, development, anatomy, and function of blood and blood-forming organs.

hematoma A collection of blood within the body's tissues.

hematuria A condition in which red blood cells are present in a patient's urine.

hemodialysis The process of diffusion across a membrane to remove toxic substances from the patient's blood while adding desirable components.

hemoglobin A complex protein-iron substance found in red blood cells that carries oxygen.

hemolysis An increased rate of red blood cell destruction.

hemolytic anemia A type of anemia that results from an abnormally shortened lifespan for mature red blood cells and the inability of the bone marrow to compensate for this occurrence.

hemophilia A A common hereditary, sex-linked disorder which affects males far more often than females, and is caused by a decreased level of Factor VIII.

hemophilia B A disease which is clinically similar to hemophilia A and occurs almost exclusively in males. Also called Christmas disease.

hemophilia C A type of hemophilia which results from a deficiency or the abnormal functioning of a specific blood coagulation factor, which is called the von Willebrand coagulation factor. Also called von Willebrand's disease.

hemostasis The arrest of bleeding, either spontaneously or by surgical means.

hemothorax A condition in which bloody fluid develops in the pleural cavity.

hepatitis An inflammation of the liver characterized by fever, malaise, loss of appetite, nausea, vomiting, abdominal pain, jaundice, and hepatomegaly.

hepatoma A common primary malignant tumor of the liver that is characterized by (1) abdominal discomfort, resulting from an enlargement or fullness in the liver, (2) fever, (3) jaundice, and (4) ascites.

hepatomegaly An enlarged liver.

hereditary disorders Disorders that are genetically transmitted from parent to offspring.

hereditary spherocytosis A dominant-gene hemolytic anemia that is characterized by the presence of abnormal, small globular red cells.

hernia The protrusion of any organ or tissue from its normal location through a weakened place, or actual opening, in the wall of the cavity that contains the organ or tissue. Also known as a rupture.

herniation of an intervertebral disk A protrusion of the nucleus pulposus which compresses the spinal cord and spinal nerves, causing pain.

herpes encephalitis (HSE) An inflammation of the brain that is caused by the herpes simplex virus, and that is characterized by headaches, fever, personality changes, disorientation, hallucinations, focal neurologic signs, and coma.

herpes simplex type I A virus that causes the common cold sore.

herpes simplex type II A sexually transmitted disease that affects the external genitalia with painful vesicles and ulcers.

HGH *See* human growth hormone.

hiatus hernia A condition in which a portion of the patient's stomach extends upward into the thoracic cavity through a weakened and dilated opening in the diaphragm. Also called a diaphragmatic hernia.

high blood pressure *See* hypertension.

high grade tumor *See* grade IV tumor.

hilum A concave indentation on the kidney where the renal artery enters the kidney.

hilus The area of the mediastinum in which the blood vessels, bronchus, and nerves enter the lung.

hinge joint A joint that permits only forward and backward motion.

Hirschsprung's disease Congenital megacolon that is a disorder of the intrinsic nervous system in the wall of the rectosigmoid area.

histology The branch of anatomy that deals with the microscopic study of tissues.

histoplasmosis A common fungal infection that affects the lungs.

HIV *See* human immunodeficiency virus.

hives *See* urticaria.

Hodgkin's disease A malignant condition characterized by painless, progressive enlargement of the lymph nodes, spleen, and general lymphoid tissue.

hordeolum A localized, red, tender, swollen abscess of the eyelid's lacrimal gland. Commonly known as a stye.

hormone A chemical substance that is produced and secreted by an organ or the cells of an organ, and that travels through the circulatory system to a target organ where the hormone elicits a response.

HSE   *See* herpes encephalitis.

human anatomy   The study of the structure of the human body, its cells, tissues, muscles, organs, blood vessels, and skeleton.

human growth hormone (HGH)   A pituitary hormone that exerts a major influence on the growth of all tissues.

human immunodeficiency virus   The virus that causes AIDS.

humerus   The bone of the upper arm. It is the longest and largest bone of the upper extremity.

hydatidiform mole   A disease in which placental cells proliferate and form small, grape-like cysts.

hydrocele   An abnormal accumulation of fluid within the sac that normally envelops the testis as it lies within the scrotum.

hydronephrosis   A pathologic condition characterized by distention of the renal pelvis and calyces with urine, as a result of obstruction of the ureter.

hydrothorax   A condition in which clear fluid develops in the pleural cavity.

hymen   A circular fold of tissue that surrounds the vaginal opening and partially closes it in virginal females.

hyperactive   Describing a condition in which a person is typically overactive, restless, and easily distractible. Also known as hyperkinetic.

hypercalcemia   A condition characterized by an increase in the serum calcium level.

hypercalciuria   A condition in which there is an increased amount of calcium in the urine.

hyperglycemia   Elevated blood glucose level.

hyperkinetic   *See* hyperactive.

hyperlipidemia   A condition characterized by elevated serum cholesterol and/or triglyceride levels.

hyperlipoproteinemia   The abnormal elevation of certain normal physiologic lipid elements in the body.

hyperopia   A condition in which rays of light are brought to a focus behind the retina resulting in farsightedness.

hyperparathyroidism   A condition characterized by an excessive amount of the parathyroid hormone.

hyperplastic polyp   An overgrowth of tissue that is not considered to be a neoplasm.

hypersplenism   A condition characterized by an enlarged spleen and a reduction of circulating red cells, white cells, and/or platelets in any combination.

hypertension   Persistently elevated blood pressure levels as determined on at least two separate occasions. Also known as high blood pressure.

hypertensive crisis A condition characterized by severe hypertension that may go on to hypertensive encephalopathy.

hypertensive encephalopathy A condition characterized by headache, confusion, and coma resulting from accelerated or malignant hypertensive effects upon the brain.

hypertensive heart disease A condition of heart hypertrophy secondary to systemic hypertension.

hypertensive retinopathy A disease of the retina that occurs in association with hypertension from any cause, and that is characterized by retinal hemorrhage and swelling and the development of exudates.

hyperthyroidism The overproduction by the thyroid gland of thyroid hormones.

hypertrophic arthritis *See* osteoarthritis.

hypertrophic cardiomyopathies A class of primary heart diseases that is characterized by hypertrophy of the left ventricle. Most cases arise as a genetic autosomal dominant disease.

hypertrophy An enlargement of any tissue.

hyperuricemia A condition characterized by an excess of uric acid in the blood.

hyperventilation A condition characterized by rapid or deep breathing in excess of that needed to maintain normal blood levels of oxygen and carbon dioxide.

hypocalcemia A condition characterized by a decrease in the serum calcium level.

hypochlorhydria A condition in which the patient's gastric mucosa produces reduced amounts of hydrochloric acid.

hypofunction A condition of diminished activity.

hypogammaglobulinemia An immunoglobulin deficiency that is characterized by recurrent bacterial infections, especially of the lung.

hypoglycemia Low blood glucose level.

hypokalemia An abnormally low concentration of potassium in the blood.

hypokinesia A reduction in the level of muscular contraction.

hypoparathyroidism A condition that is characterized by a lack of parathyroid hormone.

hypophysis *See* pituitary gland.

hypospadias A condition in which the urethra opens on the underneath, or ventral, surface of the penis.

hypothalamus An area at the base of the brain that is adjacent to and interconnected with the pituitary gland.

hypothyroidism The inadequate production by the thyroid gland of thyroid hormones.

hypoxemia   A condition in which there is a lack of oxygen in the blood.

hypoxia   A reduction of oxygen below levels necessary for proper tissue functioning despite adequate blood supply to the tissue.

hysterectomy   The surgical removal of the uterus.

hysterical personality disorder   A condition characterized by shifting emotions, susceptibility to suggestion, impulsiveness, and self-absorption.

hysterosalpingogram   The x-ray record from a hysterosalpingography. Also known as uterosalpingogram.

hysterosalpingography   A diagnostic procedure involving an x-ray study of a patient's uterine cavity and the canal of the fallopian tubes after the injection of a radiopaque substance or gas into the patient's uterus. Also known as a uterosalpingography.

hysteroscopy   The insertion into a patient's uterus of a modified fiberoptic scope, known as a hysteroscope, for visual examination of the patient's cervical canal and endometrial cavity.

idiopathic hypoglycemia   Hypoglycemia that has no known cause.

idiopathic parathyroid hyperplasia   A condition in which an abnormal increase in the number of parathyroid cells occurs for no known reason.

idiopathic thrombocytopenic purpura   A common form of thrombocytopenia which can exist in acute and chronic forms.

IGT   *See* impaired glucose tolerance.

ileocolitis   A chronic, nonspecific inflammatory disease that extends from the terminal ileum to the large intestine. Also known as Crohn's disease of the colon.

ileoileostomy   The surgical joining of two segments of ileum which does not require an opening to be created on the surface of the abdomen.

ileostomy   A surgically created opening from the ileum through the patient's abdominal wall.

ileotransverse colostomy   A procedure in which the surgeon removes a diseased portion of cecum or ascending colon and then joins the ileum and the transverse colon.

ileum   The last section of the small intestine. It connects with the large intestine.

ilium   A bone that fuses with the ischium and the pubis to form the innominate bone. The ilium forms the wide, top portion of the innominate bone.

immune complex   A protein substance that is created by the reaction of an antigen with an antibody and that usually is removed from the person's system without harm or difficulty.

immune system   A group of organs and structures, including the bone marrow, lymph nodes, spleen, thymus, tonsils and other lymphoid tissue, that defends the body against disease.

immunoglobulins Proteins secreted by the immune system that have antibody activity.

immunology The study of the body's immune system in health and disease that focuses upon the body's responses to natural infection, immunization procedures, blood transfusions, organ transplantation, cancer, and numerous other conditions.

impacted fracture A fracture that involves two bone fragments that are firmly driven into each other.

impaired glucose tolerance (IGT) A group of conditions that fall in the borderline zone between normal glucose tolerance and DM.

impetigo A skin condition that is characterized by pustular, crusted eruptions which most frequently affect the patient's face and hands.

impulsivity A condition characterized by the tendency to act before thinking, difficulty taking turns, problems organizing work, and constant shifting from one activity to another.

inappropriate secretion of antidiuretic hormone A syndrome that results from the overproduction ADH.

inattention A condition characterized by the failure to finish tasks once started, easy distractibility, seeming lack of attention, and difficulty concentrating on tasks that require sustained attention.

incarcerated hernia *See* nonreducible hernia.

incisional biopsy An open biopsy method in which a surgeon removes a small piece of tissue, usually located near the periphery of the lesion, for tissue examination.

incontinence A condition in which a person experiences loss of bowel or urinary control.

incus The middle ear bone that attaches to the malleus on one end and to the stapes on the other end.

index case The first individual who is identified as having a genetic abnormality in a family medical history.

indication Any symptom, sign, or occurrence in a disease that provides direction toward the cause, treatment, or diagnosis for the condition.

indigestion *See* dyspepsia.

infantile paralysis *See* poliomyelitis.

infantile torticollis A condition which results from an injury during birth to the muscles on one side of the infant's neck.

infectious arthritis A joint disease that results from a bacterial, viral, or other infection.

infectious mononucleosis A systemic illness caused by the

Epstein-Barr virus that generally affects young adults between the ages of 17 and 25. Also known as mono or glandular fever.

influenza   An acute viral disease that has predominately respiratory manifestations and that is characterized by fever, muscle aches, headaches, runny nose, cough, and malaise.

inner ear   The part of the ear that is encased in bone and contains three major cavities. Also known as the labyrinth.

innominate bone   The hip bone.

inspiratory reserve volume   The volume of air that, with maximum effort, can be inhaled in excess of the tidal air.

insulin   The pancreatic endocrine hormone that regulates the metabolism of sugar.

interaction   Any alteration in the effect of either of two substances because of the presence of the other.

intercostal neuritis   An inflammation of the nerves that lie between the ribs that is usually secondary to spinal cord or nerve root irritation, and that is characterized by chest pain.

intermittent claudication   A condition characterized by pain in a limb when it is exercised and relief from pain when the limb is at rest.

internal hemorrhoids   Dilated veins in the lower rectum. Also known as piles.

interstitial edema   A condition in which serous fluid from the capillaries surrounding the alveoli escapes and remains between the alveoli.

interventional radiology   Any selective catheter technique that is adopted for treatment. It includes the infusion through a catheter of therapeutic agents.

intervertebral disc   A flat plate of tissue that separates each vertebra from adjacent vertebrae.

intestinal obstruction   A major interference with the passage of intestinal contents.

intracapsular cataract extraction   The surgical removal of the entire lens.

intracerebral hemorrhage   Bleeding into the substance of the brain. It occurs from the rupture of a cerebral blood vessel, usually one that has undergone arteriosclerotic changes in its wall.

intradermal injection   The administration of any substance by injection between skin layers.

intraepithelial cancer   *See* carcinoma-in-situ.

intramuscular injection   The administration of any substance by injection in muscle tissue.

intraocular lens (IOL)   A plastic lens that a surgeon permanently inserts in a patient's eye to replace a removed cataractous lens.

intrauterine device (IUD) A small object that is surgically implanted into a woman's uterus for the purpose of preventing pregnancy.

intravenous injection The administration of any substance by injection in a vein.

intravenous pyelogram (IVP) An x-ray study of the kidney and ureters following an intravenous injection of a radiopaque dye.

intubation The insertion of a tube into a body canal or hollow organ.

intussusception An infolding or telescoping of one segment of bowel into another segment.

invasive A technique or procedure that involves the puncture of, or incision into, a patient's skin or the introduction of an instrument or foreign material into a patient's body.

invasive radiology The catheterization of blood vessels and the injection through the catheter of radiopaque contrast agents, whose circulation is observed by x-ray methods. It can also be used for therapeutic purposes.

IOL *See* intraocular lens.

iris The pigmented part of the eye. It is a circular membrane that lies in front of the lens.

iron-deficiency anemia A blood disorder characterized by low or absent iron stores, low iron concentration in the blood, low hemoglobin concentration or hematocrit, and other abnormalities.

irritable bowel syndrome A chronic functional disorder of the colon that is characterized by chronic abdominal pain and intermittent and recurrent constipation and/or diarrhea.

ischium A bone that fuses with the ilium and the pubis to form the innominate bone. The ischium forms the lower, back portion of the innominate.

islets of Langerhans Collections of cells scattered throughout the pancreas that produce insulin.

isthmus (of the thyroid) A narrow mid-portion of the thyroid that connects the right and left lobes of the gland.

ITP *See* idiopathic thrombocytopenic purpura.

IUD *See* intrauterine device.

IVP *See* intravenous pyelogram.

Jacksonian March A process in which a convulsion starts in one area of the patient's body and moves to muscle groups in other parts of the patient's body.

jaundice A condition in which the affected individual's sclera, skin, and other tissues are stained yellow by bile pigments present in excessive amounts in the patient's circulation.

jealous delusion A type of delusion in which a person is convinced without due cause that a spouse or lover is unfaithful.

jejunum   The upper two-fifths of the small intestine beginning after the duodenum and ending before the ileum.

joint   The place of union or junction between two or more bones, especially a junction that permits motion of one or more of the bones. Also known as an articulation.

Kaposi's sarcoma   A multifocal, metastasizing cancer that usually first presents as reddish blue or brownish soft nodules and tumors in the skin on the extremities.

keratitis   An inflammation of the cornea with or without ulceration.

keratoconus   A congenital or acquired disease of the cornea that often affects both eyes and is characterized by a cone-shaped protrusion of the center of the cornea.

keratoplasty   A corneal transplant.

kidneys   Lima bean-shaped hollow organs that excrete urine, and that are located in the back of the abdomen, one kidney on either side of the vertebral column.

Korsakoff's syndrome   A condition characterized by rapid mental deterioration.

kyphosis   An excessive posterior curvature of the cervical and thoracic sections of the spinal column. Commonly referred to as a hunchback.

labia   Elongated skin folds that extend down and back on either side around the vaginal opening.

labyrinth   *See* inner ear.

labyrinthine disorders   Diseases of the inner ear that are characterized by hearing loss and vertigo.

lacrimal gland   A gland in the eye that secretes just enough liquid to keep the conjunctiva clean and moist. Also known as a tear gland.

lactation   Milk production normally associated with childbirth.

lamina   The bony vertebral arch.

laminectomy   The surgical removal of the lamina.

laparoscopic cholecystectomy   The surgical removal of a gallstone during a laparoscopy.

laparoscopy   The inspection of a patient's abdominal cavity by means of a special fiberoptic instrument designed for viewing, biopsy, and surgery that a physician inserts through a small incision in the patient's abdomen.

large intestine   The tubular organ that extends from the ileum to the anus. Also known as the colon.

laryngectomy   The removal of the larynx.

laryngitis   An inflammation of the larynx.

laryngopharynx   The lower third of the pharynx. It lies behind the larynx and extends downward to the esophagus.

larynx A tubular structure that connects the oropharynx and trachea. It consists of nine cartilages that are joined by an elastic membrane. Commonly known as the voice box.

lateral meniscus A crescent shaped fibrocartilage disk that lies on the side of the knee joint.

learning disability A condition that is characterized by language problems, deficiencies in short-term memory, disordered sequencing of events in time or objects in space, or other subtle distortions in the way in which images and thoughts are processed by the brain.

leiomyoma (1) A benign tumor of smooth muscle tissue. (2) Fibroid.

lens A transparent structure in the eye that focuses light rays onto the retina.

lentigo-maligna melanoma A type of melanocarcinoma that involves a large, flat tan or brown mole that has irregularly-scattered spots.

lesion Any structural or functional alteration of tissue as a result of disease.

leukemia A cancer of the blood-forming tissue.

leukocyte One of the three types of corpuscles. Also known as a white blood cell.

leukocytosis An increase in the number of leukocytes, most commonly associated with infections.

leukopenia A decrease in the number of white blood cells, most commonly associated with infections.

leukoplakia White patches on a mucous membrane.

LH *See* luteinizing hormone.

LHRH *See* luteinizing-releasing hormone.

lichenification A thickening of the skin.

ligament Connective tissue that connects a bone to another bone.

limited scleroderma A collagen-vascular condition that involves the skin exclusively and is characterized by skin that appears tightly drawn, bound, and fixed to underlying structures, especially in the fingers where contractures may occur.

lipids Fats and fat-like substances that serve as fuel sources and important components of cell structure.

lipoma A benign growth that arises from fatty tissue.

liposarcoma A malignant tumor arising from adipose, or fatty tissue.

lithotripsy A noninvasive technique that involves the use of soundwaves to break down solid masses, such as kidney stones or gallstones, into small pieces.

liver The largest gland in the body; it lies in the upper right of the abdominal cavity and has four lobes.

lordosis   A condition characterized by excessive forward convexity in the lumbar and cervical region of the spine.

Lou Gehrig's disease   *See* amyotrophic lateral sclerosis.

low back strains   An ill-defined group of disorders that are characterized by a persistent backache that is believed to arise from stresses on the muscles and ligaments that surround and support the vertebral column.

low grade tumor   *See* grade I tumor.

lues   *See* syphilis.

lumbar puncture   A procedure in which a physician inserts a long needle between adjacent vertebrae in a patient's back and removes some cerebrospinal fluid from the subarachnoid space. Also known as a spinal tap.

lumbar vertebrae   Vertebrae that lie at the small of the back, between the chest cage and the pelvis.

lumpectomy   The surgical removal of a tumor or lump.

lung   Organ of respiration that effects the exchange of carbon dioxide and oxygen by the blood.

lung abscess   A localized lung infection that results in the destruction of tissue and the formation of pus.

lung perfusion scan   A diagnostic procedure that involves gamma camera imaging of a patient's lungs to determine the distribution of intravenously injected radioactively tagged proteins in the patient's pulmonary circulation.

lung ventilation scan   A diagnostic procedure that involves gamma camera imaging of a patient's lungs to determine the distribution of inhaled radioactively tagged gas in the pulmonary alveoli.

lupus nephritis   Glomerulonephritis that is associated with systemic lupus erythematosus.

luteinizing hormone (LH)   A pituitary hormone that initiates ovulation and stimulates the ovary to produce progesterone in females, and in males it causes the testis to secrete testosterone.

luteinizing-releasing hormone (LHRH)   A releasing factor from the hypothalmus that causes the release of LH from the pituitary.

luxation   *See* dislocation.

Lyme disease   A disease caused by an infection of a spirochete bacterium called Borrelia burgdorferi that is transmitted by a tick.

lymph   (1) lymphocyte. (2) A colorless, watery fluid which drains from between the body's cells into the lymphatic collecting system, passes through regional lymph nodes, which act as bacterial filters, and eventually reaches the blood stream.

lymph nodes   Round or oval structures that belong to the lymphatic system and are situated along the large blood vessels of the body.

lymphangioma   A benign tumor of the dermis which is composed of newly formed lymph spaces and channels.

lymphangitis   An inflammation in a lymphatic vessel.

lymphocyte   A type of leukocyte. It has a single nucleus and is involved in the production of antibodies and the destruction of cancerous cells, bacteria, and other infectious agents. Sometimes called a "lymph."

macrocytes   Abnormally large oval red blood cells present in the blood of an individual suffering from megaloblastic anemia.

macula   (1) The part of the retina directly behind the center of the lens. (2) A flat skin lesion less than two centimeters in diameter.

magnetic resonance imaging   A diagnostic technique that utilizes strong magnetic fields, radio frequency waves, and a computer to obtain images of different cross-sections of a patient's body part. Also known as MRI.

major depressive disorder   A mood disorder that occurs as syndromal episodes of depression that are generally recurrent, but may affect a patient only once during that patient's lifetime.

malabsorption syndrome   A symptom-complex associated with impaired gastrointestinal absorption of nutrients.

malaria   A widespread protozoan disease that is characterized by intermittent shaking chills and high fever.

malignant hypertension   A condition characterized by a markedly elevated diastolic blood pressure, accompanied by swelling of the optic nerve.

malignant lymphomas   A group of diseases showing neoplastic growth of the cells of the lymphoreticular system.

malignant melanoma   A malignant, darkly pigmented epithelial cancer that usually arises from a preceding mole. Also known as melanocarcinoma or melanoma.

malignant tumor   A tumor which grows autonomously, invades neighboring tissue, and spreads beyond the organ originally involved. Also known as cancer.

malleus   The middle ear bone that lies closest to the external ear.

malocclusion   The improper meeting of the teeth when the jaw is closed.

mandible   The lower jaw. It holds the lower teeth and is the largest and strongest bone of the face.

manic episode   A mental state characterized by extreme elation, overtalkativeness, extreme irritability, excitement, an unrestrained flow of ideas, and increased physical activity.

Mantoux text   A sensitive tuberculin test in which a purified protein derivative of tuberculin is injected into the patient's skin. A positive skin reaction in 48 to 72 hours indicates that the individual now has, or had in the past, active tuberculosis.

Marfan's syndrome   A congenital disorder of connective tissue characterized by abnormal length of the extremities, especially of fingers and toes, cardiovascular abnormalities, often dilation of the ascending aorta, and other abnormalities.

Marie Strumpell disease   *See* ankylosing spondylitis.

marrow   A soft tissue that occupies the central cavity of a bone.

mastoidectomy   The surgical removal of inflamed mastoid air spaces.

mastoiditis   An inflammation of the mastoid portion of the temporal bone of the skull that encloses the back side of the middle ear.

maxilla   The upper jaw. It holds the upper teeth.

MBD   *See* minimal brain damage.

MCTD   *See* mixed connective tissue disorder.

measles   *See* rubeola.

medial meniscus   A crescent shaped fibrocartilage disk that lies in the knee joint.

medical mycology   The study of fungi and how fungi may be pathogenic for humans.

medulla   The part of the brain that contains the nuclei of the cranial nerves that are not in the midbrain or pons. It also contains nerve centers for regulating heart beat and respiration rate. The medulla is an extension of the spinal cord.

megacolon   A condition in which the patient's colon is abnormally enlarged.

megaloblastic anemia   A type of anemia in which abnormally large, oval red blood cells appear in the peripheral blood and large immature red blood cells appear in the bone marrow.

megaloblasts   Large immature red blood cells in the bone marrow of an individual suffering from megaloblastic anemia.

melancholia   A general term that refers to forms of a major depressive disorder which are characterized by marked agitation, weight loss, pathologic guilt, morning insomnia, variations in mood and activity throughout the day, and the loss of the ability to experience pleasure.

melanocarcinoma   *See* malignant melanoma.

melanoma   *See* malignant melanoma.

melatonin   A pineal body hormone that suppresses the menstrual cycle.

melena   A condition characterized by the passage of stools darkened by blood.

membrane A structure in the body that consists of a surface epithelium layer supported by an underlying connective tissue that is invested with blood vessels and nerves.

Meniere's disease An endolymphatic hydrops of unknown origin in which a patient experiences vertigo, hearing loss, and tinnitus.

meninges The three membranes that protect the brain and spinal cord.

meningioma A benign tumor arising from the meninges that typically is slow-growing and is encapsulated.

meningitis An inflammation of the membranes covering the brain and spinal cord.

meningocele A sac-like herniation that contains meninges only.

meningomyelocele A protruding mass that contains meninges and spinal cord tissue.

meniscus A crescent shaped fibrocartilage disk located in a joint.

menopause A woman's last menstrual period, and the preceding years of declining ovarian activity.

menorrhagia An excessive menstrual flow.

menstruation The discharge of blood and tissues from the uterus through the vagina. This part of the menstrual cycle generally lasts three to five days every month in the absence of pregnancy.

mental retardation A condition characterized by significantly subaverage intelligence present from birth or early infancy.

mesothelioma A malignant tumor of the pleura.

MET A metabolic term that equates 3.5 milliliters of oxygen consumption per kilogram of a person's weight to one MET.

metabolism The chain of chemical processes that occur in the body to keep it functioning.

metacarpal bones The small bones of the hand.

metacarpal phalangeal joints The knuckles.

metaphysis The end of a bone.

metastasis The spread of malignant cells from a primary tumor to a distant location through lymph channels or blood vessels.

metatarsal bones The small bones of the foot.

metrorrhagia Uterine bleeding between normal menstrual periods.

microbiology The branch of biologic science that deals with the study of microorganisms such as bacteria, viruses, fungi, and protozoa.

microscopic hematuria A condition in which very small amounts of blood that can be detected only on microscopic examination are present in a patient's urine.

micturition *See* urination.

midbrain The part of the brain that contains the nuclei of some of the important cranial nerves that are not contained in the pons or medulla. It also assists in the regulation of posture and equilibrium.

middle ear   An irregular, air-filled space within the skull and medial to the external ear. Also known as the tympanic cavity.

migraine headache   A relatively common intense, paroxysmal, recurrent, vascular type of headache that is often associated with nausea and vomiting.

migrate   To move spontaneously from one location in the body to other locations in the body.

mineralocorticoid   A steroid secreted by the adrenal gland that aids in maintaining the body's sodium and potassium levels.

minimal brain damage (MBD)   A condition in which brain damage is too slight to be measured or identified clinically.

miscarriage   *See* spontaneous abortion.

mitral regurgitation   The result of failure of the mitral valve to close properly at the onset of systole, allowing blood from the left ventricle to flow back into the left atrium.

mitral stenosis   A narrowing of the mitral orifice. The narrowing impedes the flow of blood from the left atrium into the left ventricle.

mixed connective tissue disorder   A condition that presents with some manifestations of systemic lupus erythematosus, scleroderma, rheumatoid arthritis, and dermatomyositis.

modified radical mastectomy   The surgical removal of the entire breast and the associated lymph nodes in the armpit area.

mongolism   *See* Down's syndrome.

monilial vaginitis   A common fungal infection that affects the vagina.

mono   *See* infectious mononucleosis.

mononeuropathy   A functional or structural disorder affecting a single peripheral nerve.

mood disorder   Any one of several psychiatric disorders that occur when a patient's emotions, typically sadness and happiness, are overly intense and last beyond the normal response to a stressful life event.

morbid obesity   A body weight of 100 percent or more above the standard.

morphea   A localized form of systemic scleroderma that is characterized by the formation of white or pink patches, bands, or lines.

mouth   The part of the body that is located at the beginning of the digestive tract, and includes the lips, cheeks, gums, and teeth. Also called the oral cavity.

MPD   *See* myofascial pain-dysfunction syndrome.

MRI   *See* magnetic resonance imaging.

MS *See* multiple sclerosis.

mucosa A membrane that lines the cavities and passages that communicate from internal structures to the exterior of the body. Also known as a mucous membrane.

mucous membrane *See* mucosa.

mucoviscidosis *See* cystic fibrosis.

multiple fracture A fracture that involves two or more lines of fracture that are not physically connected to each other in the same bone.

multiple myeloma A malignant tumor made of plasma cells. It usually arises in the bone marrow.

multiple polyposis An uncommon, familial disease in which multiple polyps are scattered throughout the patient's large intestine.

multiple sclerosis (MS) A slowly progressive, chronic, degenerative disease that affects the brain and spinal cord, and is one of the most common causes of neurologic disability in adults.

muscular dystrophies A group of inherited muscular disorders showing progressive degeneration.

musculoskeletal system The body system that consists of the body's bones, joints, muscles, cartilage, ligaments, and tendons.

myasthenia gravis An autoimmune disorder that is characterized by muscle weakness and easy muscle fatigability.

mycobacterium A type of bacterium that, unlike other bacteria, resists decoloration by an acid-alcohol solution following an initial Gram positive staining.

mycosis fungoides A rare, chronic lymphoma that is characterized by large, firm, reddish, painful, ulcerating tumors. Also known as cutaneous T cell lymphoma.

myelocytes Cells, especially white blood cells, that contain granules.

myelography A specialized diagnostic procedure in which an oily, radiopaque dye is injected into the patient's spinal canal, and then an x-ray study is made of the movement of the dye through the canal.

myocardial infarction The death, or necrosis, of myocardium tissue resulting from inadequate blood supply. Commonly known as a heart attack.

myocardium The muscular tissue of the heart.

myoclonic seizure A seizure characterized by involuntary contractions or jerks of muscles of the patient's extremities, trunk, or face, without loss of consciousness.

myofascial pain-dysfunction syndrome (MPD) A nonarticular condition that mimics true TMJ disorders by producing pain, limitation of jaw movement, or a combination of both.

myogenic torticollis A transient condition that results from a muscle spasm caused by localized inflammation of a neck muscle.

myology The scientific study of muscles.

myoma *See* fibroid.

myomectomy The surgical removal of a fibroid.

myometrium The outer, thicker layer of muscular tissue that lines the uterine corpus.

myopia A condition in which rays of light come to a focus in front of the retina resulting in nearsightedness.

myringoplasty The surgical repair of perforations of the ear drum.

myringotomy A surgical procedure that involves an incision into a patient's ear drum to release pus behind it.

myxedema Advanced hypothyroidism.

narcolepsy A syndrome that is characterized by recurrent episodes of uncontrollable daytime sleep and abnormal nighttime sleep.

narcotics Drugs and substances that blunt the senses, relieve pain, induce drowsiness or sleep, and, when taken in large quantities, produce complete insensibility.

nasal cavity The area in the skull between the cranial cavity and the roof of the mouth.

nasopharynx The section of the pharynx that is located behind the nose and in back of and above the soft palate.

necrosis The death of tissue.

neoplasm A disturbance in the normal growth of tissue characterized by an abnormal, excessive, and uncontrolled proliferation of cells. Also known as a tumor.

nephrogenic diabetes insipidus Diabetes insipidus that results from kidney disease.

nephrolithiasis A condition marked by the presence of kidney stones.

nephron unit A glomerulus surrounded by a capsule and a tubule in a kidney.

nephropathy A general term for kidney disease.

nephrotic syndrome A condition that is characterized by low serum albumin, elevated cholesterol, massive proteinuria, and generalized edema and is seen as part of many diseases affecting the kidney.

nerve block The injection of an anesthetic agent close to a nerve to eliminate the conduction of impulses in that nerve.

nervous system The group of organs and structures that include the brain, spinal cord, and cranial and spinal nerves.

neuralgia A condition that is characterized by sudden, intense pain that extends along the course of one or more nerves.

neuritis   An inflammation of a peripheral nerve. It is associated with pain and tenderness, unusual sensations, lack of sensations, paralysis, and muscular and subcutaneous tissue wasting over the area served by the affected nerve.

neurofibroma   A tumor of the peripheral nerves that contains both nerve and fibrous tissue elements.

neurofibromatosis type I   A skin condition that has a dominant inheritance pattern and possibly involves the patient's nervous system. Also known as von Recklinghausen's disease.

neurogenic bladder   Any condition of urinary bladder dysfunction resulting from a lesion of the central or peripheral nervous system.

neuroglia   A connecting cell that is present in nerve tissue. These cells exist in the brain, spinal cord, and the cranial and spinal nerves.

neuroma   A small, benign tumor of a peripheral nerve that is often characterized by intermittent pain and abnormal sensations.

neuromuscular junction   The interface between a muscle and the nerve that stimulates that muscle.

neuron   A nerve cell that is present in nerve tissue. These cells exist in the brain, spinal cord, and the cranial and spinal nerves.

neuropathy   A general term for any abnormal function or structure involving a peripheral nerve.

neutropenia   A condition characterized by a decrease in the number of neutrophils. It is typically present in association with viral infections.

nevus   A benign tumor of the dermis commonly known as a mole.

NGU   *See* nongonococcal urethritis.

nodular melanoma   A type of malignant melanoma that involves a noticeably rapid enlargement of raised lesions.

nodular toxic goiter   The enlargement of one or several nodules of the thyroid, associated with increased secretion of thyroid hormone.

nongonococcal urethritis (NGU)   An inflammation of the urethra that is caused by a microorganism other than the gonococcus bacterium. Also known as nonspecific urethritis or simple urethritis.

non-Hodgkin's lymphomas   A heterogeneous group of malignant diseases that are characterized by the neoplastic proliferation of lymphoid cells that often spread throughout the body, but that differ histologically from Hodgkin's disease.

noninvasive   A technique or procedure that does not involve the puncture of, or incision into, a patient's skin or the introduction of an instrument or foreign material into a patient's body.

nonpsychotic psychiatric disorder   Any one of a group of conditions that have no known organic origin, and have symptoms that are distressing to the affected person and are recognized by that person as being unacceptable.

nonreducible hernia A hernia in which the protrusion remains in an unnatural location and cannot return to the customary location. Also known as an incarcerated hernia.

non-renal proteinuria A condition in which protein is present in the urine as a result of a disorder outside the organs of the urinary system, but not as the result of accidental contamination.

nonspecific urethritis *See* nongonococcal urethritis.

nontoxic goiter *See* simple goiter.

nucleus A spherical body located near the center of a cell that serves to direct all cell activities.

nucleus pulposus The soft, gelatinous central section of tissue of an intervertebral disc.

oblique fracture A fracture that occurs at a slant to the long axis of the bone.

obsession A recurrent unwanted thought that intrudes upon an individual's consciousness.

obsessive-compulsive disorder A nonpsychotic psychiatric disorder characterized by the presence of recurrent ideas and fantasies and repetitive impulses or actions that a patient recognizes as being irrational and toward which that patient feels an inner resistance.

obstetrics The branch of medicine that deals with the management of pregnancy from fertilization through labor and childbirth.

occipital lobe One of the four main lobes of the cerebrum. It sits at the back of the cerebrum and controls visual sensations.

occlusive therapy A corrective procedure in which a patient wears an eye patch over his or her good eye.

olfactory nerve The nerve responsible for transmitting nerve impulses related to the sense of smell. Also known as cranial nerve I.

oliguria A condition characterized by the reduced excretion of urine.

oncogenes Genes that may facilitate cancer development.

open fracture A fracture in which the overlying skin and soft tissues are disrupted and part of the broken bone surfaces penetrates to the outside of the body.

open head injury An injury to the skull that may include scalp lacerations and linear or depressed fractures of the skull.

ophthalmoscope An instrument that has a special illuminating system that permits an examiner to look into a patient's inner eye and to study the patient's retina.

optic disk A small, round, pale yellowish-white, slightly raised area inside the eye which contains no receptors that are sensitive to light. It lies at the point at which the optic nerve penetrates the retina.

optic nerve   A nerve composed of all of the retinal nerve fibers. This nerve is responsible for transmitting nerve impulses related to the sense of sight. Also known as cranial nerve II.

optic nerve atrophy   The degeneration and shrinking of the optic nerve. This condition is characterized by the loss of vision.

optic neuritis   A general term that refers to the inflammation or degeneration of the optic nerve.

oral cavity   *See* mouth.

oral cholecystography   A simple method of x-ray visualization of the gallbladder that follows a patient's ingestion of tablets containing a contrast agent.

oral contraceptives   *See* birth control pills.

orbit   A cavity in the skull that shelters an eyeball. Also known as an eye socket.

orchiectomy   The surgical removal of a testis.

orchiopexy   An operation in which a surgeon anchors an undescended testis in the patient's scrotum in an effort to correct cryptorchidism.

organ   A structure composed of tissues from the four major tissue groups. Each tissue serves a specialized function within the organ and all tissues work collectively for a common purpose.

organ system   A group of organs that have a similar physiologic goal.

organic brain syndrome   A general term for a group of psychological or behavioral manifestations that arise from a real or presumed physical cause, but without reference to a specific cause.

organic psychiatric disorder   Any psychiatric condition that is associated with the presence of definite brain pathology.

oropharynx   The portion of the pharynx located behind the mouth between the soft palate and the epiglottis.

orthopnea   A condition of difficult breathing except in an upright position.

orthostatic proteinuria   A condition in which protein is present in the urine only when the patient is standing.

oscilloscope   An instrument that displays images of electrical currents on the screen of a cathode-ray tube.

ossicle   One of three small, movable bones in the middle ear.

osteoarthritis   A chronic, noninflammatory, degenerative disease that usually affects several joints, particularly those, such as the knees, hips, and spine, that involve weight-bearing and daily wear-and-tear. Also known as degenerative arthritis, degenerative joint disease, and hypertrophic arthritis.

osteogenic sarcoma   A malignant primary tumor of the bone that consists of cancerous connective tissue. Also known as osteosarcoma.

osteology   The scientific study of bones.

osteoma   A benign growth that arises from bone.

osteomalacia   The abnormal mineralization of bone and cartilage in adults, whose bones have, for the most part, stopped growing.

osteomyelitis   A pus-producing infection of bone, usually resulting from staphylococcus or streptococcus bacteria.

osteonecrosis   The death of bone tissue.

osteopenia   A metabolic disease that is characterized by a decrease in the patient's bone mass.

osteoporosis   An absolute decrease in bone mass that occurs as a result of endocrine, gastrointestinal, bone marrow, or connective tissue disorders.

osteosarcoma   *See* osteogenic sarcoma.

otitis media   An infection of the middle ear.

otosclerosis   A condition of the middle ear that involves the formation of abnormal, spongy bone tissue and is characterized by loss of hearing and tinnitus.

ovary   A solid, oval, sexual gland in females in which ova, or eggs, are formed.

oviduct   *See* fallopian tube.

ovulation   A process that involves the ripening of an ovum and bursting of the follicle with the release of a mature ovum.

oxytocin   A hypothalamus hormone that causes contraction of the smooth muscle of the uterus, and is of primary importance during labor and after the delivery of a child.

pacemaker   A device used to replace the electrical components of the heart by originating electrical impulses to the atria or the ventricles, or both, in a synchronized fashion.

palliative   Affording a reduction in or relief from distressing symptoms, without providing a cure.

palpation   The application of light pressure by hand to the surface of a body in order to feel the internal body parts underneath or their movement.

palpitation   A subjective sensation of unduly rapid or irregular heart beats.

pancreas   A relatively long, narrow, and somewhat irregularly shaped gland that is located below the liver and stomach.

pancreatic juice   An exocrine substance that is secreted by the pancreas and moves through the pancreatic duct to the duodenum. It contains enzymes that assist in the digestion of protein, fat, and carbohydrate.

pancreatitis   An inflammation of the pancreas.

pancreatoduodenectomy   A surgical procedure which involves the removal of the connection between the pancreas and the duodenum.

pancytopenia   A condition which is characterized by a reduction in the number of red blood cells, white blood cells, and platelets.

panhypopituitarism   A generalized decrease in pituitary function resulting from the reduced production of all anterior lobe hormones.

Pap smear   A screening test for cervical cancer in which a physician gently scrapes the surface of a female patient's cervix and posterior vagina and places the obtained mucus on a slide.

papilledema   A noninflammatory swelling of the optic disk.

papillitis   An inflammation or degeneration of the optic nerve that is confined to the area around a patient's optic disk. Also known as anterior optic neuritis.

papilloma   A polyp-like growth that has a layer of epithelium on its surface and a connective tissue stalk for support.

papule   A raised skin lesion less than one centimeter in diameter.

paraffin block biopsy technique   A method of preparing excised tissue for microscopic examination by fixing the biopsy specimen in formalin to harden the tissue and embedding it in paraffin. From this paraffin block, the physician or technician obtains a very thin slice of tissue, mounts it on a glass slide, stains the tissue sample, and examines it though a microscope.

paranasal sinuses   Irregularly shaped air cavities that are adjacent to the nose.

paranoia   A psychiatric condition characterized by an individual's believing that someone is intent on causing him or her harm. Also known as paranoid ideation.

paranoid ideation   *See* paranoia.

paranoid personality disorder   A psychiatric condition characterized by hypersensitivity to and unwarranted suspicion of the words and behaviors of others.

paraplegia   Paralysis of the lower extremities only.

parathyroid gland   One of four tiny, flattened, oval discs that are located on the back of the thyroid gland which secrete the parathyroid hormone.

parenteral drug administration   The administration of a drug by injection.

paresthesia   A condition which involves abnormal skin sensations that have no obvious cause.

parietal lobe   One of the four main lobes of the cerebrum. It lies at the top and on the side of the cerebrum.

parietal pleura   The layer of the pleura that lines the inner surface of the chest wall.

Parkinson's disease   A chronic disorder of the central nervous system that usually first appears in patients after age 45. Parkinsonism is characterized by tremor, rigidity, and stiffness and slowness of movement.

parotid ducts   The ducts through which the parotid glands communicate with the oral cavity. Also known as Stensen's ducts.

parotids   The largest of the salivary glands. They lie upon either side of the face immediately below and in front of each external ear.

partial seizure   An epileptic seizure that originates with electrical activity in one area of the brain and may or may not spread to other areas of the brain. Also known as a focal seizure.

passive immunity   An acquired immunity that results when an individual receives a pre-formed antibody or specifically sensitized lymphoid cells.

passive-aggressive personality disorder   A condition characterized by aggression that is exhibited passively.

passive-dependent personality disorder   A condition characterized by an individual's avoidance of responsibility, lack of self-reliance, and apparent helplessness.

patch   A flat skin lesion greater than two centimeters in diameter.

patella   A flat, triangular bone located in front of the knee joint.

patent ductus arteriosus   A shunt of blood from the aorta to the pulmonary artery through an arterial connection that is normal before birth, but abnormal after birth.

pathogen   A disease-producing microorganism.

pathologic fracture   A fracture that occurs when a bone, weakened by tumor or disease, breaks during normal daily activities or minor trauma.

pathology   The study of disease.

pelvic exam   An office procedure for (1) directly visualizing a female's external genitalia, vagina, and cervix, and (2) palpating her ovaries, uterus, fallopian tubes, uterine ligaments, and rectal area for abnormalities or tenderness.

pelvic inflammatory disease (PID)   Any inflammatory infection that affects the reproductive organs in the pelvis.

pelvis   (1) The lower portion of the abdominal cavity containing the urinary bladder, sigmoid colon, rectum, and some of the reproductive organs. (2) A strong, bony ring composed of the two hip bones on the sides and front, and the sacrum and coccyx in the rear.

penis   The primary male reproductive and urinary excretion organ.

peptic ulcer   A general term for any erosion of the lining of the stomach, duodenum, or esophagus that involves a single, small, circumscribed area resembling a crater in appearance.

percutaneous transhepatic cholangiography A diagnostic procedure that allows a physician to introduce a contrast agent directly into a patient's liver through a long, thin needle inserted through the patient's skin. This procedure permits x-ray visualization of the bile ducts.

percutaneous transluminal angioplasty (PTA) An invasive procedure that involves the dilation of a blood vessel by means of a balloon-tipped catheter that is inserted through the patient's skin and into the chosen vessel.

percutaneous transluminal coronary angioplasty A procedure that is used to dilate partially occluded coronary arteries by introducing a balloon-tipped catheter into the large artery in the patient's thigh and advancing the catheter into the patient's aorta and then into the narrowed coronary artery. Also known as a PTCA.

perianal abscess *See* anorectal abscess.

pericarditis An infection or inflammation of the pericardium.

pericardium A two-layered white fibrous sac that encases the heart and the cardiac junctions of the major blood vessels.

perineum The region between the urogenital area and the rectum.

periosteum A protective fibrous membrane that coats compact bone and contains the blood vessels that supply nourishment to the bone.

peripheral iridectomy The surgical removal of a small piece of the edge of the iris.

peripheral nervous system The part of the human nervous system that contains the cranial and spinal nerves and the autonomic nervous system.

perirectal abscess *See* anorectal abscess.

peristalsis The process by which peristaltic waves propel the contents of a hollow organ.

peristaltic waves Successive, involuntary, coordinated contractions which can occur in any hollow structure.

peritoneal cavity The abdominal cavity.

peritoneum The serous membrane which lines the inner wall of the abdominal cavity and most of the structures in the abdomen.

peritonitis An inflammation of the peritoneum.

pernicious anemia A type of megaloblastic anemia caused by a deficiency of vitamin B_{12}. It is characterized by atrophy of the stomach lining, nausea, vomiting, weight loss, a faint yellow skin tint, lack of coordination, irritability, forgetfulness, dementia, and other neurologic difficulties.

persecutory delusion A type of delusion in which a person may feel conspired against, spied upon, poisoned, cheated, followed, obstructed, and/or harassed.

personality disorder   Any one of a wide group of behavior patterns that are acceptable to the affected individuals, but that produce conflict with others.

petechia   A minute, dot-like, red hemorrhage into the skin.

phalanges   The bones of the fingers or toes.

pharmacology   The study of properties of drugs and their actions in living organisms.

pharyngitis   An inflammation of the pharynx.

pharynx   A vertical, muscular, tubular structure about five inches long extending from the nasal cavity to the esophagus. Commonly known as the throat.

pheochromocytoma   A rare tumor that usually grows in the adrenal medulla, but occasionally arises in other locations. It secretes adrenaline.

phlebitis   An inflammation in a vein.

phlebothrombosis   A blood clot that develops in a vein.

phobia   A nonpsychotic psychiatric disorder characterized by irrational or exaggerated fears of objects, situations, or bodily functions.

photocoagulation   A procedure that uses an intense beam of light to coagulate tissue. It is often used to treat eye disorders.

physical dependence   A condition characterized by (1) the presence of withdrawal symptoms when a substance is withheld, and (2) tolerance to the effects of a substance. Also known as addiction.

physiology   The study of the function of the various parts of the body, how the work of one part is interrelated with the work of other structures and systems, and how a structure or organ acts when it is healthy and when it is diseased.

pia   The innermost meninge. It consists of elastic and collagenous fibers.

PID   *See* pelvic inflammatory disease.

piles   *See* internal hemorrhoids.

pineal body   A small gland in the brain that is located behind the medulla and above the cerebellum, and is connected to the substance of the brain by a small stalk.

pinkeye   *See* conjunctivitis.

pituitary gland   The master gland of the body that is involved in most endocrine activities. It is located at the base of the brain. Also known as the hypophysis.

pityriasis rosea   A skin condition that is presumed to be of viral origin and causes an itchy papular dermatitis that lasts up to three months.

placenta   An organ, found only in mammals, that provides nutrition to the conceptus throughout the pregnancy and manufactures hormones that are required in order for the pregnancy to last for the full term.

placenta previa   A condition in which the placenta lies partially or completely over the internal opening of the uterus.

plaque   A raised lesion greater than one centimeter in diameter that arises on any internal or external body surface.

plasma   The faintly-yellow liquid component of blood, in which the blood corpuscles are suspended. It is mostly water and contains mineral salts, fats, glucose, hormones, enzymes, and the waste products of cell metabolism.

plasma thromboplastin component   A type of coagulation factor found in plasma. Also known as Factor IX.

plasmapheresis   A technique in which blood is removed from a vein and transported through tubing to a blood cell separator which filters out undesirable blood components that may contribute to disease.

plastic surgery   The repair of deformities, usually superficial or external in location, in order to obtain improved appearance or function.

platelet   See thrombocyte.

pleura   A very delicate, two-layer membrane that covers a lung.

pleural cavity   The potential space between the two pleural layers.

pleural effusion   A condition characterized by the development of fluid in the pleural cavity.

pleurisy   A condition characterized by inflammation of the pleura.

pneumoconiosis   Any one of a group of lung diseases resulting from inhalation of mineral or vegetable dusts from occupational exposure.

pneumonia   An acute infection of the alveolar spaces of the lung.

pneumothorax   The presence of air or gas in the pleural cavity.

poliomyelitis   A disease of the central nervous system. It is caused by a virus that destroys the nerve cells responsible for motor activity and that affects skeletal muscles and the muscles involved with swallowing, breathing, and talking. Also known as infantile paralysis.

poly   See polymorphonuclear neutrophil.

polycystic ovary syndrome   A symptom-complex that is characterized by menstrual irregularities, obesity, sterility, and occasionally, a male type of body hair distribution. Also known as Stein-Leventhal syndrome.

polycythemia vera   A disorder of unknown cause characterized by an increase in the number of red blood cells, white blood cells, and platelets.

polygenic inheritance The interaction of several genes that have been inherited from both parents.

polymorphonuclear neutrophil The most common type of leukocyte. It has a multi-lobed nucleus. Commonly called a "poly."

polyneuropathy Any syndrome that is produced by the abnormal function or structure of multiple peripheral nerves.

polyp A protruding growth from a mucous membrane.

polyuria A condition in which the patient excretes an excessive amount of very dilute urine.

pons The part of the brain that contains the nuclei of some of the important cranial nerves that are not contained in the midbrain or medulla and provides a pathway for nerve impulses.

positional vertigo A benign, relatively common condition in which head movements or position produce the typical symptoms of vertigo.

post-concussion syndrome A condition characterized by amnesia, headache, and nausea for the period immediately following a head injury and for a short period following the patient's recovery of consciousness.

posterior cruciate A ligament that lies behind the knee joint and helps to control that joint.

postictal state A period of sleep and stupor following a tonic-clonic seizure that may last up to several hours.

postnecrotic cirrhosis A type of degenerative liver disease that results from the death of liver tissue following an attack of viral or toxic hepatitis that did not progress to complete healing.

postpartum hemorrhage The loss of excessive blood from the mother's uterine blood vessels that occurs soon after childbirth.

postpartum period The period of time following childbirth.

post-phlebitic syndrome A condition following phlebitis that is characterized by a swollen leg with skin changes.

postprandial hypoglycemia *See* reactive hypoglycemia.

Pott's disease *See* tuberculosis of the spine.

precancerous A medical designation which means that a particular condition is not a true cancer, but has a tendency to develop into a true cancer.

preeclampsia A disorder of pregnancy resulting from a metabolic disturbance that is characterized by hypertension, swelling, and proteinuria.

prefix A letter or group of letters attached to the beginning of a root.

premature infant A baby that is delivered before its organs have completed normal intrauterine development and that typically weighs less than 2500 grams.

premenstrual tension syndrome A monthly disorder of unknown cause that usually occurs during the seven to ten days prior to menstruation.

presbycusis   A physiologic loss of hearing associated with aging.

presbyopia   A condition associated with aging in which a patient has increasing difficulty seeing close objects.

primary aldosteronism   A condition characterized by the increased secretion of aldosterone. It causes hypertension and low serum potassium.

primary closed-angle glaucoma   A type of glaucoma that is characterized by a sudden and acute increase in intraocular tension. Without treatment it leads to prompt loss of vision.

primary dysmenorrhea   Painful menstruation that has no demonstrable cause.

primary hyperparathyroidism   Hyperparathyroidism that results from increased parathyroid hormone production by one or more of the four parathyroid glands.

primary hypertension   *See* essential hypertension.

primary open-angle glaucoma   A chronic, slowly progressive glaucoma that is initially asymptomatic and that typically affects both eyes.

PRL   *See* prolactin.

proctitis   A general term for an inflammation of the rectal mucosa.

prognosis   The probable course of a disease and a patient's prospect of recovery from the disease.

progressive systemic sclerosis   *See* diffuse scleroderma.

prolactin (PRL)   A pituitary hormone that stimulates the development of ducts and glands in breast tissue and is responsible for the secretion of milk.

prostate gland   A structure that surrounds the neck of the bladder and the urethra in males.

proteinuria   A condition in which a protein is present in the urine.

protozoa   A small unicellular microorganism, a few of which are pathogenic for humans.

pseudohypoglycemia   A condition in which a patient experiences the symptoms of hypoglycemia, but has normal blood sugar levels.

psoriasis   A skin condition that is characterized by itchy, raised, dull-red patches covered with thick, silvery-white scales.

psoriatic arthritis   An arthritis characterized by the presence of skin and nail psoriatic lesions.

PSS   Progressive systemic sclerosis. *See* diffuse scleroderma.

psychedelics   Drugs that produce visual hallucinations, intensified perceptions, delusions, euphoria, dream-like states, distortion of time, and other psychotic manifestations. Also known as hallucinogens.

psychiatric disorder Any one of several conditions that affect an individual's behavior and/or mental well-being.

psychiatrist A medical doctor who specializes in psychiatry and is licensed to prescribe medicine.

psychiatry The branch of medicine that deals with the study, treatment, and prevention of mental impairments.

psychoactive drugs Substances that affect the mind or senses.

psychological dependence A compulsion to continue use of a substance despite known adverse consequences. Also known as habituation.

psychomotor seizure *See* complex partial seizure.

psychopathic personality disorder *See* antisocial personality disorder.

psychosis A psychiatric disorder that is characterized by gross impairment in an individual's ability to recognize reality, as evidenced by delusions, hallucinations, incoherent speech, or disorganized and agitated behavior without apparent awareness on the part of that individual of the incomprehensibility of his or her behavior.

psychotherapy A type of treatment that is designed to produce a response by mental, rather than by physical, effects.

PTA *See* percutaneous transluminal angioplasty.

PTCA *See* percutaneous transluminal coronary angioplasty.

ptosis A condition characterized by a drooping of the eyelid.

pubis A bone that fuses with the ilium and the ischium to form the innominate bone. The pubis forms the lower, front part of the innominate.

pulmonary circulation The circulatory system that involves the network of blood vessels that transport oxygen-depleted blood from the right ventricle of the heart to the lungs for oxygenation and back again to the heart.

pulmonary edema A swelling of the lungs as the result of the escape of serous fluid from the capillaries surrounding the alveoli.

pulmonary fibrosis A pathologic condition resulting from an increase in the fibrous connective tissue in the lung.

pulmonary hypertension A condition characterized by elevated blood pressure in the pulmonary artery.

pulmonary stenosis The narrowing of the opening between the pulmonary artery and the right ventricle.

punch biopsy A diagnostic technique in which a physician uses a small metal punch to remove a piece of tissue.

pupil An opening at the center of the iris through which light enters the eye.

purpura A hemorrhage into the skin and subcutaneous tissues.

purulent meningitis   A bacterial infection of the membranes covering the brain and spinal cord.

pustule   A small irregular raised area containing pus.

PUVA   A treatment for psoriasis that consists of the oral administration of psoralen, a photosensitizing chemical, followed by exposure to high-intensity, long-wave ultraviolet light.

pyelonephritis   A bacterial infection that causes inflammation of the kidney and its pelvis.

pyloric stenosis   A permanent narrowing of the pylorus.

pyloroplasty   An incision into the pylorus in order to facilitate gastric drainage.

pylorospasm   A temporary spasm of the pylorus.

pylorus   The outlet of the stomach that communicates with the upper part of the small intestine through the pyloric sphincter.

pyoderma   An infection of the skin caused by pus-forming bacteria.

pyothorax   A condition in which pus-filled fluid develops in the pleural cavity.

pyrosis   *See* heartburn.

pyuria   A condition in which white blood cells are present in the urine.

quadriplegia   Paralysis of all upper and lower extremities.

radial keratotomy (RK)   A procedure in which a surgeon makes a series of bicycle spoke-like incisions in the patient's cornea that flatten the cornea and reduce myopia.

radiculitis   An irritation of a nerve root at the point at which the root emerges from the spinal cord.

radioisotope   A substance that emits radiation as it decays.

radionuclide   A type of radioisotope that has important diagnostic and therapeutic uses in clinical medicine and research.

radionuclide imaging   A diagnostic and therapeutic procedure in which radionuclides are administered to patients orally or intravenously after which imaging devices record the distribution of radiation the radioisotope emits.

radiopaque contrast agent   A substance that provides visible images on x-ray film.

radiotherapy   A treatment procedure that may take the form of x-rays produced by linear accelerators or of gamma rays given off by radioactive substances such as radioactive phosphorus, iodine, cobalt, and radium.

radius   The forearm bone that lies on the same side as the thumb.

Raynaud's disease   A condition of unknown cause which involves intermittent episodes of decreased bloodflow to the patient's fingers or toes. This disorder is marked by severe pallor, followed by blueness and then redness of the digits.

Raynaud's phenomenon   A condition which involves intermittent episodes of decreased bloodflow to the patient's fingers or toes. This disorder is marked by severe pallor, followed by blueness and then redness of the digits. It is secondary to an underlying cause, such as connective tissue disease, repetitive trauma, emotional stimuli, or tobacco use.

reactive hypoglycemia   A temporary condition that occurs two to four hours after the ingestion of carbohydrates. It is associated with an excessive release of insulin and, in turn, a decrease in blood sugar. Also known as postprandial hypoglycemia.

receptor   A highly specialized nerve ending that receives a sensation which is then transmitted to the brain.

recessive trait   A trait that requires the presence of the same gene on each chromosome of a pair.

rectal fissure   An open, ulcerated crevice in the mucosa of a patient's lower rectum.

rectocele   A sagging of the rectum into the vagina.

rectum   A somewhat dilated segment of the large intestine that extends from the sigmoid colon and measures about five inches in length.

red blood cell   *See* erythrocyte.

red marrow   The chief blood cell forming organ of the adult body. It is only found in the vertebrae, sternum, ribs, cranial bones, and ends of long bones.

reducible hernia   A hernia that can slip back easily into the abdominal cavity.

reducing (a bone fracture)   The act of properly aligning a fracture.

reflex sympathetic dystrophy   A disturbance in the sympathetic nervous system marked by pain, pallor, sweating, swelling, or atrophy of the skin. It typically follows trauma to a limb.

reflux   A backward flow.

reflux esophagitis   The backward flow of gastric contents, including digestive juices, from the stomach into the lower esophagus. Also known as gastroesophageal reflux.

refractive errors   Disorders of the eye in which rays of light that enter the eye are not brought into proper, precise focus on the retina.

regional anesthesia   The induced loss of sensation of a part of the body as a result of pharmacologic interruption of nerve conduction.

regional enteritis   A chronic, nonspecific inflammatory disease of the intestine that is characterized by abdominal cramps and the passage of loose stools several times daily. Also known as Crohn's disease.

Reiter's syndrome   A disorder that is characterized by urethritis, conjunctivitis, and arthritis.

releasing factors   Hypothalamus hormones that act on the pituitary gland to affect the release of pituitary hormones.

renal   Pertaining to the kidney.

renal calyces   Cup-shaped cavities that empty into the kidney pelvis.

renal colic   Acute abdominal pain produced by the passage of a stone within the urinary tract.

renal failure   A condition in which the kidney is unable to normally excrete the substances produced by metabolism.

renal glycosuria   A condition in which glucose appears in a person's urine even if that person has a normal blood glucose level.

renal proteinuria   A condition in which protein is present in the urine as a result of damage to the kidney tubules or glomeruli.

reproduction   The process by which a species creates a new generation of its own kind.

respiration   A group of processes concerned with the exchange of gases between the body and its environment.

respiratory system   The group of organs and structures that work to exchange gases between the air we breathe and our blood stream.

restrictive cardiomyopathies   A class of primary heart diseases that is characterized by a diastolic filling impairment and a normal, or near normal, systolic function and chamber size.

retina   A thin, delicate membrane at the back of the eye that is primarily composed of nerve fibers.

retinal detachment   A partial or complete separation of the retina from the choroid. This condition is characterized by (1) blurred vision or the total loss of sight or (2) the perception of flashes of light and spots before the eyes.

retinitis   An inflammation of the retina that is characterized by a reduction in the patient's visual acuity.

retinoblastoma   A malignant tumor in children arising from the cells of the retina.

retinopathy   A general term for any disease of the retina.

retrobulbar optic neuritis   An inflammation of the part of the optic nerve that lies behind the eyeball.

retrograde pyelogram   A diagnostic procedure in which a small amount of a radiopaque dye passes through a catheter into the kidney pelvis, and then a series of x-rays is obtained.

Reye's syndrome   A relatively rare acute condition that is characterized by an enlarged liver and degenerative brain disease, and that follows common viral illness, especially influenza and chicken pox, in children.

rhabdomyosarcoma A highly malignant tumor of striated muscle tissue.

rheumatoid arthritis A chronic, systemic disease characterized by inflammation in and around many joints.

rhythm method A contraceptive method that involves timing sexual intercourse around the days during each month when the woman is fertile.

rickets The abnormal mineralization of bone and cartilage in children, usually arising from vitamin D deficiency.

rickettsia A microorganism that is readily visible with an ordinary microscope and is intermediate in characteristics between a virus and a bacterium.

right and left ventriculography The x-ray visualization of the ventricles of the heart.

ringworm A common fungal infection of the skin, hair, and nails.

RK *See* radial keratotomy.

rod One of two types of highly specialized light-sensitive cells in the eye. A rod contains compounds that are responsible for vision in low light and the detection of motion.

rod bacterium A form of bacterium that has one axis which is markedly longer than the others and is cylindrical or rod-shaped.

root A complex word element that can be used as a prefix, a suffix, or the body of a longer word that is formed by the combination of the root with a prefix, suffix, or both.

rotary joint A joint that permits only rotation.

rotation Movement around an axis; a bone deformity in which the bone has turned, without any side-to-side or up-and-down movement.

rotator cuff A musculotendinous structure that surrounds the capsule of the shoulder joint, providing it with mobility and strength.

rubella A childhood viral disease, commonly known as German measles.

rubeola A childhood viral disease, commonly known as measles.

rupture *See* hernia.

sacral vertebrae Vertebrae that lie behind the pelvis.

sacrum A triangular bone that is wedged between the two hip bones.

saddle joint A joint that permits flexion, extension, abduction, and circumduction.

saliva A secretion of the salivary glands that is 98 percent water and which contains small quantities of enzymes.

sarcoidosis A predominately respiratory disorder that is characterized by the presence of a microscopic, rounded tumor-like masses of tissue in the lungs or lymph nodes. Also known as Boeck's sarcoid.

sarcoma A malignant tumor that arises from connective or muscle tissue.

scanner *See* scanning detector.

scanning detector An imaging device used for radionuclide imaging that moves back and forth across the area of the body that is under study, and radioactive patterns are recorded on paper or on x-ray film. Also known as a scanner.

scapula An irregular, flat, triangular bone that forms the rear part of the shoulder girdle. Also known as the shoulder blade.

scarlet fever An infection by streptococcal bacteria that produces a toxin which creates a red rash.

schizoid personality disorder A psychiatric condition characterized by timidity, aloofness, introvertedness, and self-consciousness.

schizophrenic disorders A group of severe emotional illnesses that are characterized by bizarre and inappropriate behavior and by a regression from a prior level of functioning in such areas as work, social relations, and self-care.

sciatic nerve The largest nerve, it arises from the sacral plexus and serves nearly all of the skin of the leg, the muscles of the back of the thigh, and the muscles of the leg and foot.

sciatica Pain which radiates down the back of the patient's leg beyond the knee along the sciatic nerve.

SCID *See* severe combined immunodeficiency disease.

scintillation camera A stationary imaging device used for radionuclide imaging. It is aimed at the area of the body being studied and displays radioactive emissions on a screen or records them as a series of "stop action" photographs.

sclera The white, fibrous tissue that forms the external coat of the eye.

scoliosis A condition characterized by one or more lateral curvatures of the spine.

scrotum An elastic external pouch that lies just below the penis and contains the testes and their accessory organs.

sebaceous gland A gland that secretes an oily, thick, semifluid substance that is formed from the disintegration of cells in the central portion of the gland.

seborrheic dermatitis A skin condition characterized by excessive oiliness of the individual's skin, particularly in areas in which sebaceous glands are highly concentrated.

secondary aldosteronism A condition in which the secretion of aldosterone in excessive amounts is stimulated by agents outside the adrenal gland.

secondary closed-angle glaucoma   A condition of increased pressure in the eye that most often results from either an intense inflammatory process that causes adhesions to form between the iris and the pupil or from some other condition that causes the lens to come into contact with the iris.

secondary dysmenorrhea   Painful menstruation that results from a known condition.

secondary hypertension   Hypertension that results from a known cause, which can often be treated successfully.

secondary open-angle glaucoma   A condition of increased pressure within a patient's eye that results from inflammation, drug use, or mechanical abnormality.

secondary polycythemia   A condition marked by an increase in the number of circulating red blood cells as a result of some other condition or factor. Also known as erythrocytosis.

sectional radiography   *See* tomography.

sedatives   Drugs that exert a calming effect, relieve irritability or excitement, ease mild pain, and, in larger doses, produce sleep.

seizure   An episode of neurologic dysfunction.

self-cauterizing   Causing the patient's affected blood vessels to clot and seal, eliminating the need for internal stitches.

sella turcica   A small bony cavity within the floor of the cranium. The pituitary gland is located in this cavity.

semen   A thick, whitish fluid that is composed of spermatozoa and secretions from the testes and other organs of the male reproductive system.

semi-rigid contact lenses   *See* gas-permeable contact lenses.

seminal vesicles   The two membranous sacs that join with the vas deferens as it opens into the urethra. These sacs produce a large part of the seminal fluid.

senile vaginitis   *See* atrophic vaginitis.

sense organs   Those structures in the body that contain highly specialized nerve endings that receive sensations and then transmit impulses to the nerve centers in the brain so that the individual can perceive the sensations.

senses   The faculties by which human beings perceive their external and internal environment.

sensitization effect   An allergic effect to a drug that is characterized by the sudden appearance of toxic signs and symptoms.

sepsis   A toxic condition resulting from the presence in the blood of chemical products of disease-causing microorganisms.

seronegative spondylarthropathies   Several forms of arthritis that are characterized by the absence of rheumatoid factor, an involvement of the spine and related bones, and at least some degree of peripheral inflammatory joint disease.

serous membrane   A membrane that lines the walls of the closed body cavities, such as the peritoneal, pleural, and pericardial cavities.

Sertoli-Leydig cell tumor   A tumor that arises from the supporting tissue of an ovary and secretes a male sex hormone.

serum   The portion of the blood that separates from a blood clot after clotting has occurred.

severe combined immunodeficiency disease   A heterogeneous group of genetic disturbances of the immune system, associated with the patient's T and B cell function, and primarily affecting infants. Also known as SCID.

sex chromosome   A chromosome that determines the gender of an individual.

sex chromosome-linked trait   *See* X-linked trait.

sex-linked trait   *See* X-linked trait.

sexually transmitted disease (STD)   Any one of several disorders that one person passes to another primarily though intimate sexual contact. Also known as a venereal disease.

shingles   A painful vesicular and papular eruption which usually affects a local area of the patient's skin. It is caused by the varicella-zoster virus.

shock   A complex failure of the circulatory system involving multiple organs including the brain, heart, lungs, liver, and kidneys.

shoulder blade   *See* scapula.

sickle cell anemia   A chronic hemolytic anemia in which red cells assume an abnormal sickle shape. It is caused by abnormalities in hemoglobin manufacture and is associated with increased red blood cell destruction. It affects blacks almost exclusively.

sigmoid colon   The part of the large intestine that assumes an S-shaped loop and which averages about 15 inches in length.

sigmoidoscopy   The inspection of the left side of the colon by means of a fiberoptic scope.

sign   A physical manifestation of a disease that can be noted by someone other than the patient.

silicosis   A type of pneumoconiosis caused by inhaling silica.

simple goiter   An asymptomatic enlarged thyroid that results from a relative or absolute deficiency in iodine. Also known as nontoxic goiter.

simple mastectomy   The surgical removal of a breast.

simple partial seizure   An epileptic seizure that is the result of an irritation of a small area of the brain. Convulsive activity associated with this type of seizure typically starts as a focal seizure in one part of the body, such as the patient's face, thumb, arm, or leg.

simple urethritis   *See* nongonococcal urethritis.

singer's nodule   An enlargement of the edge of the vocal cord.

sinus bradycardia   An alteration in the rate of normal cardiac sinus rhythm so that it is less than 60 beats per minute.

sinus node   A functionally independent and specialized piece of neuromuscular tissue that creates the electrical stimulus for each heart beat.

sinus tachycardia   An alteration in the rate of normal cardiac sinus rhythm so that it is greater than 100 beats per minute.

sinusitis   A sinus infection.

skeletal muscle   A type of muscle that comprises the bulky muscles of the body that are under voluntary control, including muscles that are attached to bone and the eye muscles. Also known as striated muscle.

skin   A complex organ that provides a tough, flexible cover for the entire body.

skin tag   A benign tumor of the dermis composed of a small cutaneous appendage, flap, or polyp.

skull   The bony framework of the head. It is composed of a series of flattened, irregular bones and lies on the top of the vertebral column.

SLE   *See* systemic lupus erythematosus.

slit lamp   An instrument with which a physician projects a beam of intense light into a patient's eye and examines the eye directly by magnifying lenses.

small intestine   The tubular organ that extends from the pylorus of the stomach to the large intestine.

smooth muscle   A type of muscle that appears in locations that are not under the voluntary control of the individual, such as the walls of blood vessels, the digestive tract, bronchi, trachea, and bladder.

sociopathic personality disorder   *See* antisocial personality disorder.

soft contact lenses   Contact lenses that consist of a malleable cover that contains a gelatinous substance.

solute   Any substance that can be dissolved.

somatic delusion   A type of delusion which is characterized by the false belief that certain parts of the patient's body are, contrary to all evidence, misshapen, ugly, or nonfunctioning.

spermatic cord   *See* vas deferens.

spermatocele   A cyst originating in the cells that connect the testis to the epididymis.

spermatogenesis   The production of sperm cells.

spermatozoa The mature male cells that fertilize the female's eggs during reproduction.

spherocyte An abnormal, small globular red blood cell.

sphincter A ring-like muscle.

sphygmomanometer A device used to measure a patient's blood pressure. Also known as a blood pressure cuff.

spina bifida A congenital disorder that results from a defect in the fetal development of a vertebra.

spinal anesthesia A special type of nerve block, used for many operations within the peritoneal cavity and on the lower extremities, that blocks the spinal nerves after their emergence from the spinal cord.

spinal column *See* spine.

spinal cord A cylindrical mass of nerve tissue that occupies the vertebral canal.

spinal tap *See* lumbar puncture.

spine A flexible series of relatively small bones that provide the primary support for the body's structures. Also known as the vertebral column, the spinal column, or the backbone.

spiral fracture A fracture that winds around the short axis of the bone.

spirochete A spiral-shaped bacterium.

spleen A fairly large organ that lies in the left upper quadrant of the abdominal cavity just below the diaphragm.

splenectomy The surgical removal of the spleen.

splenomegaly Enlargement of the spleen.

spondylolisthesis A displacement of a vertebral body over the vertebra below it.

spontaneous abortion A termination of pregnancy that occurs naturally. Also known as a miscarriage.

spontaneous pneumothorax The presence of air or gas in the pleural cavity which may result from the rupture of a superficial emphysematous air cyst or may occur in the course of some other lung disease, such as bronchiectasis, lung abscess, or tuberculosis.

sprain A condition that results from an overstretching or tearing of supporting ligaments at a joint. It generally occurs whenever movement in the joint extends beyond the normal range.

sputum A mucus-like matter that is ejected from a person's lungs, bronchi, and trachea through the mouth.

squamous cell carcinoma A type of malignancy that arises from the skin and from other locations of squamous cell epithelium.

squamous epithelium A type of epithelial tissue that is composed of thin, flat cells, and that covers the entire surface of the body and the orifices of cavities opening upon it.

staging   The evaluation of the extent of a cancer's spread from its primary site.

stapedectomy   The surgical removal of the stapes.

stapes   The innermost of the auditory bones. It attaches to the incus on one end and to the oval window of the inner ear on the other.

stapes mobilization procedure   An operation performed on otosclerosis patients in which a surgeon frees the stapes from its fixation to the oval window, giving the stapes the opportunity to vibrate more freely.

status asthmaticus   A condition that is characterized by a sudden, intense, and continuous state of asthma and the lack of response to normal therapeutic efforts.

status epilepticus   A severe form of epileptic seizures that is characterized by frequent, generalized convulsions and failure to regain consciousness between attacks.

STD   *See* sexually transmitted disease.

steatorrhea   A condition characterized by large, bulky, fatty, foul-smelling stools. It is associated with malabsorption.

Stein-Leventhal syndrome   *See* polycystic ovary syndrome.

stenosis   An obstruction to or a narrowing of a blood vessel or other hollow channel in the body.

Stensen's ducts   *See* parotid ducts.

Stevens-Johnson Syndrome   A severe, and sometimes fatal, form of erythema multiforme.

Still's disease   A subset of juvenile rheumatoid arthritis which is characterized by high spiking daily fevers, body rash, and other manifestations of systemic disease.

stomach   The most dilated part of the digestive tube. It lies just below the diaphragm.

strabismus   The deviation of an eye caused by the overrelaxation or overcontraction of a muscle that attaches to the eyeball, resulting in the failure of light rays to fall on the fovea.

strain   A condition that results from the overstretching or tearing of muscles or tendons.

strangulated hernia   A nonreducible hernia that is trapped so tightly that the blood supply to the protruding tissue is obstructed and is a surgical emergency.

striated muscle   *See* skeletal muscle.

stroke   *See* cerebral vascular accident.

stroke volume   The volume of blood each contraction of the left ventricle pumps into the aorta.

stye   *See* hordeolum.

subarachnoid hemorrhage   A condition in which the patient experiences bleeding into the space between the arachnoid and pia membranes.

subarachnoid space A tiny space that separates the arachnoid and the pia.

subclavian blood vessels Blood vessels beneath the collar bone that lead to and from the arms.

subcutaneous injection The administration of a drug by injection below the skin in subcutaneous fatty tissue.

subdeltoid bursa The bursa located between the deltoid muscle and the shoulder joint capsule.

subdural hematoma A localized collection of clotted blood lying underneath the dura, usually requiring surgical treatment.

subdural space A tiny space that separates the arachnoid from the dura.

sublingual glands The smallest of the three types of salivary glands. They are located beneath the tongue, in front of the submandibular glands.

subluxation A partial displacement of one or more bones that comprise a joint, causing a partial change in the customary alignment of these surfaces.

submandibular glands Salivary glands that lie beneath the base of the tongue in the floor of the mouth.

substance abuse The use of alcohol and other drugs and chemicals in a manner that may predictably cause harm to the user.

subtotal thyroidectomy The surgical removal of part of the thyroid.

sudden cardiac death Death within one hour of the appearance of acute symptoms of coronary artery disease.

suffix A letter or group of letters attached to the end of a root.

superficial spreading melanoma A type of malignant melanoma that involves a noticeable enlargement or discoloration of a lesion.

suprapatellar bursa The bursa located between the lower end of the femur and the tendons of the patella.

surgery Any invasive operative procedure, usually involving the physical removal of tissue or organs.

surgical diathermy A procedure that involves heating body tissues in order to disrupt them and cause the formation of exudate. Also known as electrocoagulation.

suspensory ligament (of the eye) A ligament that holds the lens in place in the eye.

sympathetic trunk One of the main nerve complexes of the autonomic nervous system. One trunk extends on one side of the vertebral column vertically through the neck, thorax, and abdomen, and the other trunk extends on the other side of the vertebral column.

symptom   A subjective phenomenon of disease that leads to a complaint by the patient.

syndrome   A set of signs and symptoms that occur together to characterize a certain abnormality.

synovial membrane   A membrane that forms the lining of movable joints.

syphilis   A veneral disease that is caused by the spirochete *Treponema pallidum*. Also known as lues.

systemic circulation   The circulatory system that includes the blood vessels that carry oxygenated blood from the left ventricle of the heart to the various organs and tissues of the body (except the lungs) and back to the heart.

systemic lupus erythematosus   A generalized connective tissue disorder that mainly affects women in the 20 to 40 age group. Also known as SLE.

systole   The period of the heart cycle during which the ventricles contract.

systolic pressure   The pressure at which the force during a heart contraction is just sufficient to overcome the pressure in a blood pressure cuff and produce a sound.

T lymphocyte   A type of lymphocyte whose tasks include both controlling and modifying the immune response to, and some of the direct cellular actions against, foreign antigens.

tamoxifen citrate   An oral antiestrogen medication that is used to treat breast cancer.

tarsal bones   The bones of the ankle.

tear gland   *See* lacrimal gland.

technetium myocardial imaging   A procedure that uses radioactive technetium to locate damaged heart tissue.

temporal lobe   One of the four main lobes of the cerebrum. It sits near the bottom and to the side of the cerebral hemisphere and has control over hearing, smell, and understanding speech.

temporal lobe seizure   *See* complex partial seizure.

temporomandibular joint (TMJ)   One of two hinge joints that connect the lower jaw bone with the side of the skull.

tendon   Connective tissue that connects a muscle to a bone.

tension headache   A headache that arises from persistent contractions of the muscles of the head and neck.

teratogenic drugs   Drugs that a pregnant woman ingests that produce physical defects in her fetus before its birth.

testicle   *See* testis.

testis   One of two egg-shaped glands in males that produce sperm cells. Also known as a testicle.

testosterone An androgen that is responsible for growth of hair in a male distribution pattern and other masculine characteristics.

tetralogy of Fallot A congenital heart condition that consists of a combination of four defects: (1) pulmonic stenosis, (2) ventricular septal defect, (3) an overriding aorta that is positioned over both right and left ventricle outlets and (4) right ventricular hypertrophy.

thalassemia A hemolytic anemia caused by abnormalities in hemoglobin manufacture. It occurs most often in people whose ethnic origins are in countries bordering the Mediterranean Sea.

thallium myocardial imaging A procedure that uses radioactive thallium to locate abnormal cardiac bloodflow or damaged heart tissue.

therapeutic abortion The deliberate interruption of pregnancy for medical reasons that usually pertain to the health of the mother or fetus.

thoracentesis The removal of pleural fluid through a needle.

thoracic cavity The conical-shaped cage that contains and protects the principal organs of respiration and circulation.

thoracic vertebrae Vertebrae that attach to the ribs and form part of the back wall of the chest cage.

thoracotomy An incision into a patient's chest wall.

thorax The chest cage. It is bounded by the thoracic vertebrae and the back of the ribs to the back, the ribs on the sides, and the breastbone in front.

threatened spontaneous abortion A condition in early pregnancy that is characterized by bleeding, menstrual-like cramps, and abdominal pain and may progress to a miscarriage.

throat *See* pharynx.

thromboangiitis obliterans *See* Buerger's disease.

thrombocyte One of the three types of corpuscles. It is an irregularly-shaped, colorless structure that has great adhesive power. Also known as a platelet.

thrombocytopenia A condition characterized by a reduction in the number of platelets in the circulating blood.

thrombocytosis A condition in which a patient's blood contains increased numbers of platelets.

thromboembolism The obstruction of a blood vessel by a blood clot, or a fragment of a blood clot, that has broken away from its initial site and has traveled through the blood stream.

thrombosed hemorrhoid A condition in which the blood within a dilated rectal vein clots.

thrombotic thrombocytopenic purpura A relatively rare form of thrombocytopenia characterized by hemolytic anemia and renal and central nervous system abnormalities.

thrombus   A blood clot.

thrush   A common fungal infection that affects the mucous membranes of the mouth.

thymus   A small gland-like body located in the upper, front chest cavity.

thyroid gland   An endocrine gland which is located in front of the trachea below the Adam's apple. The thyroid is made up of many microscopic follicles that contain the thyroid hormones.

thyroid nodules   Localized areas of enlargement in the thyroid gland that are usually painless and benign.

thyroid storm   A sudden severe attack of thyrotoxicosis.

thyroid-stimulating hormone (TSH)   A pituitary hormone that stimulates the thyroid gland to manufacture and release thyroid hormones. Also known as thyrotropin.

thyroiditis   An inflammation of the thyroid gland.

thyrotoxicosis   A general term for any condition that is characterized by the presence of excessive amounts of circulating thyroid hormones, regardless of the cause.

thyrotropin   *See* thyroid-stimulating hormone.

thyrotropin-releasing hormone (TRH)   A releasing factor that causes the release of TSH from the pituitary.

TIA   *See* transient ischemic attack.

tibia   The shin bone.

tic douloureux   *See* trigeminal neuralgia.

tidal air   The volume of air that moves during each respiration when the individual is at rest.

tinnitus   A condition characterized by the presence of a constant ringing or buzzing sound in a patient's ear.

tissue   A group of specialized cells of similar structure that are united for the performance of a particular function.

TMJ   *See* temporomandibular joint.

tomography   A noninvasive technique that sends a very narrow x-ray beam through the tissue under examination and shows detail at a predetermined level of the body while blurring the images of structures above or below the desired level. Also known as sectional radiography.

tonic convulsion   An epileptic convulsion in which all of the patient's muscles stay in a continuous state of rigid tension.

tonic-clonic seizure   A generalized convulsion that is characterized by loss of consciousness as well as tonic and clonic activity.

tonometer   An instrument that measures the pressure of the fluids in the eye.

tonsillitis An inflammation of a tonsil.

tophi Deposits of uric acid, or urate, crystals in the tissues.

topical anesthesia The induced loss of sensation of a part of the body as a result of the absorption of an anesthetic agent through an intact membrane.

torsion An act of twisting.

torticollis A condition that is caused by a spasm or contraction of the neck muscles that results in a rotation of the neck and an unnatural position of the head. Commonly referred to as wryneck.

toxic goiter An enlarged thyroid that results in the excessive manufacture of thyroid hormones, thus leading to the manifestations of hyperthyroidism.

toxic shock syndrome A bacterial infection of the genital tract that is indicated by a combination of fever, red rash, vomiting, diarrhea, and shock-like state which may be fatal.

toxoplasmosis A protozoan disease that may affect the central nervous system and may lead to blindness, brain defects, and death.

trabeculae Tiny, sharp projections in cancellous bone that form a mesh of intercommunicating spaces that are filled with bone marrow.

trachea A hollow, tubular structure located in front of the esophagus. Commonly known as the windpipe.

tracheitis An inflammation of the trachea.

tracheotomy The surgical creation of an opening in the patient's trachea to relieve airway obstruction and allow for ventilation.

trait A genetically determined characteristic that may be either dominant or recessive.

transaminase *See* aminotransferase.

transfusion reaction The destruction of a donor's red cells by antibodies in a recipient's plasma which occurs when blood is improperly matched for transfusion.

transient hypoxemia A reduction in oxygen tension in the blood.

transient ischemic attack (TIA) A brief episode in which the vascular system of the brain fails to function properly, but does not produce persistent neurological dysfunction. It may produce a stroke.

transitional cell carcinoma A type of malignancy that is found in the bladder, ureter, and renal pelvis, sites of transitional cell epithelium.

transitional epithelium A type of epithelial tissue that is composed of several layers of overlapping, large rounded cells that have the ability to stretch, and which can adapt to increases in the contents of the organs where this epithelium is found.

translation A condition in which the fragments of a fractured bone lie in totally different planes.

transplantation A surgical procedure in which tissues or organs taken from one individual are implanted in another individual to replace diseased or nonfunctioning tissues or organs.

transseptal, transsphenoidal hypophysectomy A very delicate microsurgery in which a surgeon approaches the pituitary gland through the patient's nose in order to remove a pituitary adenoma.

transurethral resection (TURP) A procedure in which the surgeon removes obstructing prostatic tissue through the patient's urethra by means of a specially designed cystoscope and an electrical cutting device.

transverse colon The part of the large intestine that bends and crosses horizontally to the left side of the body.

transverse fracture A fracture that occurs at a right angle to the long axis of the bone.

traumatic pneumothorax The presence of air in the pleural cavity caused by perforation of the chest wall, fractured ribs, crushing chest injuries, or any injury that permits air to gain access to the pleural cavity.

TRH *See* thyrotropin-releasing hormone.

trichomonas vaginalis A protozoan disease that is characterized by a copious, greenish-yellow, frothy, vaginal discharge.

trigeminal nerve The cranial nerve that serves the side of the face and head. Also known as cranial nerve V.

trigeminal neuralgia A functional disturbance of the trigeminal nerve. It is a condition of unknown cause that is characterized by sharp pain over one or more branches of this nerve. Also known as tic douloureux.

triglyceride A type of lipid that is a major metabolic component in the energy cycle of all cells, and is stored as adipose, or fatty, tissue.

TSH *See* thyroid-stimulating hormone.

TSS *See* toxic shock syndrome.

TTP *See* thrombotic thrombocytopenic purpura.

tubal ligation A surgical procedure in which a woman's fallopian tubes are constricted, severed, or crushed to prohibit the passage of sperm.

tubal pregnancy *See* ectopic pregnancy.

tuberculosis A communicable disease usually affecting the respiratory system and caused in humans by the tubercle bacillus.

tuberculosis of the spine A chronic destructive lesion of one or more vertebrae. Also known as tuberculous spondylitis or Pott's disease.

tuberculous arthritis A joint disorder resulting from tubercular infection.

tuberculous spondylitis *See* tuberculosis of the spine.

tumor A disturbance in the normal growth of tissue characterized by an abnormal, excessive, and uncontrolled proliferation of cells. Also known as a neoplasm.

tumor suppressor genes Genes that discourage the development of cancer.

TURP *See* transurethral resection.

tympanic cavity *See* middle ear.

tympanic membrane *See* ear drum.

tympanoplasty The surgical restoration of a patient's middle ear and the repair of a patient's ear drum, as well as either the reconstruction of the bony connection between the ear drum and the oval window or the replacement of one or more of the ossicles with an artificial structure.

tympanum *See* ear drum.

ulcerative colitis An inflammatory large bowel disease that is characterized by the frequent passage of stools that contain blood, pus, and mucus.

ulcerative proctitis Proctitis that occurs in association with ulcerative colitis.

ulna The longer of the two forearm bones. It lies beside the radius.

ulnar neuropathy A condition characterized by numbness in the patient's fourth and fifth fingers and weakness of certain hand muscles. It often results from injury or pressure at the point at which the ulnar nerve crosses the elbow at the ulnar notch or "crazy bone."

ultrasonography A noninvasive investigative method that utilizes sound vibrations to visualize organs by recording and displaying the reflections (echoes) of high frequency sound waves.

uncomplicated diverticulosis Diverticulosis that does not present symptoms.

urea A substance produced by the liver as the chief nitrogenous end-product of the metabolism of protein.

urea nitrogen The nitrogen component of urea.

uremia A toxic condition that is characterized by the retention of large amounts of the by-products of protein metabolism, especially urea, in the blood. It usually results from severe kidney damage.

ureter A tube that carries urine from a kidney to the bladder.

urethra The excretory duct through which urine, which has been temporarily stored in the bladder, is removed from the body.

urethritis An inflammation of the urethra.

urethrocele A sagging of the urethra and its supporting structures.

urethrogram A diagnostic procedure in which a small amount of a radiopaque dye passes through a catheter into the urethra, followed by a series of x-rays.

urinalysis The laboratory examination of a patient's urine specimen.

urinary bladder A hollow musculomembranous organ that collects and stores urine prior to excretion.

urinary system A group of organs that produce and excrete urine. Also known as the urinary tract.

urination The excretion of urine from the body. Also known as micturition.

urticaria A skin condition characterized by widely scattered, intensely itchy, slightly elevated welts, surrounded by an area of redness. Also known as hives.

uterine atony A condition in which uterine muscles lack their normal tone or strength as a result of a long labor, heavy sedation, anesthesia, multiple pregnancies, or excessive fluid within the uterus.

uterine corpus The larger, upper part of the uterus.

uterosalpingogram *See* hysterosalpingogram.

uterosalpingography *See* hysterosalpingography.

uterus A hollow, thick-walled, pear-shaped muscular organ that performs functions that are primarily related to childbearing.

vagina A hollow, elastic, muscular tube that functions as the birth canal, the passageway for the escape of menstrual fluid, and the receptacle for semen during intercourse.

vaginitis Any infection or inflammation of the mucous membrane of the vagina. It is characterized by itching and a vaginal discharge.

vagotomy A surgical procedure which involves cutting the vagus nerve pathways to the stomach and duodenum.

vagus nerve The largest of the cranial nerves, it transmits nerve impulses arising from the pharynx, larynx, trachea, bronchi, lungs, aorta, stomach, and other internal organs. Also known as cranial nerve X.

varicella A vesiculating disease, commonly known as chicken pox, that is usually mild in childhood, although it may be fatal for adults or children who have suppressed immune systems.

varicocele A dilated, elongated, tortuous network of veins that usually occur on the left scrotum.

vas *See* vas deferens.

vas deferens A continuation of the epididymis that extends through the pelvis and around the bladder, and empties into the urethra. Also known as the vas or the spermatic cord.

vascular headache A headache that results from the distention and dilation of intercranial arteries.

vasectomy The surgical removal of a portion of a man's vas deferens to prohibit the passage of sperm.

vasoconstrictor A class of drugs that constrict blood vessels.

vasodilator A class of drugs that dilate blood vessels.

veins Blood vessels that convey blood from the organs and tissues back to the heart.

venereal disease *See* sexually transmitted disease.

venous pressure The force the blood exerts on the walls of the veins.

ventricles (1) The two lower chambers of the heart. (2) Four hollow chambers inside the brain.

ventricular ectopy Extra ventricular heart beats.

ventricular fibrillation A rapid, chaotic electrical rhythm of the heart's ventricles that leads immediately to the cessation of cardiac output, shock, and death.

ventricular septal defect An abnormality that affects the septum that separates the right and left ventricles of the heart.

verruca A type of benign epidermal tumor which is caused by a virus. Also known as a wart.

vertebra Any one of the bones of the spine.

vertebral body The largest part of a vertebra. It is a solid, flat oval structure.

vertebral column *See* spine.

vertebral foramen An opening on a vertebra that contains the spinal cord and is enclosed by a vertebral body and arch.

vertigo An abnormal sensation of movement.

vesicle A small skin blister.

vestibule A centrally located cavity in the ear that has an oval window that lies next to the stapes.

virology The study of viruses, their identification, and the elaboration of their role as causative agents in disease.

virus A submicroscopic organism that lacks the capacity to reproduce itself unless it gains entrance into a cell of another living organism. Disease is the result of damage done to the host cell by the virus' use of it.

visceral pleura The layer of the pleura that covers the lung.

visual acuity The sharpness of visual perception, or "how well a person sees."

visual field The entire area within which a person can see an object while keeping his or her eye fixed upon a central point.

vital capacity The total volume of air that a person can exhale after a maximum inspiration.

vitamin K deficiency   A condition which usually occurs in individuals who fail to get an adequate amount of vitamin K from their diets or who suffer from poor vitamin K absorption from their intestinal tracts.

vitreous humor   A transparent semi-fluid, jelly-like substance that fills the chamber that lies between the lens and the back of the eye.

vocal cords   Two white fibrous bands of tissue located on the lateral walls of the larynx.

voluntary abortion   The deliberate interruption of pregnancy that is performed in the absence of a medical need.

volvulus   An obstruction resulting from the twisting of the intestine.

von Recklinghausen's disease   *See* neurofibromatosis type I.

von Willebrand's disease   *See* hemophilia C.

VSD   *See* ventricular septal defect.

vulva   The area that contains the external genital organs of a female.

wart   *See* verruca.

WBC   White blood cell. *See* leukocyte.

Wernicke's encephalopathy   A condition most often resulting from excessive alcohol consumption that is characterized by the failure of muscular coordination, double vision, the paralysis of eye movements, mental deterioration, forgetfullness, and/or delirium tremens.

Western blot test   A definitive test for the HIV antibody in which a pathologist places a blood serum or plasma sample from a person being tested and HIV antigens on opposite sides of a medium and then subjects the sample and antigens to an electric field. If HIV antibodies are present in the sample, they will migrate toward the antigens.

Wharton's ducts   The ducts through which the submandibular glands communicate with the oral cavity.

wheals   Sharply demarcated raised, slightly pink, fluid-filled areas on the skin. They develop quickly in large numbers, are very itchy, and generally remain only a few minutes to an hour or two, and then disappear without after effects.

whiplash   A heterogeneous collection of pathological conditions of the neck, typically an acute sprain or strain involving the muscles and ligaments of the cervical spine.

white blood cell   *See* leukocyte.

Wilms tumor   *See* embryonal nephroma.

withdrawal method   *See* coitus interruptus.

X-linked trait   A recessive trait that is carried by a gene located on the X chromosome in males. Also known as sex chromosome-linked trait or sex-linked trait.

zygote   *See* conceptus.

Index

Index

595

Dyspepsia, 208–9, 211, 216, see also Indigestion
Dysphagia, 204–5, 206, 207
Dysplasia, 276
Dysplastic
  cells, 276
  nevi, 84
Dyspnea, 3, 154, 160
Dystocia, 292
Dystrophy, muscular, 359, 389
Dysuria, 254, 263

E
Ear, 9, 18, 397, 412–19, 457
  canal, 332
  disorders of, 414–19
  external, 329, 351, 372
Eardrum, 166, 413, 415, 417
  perforation of, 416
Eating disorder, 435–37
Ecchymoses, 100
Echocardiography, 45, 122, 123, 126–27, 130, 131, 135–36, 144–45, 152–55, 156, 158
Echography, see Ultrasonography
Eclampsia, 291, 439
Ectopic pregnancy, 277, 278, 290, 300
Ectropion, of eyelid, 403
Edema, 47, 87, 180, 185–86, 225, 258, 259, 408, 417, 436, see also Peripheral edema
Efferent nerves, 372
Ejection fraction, 130, 155–56
Electrical
  cardioversion, 147
  stimulation technique, 344
Electrocardiography, 4, 115, 122–23, 129, 131, 135, 140, 151, 154
Electrocoagulation, 408
Electroconvulsive therapy, 424, 425, 427
Electroencephalography, 396
Electromyography, 357, 396
Electrophysiologic study, 150
Electroshock therapy, see Electroconvulsive therapy
ELISA test, 25
Embolism, 186
Embolus, 152, 155, 186, 382
  septic, 184
Embryo, 286, 287, 289
Embryonal nephroma, 260
Emphysema, 100, 180–81
  senile, 180

Empyema, 174, 175, 185
Encephalitis, 377, 386–87, 393
  viral, 15
End-stage heart disease, 119, 156
Endocarditis, 3, 108, 137, 153, 155, 157
Endocardium, 80, 108, 111, 148, 157, 177
Endocrine gland(s), 203, 235, 305, 306, 312
  cancer of, 69
  disorders of, 250, 313–27, 350
Endocrine system, 37, 305–27, 361, 365, 370
Endolymph, 414, 419
Endolymphatic hydrops, 419
Endometrial cavity, 273, 277, 300
Endometrioma, 281
Endometriosis, 276, 278, 281, 282, 290
Endometrium, 273, 275, 278, 281, 283, 284, 285, 287
Endoscopic retrograde
  cholangiography, 230
  cholangiopancreatography, 230
Endoscopy, 40–42, 230, 234, 277
Enteritis, 212, 213, 233, 457
Enthesis, 347
Entropion, of eyelid, 403
Enzyme, 199, 203, 204, 223, 231, 241, 242
Epidemic typhus, 16
Epidermis, 3, 71, 84–85, 87
Epididymis, 265, 267, 269
Epididymitis, 248, 269, 271, 300, 301
Epididymo-orchitis, 269
Epidural
  anesthesia, 367
  hematoma, 376
Epiglottis, 166, 197
Epiglottitis, 173
Epilepsy, 32, 374, 376–80, 396, 452
Epinephrine, 311, 312, see also Adrenalin
Epispadias, 252
Epithelial tissue, 8–9, 60–61, 181
Epithelium, 8, 9, 10, 263, 264, 285
Epstein-Barr virus, 59, 109
Erotomaniac delusion, 431
Erysipelas, 77
Erythema, 74, 76–77
  infectiosum, 79
  marginatum, 151
  migrans, 79
  multiforme, 76
  nodosum, 76–77
Erythroblastosis fetalis, 439

Fistula, 213, 214, 262
Flexor muscle, 340
Fluoroscopy, 52
Flutter, atrial, 147
Focal glomerulonephritis, 258
Focal seizure, see Partial seizure
Folic acid deficiency, 97, 107
Follicle, 274, 278, 285, 286, 287
Follicle-stimulating hormone, 306, 317
Forced vital capacity, 170
Fovea, 399
Fractures, 341–44, 345, 353, 354, 355
    classification, 341–342
    depressed, 375
    healing of, 343–44
    linear, 375
    treatment of, 342
Friedreich's ataxia, 32, 156
Frontal lobe, 366, 372
Frozen section biopsy method, 65–66
Functional psychiatric disorders, 425
Fundus,
    of stomach, 198, 199
    of uterus, 273
Fungus, 12, 14, 23, 157, 280, 385
Furuncle, 77

G

Galactorrhea, 316, 317
Gallbladder, 2, 9, 44, 45–46, 47, 194, 202–3, 209, 231, 234
    disorders of, 226–30
Gallstones, 98, 203, 222, 227, 228, 229, 230, 257
Ganglioneuroma, 60
Ganglions, 353
Gangrene, 218, 219, 227
Gas-permeable contact lenses, 405
Gastrectomy, 234
Gastric
    antrum, 199
    bypass, 235
    cancer, 210
    juice, 199, 210
Gastritis, 23, 42, 209, 212, 224, 234, 447, 451
Gastroenteritis, 213, 233, 385
Gastroenterocolitis, 213
Gastroesophageal
    junction, 195, 207
    reflux, 205, 206
Gastrointestinal tract, 106, 177, 182, 193, 197, 208, 212, 213, 214, 216, 300, 361, 363, 457

bleeding from, 225, 232–33, 245, 447, 453
Gastroplasty, 235
Gastroscopy, 3, 40, 41, 212
General anesthesiology, 19, 41, 228, 263, 428
Generalized seizure, 378, 380
Genes, 28, 30
Genetics, 28–34, 155, 156, 359, 428
Genital wart, 299, 302, 303
Genitourinary system, 37, 187
German measles, see Rubella
Germicidal, 4
Gestational diabetes mellitus, 324, 327
Giant cell tumor, 356, 364
Giant hives, 76
Gilbert's disease, 222
Glandular fever, see Mononucleosis, infectious
Glaucoma, 400, 401–3, 410
Gliding joint, 338
Glioblastoma, 391
Glioma, 391
Global Assessment of Function, 423
Glomerulonephritis, 27, 77, 172, 247, 254, 257, 260–61
Glomerulus, 239, 250, 254, 257–60
Glossopharyngeal
    nerve, 384
    neuralgia, 383–84
Glucocorticoid, 311
Glucose, 231, 242, 244, 268, 287, 323, 324, 326, 327, 380
    tolerance test, 231, 295, 323
Glucosteroid, 311
Glycosuria, 11, 324
Glycosylated hemoglobin, 324
Goeckerman program, 78
Goiter, 311, 316, 318–19
Gonioscopy, 400
Gonorrhea, 263, 299–302
Gout, 350–51, 353
Grading a tumor, 61–63
    Grade I tumor, 61
    Grade IV tumor, 61
Graft, 418
    of skin, 87–88
Gram stain, 12–13
Grandiose delusion, 431
Granulomatous colitis, 214
Granulosa cell tumor, 286
Graves disease, 28, 318
Gross hematuria, 248